T0345109

CLINICAL RESEARCH
in Occupational Therapy
SIXTH EDITION

CLINICAL RESEARCH
in Occupational Therapy
SIXTH EDITION

Martin S. Rice, PhD, OTR/L, FAOTA
Professor of Occupational Therapy
Dean of School of Health Sciences
Indiana Wesleyan University
Marion, Indiana

Franklin Stein, PhD, OTR/L, FAOTA
Professor Emeritus, Occupational Therapy
University of South Dakota
Vermillion, South Dakota

George Tomlin, PhD, OTR/L, FAOTA
Professor of Occupational Therapy
University of Puget Sound
Tacoma, Washington

Routledge
Taylor & Francis Group

NEW YORK AND LONDON

Clinical Research in Occupational Therapy, Sixth Edition includes ancillary materials specifically available for faculty use. Included are PowerPoints. Please visit http://www.routledge.com/9781630915094 to obtain access.

Cover Artist: Donna Trapani

First published in 2019 by SLACK Incorporated

Published 2024 by Routledge
605 Third Avenue, New York, NY 10158

and by Routledge
4 Park Square, Milton Park, Abingdon, Oxon OX14 4RN

Routledge is an imprint of the Taylor & Francis Group, an informa business

© 2019 Taylor & Francis Group

Drs. Martin S. Rice, Franklin Stein, and George Tomlin have no financial or proprietary interest in the materials presented herein.

All rights reserved. No part of this book may be reprinted or reproduced or utilised in any form or by any electronic, mechanical, or other means, now known or hereafter invented, including photocopying and recording, or in any information storage or retrieval system, without permission in writing from the publishers.

Trademark notice: Product or corporate names may be trademarks or registered trademarks, and are used only for identification and explanation without intent to infringe.

Library of Congress Cataloging-in-Publication Data

ISBN:9781630915094(hbk)
ISBN:9781003523147(ebk)

DOI: 10.4324/9781003523147

Additional resources can be found at
www.routledge.com/9781630915094

CONTENTS

Clinical Research in Occupational Therapy, Sixth Edition includes ancillary materials specifically available for faculty use. Included are PowerPoints. Please visit http://www.routledge.com/9781630915094 to obtain access.

ACKNOWLEDGMENTS

I would like to thank my colleagues and students who have supported me in this endeavor. In particular, I am grateful for the help of Chris Miller and Sara Byers for helping to keep me organized, and Joe Sharaya, Occupational Therapy Doctoral student, for helping to manage references. I am indebted to my co-authors, Franklin Stein and George Tomlin, who are a joy to work with and who are inspiring in their own right. Additionally, I would like to thank Sue Cutler for working with me as a co-author on the fifth edition of this text. Lastly, I am forever appreciative for the support, encouragement, and helpful suggestions from my wife, Carol Getz Rice, PhD, OTR/L, who provided valuable insight and suggestions for improving this current edition.

—*Martin S. Rice, PhD, OTRL, FAOTA*

I acknowledge the contributions and feedback from the many students in my classes as I was teaching research design over the years at Boston University, University of Wisconsin-Milwaukee, University of Manitoba, and University of South Dakota. I also acknowledge the help from college colleagues who have been helpful and encouraging over the years. This book has been a labor of love since I began this project in 1974 when I was a young professor in the Graduate Division in the School of Allied Health at Boston University. Occupational therapy as a profession has grown tremendously since then and clinical research has been a strong factor in demonstrating the effectiveness of the profession in improving the lives of millions of people coping with disabilities.

I am also grateful to Martin and George who have substantially improved the quality of the book. I also have to give much credit to my previous co-author, Sue Cutler, who lent her expertise in the writing and reorganization of the third, fourth, and fifth editions of the book.

—*Franklin Stein, PhD, OTR/L, FAOTA*

For this edition, I would like to thank four University of Puget Sound colleagues who helped update the list of assessments in Chapter 10: Juli McGruder, PhD, OTR/L (mental health), Tatiana Kaminsky, PhD, OTR/L (geriatrics), Anne James, PhD, OTR/L, FAOTA (physical disabilities), and Sheryl Zylstra, OTD, OTR/L, BCP (pediatrics), for their prompt and generous efforts. Also many thanks are due to Jean Deitz, PhD, OTR/L, FAOTA for her encouragement to tackle the subject of single-case experimental designs. I would also like to thank the many students I have learned with over the years, who have taught me that every discipline has its realm of knowledge, and then a parallel realm of knowledge about how to "teach" that original knowledge. Finally, I would like to express my thanks to my wife, Sybille, whose occupational therapy experience is a deep and steady sounding board for my own investigations.

—*George Tomlin, PhD, OTR/L, FAOTA*

ABOUT THE AUTHORS

Martin S. Rice, PhD, OTR/L, FAOTA, is the Dean of the School of Health Sciences, and Professor of Occupational Therapy at the Indiana Wesleyan University in Marion, Indiana. Dr. Rice received his PhD in 1996 in Motor Learning and Control and his BS in 1984 in Rehabilitation Education from the Pennsylvania State University. In 1987, he received his MS in Occupational Therapy from the Western Michigan University. Dr. Rice has served on the editorial boards and as a reviewer for several rehabilitation sciences and occupational therapy peer-reviewed journals. He has published over 50 articles and has given over 100 presentations regionally, nationally, and internationally. He completed a sabbatical at the Sheffield Hallam University where he studied safe patient handling practices within the United Kingdom.

Currently, *Franklin Stein, PhD, OTR/L, FAOTA* is Professor Emeritus of Occupational Therapy at the University of South Dakota, founding editor of *Annals of International Occupational Therapy,* and life member of the American Psychological Association. Previously, he was the Director of the School of Medical Rehabilitation at the University of Manitoba in Winnipeg, Canada, Director of the Occupational Therapy Program at the University of Wisconsin-Milwaukee, and Associate Professor, Graduate Division at Sargent College, Boston University. He is the first author with Kristine Haertl of the *Pocket Guide to Interventions in Occupational Therapy, Second Edition* (2019), the first author with Martin Rice and Susan Cutler of the textbook *Clinical Research in Occupational Therapy, Fifth Edition* (2013), *Occupational Therapy and Ergonomics* (2006) with Ingrid Soderback, Susan Cutler, and Barbara Larson, *Psychosocial Occupational Therapy: A Holistic Approach, Second Edition* with Susan Cutler (2002), *PocketGuide to Treatment in Occupational Therapy* (2000) with Becky Roose, and *Stress Management Questionnaire* (2003), as well as over 50 publications in journals and books related to rehabilitation and psychosocial research. He has also presented more than a hundred seminars, workshops, institutes, short courses and research papers at national and international conferences

George Tomlin, PhD, OTR/L, FAOTA has degrees from Massachusetts Institute of Technology, Boston University, University of Puget Sound, and the University of Washington in philosophy, international relations, occupational therapy, and educational psychology, respectively. He has enjoyed 35 years of teaching occupational therapy to students at Puget Sound, from those who grew up locally in Tacoma, Washington, to those from far away: India, Iran, Norway, Taiwan, Germany, Australia, Jordan, and the West Bank. He has brought practice experience in pediatric mental health, adult rehabilitation, and vocational rehabilitation, as well as teaching experience and research interests, to faculty, therapists, and students overseas, especially in Germany and other parts of Europe. Since 2006 he has continued a collaboration with Prof. Dr. Bernhard Borgetto, at the University of Applied Arts and Sciences, Hildesheim, Germany, advancing the ideas of the pyramid model of research evidence. From 2007 to the present he has served as a volunteer for the National Board for Certification in Occupational Therapy, first on the teams developing clinical simulations, and currently as a member of the Board of Directors. His newest project is with a group of six U.S. colleagues, investigating a more inclusive understanding of the uses of evidence in practice, and of how therapists make and justify intervention decisions.

PREFACE TO THE SIXTH EDITION

The first edition of this book, previously called *Anatomy of Research in Allied Health*, was published by Schenkman Publishing Company in Cambridge, Massachusetts, and John Wiley and Sons in 1976. As such, this text, in one form or another, has been in print for over 40 years. The original author was Dr. Frank Stein, who conceived the idea for the text and wrote the first draft of its pages during his sabbatical in Cambridge, England, in 1974 while on faculty at Sargent College, Boston University. This was the first textbook authored by an occupational therapist on research methodology. Dr. Stein wanted to write a text to demonstrate how the health science professions, including occupational therapy, were part of medical progress throughout the world. Furthermore, he believed that occupational therapy was very much tied to the knowledge base of scientific medicine. In the first edition, Dr. Stein wrote, "The overall purposes of the book are two-fold. One is to assist clinicians and students in the health fields to become effective evaluators and consumers of published research and two is to facilitate research skills by communicating the process of research and the abilities needed to plan and implement a research project" (Stein, 1976, p. viii). These goals are still relevant and appropriate today.

In this new edition, I am delighted to announce the addition of Dr. George Tomlin. Dr. Tomlin is a Professor in the School of Occupational Therapy at the University of Puget Sound. Dr. Tomlin is a leader in occupational therapy and is recognized as a profound thinker and contributor to the literature. We are fortunate to have his expertise and knowledge. I have assumed the first author's position and am grateful for the support, guidance, and input from Dr. Stein who is this edition's second author. While Dr. Tomlin and I met some years ago and have been good friends since we first met, Dr. Stein and I have known each other for 2 decades. Dr. Stein has been a good friend and mentor for all of these years and I have come to love and appreciate his love for the profession. A wise person once said, "If you want to end up like someone, become friends with that person." Not only has Dr. Stein modeled a level of professionalism that I deeply respect, his level of community involvement is remarkable and I am honored to call him friend. Dr. Stein is the epitome of a true gentleman and scholar. While not a current author, this current edition would not have been possible without the invaluable work of Dr. Sue Cutler, who co-authored several of the previous editions.

This sixth edition brings some changes, improvements, and enhancements. Some of the more noteworthy changes include the following:

- The addition of Dr. George Tomlin as the third author
- A thorough update of the published research in occupational therapy and health care
- Major revisions in all of the chapters
- The addition of a totally new chapter on single-case experimental research (Chapter 9), spearheaded by Dr. Tomlin
- Updated research boxes and contemporary examples of both quantitative and qualitative research
- Updated compilation of tests and evaluations used by occupational therapists in research studies as outcome instruments and for clinical assessments
- Revision and additions to the glossary of terms and statistics
- Updated examples of the institutional review board application forms, including an informed consent form template from Indiana Wesleyan University
- Updated landmarks in the history of occupational therapy
- Updated interfacing example with a popular statistical software, including data organization analysis and interpretation
- Updated statistical tables
- In general, the sixth edition enables the graduate student and clinical researcher to carry out a research study from the formulation of a research hypothesis to collecting, analyzing, and interpreting data in user-friendly, step-by-step procedures

—*Martin S. Rice, PhD, OTR/L, FAOTA*

INTRODUCTION

A Manifesto for a Great Clinical Research Text for Occupational Therapy

The first edition of this text was published in 1976. At that time, it was the first textbook on clinical research in the allied health professions. Since then, numerous texts have been published about research from the perspective of clinical practice in occupational therapy, physical therapy, and speech-language pathology and audiology. The current edition, the sixth, is a collaborative effort where the three authors combine their expertise as professors, researchers, and clinicians. In preparing this edition, we raised the question: What characterizes a good textbook in clinical research? In reviewing other textbooks and reexamining the strengths and weaknesses of this text, we proposed the following points:

- The textbook should be practical, well-written, and easily understood by researchers, clinicians, and students. Complex concepts should be explained carefully and presented in a logical step-by-step sequence.

- There should be a historical perspective in the text that connects the reader to other researchers who laid the foundation for research-validated practice. The development of the occupational therapy profession is a continuation of the scientific and medical revolutions that created the health professions. As health care clinicians, we are dependent on the early research in anatomy and physiology, testing and measurement, medical instrumentations, clinical medicine, and environmental health. The knowledge gained in the basic sciences strongly impact the clinical professions. As scholars, we know that current practice stands on the shoulders of the past and current researchers in basic and clinical science.

- Within the context of the text, there should be many examples from the current scientific literature, as well as hypothetical examples explaining theoretical concepts and research principles. The text should come from a pragmatic perspective that presents feasible ideas for best practice.

- The text should be a resource for further study in related areas. References should be liberally found throughout the text so that the researcher can readily locate resources in designing and implementing a research study.

- Statistical procedures and tests should be clearly explained in a stepwise procedure. The concept underlying the statistical technique should be emphasized. Although there are a number of available statistical software options, it is important for the student to understand how the statistical results are derived. The student should have a strong background in descriptive statistics before learning inferential statistics.

- In the textbook, there should be an example of a research proposal that can serve as a model for the researcher. The research proposal should be clearly described and realistically implemented.

- The textbook should be comprehensive and include several research models that are appropriate for research in occupational therapy.

- Qualitative and quantitative research models should be described with examples from the literature. Both models are appropriate and relevant. The research design is judged on its own merits as far as validity and application to clinical practice.

- An important emphasis in research is in raising relevant, significant, and feasible research questions. The researcher should be encouraged to ask questions that generate intellectual interest and curiosity. Research should be a process of discovery and intellectual excitement.

- The individual who is designing and carrying out a research study should see the relationship between one's research study and one's professional role, whether it be a clinician, administrator, educator, or researcher. Basic research and applied research are equally important in leading to effective interventions; however, collecting data alone without purpose is not appropriate.

- The research text should help the student to develop a critical view of research. The student should be able to read the literature with a critical eye and carry over this knowledge to clinical practice, especially in applying clinical reasoning. The researcher should also be able to critique the research methodology and evaluate the validity and limitations of the study.

- The researcher should have a strong appreciation of the ethical issues involved with human investigation. Researchers should be able to design an informed consent form and be able to safeguard the research participant from unnecessary psychological or physical risks.

One of the major purposes of this textbook is to link research to clinical practice. It is important that the researcher raise questions relating to clinical practice, including the practical implications, when developing the research proposal. The content of this textbook's chapters are organized comprehensively to include all the components in research: generating a significant research question, carrying out a literature review, designing a research study including the method and procedures, outlining a statistical analysis of data, and writing a scientific manuscript suitable for submission to a peer-reviewed journal.

In writing this sixth edition, the authors developed a conceptual model that serves as a rationale for the text.

- Although the medical model is an essential component of health care systems throughout the world, it is important to note that, in practice, other interventions exist that are effective and deserve research considerations. For example, alternative medicine has become a significant area of practice outside the traditional allopathic medical model. Historically, the medical model includes arriving at a diagnosis that serves as the basis of treatment. The consideration of educational, psychological, and sociological factors in treatment do not negate the medical model. Effective rehabilitation and habilitation depends on a holistic approach that often includes a combination of approaches and models.

- The goal of clinical research is to discover, through objective and systematic inquiry, the most effective interventions that can be applied to the client with a condition or disability. Research should be driven by theory and rational explanation.

- The relationship between clinical research and clinical practice is based on the premise that effective treatment depends on multiple factors, including the occupational therapist's skill, the efficacy of a treatment methodology, the suitability of the intervention given the situation and goals of the client, and the environmental factors that affect treatment. Clinical research should strive to understand the relationships among these factors in clinical treatment.

- Doing research and critically evaluating the findings help the student to become an effective clinician. Because clinical practice is dependent on clinical reasoning and decision making, the effective clinician applies the scientific method in practice. The research-oriented practitioner is able to evaluate the literature and to incorporate current research findings into clinical practice as appropriate.

1

A Short History of the Scientific Method in Medicine, Rehabilitation, and Habilitation

Supporters of evidence-based medicine say that it has many benefits:
(1) it allows clinicians to draw upon the objective experience of many researchers working with accepted
scientific standards; (2) it improves efficacy and efficiency of providers; (3) it decreases the use of ineffective
clinical practices; (4) it promises to better inform patients and clinicians about clinical practices by offering
collectively agreed upon and publicly available information about treatment options; and
(5) it provides a scientific basis for the construction of health care policy.

—Romana (2006)

OPERATIONAL LEARNING OBJECTIVES

By the end of this chapter the learner will be able to:

- Define *clinical research* and explore its primary purposes and its application to occupational therapy.
- Describe the seven stages in the history of medicine.
- Explain the cyclical nature of medical progress into the 21st century.
- Recognize the important contributions of medical researchers toward eliminating disease and improving the health of individuals.
- Understand the importance of methodological discoveries in diagnosis, assessment, prevention, and intervention.
- Describe the history and growth of occupational therapy and the allied health professions.
- Outline occupational therapy's role in the school system.
- Identify trends in rehabilitation research.

Rice, M. S., Stein, F., & Tomlin, G.
Clinical Research in Occupational Therapy, Sixth Edition (pp. 1-36).
© 2019 Taylor & Francis Group.

1.1 DEFINITION AND PURPOSES OF CLINICAL RESEARCH IN OCCUPATIONAL THERAPY WITHIN THE MODEL OF EVIDENCE-BASED PRACTICE

What is research in general and how can it best be defined? What is the relationship between clinical research and evidence-based practice? How are the results of clinical research transferred to clinical practice using the model of evidence-based practice in occupational therapy?

Research is a systematic and objective investigation utilizing the scientific method of identifying a significant problem, stating a testable hypothesis or guiding question, and objectively collecting primary data. Clinical research in occupational therapy is the systematic and objective study of treatment methods or interventions to improve health, prevent illness, and develop or restore function in individuals with disabilities. Evidence-based practice, as initially defined by Sackett, Rosenberg, Gray, Haynes, and Richardson in 1996, is "the conscientious, explicit and judicious use of current best evidence in making decisions about the care of the individual patient. It means integrating individual clinical expertise with the best available external clinical evidence from systematic research" (p. 71). In applying the concept of evidence-based practice to occupational therapy, clinical reasoning is the most important skill necessary in transferring research results to clinical practice. The occupational therapist has to weigh the validity of the research study and its relevance to practice.

Clinical research in occupational therapy has many purposes, some of which are listed in the following examples:

- *Measure effectiveness of treatment methods or interventions.* For example, a clinical researcher seeks to determine the effectiveness of sensory integration therapy in individuals diagnosed with autism (Watling & Hauer, 2015). The results of this study have direct implications for clinical practice. The results can be used to justify the application of sensory integration programs with individuals diagnosed with autism or to recommend further research.
- *Communicate to the public, third-party payers, and government agencies the effectiveness of occupational therapy interventions in improving the health of or restoring function in individuals with disabilities.* For example, the researcher decides to publish the results of a systematic review demonstrating that exercise is effective in improving cognition for people who have had a stroke (Vanderbeken & Kerckhofs, 2016). The results of this systematic review can be used to persuade third-party payers that this approach is effective and should be funded.

- *Explore and compare different strategies for interventions.* For example, clinical researchers compare the effectiveness of constraint induced movement therapy vs. motor relearning with individuals who have had a stroke (Batool, Soomro, Amjad, & Fauz, 2015).
- *Help clinicians to plan action research in site-specific environments.* For example, occupational therapists may wish to collect data on how to decrease the number of Medicare rejections in a specific hospital. In this study, occupational therapists will be collecting descriptive data and comparing it to the data published by the Centers for Medicare and Medicaid Services (https://www.cms.gov).
- *Enable clinicians to transfer the results of clinical research to practice.* For example, a clinician using splinting in hand therapy can evaluate research studies, as was done in the article "Effectiveness of Occupational Therapy Interventions for Adults With Musculoskeletal Conditions of the Forearm, Wrist, and Hand: A Systematic Review" (Roll & Hardison, 2017). This systematic review has direct clinical implications for hand therapists and can help them to select the most effective splint.
- *Develop interventions, treatment protocols, educational strategies, assessment procedures and tools, or software products that will later be evaluated for effectiveness.* For example, an occupational therapist may be interested in developing a treatment protocol to reduce anxiety in individuals with clinical depression (Krogh, Speyer, Gluud, & Nordentoft, 2015).
- *Reconstruct historical events to understand the basis for a current treatment.* For example, an occupational therapist may want to examine the historical basis for treating individuals with spinal cord injuries in the United States in the 20th century (Lifshutz & Colohan, 2004).
- *Examine reasons for improvement or failure of a specific intervention through a retrospective case study.* For example, a client with a diagnosis of multiple sclerosis (Woo, Olek, & Frohman, 2006).
- *Explore relationships between associated variables.* A clinician might want to examine the relationship between perceptual motor skills and self-care abilities or between perceptual motor skills and writing achievement in children with autism (MacDonald, Lord, & Ulrich, 2013).

The rise and development of occupational therapy as a health care profession over 100 years ago, beginning in 1917, is the direct result of the progress in medical research and practice that came before (Box 1-1). The rehabilitation professions of occupational therapy, physical therapy, speech pathology, and audiology emerged from the scientific findings in medicine that began in the 19th and 20th centuries. In this chapter, we review the seven stages in scientific medicine that are the forerunners of scientific inquiry in the rehabilitation professions.

Box 1-1. Selected International Landmarks in the History of Occupational Therapy as a Profession

1752 Pennsylvania Hospital in Philadelphia was established. Psychiatric patients were prescribed manual labor to counteract disease process.

1780 Clement-Joseph Tissot, a French physician in the cavalry, published a book prescribing the use of crafts and recreational activities for individuals with muscle and joint injuries.

1786 Philippe Pinel, a French psychiatrist in the Bicetre Asylum for the Insane, prescribed humane treatment in the care of the mentally ill, including physical exercises, manual occupation, and music.

1803 Johanann Christian Reil, a German psychiatrist, advocated that activities such as swimming, dancing, gymnastics, arts and crafts, music, and theater be part of the everyday routine for patients.

1812 Benjamin Rush, the father of American psychiatry, prescribed work, leisure activities, chess, and other board games, exercise, and theater for treatment of mental illness.

1813 Samuel Tuke, an English Quaker, founded the Retreat Asylum for the Insane in York, England. Tuke introduced the term *moral treatment,* which was the application of humane practices—including exercise, recreation, arts and crafts, gardening, and regular employment—in the maintenance of the hospital.

1833 Samuel Woodard, a physician at the Worcester State Lunatic Hospital in Massachusetts, introduced the term *occupational therapy* as a therapeutic method to keep inmates active in varied tasks and leisure activities in regular routines. The therapeutic program was clinically effective and produced a significant recovery rate.

1838 Jean Etienne Esquirol, a French psychiatrist, described the importance of corporal exercise, horseback riding, tennis, fencing, swimming, and travel for the treatment of depression.

1840 Francois Leuret, a French psychiatrist, advised that moral treatment, including arts and crafts and work, are effective in treating individuals with mental illness and intellectual disabilities.

1843 Dorothea Dix, a social reformer, worked diligently in the United States for humanistic care for individuals with mental illness, which included the use of therapeutic activities.

1854 Thomas Kirkbride, one of the founders of the American Psychiatric Association advocated a highly structured regimen for patients that included exercise, lectures, music, arts and crafts, and entertainment.

1895 William Rush Dunton, a psychiatrist and innovator in applying occupational therapy, used arts and crafts activities at Sheppard and Pratt Asylum in Baltimore, Maryland.

1895/ 1922 Adolf Meyer, a strong advocate of occupation, believed in a holistic approach to treatment centering on sleep habits, nutrition, work, play, and socialization.

1895 Mary Potter Meyer, a social worker and wife of Adolf Meyer, used arts and crafts activities in the State Hospital in Worcester, Massachusetts.

1904 Herbert Hall, a physician, prescribed occupation as a medicine to regulate the life and direct interests of the patient. He called this the *work cure.*

1905 Susan Tracy, a nurse, applied occupational therapy activities in working with individuals with mental illness while she was director of the Training School for Nurses at the Adams Nervine Asylum in Boston, Massachusetts.

1906 Herbert Hall was awarded a grant of $1000 by Harvard University to study the application of activities and graded manual occupation in the treatment of psychiatric disorders.

1908 Training courses in occupations for hospital attendants were initiated at Chicago School of Civics and Philanthropy.

1909 Clifford Beers, founder of the National Committee for Mental Hygiene, described his emotional illness in the book, *A Mind that Found Itself* (Beers, 1908). Beers reinforced the application of therapeutic activities in treating individuals with mental illness.

1910 Susan Tracy authored the first book on occupation studies, *Studies in Invalid Occupations: A Manual for Nurses and Attendants* (Tracy, 1910).

(continued)

Box 1-1. Selected International Landmarks in the History of Occupational Therapy as a Profession (continued)

1911 Susan Tracy initiated the first course on occupation in a general hospital at Massachusetts General Hospital in Boston.

1911 Eleanor Clark Slagle, a social worker, established an occupation department at Phipps Psychiatric Clinic at Johns Hopkins University in Baltimore.

1914 George Edward Barton, an architect who had contracted tuberculosis, reintroduced the term *occupational therapy* at a meeting in Boston of hospital workers.

1917 The National Society for the Promotion of Occupational Therapy was founded in Consolation House in Clifton Springs, New York. The charter members included George Barton, an architect; Eleanor Clark Slagle, a social worker at Hull House in Chicago, Illinois; Thomas Kidner, a vocational specialist from Canada; William Rush Dunton, a psychiatrist at Sheppard and Pratt Hospital in Baltimore, Maryland; Susan Cox Johnson, an arts and crafts instructor from New York City; Isabel Gladwin (Newton) Barton, first Secretary of the Society ; and Susan E. Tracy, a nurse at the Adams Nervine Asylum in Boston, Massachusetts. This meeting led to the occupational therapy profession in the United States.

1917 Reconstruction aides were recruited to serve in U.S. army hospitals during World War I, applying arts and crafts and exercises in the treatment of physical and mental disorders.

1918 Formal educational training programs in occupational therapy were established at the Henry B. Favil School in Chicago, Teachers College of Columbia University, and the Boston School of Occupational Therapy.

1919 Bird T. Baldwin authored the *U.S. Army Manual on Occupational Therapy* (Baldwin, 1919), which included information on evaluation and treatment procedures for the restoration of physical function.

1919 George Barton (1919) wrote the book *Teaching the Sick, A Manual of Occupational Therapy as Reeducation*.

1922 The *Archives of Occupational Therapy* was published and became the official journal of the American Association of Occupational Therapy.

1925 *Occupational Therapy and Rehabilitation* was first published.

1928 Six programs were available to prepare occupational therapists: Boston School, Philadelphia School, St. Louis School, Milwaukee-Downer College, University of Minnesota, and the University of Toronto

1931 National registry for the American Occupational Therapy Association was established.

1933 The American Medical Association (AMA) began the accreditation of occupational therapy educational programs

1934 Essentials of an acceptable education curriculum in occupational therapy was adopted by the American Medical Education Council on Medical Education and Hospitals.

1939 Among all AMA-approved hospitals, 13% employed occupational therapists.

1943 The Barden-LaFollette Vocational Rehabilitation Act was passed by Congress providing coverage of medical services, including occupational therapy, for individuals in vocational rehabilitation programs.

1945 Eighteen approved occupational therapy programs were available in the United States, compared with five in 1940.

1947 First national registration examination for U.S. occupational therapists was given.

1947 Advanced master's degree in occupational therapy was offered at the University of Southern California and New York University.

1947 Helen Willard and Clare S. Spackman, occupational therapy educators, authored the first textbook in occupational therapy.

1952 The World Federation of Occupational Therapy (WFOT) was established. The 10 founding member countries were Australia, Canada, Denmark, Great Britain, India, Israel, New Zealand, South Africa, Sweden, and the United States.

1958 Essentials and Guidelines for an approved Educational Program for Occupational Therapy Assistant in the U.S. adopted.

(continued)

Box 1-1. Selected International Landmarks in the History of Occupational Therapy as a Profession (continued)

1964 Certified occupational therapy assistant (COTA) certifications were available in the United States.

1964 The first entry-level master's program in occupational therapy was established at the University of Southern California. Shortly thereafter, basic master's programs were begun at Boston University and Virginia Commonwealth University.

1965 The American Occupational Therapy Foundation (AOTF) established as a philanthropic organization for advancing the science of occupational therapy.

1965 Lyndon B. Johnson signed Medicare into law on July 30, 1965.

1973 The Rehabilitation Act passed by Congress protecting the rights of persons with disabilities. Section 504 of the Rehabilitation Act of 1973 prohibits discrimination based on disability in programs or activities receiving federal financial assistance. (See http://www.access.gpo.gov/nara/cfr/waisidx_99/34cfr104_99.html and http://www2. ed.gov/policy/speced/reg/narrative.html)

1974 New York University developed the first doctoral program in occupational therapy.

1975 Education for All Handicapped Children Act (EHA; PL. 94–142) facilitated free appropriate public education services for students with disabilities at all levels and provided funding for these services. The concept of least restrictive environment, inherent in the law, specifies that students with disabilities are educated with typical students "to the maximum extent possible."

1976 Support was given to students for development of their organization on a national level, which was later named the American Student Occupational Therapy Alliance.

1979 "Uniform Terminology System for Reporting Occupational Therapy Services" developed and adopted by the Representative Assembly (RA).

1980 AOTF published the *Occupational Therapy Journal of Research.*

1981 Entry-level role delineation for OTRs and COTAs adopted by RA.

1986 Medicare amendments expanded coverage for occupational therapy services under Part B in the United States.

1990 The Americans with Disabilities Act (ADA; PL 101–336; [42 USC 12101]) was passed by Congress and signed by President George H. W. Bush. The ADA guarantees equal opportunity for individuals with disabilities in employment, public accommodations, transportation, governmental services and telecommunications (Family Center on Technology and Disability, 2010). (See also http://www.usdoj.gov/crt/ada/cguide.htm#anchor62335 and http://www.ada.gov)

1990 PL 94–142 reauthorized and renamed the Individuals with Disabilities Education Act (IDEA). This law continued federal funding from 94–142, and increased services by adding related services, transition from school to work, and parental involvement. Under this act, occupational therapy is considered a related service in helping students with disabilities in public schools.

1991 The AOTA RA approved a physical agent modalities (PAMs) position paper that recommended the use of PAMs as an adjunct to purposeful activity to enhance occupational performance.

1994 *Occupational Therapy International* is founded as the first refereed journal publishing manuscripts by occupational therapists throughout the world

1997 The Balanced Budget Act (BBA; PL 105–33) significantly changed the procedures for payment of services for rehabilitation personnel affecting the quality of care, especially in home health.

1998 The Assistive Technology Act (PL105–394 [29 USC 2201]) passed. This legislation provides funds to the States to support the establishment of assistive technology (AT) demonstration centers, information centers, facilities, referral services, and advocacy services to help people with disabilities access AT services. The act also provides low interest loans to purchase AT (FCTD, 2010). (See also http://www.ataporg.org/atap/index.php and http://www. assistivetech.net/webresources/stateTechActProjects.php for information regarding State projects)

(continued)

Box 1-1. Selected International Landmarks in the History of Occupational Therapy as a Profession (continued)

1998 Carl D. Perkins Vocational and Technical Education Act Amendments of 1998 (PL105–332 Section 1 (b) [20 USC 2302]). This act requires schools to integrate academic, vocational, and technical training; increase technology use; provide professional development opportunities; develop, implement, and expand quality programs; and link secondary and post-secondary vocational education (FCTD, 2010). (See also http://www.ed.gov/offices/OVAE/CTE/legis.html)

1999 The AOTA RA passes a resolution to mandate that entry-level education in occupational therapy should be at the post-baccalaureate level.

2001 The *International Classification of Functioning, Disability and Health*, known more commonly as ICF, is a classification of health and health-related domains. These domains are classified from body, individual, and societal perspectives by means of two lists: a list of body functions and structures, and a list of domains of activity and participation. As an individual's functioning and disability occur in a context, the ICF also includes a list of environmental factors. The ICF is the World Health Organization's (WHO) framework for measuring health and disability at both individual and population levels.

2002 No Child Left Behind (NCLB; PL 107–110; http://www2.ed.gov/policy/elsec/leg/esea02/index.html) enacted. As part of the need to improve education, the law focused on requiring each state to develop and implement a statewide accountability system that insured adequate yearly gain for all schools in reading and math. It is based on the concept that setting standards and measurable educational goals can improve academic performance in the classroom.

2002 The *Occupational Therapy Practice Framework: Domain and Process* was developed in response to current practice needs, intended to "more clearly affirm and articulate occupational therapy's unique focus on occupation and daily life activities and the application of an intervention process that facilitates engagement in occupation to support participation in life" (AOTA, 2002, p. 609).

2004 The Individuals with Disabilities Education Improvement Act of 2004 (IDEIA; PL108–556; http://idea.ed.gov/) is the reauthorization of PL 94-142 enacted in 1975. The law ensures that services to more than 6.5 million eligible infants, toddlers, children and youths with disabilities throughout the nation. With this reauthorization, IDEA-2000 was aligned with NCLB. In addition to funding, IDEIA governs how states and public agencies provide early intervention, special education and related services.

2004 The fourth edition of the Canadian Occupational Performance Measure (COPM; Law et al., 2005) is published. It is an individualized, client-centered measure designed for use by occupational therapists to detect change in a client's self-perception of occupational performance over time. It is designed to be used as an outcome measure. The COPM is designed for use with clients with a variety of disabilities and across all developmental stages. The COPM has been used in more than 35 countries and has been translated into over 20 languages.

2008 *Occupational Therapy Practice Framework: Domain and Process, Second Edition* is published (AOTA, 2008; Roley et al., 2008).

2009 New emerging areas of occupational therapy practice in the United States identified by the AOTA: psychosocial needs of children and youth, health and wellness, driver rehabilitation, low vision services, ergonomics, community health, welfare to work, and technology and assistive device development and consulting.

2009 Americans with Disabilities Act Amendment (PL 110–325; http://www.judiciary.state.nj.us/legis/110-325_Law. pdf), signed on September 25, 2008 by President George W. Bush and went into effect on January 1, 2009. Under the Amendment, millions more Americans qualify as disabled and fall under the Act's protections. Under the Amendment, the definition of disability was modified so that the individual may be regarded as having an impairment, without regard to whether it substantially limits a major life activity. The Amendment also expands the phrase "major life activities" as "caring for oneself, performing manual tasks, seeing, hearing, eating, sleeping, walking, standing, lifting, bending, speaking, breathing, learning, reading, concentrating, thinking, communicating, and working." Another important change requires that impairments that are episodic or in remission qualify as a disability if they would qualify in their active stage.

2010 World Federation of Occupational Therapists (WFOT) meets in Santiago, Chile for its 15th Congress. There are 70 member countries of the WFOT.

(continued)

BOX 1-1. SELECTED INTERNATIONAL LANDMARKS IN THE HISTORY OF OCCUPATIONAL THERAPY AS A PROFESSION (CONTINUED)

2010 On March 23, President Barack Obama signed the Affordable Health Care for America Act (PL 111–148; http://democrats.senate.gov/reform/patient-protection-affordable-care-act-as-passed.pdf). The general principle is to ensure that all Americans have access to quality, affordable health care. It is projected that the Act will provide health care coverage to 95% of Americans. (See http://www.aota.org/Practitioners/Advocacy/Federal/Highlights/Reform.aspx for the impact of the Act on occupational therapy)

2014 The third edition of the *Occupational Therapy Practice Framework: Domain and Process* is published by the AOTA (2014).

2014 WFOT meets in Yokohama, Japan for its 16th Congress.

2014 The fifth edition of the Canadian Occupational Performance Measure is published (Law et al., 2014). The COPM is now used in over 40 countries and has been translated into more than 35 languages.

2017 AOTA celebrates its 100th Anniversary in Philadelphia, Pennsylvania during the Annual Conference.

2018 WFOT meets in Cape Town, South Africa. There are now over 92 member organizations and approximately 400,000 occupational therapists internationally.

1.2 HISTORICAL REVIEW OF RESEARCH IN MEDICINE, REHABILITATION, AND HABILITATION

Before the beginnings of modern science in the latter half of the 19th century, relationships between causes and effects still retained explanations that bordered on the supernatural. Vitalism, a recurrent movement in medicine, was typified by the 18th-century physician who ascribed mysterious substances in the blood to life functions. This theory was an outcome of the prescientific thinking that gave way to the systematic and orderly explanations that we now associate with modern scientific research. The understanding of the disease process began with the laboratory experimentation of Pasteur (1822–1895), who served as a model for the medical scientist. The impact of scientific technology in the treatment and rehabilitation of the sick and the disabled has been a remarkable record in human progress. In few other areas of knowledge has humanity made greater strides.

The analysis of the progress in medical science and rehabilitation is divided into the seven stages identified in Table 1-1. These seven stages are progressive, interactive, and dynamic. For example, basic research in biological and chemical processes in Stage I continues to be important as evidenced by the investigations of DNA and RNA as the building blocks in protoplasm. Similarly, methodological research is in the forefront by the integration of high technology with clinical practice, as demonstrated in the areas of robotics, prosthetics, transplant operations, kidney dialysis techniques, and artificial replacement of bodily organs. Medical scientists are constantly refining treatment and preventive methodologies. Immunologists who formerly sought chemicals to destroy harmful bacteria and viruses have led the way for present-day investigators searching for vaccines to prevent cancerous growths and life-threatening diseases, such as AIDS.

Progress in science is cyclical and cumulative. As knowledge grows, medical scientists refine their methods of research. Stages of development in medicine point to the cumulative process of obtaining knowledge and to the evolutionary process of scientific methodology and its impact on clinical practice.

1.3 BIOLOGICAL DESCRIPTION: STAGE I

1.3.1 The Growth of Scientific Anatomy and Physiology

The earliest medical research started with the discovery of the physiological processes and anatomical systems of the body. Biological description: Stage I, the evolution of medical research, is outlined in Table 1-2. Knowledge of the anatomical structure of animals during the Middle Ages and the Renaissance was greatly influenced by Galen (AD 138–201), who experimented on lower mammals; Leonardo Da Vinci (1452–1519), who made precise drawings of human anatomy; and later by Vesalius (1514–1564), who, through careful dissection, described human anatomy. Identifying and describing the anatomical structures of the body led to increased knowledge about relationships between systems and the interrelationships of cardiovascular, respiratory, and genitourinary functions. For example, Harvey's (1578–1657) concept of the circulation of blood led the way

TABLE 1-1

SEVEN STAGES IN THE HISTORY OF MEDICINE, HEALTH, AND REHABILITATION

STAGE I		STAGE II
Biological Description		*Methodological*
Accurate description of anatomical structure and physiological processes, producing a basic understanding of the bodily organs and systems.		Development of instruments, procedures, and tests to produce valid and reliable methods in evaluation, diagnosis, and treatment.
STAGE III	**STAGE IV**	**STAGE V**
Etiology	*Prevention*	*Treatment*
Understanding of the disease process and cause-effect relationships to produce a science of medicine and universal agreement in diagnosing diseases.	Development of medical technology to prevent initial onset of disease, resulting in the science of immunology and public health.	Application of treatment techniques based on a theoretical understanding of disease processes, leading to the growth of chemical intervention, antiseptic surgery, and nursing care in hospitals.
STAGE VI		**STAGE VII**
Rehabilitation		*Habilitation and Special Education/ Programming Interventions*
Development of therapeutic techniques and restoration of maximum function for individuals with chronic disabilities, leading to the evolution of allied health professions.		The identification of treatments for the developmental and social disabilities applying specialized educational and psychological techniques to populations at risk.

TABLE 1-2

THE EMERGENCE OF THE MEDICAL SCIENTIST—STAGE I

MEDICAL EVENTS	DISCOVERY DATES	SCIENTISTS	IMPLICATIONS
Hippocratic writings	400–500 BC	Hippocrates (500 BC)	Provided a model for medical practitioners based on ethical and humane treatment
Systematic study of bodily processes	AD 169–180	Claudius Galen (AD 129–199)	Influenced medical practice for 1300 years, presenting an eclectic synthesis of prior knowledge
The Canon of Medicine	translated 1187	Avicenna (980–1037)	Significant figure of Arabic medicine whose work was dogma during the Middle Ages
Paragranum: The four pillars of medicine: philosophy, astronomy, chemistry, and virtue	1530	Paracelsus (1493–1541)	Created the foundation for general medical practice based on a knowledge of pharmaceutical chemistry

(continued)

TABLE 1-2 (CONTINUED)			
THE EMERGENCE OF THE MEDICAL SCIENTIST—STAGE I			
MEDICAL EVENTS	DISCOVERY DATES	SCIENTISTS	IMPLICATIONS
Atlas of Anatomy (*De humani corporis fabrica*)	1543	Andreas Vesalius (1514–1564)	Made descriptive anatomy the basis of medicine and replaced aspects of Galen's work
Manual of Surgery	1543	Ambroise Pare (1510–1590)	Generated surgical innovations based on accurate anatomical knowledge
Discovery of the circulation of the blood, *Exercitatio*	1628	William Harvey (1578–1657)	Integrated anatomy with physiological knowledge of blood circulation
Digestive system, *Experiments and Observations of Gastric Juice and the Physiology of Digestion*	1833	William Beaumont (1785–1853)	Used objective observation in discovering the process of digestion

to an understanding of the physiological mechanisms in the body. Galen, Da Vinci, and Harvey were among the first scholars to accurately describe the human body; however, the ancient Greeks initially brought rational thought to an evaluation of health and disease. The Hippocratic writings reflect the depth of Greek thought.

1.3.2 The Hippocratic Writings

The first stage in the history of medicine was essentially clinical observation. The healer, applying Hippocratic methods, used himself as a measuring instrument, carefully noting what he saw, felt, smelled, and heard. He used rational thought regarding the causes and treatments of diseases based on these observations. In the ancient Greek civilization, scholars were allowed the freedom to speculate on all aspects of human life. Thus, the model for the Western physician emerged. Hippocrates, who is traditionally called the *Father of Medicine*, was probably representative of several individuals. It is more accurate to speak of the "Hippocratic writings" than to attribute all ancient Greek medicine to one individual. The Hippocratic writings cover many areas of medicine, including ethics, disease etiology, anatomy, physiology, and treatment. These writings are not a consistent work linking theory to practice, but a compendium of clinical histories and a description of Hellenistic medicine.

We know little about Hippocrates' life, except that he lived during the 5th century BCE in Cos, an island off the Greek mainland, and that he was a famous practitioner and teacher of medicine. The following excerpt from the Hippocratic writings, *On the Articulations* (ca. 400 BC/1952) translated by Francis Adams, demonstrates the method of clinical observation used to diagnose a dislocation of the shoulder joint and the importance of individual differences in human anatomy:

A dislocation may be recognized by the following symptoms: Since the parts of a man's body are proportionate to one another, as the arms and the legs, the sound should always be compared with the unsound, the unsound with the sound, not paying regard to the joints of other individuals (for one person's joints are more prominent than another's), but looking to those of the patient, to ascertain whether the sound joint be unlike the unsound. This is a proper rule, and yet it may lead to much error; and on this account it is not sufficient to know this art in theory, but also by actual practice; for many persons from pain, or from any other cause, when their joints are not dislocated, cannot put the parts into the same positions as the sound body can be put into; one ought therefore to know and be acquainted beforehand with such an attitude. But in a dislocated joint the head of the humerus appears lying much more in the armpit than it is in the sound joint; and also, above, at the top of the shoulder, the part appears hollow, and the acromion is prominent, owing to the bone of the joint having sunk into the part below; there is a source of error in this case also, as will be described and also, the elbow of the dislocated arm is farther removed from the ribs than that of the other; but by using force it may be approximated, though with considerable pain; and also they cannot with the elbow extended raise the arm to the ear, as they can the sound arm, nor move it about as formerly in this direction and that. These, then, are the symptoms of dislocation at the shoulder. (as cited in Hutchins, 1952, pp. 94-95)

With their emphasis on dietetics, exercise, and natural methods, the Hippocratic writings were the complete holistic guide for the ancient physician.

1.3.3 Galen

Greek medicine provided the foundation for medical practice in the Western world. Galen, a product of the Roman civilization, was the next link in the chain of medicine. He was born in Pergamum, Greece, in the 2nd century CE when Roman civilization controlled much of the Western world. Galen was educated in philosophy, mathematics, and natural science. He learned medicine by traveling to places where the great physicians practiced. After acquiring knowledge steeped in the Hippocratic tradition, he became a doctor to the gladiators who performed in the Roman arenas. Galen became an acclaimed practitioner in Rome and later spent his time writing extensively. He is a model for the medical scientist who engages in clinical practice, teaching, and scholarly publication. Galen's genius was in his ability to integrate prior knowledge with his clinical observations of disease. Unfortunately, his writings on medicine became the authoritative dogma from the Middle Ages to the time of the rebirth of scientific inquiry in the Renaissance. The following excerpt from Galen (ca. AD 192/1971) typifies his skill in teaching anatomy, as well as his careful methods of observation:

> Since therefore, the form of the body is assimilated to the bones, to which the nature of the other parts corresponds, I would have you first gain an exact and practical knowledge of human bones. It is not enough to study them casually or read of them in a book; no, not even in mine, which some call Osteologia, others Skeletons, and yet others simply On Bones, though I am persuaded that it excels all earlier works in accuracy, brevity, and lucidity.
>
> Make it rather your serious endeavor not only to acquire accurate book-knowledge of each bone, but also to examine assiduously with your own eyes the human bones themselves. This is quite easy at Alexandria because the physicians there employ ocular demonstration in teaching osteology to students. For this reason, if for no other, try to visit Alexandria. But if you cannot, it is still possible to see something of human bones. I, at least, have done so often on the breaking open of a grave or tomb. Thus once a river, inundating a recent hastily made grave, broke it up, washing away the body. The flesh had putrefied, though the bones still held together in their proper relations. It was carried down a stadium (roughly 200 yards), and reaching marshy ground, drifted ashore. This skeleton was as though deliberately prepared for such elementary teaching.
>
> If you have not the luck to see anything of this sort, dissect an ape and having removed the flesh, observe each bone with care. Choose those apes likest man

with short jaws and small canines. You will find other parts also resembling man's, for they can walk and run on two feet. Those, on the other hand, like the dog-faced baboons with long snouts and large canines, far from walking or running on their hindlegs, can hardly stand upright. The more human sort have a nearly erect posture; but firstly the head of the femur fits into the socket at the hipjoint rather transversely, and secondly, of the muscles which extend downward to the knee, some go further (than in man). Both these features check and impede erectness of posture, as do the feet themselves, which have comparatively narrow heels and are deeply cleft between the toes.

> I therefore maintain that the bones must be learnt either from man, or ape, or better from both, before dissecting the muscles, for those two (namely bones and muscles) form the ground-work of the other parts, the foundations, as it were, of a building. And next, study arteries, veins, and nerves. Familiarity with dissection of these will bring you to the inward parts and so to a knowledge of the viscera, the fat, and the glands, which also you should examine separately, in detail. Such should be the order of your training. (as cited in Wightman, 1971, pp. 32-33)

1.3.4 Renaissance Medicine in the Sixteenth and Seventeenth Centuries

The history of medicine parallels, in many ways, the rise of Western civilization. The Middle Ages in Europe was a sterile period for the growth of new ideas and experimentation. Medical practice existed then as dogma, closely linked to the practices and beliefs of the Church. Although Medieval Europe adhered to rigid doctrine, medical practice flourished in the Middle East, as represented by the Arab physician, Avicenna (980–1037). With the onset of the Renaissance, scientists performed experiments on humans using dissection under great risk of public denouncement and physical punishment. Despite this, a psychological climate was established in the 16th century that allowed medical scholars and scientists to seek the truth by experimentation. Physicians made great strides in integrating laboratory observations with clinical practice.

Renaissance physicians rekindled the torch of medical science that had been stagnant for approximately 1000 years. The scientists of the Renaissance were scholars familiar with Greek and Roman writings who questioned all knowledge and accepted little dogma. Furthermore, they reexamined the anatomical knowledge of Galen, experimented in chemistry, and sought explanations for the life processes in humans. In short, their work marked the beginning of the science of physiology.

1.3.5 Andreas Vesalius and the Refinement of Human Anatomy

The most important medical anatomist of the Renaissance was Andreas Vesalius. He was the first medical specialist in human anatomy. By critically examining the work of Galen, he realized that Galen's observations of anatomy were not based on human dissection but rather were descriptions of the bodily structures of monkeys, pigs, and goats. From 1537 to 1542, Vesalius worked on an anatomical atlas, *De humani corporis fabrica libri septea*, which was published in 1593. The book contained 663 folio pages. Vesalius' research on human anatomy became the basis of medical science and provided the necessary knowledge for the surgeon. The interplay between laboratory observations and clinical practice provided scholars with the data they needed for readjusting theory to practice and practice to theory. The model for obtaining anatomical knowledge in the medical sciences was forged in the 16th century.

1.3.6 Paracelsus the Medical Chemist

The next great development in medicine was in physiology. Chemistry and physics are the bases of physiology. The understanding of human physiology awaited great discoveries in these areas. The first physician to apply chemistry to an understanding of biological processes was Paracelsus. He advocated using pharmaceutical agents, singly or in combination, to treat specific illnesses. He used sulphur, lead, antimony, mercury, iron, and copper as therapeutics. Paracelsus emphasized the relationship between practical clinical experience and scientific experimentation, as evidenced in the following quotation from his work *Paragranum* (as cited in Wightman, 1971):

> The doctor must therefore be practiced in Experienz; and medicine is nothing but a wide, certain, Experienz, namely that every procedure is based in Experienz. And that is experientia which is correctly and truly founded. Anyone who has learnt his stuff without Experienz is a doubtful doctor.

> Experientia is like a judge; and whether a procedure is undertaken or not depends on its approval; wherefore Experienz ought to keep pace with science, for without science Experienz is nothing. Similar an Experiment grounded in Experienz is well founded and its further use understood. ... Experiment divorced from science is but a matter of chance. (pp. 50-51)

1.3.7 William Harvey

In the publication *Exercitatio* in 1628, William Harvey described the circulation of the blood accurately for the first time. Harvey, an English physician, was trained in Padua, Italy, where Vesalius had taught human anatomy. After mastering the physiological theories of his time, he proposed questions, such as:

- What is the pulse?
- How does breathing affect the actions of the heart?
- How does the blood move?

These questions directed Harvey's experimental procedures. First, he systematically stated a testable hypothesis on the circulation of the blood, and then he proceeded with rigorous experimental observation. He used precise measurements in recording pulse rate and the volume of blood ejected by the heart over time. He observed the movements of the heart and blood in living animals. He also analyzed the blood circulation of the fetus to support his theory. By using the scientific method, Harvey discovered the most vital process in human life. He did this by (a) presenting a researchable question, (b) mastering the published literature on blood flow, (c) using accurate observations, (d) being guided by predictive hypothesis, (e) using rigorous procedures for collecting data, (f) applying measurement to the process of blood flow, and (g) making a deductive analysis and conclusions.

Harvey's achievement in describing the circulation of the blood ranks with Newton's discovery of gravity as one of the greatest scientific accomplishments in the seventeenth century. Harvey's work at first was met with the jealousy and suspicion that many times accompanies an important discovery or change of thinking. In the first chapter from *Exercitatio* entitled "The Author's Motives for Writing" (1628/1952), Harvey (1938) explained his reasons for publishing his findings and his desire to bring objective criticism to his work.

> I have not hesitated to expose my views upon these subjects, not only in private to my friends, but also in public, in my anatomical lectures, after the manner of the Academy of old.

> These views as usual, pleased some more, others less; some chide and calumniated me, and laid it to me as a crime that I had dared to depart from the precepts and opinions of all anatomists; others desired further explanations of the novelties, which they said were both worthy of consideration, and might perchance be found of single use. At length, yielding to the requests of my friends, that all might be made participators in my labors, and partly moved by the envy of others, who receiving my views with uncandid minds and understanding them indifferently, have essayed to traduce me publicly. I have moved to commit these things to the press, in order that all may be enabled to form an opinion both of me and my labours. (pp. 273-274)

By the end of the 17th century, the medical scientist was emerging. At this point in history, medical practice was not at all consistent, yet there was a body of knowledge being created that served as the basis for later discoveries and practices. Medical schools were founded in Europe during the 17th century, but it was not until the latter half of the 19th century that medical education was rigorously evaluated. These discoveries occurred in a comparatively short period of intense activity from the 19th century to the present. The early research describing the human organism served as a foundation of scientific knowledge that was later expanded and incorporated into clinical practice.

1.4 METHODOLOGICAL PROCESS: STAGE II

1.4.1 Development of Medical Technology in the Eighteenth and Nineteenth Centuries

The second stage in medical research was the development of precision instruments and test procedures that enabled the medical scientist to examine and measure the internal processes in the body. Typical among early scientific inventors in medicine was Laennec (1781–1826) who, by watching children playing with hollow cylinders, invented the stethoscope. Methodological research over the centuries has brought about technological advances such as the electroencephalogram (EEG), electrocardiogram (ECG), radiograph, procedures for urine analysis, positron emission tomography (PET), single photon emission computed tomography (SPECT), computed tomography (CT) scan, magnetic resonance imaging (MRI), and other important instruments and procedures that have become basic tools in clinical medicine. Moreover, technology is continually being refined and updated.

Methodological research is unique in its application of industrial technology to the problems of diagnosis and treatment. Initially, the great advances in methodology coincided with the rise of the industrial revolution in the 18th century. Medical scientists working with engineers were able to create objective medical tests that were the bases of modern medicine. Many of these advances were examples of interdisciplinary research where investigators from diverse professions applied their special knowledge to a specific research problem.

Norbert Wiener (1948), who proposed the theory of cybernetics that led to computers, used interdisciplinary seminars as a means of generating new ideas and stimulating creative thinking. Presently, engineers are working in conjunction with medical scientists to create artificial materials and devices that can replace organs in the body. Biomedical engineering is a direct application of methodological research to medicine. Prosthetics, self-help devices, and orthotics are examples of methodological research applied to the field of rehabilitation. Table 1-3 summarizes

the major methodological inventions that have impacted medical care.

1.4.2 The Practice of Medicine in the First Half of the Nineteenth Century

The latter half of the 19th century was a golden period in the history of medicine. During this time, medical schools were given the legal authority to certify physicians. Examinations were required for anyone who practiced medicine in the United States and Europe. In England, for example, a Medical Register was established in 1858. Atwater (1973) in an article documenting the medical profession in Rochester, New York, from 1811 to 1860, described the current state of medical knowledge available to general practitioners. Table 1-4 contains an abstracted description of the advances in medicine made during the prior three centuries according to Atwater (1973).

Although medicine had achieved great gains up until this period, most contagious diseases, except for smallpox, were untreatable. Surgeons worked at a great disadvantage without antiseptic techniques, and hospitals did not provide the care we associate with excellent nursing. Medical advances would have to wait for Pasteur, Lister, Morton, and Nightingale to provide the revolutionary innovations in antiseptic medicine.

1.5 ETIOLOGICAL ADVANCES: STAGE III

1.5.1 Medical Research in the Latter Half of the Nineteenth Century

The third stage in medical research was the integration of physiology and pathology with the use of a reliable methodology to arrive at a diagnosis. The evolution of the dynamic understanding of the disease process is described in Table 1-5. During this stage, an understanding of the etiology of a disease through experimental laboratory research was used to verify cause-effect relationships. This breakthrough in treating disease on a scientific basis started with Pasteur's discovery of the germ theory. From Pasteur's work, laboratory scientists could investigate disease processes by identifying a specific microorganism. The age of chemotherapy was initiated. For every microorganism causing a disease, which was isolated in the laboratory, researchers sought a chemical substance harmless to the body to counteract the germ. From 1850 to 1910, the process of identifying the germ responsible for a disease and the discovery of a chemical to eliminate the germ was the basis for the rapid conquest of many communicable diseases. The elimination of many communicable diseases would not have occurred without the microscope and the laboratory

TABLE 1-3

METHODOLOGICAL ADVANCES—STAGE II

MEDICAL EVENTS	DATES	SCIENTISTS	IMPLICATIONS
Clinical thermometer	1614	Santotio Santorio (1561–1636)	Physical examination in clinical medicine
Microscopical anatomy	1661	Marcello Malpighi (1628–1694)	Diagnostic studies of the blood
Clinical microscope	1695	Antony Van Leeuwenhoek (1632–1694)	Refinement of microscope
Technique of thoracic percussion	1761	Leopold Auenbrugger (1722–1809)	Diagnosis of respiratory disorders
Stethoscope	1819	Rene Laennec (1781–1826)	Diagnosis of circulatory disorders
Hypodermic syringe	1853	Alexander Wood (1817–1884)	Blood transfusions
Method for testing the quantity of sugar in urine	1848	Herman von Fehling (1811–1885)	Diagnosis of diabetes mellitus
X-ray	1895	Wilhelm Roentgen (1845–1923)	Detection of tuberculosis, fractures, and dislocations
Ophthalmoscope	1851	Hermann von Helmholtz (1821–1894)	Detection of morbid changes in the eye
Cystoscope	1890	Max Nitze (1847–1907)	Disease of urinary system
ECG	1903	Willem Einthoven (1860–1927)	Coronary functioning
EEG	1929	Hans Berger (1873–1941)	Cerebral dysfunction
Magnetic resonance phenomena used in MRI	1952	Edward M. Purcell (1905–1983) Felix Bloch (1912–1997)	Diagnostic assistance
CT scan	1972	Allan Cormack (1924–1998) Sir Godfrey Hounsfield (1919–2004)	Diagnostic assistance
Pulsed neuromagnetic resonance and MRI	1975	Richard Ernst (1933–)	Diagnostic assistance
PET	1970s	William H. Sweet (1930–2001) Gordon Brownell (1922–2008)	Diagnostic assistance
SPECT	1970s	R. Q. Edwards (1921–1976) D. E. Kuhl (1929–2017)	Diagnostic assistance

techniques of microbiology and biochemistry. The technology for protecting the individual from infectious diseases was a direct result of the understanding of human physiology and cellular theory. Septic techniques for surgery were later developed by Lister (1827–1912), who was greatly influenced by the work of Pasteur, and Semmelweis (1818–1865), an obstetrician who recognized the importance of hospital surgeons using prophylactic techniques during childbirth to prevent infection.

The knowledge of cellular activity by Virchow (1821–1902) was another line of evidence verifying the germ theory of disease. According to Virchow, the cause of disease was a result of changes at the cellular level.

Virchow's cellular theory of disease compelled pathologists to use microscopes in searching for lesions and abnormalities within the cells. Metchnikoff (1845–1916) discovered phagocytosis, recognizing that white blood corpuscles in the body counteract disease. The understanding of the dynamics of disease led to the science of clinical medicine.

Physicians were then able to diagnose disease through laboratory microscope techniques, thus replacing vitalism and metaphysics as explanations for the onset of communicable disease. Probably the most important work on medical research in the 19th century was Claude Bernard's *Introduction to the Study of Experimental Medicine* published in 1865. Pasteur acknowledged Bernard as an

TABLE 1-4
PROGRESS IN SURGERY, CLINICAL MEDICINE, AND PUBLIC HEALTH UP TO PASTEUR'S FORMULATION OF THE GERM THEORY IN 1878

SURGERY	DIAGNOSIS AND TREATMENT	PUBLIC HEALTH
• Use of ether and chloroform as anesthetics • Setting of broken bones and reduction of dislocated joints • Removal of superficial diseased tissue and kidney stones • Widespread practice of obstetrics and gynecology	• Use of microscope, auscultation, and stethoscope in diagnosis • Dynamic understanding of anatomy and physiology • Isolation of patients with contagious diseases • Relief of local pain pharmacologically	• Construction of municipal sewers • Recording of vital statistics • Custodial care of people who are mentally ill, intellectually impaired, poor, or homeless • Prevention of smallpox through vaccination

TABLE 1-5
DYNAMIC UNDERSTANDING OF DISEASE PROCESSES—STAGE III

MEDICAL EVENT	DATE	SCIENTIST	IMPLICATIONS
Clinical physiology	1857	Claude Bernard (1813–1878)	Treatment of physiologic and metabolic disorders through pharmacology
Cell theory	1858	Rudolf Ludwig Virchow (1821–1902)	Cellular pathology as the basis of treatment
Germ theory	1878	Louis Pasteur (1822–1895)	The role of microorganisms in disease established
Bacteriology	1882	Robert Koch (1843–1910)	Treatment of bacterial infections could be controlled by the physician
Role of filterable viruses	1888	Pierre Roux (1853–1933)	Identification of viruses resulted in the search for preventative measures
Immunization process	1892	Elie Metchnikoff (1845–1916)	Understanding of the body's phagocytosis defense mechanisms against disease was recognized
Chemotherapy	1899	Paul Ehrlich (1854–1915)	Specific chemical compounds used to treat communicable diseases

important influence in his own work. Bernard's major contributions to understanding disease included physiology of digestion, neurophysiology, pharmacology, and organic chemistry. Bernard's work has had a profound influence in medical science. Concepts such as homeostasis and stress, introduced by Cannon (1932) and Selye (1956), respectively, are based on Bernard's experimental findings on the internal gastrointestinal environment. Bernard, through his experimental methodology, established the future direction of medical research based on rigorous observation, repeated replication, and the acceptance or rejection of a hypothesis.

"Scientific generalization must proceed from particular facts or principles" (Bernard, 1957, p. 2). This simple statement is the foundation of 20th century medical research.

With a refined scientific methodology and a comprehensive theory of disease, medical researchers from about 1880 to 1910 made dramatic progress in identifying disease agents. This advance is exemplified by Koch's work in tuberculosis in 1890, von Behring's work in diphtheria in 1900, and Ehrlich's persistent search for a chemical to counteract syphilis, culminating in the discovery of the drug Salvarsan in 1910 after 606 experimental clinical trials.

TABLE 1-6			
CONTROL OF COMMUNICABLE DISEASES THROUGH IMMUNIZATION			
DISEASE	CAUSATIVE AGENT	MEDICAL RESEARCHER	DISCOVERY DATE
Bubonic plague	Bacterium	Shibasaburō Kitasato Alexandre Yersin	1893–1894
Cholera	Bacterium	Robert Koch	1884
Diphtheria	Bacterium	Emil Von Behring	1890
Measles	Virus	Francesio Cenci	1901
Poliomyelitis	Virus	Jonas Salk	1954
Rabies	Virus	Louis Pasteur	1885
Rocky Mountain spotted fever	Virus	Howard Ricketts	1909
Smallpox	Virus	Edward Jenner	1796
Tuberculosis	Bacterium	Albert Calmette Camille Guerin	1921
Typhoid fever	Bacterium	Almroth Wright	1906
Typhus	Virus	Charles Nicolle	1910
Yellow fever	Virus	Max Thieler	1936

1.6 PREVENTION: STAGE IV

1.6.1 Preventive Medicine in the Twentieth Century

The advances in medical research that have had the most dramatic effect in eliminating diseases can be attributed to primary prevention, including public health techniques and mass vaccinations. Public health measures, such as purification of water, elimination of human waste products, and protection against food spoilage, were used by ancient civilizations, such as the Egyptians, Greeks, and Romans. However, when superstition prevailed over using prophylactic methods, as during the Middle Ages in Europe, epidemics and widespread disease occurred. Throughout the world, the potential for epidemics still exists in underdeveloped countries or in war and disaster zones where public health measures have been disregarded. The elimination of typhus, cholera, bubonic plague, polio, and smallpox in areas with access to modern medicine has been accomplished through the combination of medical advances and public health practices. Vaccination as a way of preventing disease has provided the means to control widespread epidemics that dramatically reduced populations in the past. The first physician to conceive of the use of vaccinations to prevent disease was Jenner (1749–1823), who experimented with cowpox infection, a mild disease, as a means of protecting against smallpox, one of the leading causes of death in the 18th century. Jenner noted that dairymaids who contracted cowpox by milking infected cows developed a natural immunity to smallpox. This observation led him to believe that if people were deliberately infected with cowpox, they would escape the dreaded smallpox. In 1798, Jenner published his findings, which included 23 case histories of individuals inoculated with cowpox.

Initially, Jenner's work was not accepted by the medical community in England. He gradually gained recognition after his work was replicated by other physicians. Jenner's original research on vaccinations remained singularly unique until Pasteur's discovery of the germ theory about 100 years later in 1878. Jenner's method of inoculation to prevent disease was rediscovered by medical researchers who were later able to isolate pathogenic bacteria and viruses. Table 1-6 lists many of the communicable diseases that are now controlled by vaccination.

Presently, the concept of preventive medicine includes the following health procedures:

- Inoculation to prevent communicable diseases
- Environmental health to reduce atmospheric and water pollution
- Prenatal care to prevent birth defects
- Mental health community services to prevent institutionalization
- Family planning and population control
- Supervision of food handling and processing of foods to prevent botulism

- Prevention of industrial accidents through ergonomics
- Sanitary engineering to prevent typhus and cholera

Until the 20th century, physicians could do little for a patient who was severely ill. The introduction of chemotherapy, aseptic surgery, and efficient hospital care changed the course of medical practice.

1.7 Chemotherapy, Surgery, and Hospital Care—The Bases of Treatment: Stage V

1.7.1 Chemotherapy

As knowledge about anatomy and physiology progressed, technology was developed to improve the diagnoses of illnesses. The foundations, created to produce a body of knowledge underlying therapeutics, resulted in chemotherapy, surgery, and hospital care as the bases of modern-day treatment. Although ancient civilizations and primitive cultures existing today have used various effective treatments, the causes of diseases and the rationale for understanding the processes were veiled in mystery. For example, rauwolfia serpentine was used in India (100 AD) as the "medicine of sad men" (Thorwald, 1963, p. 205) without the present understanding of the biochemical process of a tranquilizer. Ancient Egyptian doctors used mud and soil in the treatment of eye diseases. This type of "sewerage pharmacology" was not understood until 1948 when Dr. Benjamin M. Dugger, a professor of plant physiology at the University of Wisconsin, discovered the drug aureomycin, a chemical similar to natural substances found near the Nile River. Aureomycin has been highly effective in the treatment of trachoma.

For centuries, practical treatment for many disabilities, diseases, and illnesses has been applied by trial and error without an understanding of the theoretical dynamics of the disease processes. Healers, such as shamans and witch doctors, intersperse treatment with superstition, sometimes attaining positive results. The important difference between applying therapeutics in modern science and in prescientific civilizations is in the explanation of why a specific treatment cures a disease. The search for cures to diseases, beginning with the germ theory of Pasteur and continuing through Alexander Fleming's discovery of penicillin in 1928 and Selman A. Waksman's discovery of streptomycin in 1944, spurred the corporate growth of therapeutic pharmaceutics. Modern medicine is heavily dependent on the availability of various drugs to control abnormal physical conditions, such as hypertension, arteriosclerosis, blood clotting, edema, and emotional illness. Hormone therapy and uses of vitamins and dietetics are other common methods akin to chemical therapy as forms of treatment.

1.7.2 Surgery

Surgical interventions in the 21st century continue to make dramatic gains in improving health care throughout the world. From 1992 to 2012, the total number of surgeries at community hospitals in the United States increased by 17% to about 26.8 million surgeries. Outpatient surgeries represented a growing share (65%; 17.3 million) of all surgeries at community hospitals in the United States in 2012, up from 54% (12.3 million) in 1992 (Healthcare Cost and Utilization Project [HCUP], 2019). Surgery is increasingly used as an outpatient procedure that has reduced the time in surgery and the time for patient recuperation. There was a 300% increase in the rates of visits to free standing ambulatory surgery centers from 1996 to 2006. A list of the most frequent surgical procedures performed in the United States is shown in Table 1-7 (Cullen, Hall, & Golosinskiy, 2009). Surgery as an advanced medical intervention has a long evolution in the history of humanity. Ancient civilizations, such as the Incas of Peru in 200 BCE, used trepanation (removing parts of a skull) as a method to relieve epileptic fits and intractable headaches (Ellis, 2001). The ancient Romans (ca. 70–200 BCE) used up to 200 different surgical instruments in various operations. In addition, ligature of blood vessels was performed; obstetric surgery, specifically Caesarean section, was known; and even anesthesia was used (Martí-Ibáñez, 1962).

Modern surgery as an effective and safe method was the result of two important events: the development of antiseptics by Lister in 1867, who tested the capacity of carbolic acid in preventing infection in general surgery; and the discovery of ether anesthesia as a practical method by William Morton, a dentist, in 1846 (Ellis, 2001; Haeger, 1988).

1.7.3 Hospital Care

The third component in the development of modern treatment, parallel to chemotherapy and surgery, was the rise of hospital nursing care. Florence Nightingale's role in developing the nursing profession is legendary. Singlehandedly, she aroused world public opinion about the plight of hospital patients, who were often left to die because of neglect. The story of Nightingale's success is well-known. During the Crimean War of 1854, she organized a group of nurses to tend wounded British soldiers. Her experience gave her the insight into the need for clean, efficient hospitals. Reform in hospital care became a national issue in England after the Crimean War, and social legislation was enacted to provide governmental support. Florence Nightingale also started the first school of nursing at St. Thomas' Hospital, London, in 1860. With hospital reform enacted through legislation and a nursing school started, the foundation for progress in the treatment of the hospitalized patient was established.

The following is a short outline of the historical development of hospitals as documented by Rene Sand (1952):

TABLE 1-7		
MOST FREQUENT SURGICAL PROCEDURES IN THE UNITED STATES IN 2012		
PROCEDURE	NUMBER	RATE PER 100,000 POPULATION
Knee arthroplasty	700,100	223.0
Percutaneous coronary angioplasty	534,600	170.3
Laminectomy, excision intervertebral disc	468,200	149.1
Hip replacement, total and partial	468,000	149.1
Spinal fusion	450,900	143.6
Cholecystectomy and common duct exploration	406,300	129.4
Partial bone excision	338,000	107.7
Hysterectomy, abdominal and vaginal	312,100	99.4
Colorectal resection	305,900	97.4
Excision, lysis peritoneal adhesions	305,800	97.4

Note: Includes only nonmaternal and nonneonatal stays. All-listed operating room procedures were identified using Clinical Classifications Software procedure categories. Procedures designated as Other are not reported.

Adapted from Agency for Healthcare Research and Quality (AHRQ), Center for Delivery, Organization, and Markets, Healthcare Cost and Utilization Project (HCUP), National Inpatient Sample (NIS), 2012. This publication is available through https://www.hcup-us.ahrq.gov/reports/statbriefs/sb186-Operating-Room-Procedures-United-States-2012.jsp

- *Ancient Greece, 6th Century, BC*: A large open building was provided for the Greek physician. It comprised a waiting room, consulting room, and theater for operations and dressings.
- *Ancient Rome, 1st Century, AD*: Sick bays were attached to the family estates of the wealthy.
- *Early Medieval Europe, 4th Century, AD*: Early Christians established *hospitia* for travelers, abandoned children, and the sick who were traveling on their way to pilgrimages. Care was under the direction of monastic and sisterly orders.
- *Middle East, 12th Century, AD*: Muslims in Baghdad founded the first hospitals where physicians cared for the ill. Special wards for mental illness, blindness, and leprosy were established.
- *Later Middle Ages, Europe, 5th to 14th Centuries*: Hostelries under the jurisdiction of the Roman Catholic Church provided care for the sick. Brothers and sisters of the Roman Catholic Church in attached ecclesiastical hospitals provided treatment remedies, performed simple operations, and attended those with serious illnesses.
- *Renaissance Europe, 15th Century*: For the first time in the Western world, physicians and midwives treated the sick in hospitals. Terminal patients were segregated from the acutely ill.
- *Europe, 18th Century*: Gradually hospitals began to treat emergency care patients, outpatient departments grew, and hospitals served as training facilities for medical students.
- *Europe and America, 19th Century*: Nursing care was established in hospitals. Antiseptic surgery, anesthesia, and improvement in general care of the hospitalized patient were initiated.
- *Worldwide, 20th Century*: The growth of specialized hospitals, regional planning, and national health services. A world movement exists in extending health care to underdeveloped countries under the auspices of the United Nations, WHO.

Current medical treatment is based on the principle of healing—stopping the progression of a disease and promoting natural bodily processes. Chemotherapy, surgery, and nursing care are the three basic methods that have made medical practice effective in treating many communicable diseases and physiological disorders and anatomical defects. However, there are still limitations of medical treatment for individuals with severe chronic disabilities, such as schizophrenia, arthritis, cardiovascular disease, and cerebrovascular accident. Medical treatment alone is effective only when the disease process can be narrowed down to a specific etiology. Chronic diseases present problems of multiple etiologies and treatment requiring complex solutions and interdisciplinary efforts. The search for solutions to the chronic disabilities led to the rehabilitation movement.

Table 1-8

Historical Factors Leading to the Rehabilitation Movement

- Incorporation of scientific methodology into clinical medicine
- Industrialization and its impact on clinical procedures for diagnosis and treatment
- Large population of veterans with disabilities from World War I
- The availability of financial resources through Social Security and National Health Insurance
- Medical specialties and the development of allied health professions
- Public acceptance that individuals with disabilities can be restored to independence through rehabilitation
- Public acceptance of individuals with disabilities in social and work situations

1.8 Rehabilitation Movement: Stage VI

The emergence of rehabilitation as a distinct entity in the health care system began in 1916 during World War I. The aftermath of World War I and the devastation it brought saw the beginning of the rehabilitation movement, coinciding with the need for restoring function to those who were permanently disabled. One may ask why the rehabilitation field developed at that time and not in prior periods of recovery from war. The historical factors that led to the rehabilitation movement are outlined in Table 1-8. Until the 18th century, chronic illness and permanent disability in general were not always considered medical problems. For instance, psychiatric illness and epilepsy were considered problems of morality and satanic possession. Treatment of psychiatric illness, if any, was stark, brutal, or radical. Before the rise of large institutions providing custodial care for patients, the attitude toward chronic mental illness was at best benign neglect and at worst rejection and punishment. In a related area, birth injuries, such as cerebral palsy, were misunderstood by ancient cultures. Not until 1862, when W. T. Little, an English orthopedic surgeon, described the relationship between birth injury and neurological disorders, was there any dynamic understanding of this disability. Individuals with other chronic disabilities, such as arthritis, emphysema, stroke, cardiovascular disease, and spinal cord injuries, were left either to the custodial care of the family, or worse, were placed into the hands of charlatans who promised miraculous cures.

1.8.1 Social Welfare and Rehabilitation

The change from custodial care to therapeutic treatment of the individual with chronic disabilities occurred at a period of time in history when social welfare had become a worldwide concern. Social security was the forerunner in public health and medicine for the indigent with chronic disabilities. Germany, in 1883, and England, in 1897, were the first countries in Europe to enact legislation providing worker's compensation to cover disability and illness resulting from occupational accidents. The progress toward social and occupational health and safety is described in Table 1-9. Governmental financial support, resulting from national policies on health and welfare, was necessary because of the enormous hospital resources and health personnel required in the rehabilitation of individuals with disabilities. In the United States, social security legislation, first enacted in 1935, has been a major impetus for the development of the rehabilitation movement. Change in societies' attitudes toward the individual with chronic disabilities, as evidenced in the social welfare movement, has encouraged the growth of the allied health professions.

1.8.2 Development of Allied Health Professions: Phase I

Three major phases in the history of rehabilitation have affected the growth of the allied health professions. The first phase occurred shortly after World War I. During this period, the need for physical and social rehabilitation of individuals with disabilities was recognized by the medical community. Casualties from the war included individuals with lower extremity amputation, victims of poisonous gas (resulting in neurological disabilities), and soldiers with psychiatric disabilities caused by the horrors of war. At that time, these veterans of the war needed assistance in readjusting to community living. Reconstruction workers recruited from nursing staffs were the first health personnel in rehabilitation. Immediately after World War I, the goal of rehabilitation was primarily humane and supportive to the medical treatment. There was no direct effort by the rehabilitation workers to change the course of a disability or to make the individual with disabilities more functional. During the late 1920s, rehabilitation departments were established for the first time in hospitals. The health personnel recruited to work in these departments were, on the whole, dedicated people who applied caring support and activity to facilitate the patient's readjustment to the community.

1.8.3 Education and Professionalization: Phase II

The second phase of rehabilitation, during the 1930s, 1940s, and 1950s, can be identified as the *educational*

TABLE 1-9		
PROGRESS TOWARD SOCIAL REFORM IN OCCUPATIONAL HEALTH AND SAFETY		
ANTIQUITY • Manual labor and tradesmen neglected • Occupational diseases ignored	**MEDIEVAL GUILDS** • Voluntary associations formed for mutual aid protection of tradesman • Assist worker with disabilities • Assist in funeral expense	**SOCIETY OF ARTIFICERS** • Established apprenticeship system • Workday regulated 12 to 13 hours
PROTECTION OF MINERS • 16th century • Ventilating machines for mines	**OCCUPATIONAL MEDICINE** • Established 17th century • Relationship between occupation and disease investigated medically • Prevention measures introduced (e.g., rest intervals, positioning, cleanliness, protective clothing)	**COMPILING OF VITAL STATISTICS ON OCCUPATIONAL DISEASE** • 18th century • Use of medical inspectors
PROTECTION OF VULNERABLE WORKERS IN DANGEROUS TRADES • 19th century • Public health legislation to regulate child labor • Work day reduced to 10 hours	**WORKMEN'S COMPENSATION** • 1890 to 1910 • Compensate workers for occupational accidents and diseases	**NATIONAL WOMEN'S TRADE UNION** • 1920 • Protection of women from dangerous industries
WORKER HEALTH BUREAU • Established 1927	**SOCIAL SECURITY LEGISLATION** • 1930s • Place safety and health activities within Labor Department	**OCCUPATIONAL SAFETY AND HEALTH AGENCIES** • Established 1970 • Onsite inspections, regulations, and enforcement of laws relating to dangerous and unhealthy conditions in all industries
THE NATIONAL INSTITUTE FOR OCCUPATIONAL SAFETY AND HEALTH • Established 1970 • Provide information through research, information, education and training to aid in improving safe and healthful working conditions	**SCIENTIFIC INVESTIGATIONS OF PREVENTION AND TREATMENT OF OCCUPATIONAL INJURIES AND DISEASES** • 1980s • Application of ergonomics and rehabilitation of principles	**FUTURE TRENDS IN OCCUPATIONAL MEDICINE** • Occupational health teams: ergonomist, occupational therapist, physician, industrial hygienist, physical therapist, safety officer, and nurse • Investigation of physical, chemical, biological, and psychological factors in work environment that may cause or aggravate disease in individuals who are vulnerable • Investigation of long-term effects of exposure to toxic chemicals, repetitive motion, vibration, excessive noise, extreme temperature, radiation, dust, bacteria • Prevention of accidents or disease

TABLE 1-10			
EARLY LANDMARKS IN REHABILITATION MOVEMENT—STAGE VI			
REHABILITATION EVENTS	**DATES**	**CONTRIBUTORS**	**SIGNIFICANCE**
First comprehensive rehabilitation	1946	Howard Rusk	Served as model for physical medicine programs in a general hospital rehabilitation team approach
Physical therapy methods	1949	H. O. Kendall F. P. Kendall	Basis for physical therapy techniques for muscle testing and patient evaluation
Retraining methods of ADLs	1956	Edith Buchwald Lawton	Provided functional rehabilitation methods for increasing independence
Vocational rehabilitation	1957	Lloyd H. Lofquist	Established the role of the rehabilitation counselor
Aphasia rehabilitation	1955	Martha L. Taylor M. Marks	Provided rehabilitation techniques for speech therapy
Prosthetics	1959	M. H. Anderson C. O. Bechtol R. E. Sollars	Led to cooperative research by physicians, engineers, and prosthetists in the design of artificial limbs
Orthotics	1962	Muriel Zimmerman	Led to the development of self-help devices for the homemaker and worker with physical disabilities

and professionalization phase. Table 1-10 lists the early landmarks in physical rehabilitation. During this time, programs in colleges and universities were initiated, professional associations grew, and rehabilitation services evolved. The training of allied health specialists who had a unique combination of knowledge in the application of activities and rehabilitation techniques, understanding of medical treatment, and a background in the social sciences were considered necessary preparation for working in a hospital setting. The concepts underlying rehabilitation at that time were taken from other clinical and applied disciplines, such as anatomy, physiology, nutrition, language development, psychology, clinical medicine, and education.

1.8.4 Physical Medicine and Rehabilitation

The first rehabilitation medical service in a general hospital was created in 1946, in Bellevue Hospital, New York City, New York (Rusk, 1971). This unit served as a model for the interdisciplinary rehabilitation team. In addition, the physiatry specialty in rehabilitation medicine was started. Conceptually, rehabilitation was defined as restoring the individual to the highest level of cognitive, physical, economic, social, and emotional independence. This process, involving a team evaluation of the patient's functions, the establishment of treatment goals and priorities, and an interdisciplinary approach to treatment, became the model for rehabilitation. This process is listed in Table 1-11.

Parallel to the evolution of a medical rehabilitation team was the involvement of federal and state governments in providing vocational rehabilitation services that resulted from the Vocational Rehabilitation Act of 1954. Sheltered workshops (e.g., Abilities, Inc., in New York City; Epi-Hab in Phoenix, Arizona, and Los Angeles, California; Community Workshops in Boston, Massachusetts; and Goodwill Industries) provided the vocational training component and the specialized employment placement that helped reemploy individuals with disabilities.

1.8.5 Allied Health Treatment Technologies

As the training of allied health professionals developed during the 1940s and 1950s, a treatment technology emerged, especially in physical therapy. Methods for objectively assessing muscle function were established (Daniels, Williams, & Worthingham, 1956; Kendall & Kendall, 1949). Electrodiagnosis of muscle function, measurement of range of motion, and techniques for improving muscle and joint action through heat, ultraviolet rays, electrical stimulation, whirlpool, and cold packs were developed through trial and error and clinical practice. These techniques were a major part of the physical therapist's treatment procedures (Downer, 1970). The need for retraining patients in ADLs

TABLE 1-11		
THE PROCESS OF PHYSICAL MEDICINE AND REHABILITATION		
CHRONIC DISABILITY	**EVALUATION OF FUNCTION**	**TREATMENT**
• Amputee • Arthritis • Degenerative disease of the central nervous system • Emphysema and pulmonary disease • Epilepsy • Spinal cord injury • Stroke	• ADLs • Ambulation • Diet • Leisure activities • Muscular and joint function • Neurological processes • Psychological factors • Speech and language • Vocational adjustment	• Chemotherapy • Dietetics • Nursing care • Occupational therapy • Orthotics • Physical therapy • Prosthetics • Psychological counselling • Social work • Speech therapy • Surgery • Vocational rehabilitation
Rehabilitation is the process of restoring function in individuals with severe disabilities. Assessment of the physical, cognitive, psychosocial and vocational factors are carried out before intervention is planned and implemented.		

was recognized by therapists as an important area for intervention. Lawton (1956), working with Howard Rusk at the Institute of Physical Medicine and Rehabilitation, published a manual for therapists describing methods to retrain patients to become functionally independent in their everyday activities. The need to retrain patients with aphasia to regain their use of language as the result of a stroke or brain injury led to the development of sequentially programmed techniques (Sarno & Marks, 1955).

Another important component of rehabilitation was in the area of vocational rehabilitation. Lofquist (1957), McGowan (1960), and Patterson (1958) were some of the early workers who defined the role of the rehabilitation counselor in prevocational evaluation, special placement, and vocational training. Occupational therapy progressed as an integral part of the rehabilitation movement in a more general direction than physical or speech therapy. The use of activities as treatment modalities in work, leisure, and ADLs was applied to a broader spectrum of disabilities. Occupational therapists worked mainly in rehabilitation departments, psychiatric state hospitals, Veterans Affairs facilities, and state schools for those with physical and mental disabilities (Willard & Spackman, 1971). As the rehabilitation movement gained momentum in the 1950s, biomedical research in the replacement of limbs and joints led to the field of prosthetics. The design of component parts, fitting of the prosthesis, and gait training gave rise to another member of the physical rehabilitation team, the prosthetist (Anderson, Bechtol, & Sollaris, 1959). Specialization in rehabilitation also occurred at a rapid rate within the fields of nutrition, social work, psychology, and nursing.

1.8.6 Psychiatric Rehabilitation

In comparison with physical rehabilitation techniques, psychiatric treatment has lagged behind in developing the techniques to treat the individual with mental illness. The initial optimism from 1930 to 1950 that was generated by biological interventions, such as electric convulsive therapy, insulin therapy, metrazol treatment, and psychosurgery, has faded. From the 1960s to the 1990s, psychiatric treatment remained in a state of disarray. The onset of neuroleptic drugs and the community mental health movement in the 1960s led to the dismantling of large psychiatric hospitals that served as custodial "warehouses" for the patients who were chronically mentally ill.

Since the 1960s, the length of hospitalization for patients with psychiatric disorders has been drastically reduced, but the number of individuals with mental illness living in the community and homeless without treatment has increased. Current enlightened psychiatric treatment emphasizes early return to the community in combination with outpatient vocational rehabilitation. In many state hospitals for those with mental illness, a large percentage of elderly patients form a residual population from the custodial period. This population is mainly rejected, untreated, and provided mostly with maintenance care. Other individuals with mental illness are in nursing homes, custodial care facilities, or prison facilities or are left untreated in large cities as members of homeless populations.

Evaluation of psychiatric treatment remains a fertile area for clinical researchers. Apart from descriptive observations, few comprehensive studies have analyzed treatment techniques in depth. Although many clinicians believe that what they are doing is beneficial, there is little systematically collected empirical evidence to support their claims.

Why has psychiatric rehabilitation lagged compared to other areas of medical progress? First, there has been wide disagreement in identifying, diagnosing, and treating mental illness despite the attempt to classify it as exemplified in the *Diagnostic and Statistical Manual of Mental Disorders, Fifth Edition* (American Psychiatric Association, 2013). Theorists have differed widely in their approaches in psychiatry, advocating specific treatment techniques for the broad spectrum of mental illness. Many clinical researchers have failed to recognize the individual needs of patients and the differential effects of treatment. A second reason for the lag in scientific progress in psychiatric rehabilitation is the lack of comprehensive studies. Psychiatric research has been fixed at the 19th century, two-variable research stage model, which assumed a single-factor cause for mental illness. If progress in psychiatric rehabilitation is to occur, multidisciplinary efforts must investigate mental illness on a broad front, using a biopsychosocial model, rather than using narrow, one-dimensional research. The promise in psychiatric rehabilitation lies in a holistic approach, the incorporation of a community mental health model relying on halfway houses, vocational programs, and support groups, with an individualized approach to evaluation, education, psychotherapy, counseling, and drug treatment.

1.8.7 Third Phase of Allied Health—1950 to Present

This development led to the present period of rehabilitation, which has been characterized by various treatment theories. Unfortunately, these theories have become so specialized that professionals in allied health fields can no longer change from one disability area to another without familiarizing themselves with a vast amount of knowledge and technology. For example, allied health professionals have specialized in diverse areas such as constraint therapy, augmentative communication, computer technology, sensory integration therapy, neurodevelopmental therapy, robotics, telemetry, cinematography, and biofeedback. These areas of rehabilitation are unique. They are interdisciplinary in nature and incorporate theories and findings from the physical and social sciences. Table 1-12 shows the rapid growth of the allied health professions from 1950 to the present.

The extraordinary growth of the allied health professions since 1950 is apparent if one examines the percentage increase in the number of active practitioners and the number of professional schools. In comparison with the United States' population increase from 150 million in 1949 to 210 million in 1972, one would have expected the professions to increase about 40%. We find, however, that professions such as occupational and physical therapy increased 300%

during the same period. The number of radiologic technologists increased 685%, registered nurses increased 149%, and physicians increased 58% during this period. On the other hand, the smallest increases were in the numbers of chiropractic, osteopathy, optometry, and pharmacy professionals. The growth of the allied health professions has continued into the 1980s and 1990s with forecasts of continued growth far into the 21st century.

Another indication of the rapid expansion of the allied health professions is the emergence of new fields that did not exist 40 years ago. *The Occupational Outlook Handbook* from 1951 did not include many allied health professions, which appeared in later editions, starting with 1972 (Table 1-13).

1.8.8 Rehabilitation Research Trends (1950 to 1975)

In an analysis of rehabilitation research, Goldberg (1974) identified 10 areas that are related to clinical practice:

- *Program evaluation*: The assessment of the effectiveness of a clinical program in reaching stated objectives or meeting a list of criteria
- *Management*: The study of factors related to health manpower, cost effectiveness, and comprehensive planning in providing health care to those in need of services
- *Dissemination*: The process of communicating research findings over a wide area, including to professional and lay persons
- *Involvement of consumer groups*: The identification of research problems
- *Chronic severe disability*: Functional problems as a major focus of research in rehabilitation
- *Social problems*: Alcoholism, adult crime, drug addiction, and juvenile delinquency as areas included under health-related problems instead of correctional problems
- *Functional assessment methods*: Targeted to the individuals with severe disabilities who are in supported employment and working at home
- *Need for follow-up and follow-along research*: Evaluation of the continuity of care
- *Rehabilitation utilization*: Incorporation of rehabilitation research in clinical practices
- *Rehabilitation engineering*: Interdisciplinary research in solving practical rehabilitation problems especially in the fields of prosthetics, orthotics, communication, mobility, and independent living

These trends continued to have an impact on current rehabilitation research in the 1990s. From the initial emphasis on the physical restoration of the individual, researchers are now turning to the more complex chronic social problems that are associated with poverty, substandard housing,

TABLE 1-12					
THE GROWTH OF HEALTH PROFESSION, 1950 TO 2014					
HEALTH SPECIALTY	**POSTSECONDARY TRAINING (YEARS)**	**ACTIVE PRACTITIONERS**			
		1950	*1972*	*1992*	*2014*
Audiologist[a]	6 to 8	—	—	—	13,200
Chiropractor	6 to 8	14,000	16,000	46,000	42,200
Dentist	8	75,300	105,000	183,000	151,500
Dietitian and nutritionists	4 to 5	15,000	33,000	50,000	66,700
Occupational therapist	5 to 6	2,300	7,500	40,000	114,000
Optometrist	7 to 8	17,000	18,700	31,000	40,000
Pharmacist	6 to 7	100,000	131,000	163,000	207,100
Physical therapist	6 to 7	4,500	18,000	90,000	210,900
Physician and surgeon[b]	8 to 16	200,000	316,500	556,000	708,300
Physician assistant[c]	4 to 6	—	303	22,305	94,400
Podiatrist	10 to 12	6,400	7,300	14,700	9,600
Psychologist	9 to 10	10,000	57,000	144,000	173,900
Registered nurse	3 to 5	300,500	750,000	1,835,000	2,751,000
Respiratory therapist	2 to 4	—	17,000	74,000	120,700
Speech-language pathologist	6	2000	27,000	73,000	135,400
Social worker	4 to 8	100,000	185,000	484,000	649,300

[a]Audiologists were included with speech-language pathologists until 2008.

[b]Surgeons were added in 2008.

[c]Physician's assistant programs were started in 1967.

Note: The information contained in this table is based on data from U.S. Department Labor, *Occupational Outlook Handbook* (1951, 1974–1975, 1982–1983, 1992–1993, 1994–1995, 1998–1999, 2010–11, 2017). Retrieved from http://stats.bls.gov/oco/ and from information obtained from professional societies.

undernourishment, alienation, and addiction. Evidence is present that severe chronic disabilities from diagnoses such as polio, tuberculosis, stroke, emphysema, and coronary thrombosis can be alleviated or reduced through public health immunization programs, balanced nutrition, exercise regimes, and self-monitoring of symptoms. The cost of preventing chronic illnesses is much less than the cost of rehabilitation. Primary, secondary, and tertiary prevention have begun to make an impact in the work of allied health professionals. Research has an important part in justifying the efficacy of treatment intervention, either in restoring function or preventing chronic disability.

Current trends in rehabilitation research are listed in Table 1-14, whereas Table 1-15 gives some examples of current review of rehabilitation and habilitation research.

1.9 HABILITATION AND SPECIAL EDUCATION: STAGE VII

The success of the rehabilitation movement led to the field of habilitation, which goes beyond the medical model. While the medical model traditionally relies on etiology, diagnosis, and treatment, habilitation includes the integration of psychological, sociological, and educational fields of knowledge emphasizing research in developmental theory and educational technology. Rehabilitation is traditionally defined as the restoration of function and the maximization of abilities in individuals with chronic disabilities. In contrast, habilitation is defined as the development of functions and capabilities in individuals with disabilities

Table 1-13

Growth of Selected Health Professions of Technologists and Assistants, 1972 to 2014

HEALTH FIELD	1972	1986	1996	2014
Dental hygienist	17,000	87,000	133,000	200,500
ECG technician	10,000	18,000	15,000	112,000
Medical record technician	8000	40,000	87,000	188,600
Nuclear medicine technologist	—	9700	13,000	20,700
Occupational therapy assistant	6000	9000	16,000	41,900
Physical therapist assistant	10,000	12,000	84,000	128,700
Radiology and MRI technologist	55,000	115,000	174,000	230,000
Respiratory therapist	17,000	56,000	82,000	120,700
Surgical technician	25,000	37,000	49,000	99,800

Note. Data are taken from the U.S. Department of Labor, *Occupational Outlook Handbook* (1972–1973, 1988–1989, 1992–1993, 1998–1999, 2010–2011, 2016-2017), retrieved from https://www.bls.gov/ooh/, and from professional associations.

Table 1-14

Current Trends in Rehabilitation Research, 2017

- Development of standardized (norm- and criterion-referenced) outcome measures that have acceptable coefficients of reliability and validity
- Evaluation of treatment techniques using prospective designs
- Operational definitions of treatment methods that can be replicated in clinical practice
- Controlled observation of normal developmental landmarks that serve as reference points for populations with disabilities
- Fundamental investigations of the biopsychosocial nature of disease and underlying dynamics
- Survey of the perceptions of patients with chronic disabilities toward their disability and their evaluation of treatment techniques
- The incorporation of high technology instrumentation in evaluation and treatment (e.g., microcomputers, cinematography, psychophysiological measures)
- Qualitative research and action research methods
- Application of research findings to evidence-based practice
- Meta-analyses of evidence-based practices

occurring at birth, during childhood, or during a traumatic incident (e.g., traumatic brain injury, posttraumatic stress). The process of habilitation is presented in Table 1-16. The child with intellectual disabilities, the individual who is congenitally blind or deaf, the child born with a missing limb or with cerebral palsy, the child with autism, and the child who is extremely disadvantaged have needs that are different from adults who acquired a physical disability. Helping the child develop independence, coping skills, and physical and mental capabilities to adapt to societal demands requires specialized techniques. The child who is developmentally delayed, unlike the adult with a disability, has not lost a capacity or skill that requires remedial education, sensory retraining, or vocational readjustment. Instead, the child with a disability needs special education, sensorimotor or language training, occupational preparation, and training for ADLs basic to the habilitation process. Special education services, available for individuals with special needs, have been developed to provide training and instruction in functional skills necessary for independent living and self-support. What were the early historical precursors to the field of habilitation?

TABLE 1-15
EXAMPLES OF CURRENT REVIEWS OF RESEARCH IN REHABILITATION AND HABILITATION FROM PUBLISHED ABSTRACTS

ANXIETY AND DEPRESSION

Ravindran, A. V., Lam, R. W., Filteau, M. J., Lespérance, F., Kennedy, S. H., Parikh, S. V., & Patten, S. B. (2009). Canadian Network for Mood and Anxiety Treatments (CANMAT). Clinical guidelines for the management of major depressive disorder in adults. V. Complementary and alternative medicine treatments. *Journal of Affective Disorders, 117*(Suppl 1), S54-S64.

***Abstract:* Background**: In 2001, the Canadian Psychiatric Association and the Canadian Network for Mood and Anxiety Treatments (CANMAT) partnered to produce evidence-based clinical guidelines for the treatment of depressive disorders. A revision of these guidelines was undertaken by CANMAT in 2008–2009 to reflect advances in the field. There is widespread interest in complementary and alternative medicine (CAM) therapies in the treatment of major depressive disorder (MDD). **Methods**: The CANMAT guidelines are based on a question-answer format to enhance accessibility to clinicians. An evidence-based format was used with updated systematic reviews of the literature and recommendations were graded according to Level of Evidence using pre-defined criteria. Lines of Treatment were identified based on criteria that included evidence and expert clinical support. This section on "Complementary and Alternative Medicine Treatments" is one of 5 guideline articles. **Results**: There is Level 1 evidence to support light therapy in seasonal MDD and St. John's wort in mild to moderate MDD. There is also some evidence for the use of exercise, yoga and sleep deprivation, as well as for omega-3 fatty acids and SAM-e. Support for other natural health products and therapies is still limited. **Limitations**: The evidence base remains limited and studies often have methodological problems, including small samples, variability in dose, short duration of treatment, unknown quality of the agent and limited long-term data. Safety data are also sparse with little information about drug interactions. **Conclusions**: Some CAM treatments have evidence of benefit in MDD. However, problems with standardization and safety concerns may limit their applicability in clinical practice.

AUTISM

Cotugno, A. J. (2009). Social competence and social skills training and intervention for children with Autism spectrum disorders. *Journal of Autism and Developmental Disorders, 39*, 1268-1277.

Abstract: This study examined the effectiveness of a 30-week social competence and social skills group intervention program with children, ages 7 to 11, diagnosed with Autism Spectrum Disorders (ASD). Eighteen children with ASD were assessed with pretreatment and posttreatment measures on the Walker-McConnell Scale (WMS) and the MGH YouthCare Social Competence Development Scale. Each received the 30-week intervention program. For comparison, a matched sample of ten non-ASD children was also assessed, but received no treatment. The findings indicated that each ASD intervention group demonstrated significant gains on the WMS and significant improvement in the areas of anxiety management, joint attention, and flexibility/transitions. Results suggest that this approach can be effective in improving core social deficits in individuals with ASD.

PEDIATRIC DISORDERS

Parsons, T. D, Rizzo, A. A., Rogers, S., & York, P. (2009).Virtual reality in paediatric rehabilitation: A review. *Developmental Neurorehabilation, 12*, 224-238.

***Abstract:* Objective**: To provide a narrative review of studies regarding the outcomes of Virtual Reality (VR)-based treatment and rehabilitation programmes within the paediatric population. **Methods**: Studies related to the use of VR across a number of paediatric areas (e.g., cerebral palsy, autism, foetal alcohol syndrome and attention deficits) were identified and summarized. **Results**: Outcomes from the studies reviewed provide preliminary support for the use of VR. **Conclusion**: VR may be an effective treatment method for specific disorders, although the generalizability of this literature is hindered by several methodological limitations, such as small samples and the absence of appropriate control participants.

(continued)

TABLE 1-15 (CONTINUED)

EXAMPLES OF CURRENT REVIEWS OF RESEARCH IN REHABILITATION AND HABILITATION FROM PUBLISHED ABSTRACTS

SCHIZOPHRENIA

Taylor, T. L., Killaspy, H., Wright, C., Turton, P., White, S., Kallert, T. W., . . . King, M. B. (2009). A systematic review of the international published literature relating to quality of institutional care for people with longer term mental health problems. *BMC Psychiatry, 9*, 55. doi:10.1186/1471-244X-9-55

Abstract: **Background**: A proportion of people with mental health problems require longer term care in a psychiatric or social care institution. However, there are no internationally agreed quality standards for institutional care and no method to assess common care standards across countries. We aimed to identify the key components of institutional care for people with longer term mental health problems and the effectiveness of these components. **Methods**: We undertook a systematic review of the literature using comprehensive search terms in 11 electronic databases and identified 12,182 titles. We viewed 550 abstracts, reviewed 223 papers and included 110 of these. A "critical interpretative synthesis" of the evidence was used to identify domains of institutional care that are key to service users' recovery. **Results**: We identified eight domains of institutional care that were key to service users' recovery: living conditions; interventions for schizophrenia; physical health; restraint and seclusion; staff training and support; therapeutic relationship; autonomy and service user involvement; and clinical governance. Evidence was strongest for specific interventions for the treatment of schizophrenia (family psychoeducation, cognitive behavioural therapy (CBT) and vocational rehabilitation). **Conclusion**: Institutions should, ideally, be community based, operate a flexible regime, maintain a low density of residents and maximise residents' privacy. For service users with a diagnosis of schizophrenia, specific interventions (CBT, family interventions involving psychoeducation, and supported employment) should be provided through integrated programmes. Restraint and seclusion should be avoided wherever possible and staff should have adequate training in de-escalation techniques. Regular staff supervision should be provided and this should support service user involvement in decision making and positive therapeutic relationships between staff and service users. There should be clear lines of clinical governance that ensure adherence to evidence-based guidelines and attention should be paid to service users' physical health through regular screening.

SPINAL CORD INJURY

Cooper, R. A., & Cooper, R. (2010). Quality-of-life technology for people with spinal cord injuries. *Physical Medicine and Rehabilitation Clinics of North America, 21*, 1-13.

Abstract: Technology plays a critical role in promoting well-being, activity, and participation for individuals with spinal cord injury (SCI). As technology has improved, so has the realm of possibilities open to people with SCI. School, work, travel, and leisure activities are all facilitated by technology. Advances in materials have made wheelchairs lighter, and developments in design have made wheelchairs that fit individual needs. Software has made computer interfaces adaptive and in some cases intelligent, through learning the user's behavior and optimizing its structure. As participatory action design and aware systems take greater hold, transformational change is likely to take place in the technology available to people with SCI.

(continued)

TABLE 1-15 (CONTINUED)

EXAMPLES OF CURRENT REVIEWS OF RESEARCH IN REHABILITATION AND HABILITATION FROM PUBLISHED ABSTRACTS

STROKE

Carter, A. R., Connor, L. T., & Dromerick, A. W. (2010). Rehabilitation after stroke: Current state of the science. *Current Neurology and Neuroscience Reports, 10*, 158-166.

Abstract: Stroke rehabilitation is evolving into a clinical field based on the neuroscience of recovery and restoration. There has been substantial growth in the number and quality of clinical trials performed. Much effort now is directed toward motor restoration and is being led by trials of constraint-induced movement therapy. Although the results do not necessarily support that constraint-induced movement therapy is superior to other training methods, this treatment has become an important vehicle for developing clinical trial methods and studying the physiology underlying activity-based rehabilitation strategies. Other promising interventions include robotic therapy delivery, magnetic and electrical cortical stimulation, visualization, and constraint-driven aphasia therapies. Amphetamine has not been demonstrated to be effective, and studies of other pharmacologic agents are still preliminary. Future studies will incorporate refinements in clinical trial methods and improved activity- and technology-based interventions.

TRAUMATIC BRAIN INJURY

Devine, J. M., & Zafonte, R. D. (2009). Physical exercise and cognitive recovery in acquired brain injury: A review of the literature. *PM & R: The Journal of Injury, Function, and Rehabilitation, 1*, 560-575.

Abstract: Objective: Physical exercise has been shown to play an ever-broadening role in the maintenance of overall health and has been implicated in the preservation of cognitive function in both healthy elderly and demented populations. Animal and human studies of acquired brain injury (ABI) from trauma or vascular causes also suggest a possible role for physical exercise in enhancing cognitive recovery. **Data Sources**: A review of the literature was conducted to explore the current understanding of how physical exercise impacts the molecular, functional, and neuroanatomic status of both intact and brain-injured animals and humans. **Study Selection**: Searches of the MEDLINE, CINHAL, and PsychInfo databases yielded an extensive collection of animal studies of physical exercise in ABI. Animal studies strongly tie physical exercise to the upregulation of multiple neural growth factor pathways in brain-injured animals, resulting in both hippocampal neurogenesis and functional improvements in memory. **Data Extraction**: A search of the same databases for publications involving physical exercise in human subjects with ABI yielded 24 prospective and retrospective studies. **Data Synthesis**: Four of these evaluated cognitive outcomes in persons with ABI who were involved in physical exercise. Three studies cited a positive association between exercise and improvements in cognitive function, whereas one observed no effect. Human exercise interventions varied greatly in duration, intensity, and level of subject supervision, and tools for assessing neurocognitive changes were inconsistent. **Conclusions**: There is strong evidence in animal ABI models that physical exercise facilitates neurocognitive recovery. Physical exercise interventions are safe in the subacute and rehabilitative phases of recovery for humans with ABI. In light of strong evidence of positive effects in animal studies, more controlled, prospective human interventions are warranted to better explore the neurocognitive effects of physical exercise on persons with ABI.

TABLE 1-16

THE PROCESS OF HABILITATION, OR DEVELOPMENT OF FUNCTION

CHILDHOOD DISABILITIES RELATED TO GENETIC, EMBRYOLOGIC, OR TRAUMA INJURY	EVALUATION OF FUNCTION	EDUCATIONAL AND TREATMENT TECHNIQUES
• Attention-deficit/hyperactivity disorder (ADHD) • ASD • Cerebral palsy • Childhood amputee • Dyslexia • Epilepsy • Fetal alcohol spectrum disorders • Hearing impairment • Intellectual disabilities and developmental delay • Juvenile arthritis • Learning disabilities • Neuromotor Impairments • Orthopedic impairments • Sensory integration disorder • Traumatic brain injury • Visual Impairments	• Academic • ADLs • Cognitive • Leisure interests • Neuromuscular • Mental health • Memory • Neuropsychological • Prevocational • Psychosocial • Sensory	• Augmentative and alternative communication • Braille • Community-based instruction • Computer-assisted instruction • Explicit or direct instruction • Inclusive education • Individualized learning • Medical treatment • Motor therapy (occupational and physical therapy) • Orientation and mobility • Psychological counseling • Response to intervention • Self-care skills • Sensorimotor training • Sign language • Speech-language therapy • Strategic teaching • Vocational development
Children with special needs are evaluated and then taught using appropriate educational and treatment techniques.		

1.9.1 Initial Concern for Those With Disabilities

Although prior to the twentieth century some services were available for individuals with disabilities, these services were minimal, generally no more than custodial care and assistance through the efforts of religious orders and voluntary charities. The earliest report of attempts to treat and educate the blind was the establishment of a hospital in 1260 (Hallahan & Kauffman, 1994). Rousseau (1712–1779), a philosopher and theorist, petitioned in his treatise "Emile" for the study of children directly rather than using what was known about adults and applying that knowledge to children. "Nature intends that children shall be children before they are men. …Treat your pupil as his age demands" (Rousseau, 1883, pp. 52, 54)

During the mid-1800s, Jacob Rodreques Pereire (1715–1780), a Spanish medical doctor living in France,

developed an oral method to teach individuals with severe hearing loss to read and speak. At the same time, a Frenchman, Abbé de l'Epée (1712–1789), developed a manual sign language for "deaf-mutes." "The natural language of the Deaf and Dumb is the language of signs; nature and their different wants are their only tutors in it: and they have no other language as long as they have no further instructors" (Epée, 1784/1820, as cited in Lane, 1976, p. 79).

Sicard (1742–1833), a French medical doctor influential in the education of the deaf expanded Epée's methods, producing a way to teach deaf people to read and write:

[Epée] saw that the deaf-mute expressed his physical needs without instruction; that one could, with the same signs, communicate to him the expression of the same needs and could indicate the things that one wanted to designate: these were the first words of a new language which this great man has enriched, to the astonishment of all of Europe. (Sicard, 1795, as cited in Lane, 1976, p. 79)

1.9.2 Itard's Influence

The earliest reported case of enlightened intervention with children identified as being intellectually disabled was Jean-Marc Gaspard Itard's (1774–1838) work with Victor, "the wild boy of Aveyron" (Lane, 1976). Victor (ca. 1785–1828), who emerged from the forests of Aveyron between 1797 and 1800, was thought to have been abandoned by his parents as an infant or young child. Itard, a young physician, was assigned the responsibility to teach Victor. Itard applied methods developed earlier by Epée and Sicard. These methods included breaking up each task into small segments and using techniques that had been successful for deaf people. In this way, Itard believed that he could teach Victor to be social and use language (Lane, 1976; Winnie, 1912). After 6 years, even though Itard considered his work a failure, Victor had developed some social skills and could read a few words. On the other hand, Itard's work with Victor inspired him to further his methods for teaching deaf people:

> The child, who was called the wild boy of Aveyron, did not receive from my intensive care all the advantages that I had hoped. But the many observations that I could make and the techniques of instruction inspired by the inflexibility of his organs were not entirely fruitless, and I later found a more suitable application for them with some of our children whose mutism is the result of obstacles that are more easily overcome. (Itard, 1825, as cited in Lane, 1976, p. 185)

Several authors in education (Forness & Kavale, 1984; Hunt & Marshall, 1994; McDermott, 1994; Smith & Tyler, 2010) have recognized the significant contribution of Itard's work with Victor to present-day methods used in special education classes. In his effort to teach Victor, Itard developed methods that encompassed multiple senses (auditory, visual, kinesthetic) and demonstrated that individual instruction could be successful. Eduardo Séquin (1812–1880), a student of Itard, advanced these methods. He opened the first school for the "intellectually deficient" in 1837 and demonstrated that they could be systematically trained and educated. Finally, as a physician involved in the education and treatment of individuals with disabilities, Itard played a significant part in the development of educational and treatment services for individuals with disabilities (Forness & Kavale, 1984). Initially, the emphasis of special education relied on a medical model using etiology, symptomology, differential diagnosis, and specialized treatment. This resulted in an educational system based on classification and segregation, rather than a system based on community participation and mainstreaming in general education. It is notable that Itard's work using a single case study has lead to the development of general methods for teaching children with disabilities (Kirk & Gallagher, 1989).

1.9.3 Montessori's Contribution to Special Education

The following quote is from Marie Montessori who, as a physician and teacher, established the basis for special education in Italy at the end of the nineteenth century. "In this method the lesson corresponds to an experiment, the more fully the teacher is acquainted with the methods of experimental psychology, the better will she understand how to give the lesson" (Montessori, 1912, p. 107)

Montessori advocated that the special education teacher of individuals with intellectual disabilities should use observation and experimentation in sequencing pedagogical activities. Montessori, who acknowledges the influence of Itard and Séquin, was a forerunner in the movement to provide special education methods through perceptual-motor training to the child with disabilities. These materials and methods were based on concrete, three-dimensional manipulatives (hands-on activities) that allowed exploration and learning through discovery. Today these methods are used with populations of typical children and children with special needs (Shea & Bauer, 1994).

Theoretically, Montessori's method changed the direction of treatment from a medical model to a model based on education, psychology, and child development. This approach was not limited to the child with intellectual disabilities. For example, Louis Braille, who was blind, developed a system of reading for the blind over a period from 1825 to 1852 (Illingworth, 1910). This method of teaching was the basis of special education for the blind in the early 1900s. Analogous to Braille as a method for teaching the blind was sign language for the deaf, devised by Abbé de l'Epée around 1755 (Winnie, 1912). The oral method was later practiced in Germany by Heinicke and Hill, who felt that speech development in the deaf child should parallel normal speech development (Winnie, 1912). Because of the complexity in educating children who are blind and deaf, special schools that segregated them from the public schools were founded. The significance of the Montessori method for those with intellectual disabilities, of the Braille system for the blind, and of sign language for the deaf is that these methods compensate for the child's inability to learn in a typical classroom. They are specific, technological advances designed to help the child to learn. These methods have allowed special education to be effective for children who are blind, deaf, or intellectually disabled.

1.9.4 Early Services in the United States

Séquin's contribution to the education of individuals with disabilities extended to the United States. Through the efforts of Samuel Gridley Howe, Séquin immigrated to the United States in 1848 where he shared his knowledge of educational methods for teaching individuals with intellectual disabilities. He was later instrumental in founding the American Association on Intellectual and Developmental Disabilities (AAIDD), formerly known as the American Association on Mental Deficiency. This association "promotes progressive policies, sound research, effective practices and universal human rights for people with intellectual and developmental disabilities" (AAIDD, 2017, para 1).

In the United States, Reverend Thomas Gallaudet, Horace Mann, and Samuel Gridley Howe were pioneers in the early development of special schools for children with disabilities. In 1817, in Hartford, Connecticut, Gallaudet, assisted by Clerc, a deaf person trained by Sicard, founded the first residential school for the deaf (Lane, 1976). This outstanding school still exists. Gallaudet University, located in Washington, DC, is the only liberal arts college established for students with hearing impairments. The university was founded by Gallaudet's grandson in 1864 (Lane, 1976). In 1829, Howe opened the Perkins Institute at Watertown, Massachusetts, a residential school for students with visual impairments. This school is well known because Anne Sullivan, teacher of Helen Keller, was trained there. Fernald State School, the first institution for individuals with intellectual disabilities, was opened in 1848, with the Commonwealth of Massachusetts assuming full financial responsibility (Sigmon, 1987). In addition to Séquin and his work in intellectual disabilities, individuals such as Louis Braille and Alexander Graham Bell, who was instrumental in the amplification of sound for the hearing impaired, greatly influenced the teaching methods used in these early institutions (Kirk & Gallagher, 1989).

A major change in educational practices in the United States occurred when individual states mandated compulsory education between 1852 and 1918. Although some students with disabilities were taught in the general education program, the degree of severity in these individuals resulted in the creation of residential institutions, segregated day schools, and special classes. The first special education day school in the United States, the Horace Mann School, was opened in 1868 in Roxbury, Massachusetts. In 1911, New Jersey was the first state to mandate programs for students with disabilities (Sigmon, 1987). Individuals confined to wheelchairs or with severe disabilities continued to be excluded from public schools until the 1960s and 1970s. The right for children with disabilities to be educated in a public school was mandated by court decisions such as *Pennsylvania Association of Retarded Citizens (PARC) v. Pennsylvania* (1971) and *Mills v. Board of Education, Washington, D.C.* (1972). Decisions from these judicial cases supported the position that individuals with disabilities were entitled to a free and appropriate public education regardless of the degree of severity or educational need (Turnbull & Turnbull, 1998).

1.9.5 Special Education Assessment and Programming

In 1905, Alfred Binet (1857–1911), a French psychologist, was commissioned by the French Government to provide a useful assessment tool that would identify those children who needed special techniques to learn. Binet began working to develop methods of assessing intelligence in 1886. His first book, published at that time, was entitled *Psychologie du Raissonnement* (*The Psychology of Reasoning*; 1899/1912). This was the beginning of intelligence testing as we know it today. (More information regarding Binet and the development of intelligence tests can be found in Chapter 10 in the discussion on intelligence testing.) In the United States, Lewis Terman (1877–1956) and Henry Herbert Goddard (1866–1957), strongly influenced by Binet, continued the development of intelligence tests. Both believed that intelligence was inherited, stable, and did not change over time. A student's failure in the general education curriculum was explained by his or her inadequate intellectual level, not by methods of teaching or environmental factors. As a result, in the first half of the twentieth century, institutionalization and segregation of those individuals with severe intellectual deficits and physical disabilities became the norm. It was not until the 1960s when there was a major push toward normalization (Wolfensberger, Nirje, Olshansky, Perske, & Roos, 1972) and deinstitutionalization that individuals with intellectual disabilities and physical impairments were returned to the community and local school programs.

Historically, the habilitation of those with mild intellectual disabilities, blindness, and deafness has been more successful than the habilitation of individuals with brain damage, learning disabilities, autism, or social deprivation. One reason for these differences has been in the specialized educational curricula that have been developed to compensate for the child's disability. Methods for educating students with brain damage, learning disabilities, autism, or social deprivation were slower to develop.

During the latter half of the nineteenth century and the beginnings of the twentieth century, physicians such as James Hinshelwood (1917) and Samuel T. Orton (1879–1948) used adult models to understand reasons for learning difficulties in children who were not deaf, blind, or intellectually disabled. Both clinicians developed a multisensory method for teaching reading. Later, their ideas were expanded by special educators. The methods developed are still used today in many classrooms (Mercer, Mercer, & Pullen, 2011).

The aftermath of World War I was another turning point in the development of educational programs for individuals with brain injuries. Kurt Goldstein (1878–1965), in his experimental work with soldiers who had sustained head injuries during battle, contributed much to the understanding of the consequences of brain damage. His work inspired Alfred Strauss and Heinz Werner (1943) to study children with brain damage during the 1930s and 1940s at Wayne County Training School in Michigan. Their findings led to the identification of a group of children with brain damage. Although these children appeared to be intellectually disabled, the cause of the disability was not genetic. Moreover, their behavioral characteristics were similar to the symptoms displayed by soldiers with brain injuries, such as perseveration, distractibility, inattention, and memory problems (Mercer, 1983). In their classic book, *Psychopathology and Education of the Brain-Injured Child*, Strauss and Lehtinen (1947) described symptoms and behaviors of the child with brain injury and justified special education methods for teaching this group of children. Prior to the published works by Strauss and collaborators (Strauss & Kephart, 1940; Strauss & Lehtinen, 1947; Strauss & Werner, 1941; Strauss & Werner, 1941), treatment for the child with brain damage was undifferentiated. Strauss and Lehtinen (1947) described the problem as follows: "The response of the brain-injured child to the school situation is frequently inadequate, conspicuously disturbing, and persistently troublesome" (p. 127).

Luria (1961) and Vygotsky (1934/1961), Russian neuropsychologists, were influential in the understanding of brain functioning and language development. Luria believed that the brain was made up of three functional units: the brainstem, involved with arousal and attention; the posterior portion, involved with taking in and processing of sensory information; and the anterior portion, implicated in planning, monitoring, and verifying one's performance. Luria and Vygotsky postulated that the development of language played an important part in one's ability to organize tasks involving planning, self-monitoring, and self-regulating. Individuals with brain damage who no longer use language for organization manifest extreme difficulties in self-regulatory and self-monitoring activities. Likewise, children who do not use language for organization do not develop self- regulation or planning skills. These ideas of Luria and Vygotsky have influenced the way we teach all students in developmentally appropriate early childhood classes.

Until recently, children with autism faced an even more uncertain future because of the lack of effective methods to compensate for their disability. For example, Bettelheim (1967) described the initial reaction to the orthogenic school and the problems of communication in an 11-year-old girl with autism:

> At first what little speech she had consisted of very rare, simple, highly selective and only whispered echolalia. For example, when we asked her if she wanted some candy she would merely echo "candy."

She would say "no" but never "yes."… It was not our language she used, but a private one of her own. (p. 162)

Currently, programs such as Treatment and Education of Autistic Children and Communication Handicapped Children at the University of North Carolina in Chapel Hill, North Carolina, provide expertise and technical assistance in diagnosis and treatment to teachers and parents of students with autism (Edwards & Bristol, 1991).

As with the child with brain damage or autism, the child who is socially disadvantaged has been an enigma in the classroom. Gordon (1968) characterized the child who is socially disadvantaged as unprepared for a normal educational experience. He wrote: "As a consequence, these children show in school disproportionately high rates of social maladjustment, behavioral disturbance, physical disability, academic retardation and mental subnormality" (p. 6). Many of the children formerly characterized as socially disadvantaged are now diagnosed with attention deficit hyperactivity disorder (ADHD).

In 1963, at the first national meeting of what later became the Association for Children with Learning Disabilities (now named the Learning Disabilities Association of America), the term *learning disabilities* was identified by Samuel A. Kirk (1963):

> Recently I have used the term 'Teaming disabilities" to describe a group of children who have disorders in development, in language, speech, reading, and associated communication skills needed for social interaction. In this group I do not include children who have sensory handicaps such as blindness or deafness, because we have methods of managing and training the deaf and the blind. I also exclude from this group children who have generalized mental retardation. (p. 3)

Another impetus for the development of appropriate educational programs for individuals with disabilities was the formation of various organizations, such as the March of Dimes, National Easter Seal Society, and United Cerebral Palsy, designed to provide community-based services. Although these organizations originally provided resources for equipment and medical care for children with disabilities, parents of these children became politically proactive in obtaining rehabilitation hospitals and clinics, special education programs, community services, and barrier-free environments. These organizations have been instrumental in the development of support groups for families and in the publication and distribution of educational materials on the prevention and treatment of disabilities.

Compared with children who have disabilities that cause severe problems in communication and learning; children with physical impairment who have normal language and sensory functions present different problems in habilitation. Physical barriers present problems in architectural design. Emotional and social adjustment is affected by the self-concept of children with disabilities, as well as by their feelings of competence. Other chronic disabilities of childhood such as juvenile arthritis, ulcerative colitis, childhood diabetes, heart defects, and epilepsy, profoundly affect the child's development and require adaptive or specialized treatment methods.

1.9.6 Services for Individuals With Disabilities

Since the passing of Section 504 of the Rehabilitation Act in 1973, the Education for the Handicapped Act (EHA; Public Law 94-142) in 1974, the reauthorization and amendment of EHA as Public Law 99-457, the passing of the Americans with Disabilities Act (1990), the reauthorization and amendment of EHA as Public Law 101-456 (also known as Individuals with Disabilities Education Act [IDEA]) in 1990, the Individuals with Disabilities Education Act Amendments of 1997 (Public Law 105-17), No Child Left Behind (NCLB; Public Law 107-110) in 2002, and the reauthorization of IDEA through the Individuals with Disabilities Education Improvement Act (IDEIA; Public Law 108-446) in December 2004, programs for students with special needs have grown by leaps and bounds. For example, in 1976–1977, approximately 3.5 million students, ages 6 to 18, were served in special education. By 1987–1988, this number had increased to 4.1 million, and by 1996–1997, there were 5.3 million students, ages 6 to 21, or approximately 8.5% of the population (U.S. Department of Education, 1998). In 2004, there were approximately 6 million students, ages 6 to 21, or approximately 9.2% of the population served in special education. This increase is a result of the increased number of students identified as autistic and ADHD since 1995. Additionally, the number of students ages 3 to 5 served in special education during the period 1995–2004 has increased 28% (U.S. Department of Education, Office of Special Education and Rehabilitative Services, Office of Special Education Programs, 2009).

Approximately 13,100 occupational therapists were employed in educational and school settings during the 2007–2008 school year (Bureau of Labor Statistics, 2009). Treatment and educational services are provided by public schools for any student from birth to age 21 who is at risk or is disabled. In addition, a continuum of services is available that ranges from consulting with the general education teacher about a student's needs to providing an intense, restrictive residential setting for a student. Augmentative communication, life-skills training, and assistive technology are provided to the student when needed (Meyen & Skrtic, 1988; Smith & Tyler, 2010).

During the 1950s, 1960s, and 1970s, services for students with special needs were available primarily in residential institutions, special day schools, or special classes that were often physically isolated and segregated from the mainstreamed students. The concept of LRE, delineated in EHA (Public Law 94–142), states that each student will be educated in the program that allows him or her to be educated with his or her own peers to the maximum extent possible. Efficacy studies examining the effectiveness of special classes show mixed results. Earlier studies (Dunn, 1968; Epps & Tindall, 1987; Haynes & Jenkins, 1986) found special education to be ineffective; however, more recent studies have suggested that students with learning disabilities and behavior disorders often show greater improvement in the special education classroom (Fuchs, Fuchs, & Fernstrom, 1993; Marston, 1987-1988). Madeline Will (1986), the Assistant Secretary of Education, strongly recommended that students with mild disabilities be returned to general education. She argued that general educators should take more responsibility for teaching these students. This position, originally called the Regular Education Initiative, is now known as the General Education Initiative. Although some individuals, such as Sailor (1991) and Stainback and Stainback (1992) proposed total inclusion (i.e., placement of all students, regardless of their educational needs, into their home schools and into the regular classroom), others (Vergason & Anderegg, 1992) encouraged a range of inclusiveness, with each student's placement based on individual needs and related to specific long-term goals. This latter stance appears to be more in accord with the concept of LRE as stated in IDEA.

Two factors have influenced changes in how services are provided to students in special education. First, NCLB mandated that students with special needs have access to the general education curriculum. Second, following the passage of IDEA (2004), the Office of Special Education and Rehabilitation mandated the "implementation of a process known as response to intervention" (Reynolds, 2008, p. 15) be used with students with learning disabilities. As a result, more than half of the students in special education are taught in the general education classroom with supports provided as needed (U.S. Department of Education, 2009). With the increase in inclusive classes, additional training in collaborative techniques has been provided for general educators, special educators, occupational therapists, physical therapists, speech-language pathologists, school psychologists, and audiologists. Students with severe disabilities may continue to receive educational services in special class placements, especially when the educational needs include self-care and independent living skills.

Although much has been achieved in the development of programs and services for those individuals with special needs, there is much more to accomplish. There continues

TABLE 1-17		
COMPUTER APPLICATION IN DIAGNOSIS AND TREATMENT		
BODILY PROCESSES	**MACHINE MONITORING**	**COMPUTER DIAGNOSIS**
• Circulatory • Gastrointestinal • Neurophysiological • Genitourinary • Skeletal-muscular • Respiration	• ECG • EEG • Respirator • MRI • CT scan	• Aids health professionals in diagnosis and prescription of treatment

to be a greater percentage of students from minority groups placed in special education than those from the majority population. We are only beginning to understand how to remediate and improve cognitive deficits. Augmentative communication, assistive technology, and the use of computer-assisted instruction in education and training are still in the infancy stage of development. Although increased medical technology has made it possible to keep infants and patients with severe disabilities alive, we have only just begun to develop educational and training needs for these individuals.

Habilitation is the latest frontier in health research. Much research remains to develop the knowledge and technology that will facilitate growth and learning in the child with disabilities. The progress that has been made is the result of the persistent efforts of investigators devoting a lifetime of work to specific problems.

1.10 RESEARCH AND THE FUTURE OF HEALTH CARE

What are the future directions and goals of health care? The physician, an individual educated in the arts and science of healing, historically has been the primary health practitioner. At first, education of the physician was "at the foot of a master"; later, formal training permitted one to legally practice medicine. It is only in the last 100 years that medicine has become a science with reliable and valid methods. The science of modern medicine began with Claude Bernard and Louis Pasteur, who provided the research methods and theory of disease that underlie clinical practice. Progress has been dramatic since the late 1800s, culminating with the elimination of many major diseases through vaccination, chemotherapy, surgery, and effective hospital care. Preventive medicine is now the cornerstone of health maintenance. At the beginning of the 21st century, researchers are mobilizing their efforts to discover means to prevent premature deaths from heart disease, stroke, cancer, arthritis, emphysema, and AIDS.

Ironically, chronic disabilities continue to persist as people live longer. As new diseases emerge (e.g., Ebola virus), they present new challenges for medical and rehabilitation researchers.

A second trend in medical progress is toward self-regulation of health care through education and monitoring of bodily symptoms. The individual's understanding of one's own anatomical, physiological, and psychological makeup through public health education continues to play an increasingly important role. Present trends have included wellness as part of the curriculum. Educating the public toward an understanding of the relationship between mind and body is an example of the wellness movement. The trend toward self-regulation in health will lead to more responsibility for one's own well-being in preventing illness through activities such as exercise, stress management, diet, and complementary medicines. Scientific research is beginning to explore the effectiveness of these methods.

Another trend in health care is the growth of specialized health professions. Up until 1920, the doctor and the nurse were the main health care providers. More than 100 health-related professions now exist. These new positions, such as cardiovascular technologist, respiratory therapist, nuclear medicine technologist, sanitarian, and public health educator, are the result of progress made in medical technology and the advancement of public health methods. New professions will continue to emerge from advanced technology. As research refines the diagnosis and treatment of illness, there will be a parallel growth in specialized health professions.

The medical practice of the future may well be dominated by machines that monitor physiological changes; control the heart rate; stimulate nerves, muscle, and skin; replace bodily organs; and, in general, receive and transmit information to and from the body (Longmore, 1970). These medical machines will be designed to adapt to the internal organism of the body. Computers connected to the machines will be programmed to interpret accurately the information received. This relationship is shown in Table 1-17.

Another trend in rehabilitation medicine is the merging of technology in assisting individuals with disabilities. For many years, professionals in rehabilitation have recognized the need to develop devices and apparati to help individuals with disabilities maximize their independence and functional activities. The growth of the fields of orthotics (i.e., braces and splints), self-help devices, prosthetics (i.e., design of artificial limbs), and assistive technology is a direct result of this vision. Methodological research in health care is an example of interdisciplinary cooperation between scientists. Biomedical engineering, which emerged as a complex multidisciplinary field incorporating medicine, engineering, psychology, economics, computer technology, law, sociology, and the environmental sciences, has grown rapidly in the last 60 years. Rushmer (1972), a researcher at the Center for Bioengineering, University of Washington, in Seattle, Washington, was one of the first to describe the interaction of these multidisciplines. Table 1-18 is adapted from his description.

The Defense Advanced Research Projects Agency launched an initiative to develop technologically sophisticated upper extremity prosthetic devices. Titled *Revolutionizing Prosthetics 2007* and *Revolutionizing Prosthetics 2009*, the goals were to develop prosthetic devices that could mimic the functioning of a normal healthy upper extremity, including having five dexterous fingers, as well as an articulating wrist with normal motion, including flexion, extension, abduction, adduction, supination, and pronation. The limb is required to have an elbow strong enough to lift weight, and a shoulder with range of motion to allow flexion above the head and internal rotation to reach behind the back. Additionally, the device is required to have a power source to last an entire day, be waterproof, have normal looking skin, and weigh no more than 8 pounds (Beard, 2008).

The merging of medicine with the social sciences to find solutions to the complex problems of mental illness, alcoholism, drug addiction, and criminology is inevitable. Interdisciplinary approaches to prevention and rehabilitation will result in the merging of the physical and social sciences. The study of the relationship between psychology and physiology and the immune system has lead to the field of psychoneuroimmuniology. The relationship of poverty, alienation, malaise, and hopelessness, which are social variables, to the onset of disease, self-destruction, and social aggression have attracted the attention of health researchers who work closely with social scientists.

The controversy in the United States during the 1990s regarding the creation of a national health care system was influenced by the health consumer's concern about being denied the right to choose a health plan. The rise of health maintenance organizations and managed care in the 1990s brought attention to the issue of quality health care.

The Health Care Reform Bill of 2010 was signed into law by President Obama on March 23, 2010 (Meckler & Hitt, 2010). This bill provides many substantial changes to the health care system in the United States. Some of these changes will begin to take place in a graded fashion for several years after being signed into law:

- In 2010, subsidies were made available to small businesses to help offset the cost of providing health insurance coverage for their employees. A notable change during 2010 was that insurance companies were barred from denying health insurance coverage for children with preexisting illnesses. Additionally, children were allowed to stay on their parent's health insurance until the age of 26 years.

- During 2011, a long-term care program initiative will begin where people who pay premiums into the long-term care program will become eligible for long-term care support payments if they require assistance in daily living.

- In 2014, "exchanges" will be created where individuals without employer health care insurance, as well as small businesses, can shop for health care coverage. Another significant change for 2014 is that insurance companies are barred from denying health insurance coverage to anyone with preexisting conditions. Additionally, 2014 is the year where most people are required to have health insurance. People at or below 133% of the federal poverty level will be required to pay a maximum of 3% of their income for coverage; people at 400% of the poverty level will be required to pay up to 9.5% of their income for coverage (the poverty level in 2010 for a family of 4 is $22,000). 2014 also marks the year when Medicaid expands to Americans, in states where the expansion was accepted, with income up to 133% of the federal poverty level. Additionally, subsidies will be available for small businesses to provide health care insurance coverage.

The plan to finance these changes involves a combination of cost-saving Medicare policies, increased Medicare wage taxes, a new tax on unearned income, annual fees for pharmaceutical and insurance companies (in the billions of dollars), other taxes, and fines/penalties for those who do not carry health care coverage. In summary, the Health Care Reform Bill of 2010 promises that more people will have health insurance coverage regardless of preexisting illnesses. While there is some controversy over this bill (e.g., the magnitude of changes and its associated costs), it does increase accessibility of health care insurance to many individuals who otherwise would and have gone without such health care insurance (Meckler & Hitt, 2010).

TABLE 1-18

THE CURRENT SCOPE OF BIOMEDICAL ENGINEERING: POTENTIAL AREAS OF INTERACTION BETWEEN LIFE SCIENCES AND ENGINEERING

APPLIED BIOENGINEERING

Technological Development	*Therapeutic Techniques*	*Health Care System*	*Environmental Engineering*
Research Tools • Physical measure • Chemical composition • Microscopy • Isotope Clinical Interventions • Audiology • Cardiology • Gastrointestinal • Genitourinal • Musculoskeletal • Neurology • Respiratory Diagnostic Data • Automation • Chemistry • Microbiology • Pathology • Multiphasic screening Computer Applications • Data processing • Analysis • Retrieval • Diagnosis	Therapies and Services • Assistive technology • Occupational therapy • Physical therapy • Radiation therapy • Respiratory treatments • Special education • Speech-language therapy • Surgical interventions Monitoring • Intensive care • Surgical, postoperative • Coronary care • Ward supervision Artificial Organs • Sensory aids • Heart-lung machine • Artificial kidneys • Artificial extremities (e.g., myoelectric prostheses, mechanical arms, legs) Transplants • Liver • Heart • Blood vessels • Kidneys	Components • Organization • Medical economics • Long-range planning Methods and Improvements • Support functions • Service functions • Nursing • Facilities design • Medical care • Community care • Independent living Operations Research • Optimization of laboratories • Support functions • Personnel • Processing • Scheduling Cost-Benefit Analysis • Cost accounting • Evaluation of results • Beneficial economy	Focus Areas • Pollution • Air • Water • Noise • Solid waste • Food • Human fertility • Population control Aerospace • Environment control • Closed ecological systems • Physiological adaptation Underwater Compression Effects • Heat conservation • Communication

Adapted from Rushmer, R. F. (1972). *Medical engineering: Projections for health care delivery.* Cambridge, MA: Academic Press.

Currently, health care is dominated by a biomedical model in which prescription drugs have dominated treatment. The over-prescribing of drugs such as Prozac (fluoxetine), Ritalin (methylphenidate), and Tagamet (cimetidine) and the overuse of drugs such as ibuprofen by the general public have led many health care consumers to prescribe alternative medicines. It is hoped that research will resolve the conflict between the biomedical model and alternative medicine, promoting a holistic approach to health care.

A delicate balance between governmental intervention and the respect for the sanctity and privacy of the individual must be maintained. The right of every individual to have the very best health care should be among the most important priorities for every nation. In evaluating and treating clients, occupational therapy and special education should be guided by the application of sound research. In the following chapters, the methods and procedures intrinsic to scientific research applied to occupational therapy and special education are presented.

2

The Scientific Method and Research Models

Scientific research is a systematic, controlled, empirical, and critical investigation of hypothetical propositions about presumed relations among natural phenomena.

—Kerlinger (1973, p. 11)

Research is defined as multiple, systematic strategies to generate knowledge about human behavior, human experience, and human environments in which the thinking and action processes of the researcher are clearly specified so that they are logical, understandable, confirmable, and useful.

—DePoy & Gitlin (2016, p. 3).

Operational Learning Objectives

By the end of this chapter, the learner will be able to:

- Define *research*, *theory*, *scientific method*, *independent* and *dependent variable*, *associational* or *statistical relationship*, and *hypothesis*.
- Give examples of common fallacies in scientific thinking.
- Outline and analyze the components of a research article.
- Identify overall objectives of the researcher.
- Contrast the nomothetic and idiographic methods of scientific inquiry.
- Compare and contrast research models.
- Compare and contrast quantitative, qualitative, and action research.

Rice, M. S., Stein, F., & Tomlin, G.
Clinical Research in Occupational Therapy, Sixth Edition (pp. 37-54).
© 2019 Taylor & Francis Group.

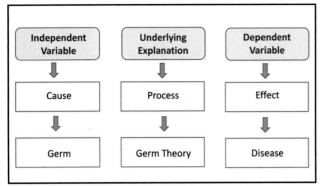

Figure 2-1. Relationship between the independent and dependent variable.

2.1 SCIENCE, RESEARCH, AND THEORY

The concept of the scientific method was first introduced by the ancient Greeks, who proposed that knowledge is enacted by formulating a hypothesis that leads to observation and logical reasoning (Northrop, 1981). The scientific method is founded upon an empirical view of the world. The scientific method can be summarized in four steps:

1. A hypothesis that is testable is proposed, preferably based on a proposed theory.
2. Objective observations are collected.
3. Results are analyzed in an unbiased manner.
4. Conclusions proposed are based on the results of the study and previous knowledge.

The dictionary definition of *research* is "systematic knowledge of the physical or material world gained through observation and experimentation" (Webster's College Dictionary, 1992, p. 1201). *Science* is defined as the "systematic, objective study of empirical phenomena and the resultant bodies of knowledge" (Gould & Kolb, 1964, p. 620). Research and science are almost identical in definition; both imply systematic objective inquiry resulting in knowledge. Scientific *theory*, on the other hand, is a comprehensive explanation of empirical data. Theory predicts what will be observed under certain conditions. A theory, formulated by induction from empirical data, represents a *proposed method* of understanding the world. It predicts causal relationships in nature. Theories are developed by considering underlying processes, linking an observed cause with an effect.

For example, when medical scientists investigated the relationship between a specific bacteria and the cause of a disease, a theory was proposed to explain this relationship. The theory served as the *underlying explanation*—that is, the link between the *independent variable* (presumed cause) and *dependent variable* (presumed effect). This relationship is schematically diagrammed in Figure 2-1.

2.1.1 Theory Building

Theory building is a key part of research. Many assumed cause-effect relationships instead may be in actuality *associational* or *statistical relationships* where a direct connection between cause and effect does not exist. Instances of associational relationships are those phenomena in nature that may occur together, such as precipitation in India and an increased birth rate, or solar activity and wars. By proposing a theory, however, a researcher seeks to explain the direct relationship between observed causes and effects. Theory building is a way of distinguishing those relationships that are interdependent. Theories are developed by scientists who have systematically collected data. Proposed scientific theories generate research by inviting studies to support or refute them.

2.1.2 Characteristics of a Theory

A theory is defined "as a set of interrelated constructs (concepts), definitions and propositions that present a systematic view of phenomena by specifying relations among variables, with the purpose of explaining and predicting phenomena" (Kerlinger, 1986, p. 9). Scientific theories are characterized by certain assumptions:

- *Technical vocabulary, language, or terms are generated by a theory.* For example, Piaget, in developing a theory of cognitive development, introduced the terms *assimilation*, *accommodation*, and *differentiation*. Theorists now use these terms in child development to explain how a child thinks. Freud, in introducing the theory of psychoanalysis, gave new meaning to familiar terms such as *ego*, *id*, *super ego*, *unconscious*, *libido*, and *catharsis*. Sometimes these terms lose their ordinary connotations and take on the precise meanings of the theorist.

- *Natural phenomena or behavior can be explained by a theory.* For example, Darwin's theory of evolution was shaped by his observations of animals and the examination of fossils. He formulated a theory from years of painstaking field observation. The pieces of evidence he amassed on animal and plant evolution were mosaics that he composed to form a theory. His research expeditions were guided by questions about the wide variations in animal structure and behavior that he observed in his expeditions to South America and the Pacific Islands.

- *A theory is a tentative set of beliefs that can be supported or undermined by scientific research.* Pasteur, in 1863, proposed the germ theory after proving that the processes of putrefaction and fermentation were caused by microorganisms. In 1880, Koch built on the work of Pasteur by completing scientific laboratory investigation of tuberculosis and cholera, thus demonstrating the validity of the germ theory. Koch's (1880) postulates were an example of deterministic causality.

Figure 2-2. Relationship between theory and law. A theory can become a law only through accurate and systematic research resulting in repeated confirmatory findings.

To claim that an organism causes a disease, he required that (a) the organism must be isolated in every case of the disease (i.e., be necessary); (b) the organism must be grown in pure culture; (c) the organism must always cause the disease when inoculated into an experimental animal (i.e., be sufficient); and (d) the organism must then be recovered from the experimental animal and identified.

- *A theory predicts events that can be simulated in the laboratory or observed under controlled conditions.* The theory of genetic determinacy predicts that a child born with a chromosomal deficit, such as Down syndrome, may likely develop intellectual disabilities. An infant is diagnosed with Down syndrome when an extra chromosome 21 is detected through genetic screening.

- *A theory gives a researcher tools to interpret results and to form conclusions.* Konrad Lorenz (1937/1957), an ethnologist who received the Nobel Prize in Medicine, studied instinctive behavior patterns and proposed a theory of aggression. This theory seeks to explain the presence of conflicts and wars throughout human history.

- *A theory organizes knowledge and leads to the development of further theories.* Gesell's (1928) theory of development predicted that normal human growth is based on sequential, hierarchical stages that unfold at critical ages. Other theorists, such as Erikson (1950; eight stages of psychosocial development), Kohlberg (1981; theory of moral reasoning), and Brofenbrenner (1979; theory of ecological systems), were greatly influenced by Gesell's work in the 1920s.

- *A theory can be completely or partially accurate or completely inaccurate.* When Freud proposed the psychoanalytic theory at the turn of the 20th century, many of his colleagues rejected his work as unsubstantiated, based on clinical speculation. Psychoanalysis was later incorporated into psychiatric treatment programs, especially in the United States, from early in the 20th century until about 1960 when criticism started to appear in professional journals. Many parts of Freud's theory, such as the terms he defined, are widely used in many studies of psychotherapy. Does psychoanalysis retain any accuracy as a theory of behavior? This question is still unresolved.

For clinical research, theories are a critical component in a study. To paraphrase Lewin (1939), nothing is so practical as a good theory. A scientific theory implies that phenomena or events in the world can be explained in a logical or rational way. Theories are the engines for scientific research that relies on an inductive-deductive system of knowledge formation. Data, which are collections of facts or information, result from research and, in turn, can give rise to scientific theories. The systematic collection of data entails procedures for the review of previous results, the selection of research subjects, and the use of measuring instruments.

The relationship between theories and laws is diagrammed in Figure 2-2. In all scientific research, the objectivity and scientific competence of the investigator are the most crucial variables. How a clinician or practitioner gains knowledge is often through the process of constructivism. Proponents of this paradigm of learning (constructivism) believe that a person gains knowledge through relating a personal experience to what he or she already knows. Constructivism is learner-driven rather than teacher-initiated (Piaget, 1977; Steffe & Gale, 1995; Vygotsky, 1986). A person can construct his or her knowledge base in several ways. Figure 2-3 describes major factors that promote constructivism.

Figure 2-3. Factors that promote constructivism or the construction of one's knowledge base.

2.2 FALLACIES RELATED TO RESEARCH

Before the development of scientific research at the turn of the 20th century, our knowledge of medicine rested on a combination of trial and error methodology and deductive reasoning based on a priori assumptions. Fallacies growing out of the acceptance of invalid methods of treatment were common during times of superstition, such as in the Dark Ages in Europe and in primitive societies. These fallacies are incorrect arguments that are psychologically persuasive and, in many societies, continue to influence health practices. For example, contemporary practitioners who treat patients with methods that have no theoretical foundation act as if there were data supporting their methods. Some clinicians advocate a particular treatment method or drug based on the fallacious premise that a disease is highly prevalent, and therefore, any treatment is better than no treatment. A specific example of this may be the use of antibiotics to treat the cold virus. Also, explanations by authorities in the field are used to support therapeutic applications. In the past, experimentation with radical procedures, such as the use of psychosurgery with psychiatric patients, was rationalized as relevant to treatment merely because the patients were severely psychotic and considered hopeless. To cite another fallacy, people refuse to accept data linking smoking to lung cancer and heart disease because they assume it cannot happen to them, but only to other people. Knowledge of the more common fallacies is helpful to analyze objectively the validity of published studies. Gambrill (2012) proposed common fallacies that can occur

in scientific research. These fallacies and others applied to health research and clinical practice are listed here.

2.2.1 Irrelevant Conclusion

This fallacy is evident when an investigator intends to establish a particular conclusion by shifting his or her argument to another conclusion. For example, a clinician seeks support for a treatment method for patients with arthritis by arguing that arthritis is a crippling disease affecting millions of individuals. The fallacy in this argument is that the clinician proposes the acceptance of a treatment method based on the irrelevant fact that a specific disease is widespread. In this case, the specific treatment method that is introduced requires objective data to support its use irrespective of the pressing need to help patients with arthritis. Another example of this fallacy in research is the use of unreliable or invalid tests because no other tests for measuring a specific variable exist. For example, a test written in English is given to a speaker whose first language is Navajo because there are no tests written in Navajo. Results obtained are questionable and probably invalid. If a test is invalid or unreliable, it should not be used to measure function.

2.2.2 Appeal to Authority

It is fallacious for a researcher to accept the opinions of respected scientists on the sole basis of their reputation but without any supporting data. For example, in recognizing an authority's knowledge of nutrition, an investigator may use his or her opinions to support a position that megavitamins are an effective treatment for patients with schizophrenia. The authority on nutrition may not have any research data to support or negate this position. A respected authority's personal opinion is not valid scientific evidence. Researchers who appeal to authorities as supporting evidence fail to separate a scientist's previous reputation from his or her current opinion. In an age of specialization, scientists are no longer encyclopedists who are knowledgeable in all areas. The intensive study required for excellence in one area makes it almost impossible to have expertise in other areas, even in related ones. When a researcher uses greatly respected scientists' opinions as supporting evidence, especially outside their area of competence, he or she is committing the fallacy of appeal to authority.

2.2.3 False Cause

This fallacy is common in societies where superstition and ignorance of cause and effect exist. Curing diseases through special amulets, magical words, or patent medicines are examples of the use of false cause. It also exists in some nonexperimental research where correlational relationships are observed. For example, it may be noted that a full moon is associated with an increase in admissions to psychiatric hospitals. The relationship between the full moon and insanity (Raison, Klein, & Steckler, 1999) is then fallaciously transposed to the conclusion that a full moon causes insanity. A cause-and-effect relationship is not established by correlational data.

In the absence of valid causes of a disease, simple and reductive explanations often are accepted. For example, a researcher investigating a complex variable, such as a learning disability, may accept *prima facie evidence* that the learning disability is caused by hyperactivity. The researcher bases this conclusion on correlational evidence that children with a learning disability are also hyperactive. The fallaciousness of the argument is illustrated in Figure 2-4.

In this hypothetical example, not all individuals with ADHD have a learning disability, although a large number of individuals with a learning disability do have ADHD. Nonetheless, there is no evidence to support the conclusion that ADHD causes a learning disability or that a learning disability causes ADHD. The very nature of a complex variable presupposes multiple causes and interactional effects among variables.

Another example of false cause in clinical practice is observing the effectiveness of a treatment method without adequately explaining the direct effect of treatment on improvement. Even though a treatment method is associated sequentially with improvement, it does not logically follow that it alone changed the condition of the patient. There may be other factors in a patient's experience or in the research conditions that could have contributed to a patient's or subject's improvement. These potential factors, which could affect the result of an experiment, must be controlled before a researcher can conclude that a specific treatment affects improvement. For example, the *placebo*

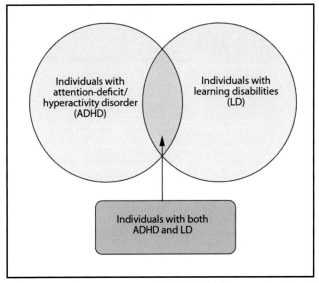

Figure 2-4. The diagram depicts the fallacy of the argument that all individuals with ADHD are learning disabled. In fact, there are two populations: individuals with ADHD and those with learning disabilities. A few of the individuals have both conditions.

effect (or "dummy treatment") is widely recognized in drug research as a change in a condition brought about seemingly by a drug but in reality by the power of suggestion that is attached to a drug. The *Hawthorne effect* is another example of a camouflaged relationship between cause and effect. In the Hawthorne effect, the change in behavior is produced by the attention of the researcher or clinician to the subjects or patients rather than solely by the specific treatment method applied. False cause is a fallacy based on traditional thinking or superstition and without supporting research evidence.

2.2.4 Ambiguity

The lack of rigor in operationally defining terms and variables used in research produces the fallacy of ambiguity. When researchers compare outcome studies of wellness, perception, functional capacity, or weight loss, false conclusions may result if their comparisons fail to acknowledge the differences in defining and measuring these variables. Wellness can be defined in multiple ways and is measured by various tests and outcome measures. How the researcher defines and measures wellness will affect the conclusions and comparisons made. When a researcher states that there is a direct relationship between healthy living and wellness, one must denote how these variables were operationally defined. Otherwise one may be operating on a simplistic and false basis that fails to take into consideration the various ways of operationally defining wellness.

For the purpose of explanation, let us examine a hypothetical example of ambiguity as shown in Table 2-1. In this example, if the researcher did not state how these two variables—healthy living and wellness—are operationally defined, then there is no basis for comparing the results.

TABLE 2-1
OPERATIONALLY DEFINING AMBIGUOUS TERMS

PRESUMED CAUSE: HEALTHY LIVING	PRESUMED EFFECT (OUTCOME MEASURE): WELLNESS
• Balanced diet • Adequate exercise • Reduction of stress • Positive interpersonal relationship	• Trips to a physician • Self-report • Findings from a physical examination • Standardized test of wellness

In actuality, there are many different studies measuring the relationship between these two abstract variables. For example, in one study the researcher could examine the effects of nutrition on the four outcome measures; in another study, exercise could be substituted for nutrition. Each of these presumed causes and effects will need to be elaborated on further so that another researcher can replicate the study.

Complex abstract variables that are investigated by researchers must be operationally defined; that is, the measuring instrument or procedure must be clearly identified before studies can be compared and conclusions proposed. Ambiguity is an example of comparing apples with oranges. For example, an investigator decides to use diet therapy as an independent variable (presumed cause) and weight reduction as the dependent variable (presumed effect); however, the specific method employed in diet therapy and the method used in measuring weight reduction are the variables that are, in fact, being investigated, not diet therapy or weight reduction per se. Clearly, operationally defining variables is important in eliminating the fallacy of ambiguity.

2.2.5 Generalization

Much quantitative scientific research involves collecting group data from a representative sample of a target population. Group data represent the average of all individual scores. Also, the data imply a range of scores from high to low on specific measured variables. The fallacy of generalization occurs when a researcher applies group data to a specific individual subject. For example, a researcher collects evidence of a statistically significant relationship between the absence of epilepsy and the occurrence of schizophrenia. The researcher concludes this from a study of seizures in which there were fewer individuals with epilepsy among patients with schizophrenia compared to the general population. However, the statistics are based on probability factors, not on a one-to-one relationship. The investigator can conclude only that there are fewer individuals with epilepsy in a population of individuals also exhibiting schizophrenia than in the general population, but not that every individual with epilepsy will not become schizophrenic nor that every individual with schizophrenia

will not be epileptic. Nor can one conclude that if epilepsy is produced through electric shock, schizophrenia can be prevented or treated. This is a fallacy where group data describing a population is generalized to every individual in the population. The error variance in probability makes it impossible to make predictions about the specific individual from group data. One can only describe the general characteristics of groups, not the individual subjects that comprise the group. From probability statistics we can describe groups of patients, students, hospitals, or schools, but we are unable to predict the individual case with any confidence. For example, Alberg and Samet (2003), in reviewing the literature, reported that 90% of people who get lung cancer are smokers; however, we cannot predict which of those individuals who smoke will actually develop lung cancer.

Another example of generalization fallacy is in the selection of students based on entry examinations, such as the SAT or Graduate Record Examination. For example, a researcher interested in predicting academic success in an occupational therapy program may find a positive correlation of $r = .73$ between aptitude test scores and grade point averages. This is not a perfect correlation; however, it indicates only that many students with high aptitude test scores will attain relatively high grade point averages. If a program director has to predict a specific individual's success or failure, the data cannot support complete accuracy. In fact, the chance of error in predicting a specific individual's grade point average is high, although there may be accuracy in predicting a group's success in a program.

An example of the fallacy of generalization applied to clinical treatment is the *Procrustean bed*. In this case, clinicians who advocate a specific treatment method apply this method as a panacea to all patients regardless of individual differences. The clinician falsely applies the treatment method as a cure-all. For example, in the 15th and 16th centuries, tobacco was thought to have several therapeutic purposes and was considered to be a panacea for health. In the mid-20th century, the harmful effects of tobacco were established (Fraga, 2010). Good treatment implies fitting the best available treatment method to the individual based on his or her needs rather than fitting the patient to a panacea.

Despite the strong arguments used by researchers to convince clinicians to accept the findings of a study or the efficacy of a treatment method, the fallacies of irrelevant conclusion, appeal to authority, false cause, ambiguity, and generalization must be recognized by consumers of research as totally unacceptable means of advancing knowledge. The following discussion includes positive guidelines for analyzing the research process and the qualities of the researcher.

2.3 CRITICAL ANALYSIS OF THE RESEARCH PROCESS

How is a research study judged to be either adequate or valid? How does one analyze the components of research and detect the biases of the investigator, the limitations of the design, and the deficiencies of the sampling procedure? The consumer of research must critically evaluate the methodology of a study before feeling confident in the results and conclusions. Many times, the results of a study are reported in mass media without an evaluation of the methodology. The results of research can play a prominent role in supporting or undermining a particular theory or social action. Governmental policies affecting funding patterns and priorities of social programs are influenced by the results of research studies. For example, continued funding of the children's television program *Sesame Street* is dependent on data that support the position that the program has educational value. Early childhood programs, such as Head Start, manpower retraining, state mental health systems, and graduate training programs in the occupational therapy profession are examples where evaluation research was used to justify federal grant support. The unfortunate policy of "benign neglect" toward minority groups during the latter half of the 1960s and 1970s was a result of government-sponsored research that supported the discontinuance of many antipoverty programs. When research is used as evidence to initiate or discontinue social programs, there is an obvious need to evaluate methodology before accepting or rejecting the conclusions. Research is not acceptable merely on the basis of social appeal, no matter how desirable the conclusions. Political considerations are one of the abuses of research that confront investigators of controversial social issues, such as community health programs or family planning.

Despite the diversity in content and the differences in application to treatment, all research has a common methodological format. When a researcher poses a question, the process of research is initiated. The question generates a search of the literature, predictions of results, and for quantitative research, a controlled objective procedure for collecting data. Background questions are generated by an investigator to help lead into specific research questions.

This is a way of helping students to discover research topics of interest to them and to narrow a research study to feasible dimensions.

Raising background questions is a brainstorming tactic to lead one into a review of the literature. The student or clinical investigator is encouraged to list as many basic questions as possible to initiate a study. For example, if the goal of a clinical study is to determine the most effective treatment methods for children with traumatic brain injury (TBI), the background questions related to TBI would include the following:

- How is TBI operationally defined?
- What are the diagnostic tests to identify TBI?
- What are the prevalence and incidence rates of TBI?
- What are the most common treatment methods for children with TBI?
- What are the research data supporting treatment interventions for TBI?
- What are outcome measures used to measure treatment effectiveness?
- What is the typical course of the disability?
- What is the prognosis of TBI?
- How can vocational rehabilitation be used to treat individuals with TBI?
- How are functional capacity evaluations applied?

The investigator uses a literature review to answer some of these background questions. This process enables the investigator to become familiar with the research literature and to begin narrowing the study. In general, research is a process of systematically accumulating knowledge. What has been done previously is incorporated into current research. Background questions generate the research process and set in motion the beginning stages of completing a research study. Figure 2-5 describes this process.

The following outline of a quantitative research study is based on the scientific method. It is a systematic and objective way to investigate a topic.

I. A *title* includes variables investigated, populations studied, and the setting to which the results can be generalized, such as a hospital or outpatient clinic.

II. An *abstract* is usually between 150 and 300 words, contains 1 or 2 sentences from each section of the research study, and summarizes the findings, limitations of the methods, and recommendations for further research.

III. The *problem* includes the research questions examined and the stated need and significance of the study.

IV. A *literature review* contains the findings of related studies that are obtained through a systematic search.

V. *Stated hypotheses* include the operationally defined variables and research predictions.

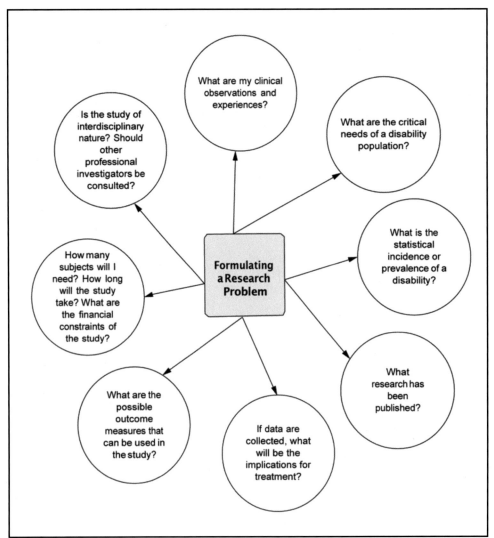

Figure 2-5. Raising basic questions, such as those in this figure, lead to a review of the literature as the beginning of a research study.

VI. A *methods section* includes obtaining approval from a human ethics review board, procedures for selecting subjects, screening criteria, measuring instruments, data collection procedures, and a plan for statistical analysis.

VII. *Results* include objective findings that are organized into tables, charts, and graphs and are statistically analyzed.

VIII. *Discussion, conclusions, limitations, and recommendations* include the significance of the findings related to previous research and the implications for further investigations.

Each of the subsections can be analyzed by posing specific questions relating to the objectivity of the investigator and the validity of the methods:

I. Title
  a. Does the title of the study clearly define what was actually done by the investigator or does it refer only to a segment of the study?
  b. Can the results of the study be generalized to the population identified by the title?
  c. Are the variables stated in the title identifiable and unambiguous?

II. Abstract
  a. Are the number of words between 150 and 300?
  b. Does the abstract include the highlights from each section of the study?
  c. Does the abstract summarize the results of the study?
  d. Are implications or recommendations for further research summarized?

III. Problem or research question
  a. Are the purposes or objectives of the study stated clearly?
  b. Are the research questions clearly identified?
  c. Is the study justified in relation to social need, importance, or potential contribution to occupational therapy?

d. Are statistics used to support the incidence and prevalence of a disability or to justify the investigation?

e. What is the relationship of the study to occupational therapy?

f. Does the study have a potential significant contribution to evaluation methods, treatment techniques, student training, or program administration?

g. Are the projected results of the study practical so they can be implemented into practice?

h. Is the researcher being objective in selecting a specific problem for investigation or is there evidence that personal biases will affect the results?

IV. Literature review

a. What information retrieval systems and primary sources of data did the investigator use in systematically reviewing the literature?

b. Are there theoretical assumptions that are unstated but are tacitly accepted?

c. What major areas were reviewed?

d. Was the literature search exhaustive in regard to the research problem?

e. Did the investigator use primary or secondary sources of information?

f. Was the investigator objective in listing results from studies that refute the stated hypotheses, as well as those studies that support the hypotheses?

g. How were previous studies reported? Did the investigator describe the number and characteristics of subjects and tests used when reporting the results of studies?

h. Are references up to date?

i. Did the researcher review a wide range of computer databases and journals related to the research topic?

V. Stated hypotheses

a. Are independent and dependent variables identifiable?

b. Are variables operationally defined?

c. Did the investigator present guiding questions?

d. Were hypotheses generated from a review of the literature, and did the investigator cite previous findings?

e. Were the hypotheses stated in null form or directionally?

VI. Research methods

a. How were the subjects selected for the study: randomly, convenience sample, or volunteers (e.g., they responded on their own to a mass communication)?

b. Were screening criteria used in selecting a representative sample (this may not be appropriate for all research designs)?

c. Were subjects a representative sample for a specified target population?

d. How were the measuring instruments selected?

e. Did the investigator state the reliability and validity of measuring instruments?

f. Do the measuring instruments have a test manual including standardized procedures for data collection and scoring?

g. How did the researcher inform subjects of risks and benefits in the study?

h. How easily could the research study be replicated?

i. Did the investigator carefully outline the procedure for data collection?

VII. Results

a. What statistical techniques were used in analyzing the data?

b. How were the results reported?

c. At what level of statistical significance were results reported? .

VIII. Discussion, conclusions, limitations, and recommendations

a. Were the findings compared to or contrasted with previous literature?

b. Were conclusions justified from reported results?

c. Is researcher bias evident in interpreting results or "rationalizing away" results?

d. Were there unforeseen events that influenced results?

e. Are results omitted that contradict the hypothesis?

f. Were limitations of the study presented?

g. Is further research indicated?

2.4 Qualities of a Researcher

What are the qualities of a researcher? Scholars analyzing the process of research consider that the attitudes and integrity of the researcher are sometimes more important than the rigor of the methodology and the veneer of scientism. The following has been enlarged from Gee's (1950) discussion of the qualities of a researcher.

2.4.1 Dissonance

The researcher feels uncomfortable with an aspect of the world and the problem serves as the motivation for carrying out the research. Research is perceived as problem oriented. For example, Semmelweis's concern over the large number of maternal deaths after pregnancy in the 19th century spurred him to initiate research into the causes of puerperal fever. Salk's experimenting with a vaccine to prevent polio was concerned with the alarming incidence of polio world wide. These are two examples of medical researchers who were motivated by dissonance. Investigators starting with a problem, such as delinquency, malnutrition, AIDS, cancer, or homelessness, are energized and moved to action by the amount of pain, anxiety, and degradation that a problem produces in society and arouses public empathy.

2.4.2 Objectivity

This quality enables an investigator to follow the data where it takes one instead of arriving at a conclusion first and then collecting data to support personal biases. Objectivity many times leads to accidental discoveries made through serendipity and happenstance. The researcher is open to accepting whatever the data reveal. Accidental discoveries of major significance are numerous in the history of science and technology: Bell's discovery of the telephone; Edison's stumbling upon the phonograph; Goodyear's accidentally inventing a process to vulcanize rubber; Roentgen's noticing chemical changes on paper, which led to the discovery of the x-ray; and Fleming's discovery of penicillin.

2.4.3 Perseverance

The scientist's persistence and dedication to an area of research is prominent in medicine. The history of medical research is filled with researchers, such as the Curies, who devoted their entire professional lives to uncovering the properties of radium. Perseverance and persistence are necessary qualities if a researcher wants to uncover ample evidence before publishing findings. The pressure on the contemporary researcher to rush to publish results discourages persistent and painstaking efforts to accumulate an abundance of evidence. The tendency to release findings prematurely, such as in pharmaceutics, has led to medical calamities, such as the effects of the drug thalidomide on fetal development. The need still remains for the researcher to persevere in the face of the pressure to publish.

2.4.4 Intellectual Curiosity

The scientist pursues a topic not only for the practical benefits that may result from the study, but also because of the desire to know. Basic research is ordinarily carried out because of the intellectual curiosity of the investigator. The basic research that produced the breakthrough in understanding the anatomy and physiology of humans came about because of Renaissance scientists' need to know. How does the body function? What are the basic processes in cell division? What is the basic chemistry of living protoplasm? Questions regarding the essential nature of the universe and matter can be answered only by research conducted by individuals with intellectual curiosity. The researcher who earnestly seeks knowledge is likely to be diligent and persevere in attaining some significant goal.

2.4.5 Self-Criticism

The investigator pursuing an area of interest needs to evaluate work critically by redesigning problems, reworking hypotheses, and initiating new methods for collecting data. The ability to examine one's work critically is important in preventing stagnation. Research involves a continual process of questioning, obtaining evidence, and re-questioning. The data from research serve as feedback for the reformulation of hypotheses only if the researcher is able to criticize oneself objectively.

2.4.6 Creativity

Being creative does not necessarily mean being novel or different. The creative researcher juxtaposes different ideas and integrates previous knowledge with contemporary issues. The qualities of risk, innovation, and independence are aspects of creativity. At odds with creativity are conformity and the need to please others while denying one's own ideas. Creativity may be a necessary quality in the researcher who desires more than fulfilling the needs of a corporate body or serving as a data collector for someone else's mission. Formulation and planning a research design is a creative act. The process of identifying a research problem and designing an objective method to test a hypothesis demands a creative quality.

2.4.7 Integrity

The researcher represents an attitude of mind. In applied health and educational fields, the researcher must be guided by ethical principles that involve a respect for the rights of participants and the honesty to bide by one's own research design and report data as found. The researcher who engages in human research is ethically bound not to abuse participants. The demand by social action groups and consumer advocates for formalized regulations in regard to the use of human subjects (especially in institutional environments, such as prisons, psychiatric centers, and former chronic disease hospitals, as well as state schools for individuals with intellectual disabilities) reflects the past abuses in human research. An informed consent contract between researcher and subject must be included in every research design. The contract shall include the following considerations:

- The exact procedure to be carried out must be explained in language that is understandable to the participants. Jargon and technical terms should be avoided.
- The possible physical and psychological side effects in the study and the steps taken by the researcher to prevent harm to the participants should be stated.
- The participant's time commitment in the study, procedures involved, and place of study should be clearly stated.
- If the participants are mentally or physically incompetent or under age, then legal guardians or parents must be asked to provide written consent for the participants' inclusion in a study.

- If the researcher requires that the purposes of the study not be revealed to the participants, then the researcher should explain this openly to the participants and debrief them as soon as possible after the data collection as to the true purpose of the study.
- The researcher should not use coercion through any means that implies social disapproval or by penalizing the participants for not participating in the study.
- If participants are paid for participation in an experiment, it should be based on work and time considerations, not as a camouflaged attempt to disguise the risks involved in being a participant or as an inducement to vulnerable individuals.
- The findings of the research are to be treated as confidential; an individual participant's data should not be identified. Ongoing research data should be stored in a locked cabinet or a password-protected computer located in a secure area.

No research is so important that it may justifiably disregard the rights of participants. The practices during World War II by the Nazis who engaged in human research without any regard for human rights (Lifton, 2017) is an extreme example of the abuse of research done with fanaticism and conformity to political goals. A researcher's integrity should be within the confines of an ethical code that must go beyond the mere search for data. Research with human subjects is not a pure or amoral theoretical activity.

Integrity in research also involves honesty in abiding by a research design and in reporting data accurately. Often, overzealous researchers are eager to present a theory of treatment or a technological advance without having conclusive evidence. The pressure to present significant or dramatic findings sometimes is a result of the career ambitions of the researcher. Unfortunately, it may become more important for the researcher to gain personal distinction than to report one's data honestly. The scientific community frequently has witnessed personality struggles in which rival researchers engaged competitively while striving for national recognition (Watson, 1968). The research in heart transplants, cancer, and DNA have been marked by personality conflicts.

2.4.8 Replication

Scientific research does not exist in a vacuum, nor is it usually the product of a single individual. When researchers investigate something, they typically build on the work of others. Even the giants of science, such as Newton, Einstein, Pasteur, and Edison, were vitally aware of previous research findings in the literature. Replication means that the researcher is able to repeat an experiment that was reported previously. The researcher who initially carries through an experiment must be able to describe the methodology in sufficient detail to allow other researchers to repeat the experiment. Research is not a mysterious activity carefully guarded and left to mystics. It is an open activity in which a scientific community of scholars engages. Without replicability, knowledge would be stagnant, as in the Dark Ages when researchers carefully hid their methods of alchemy and magic. In clinical research, it is vital that investigators share their findings with the clinical community and receive feedback from clinicians who undertake pilot studies of new practices and treatments.

2.5 Nomothetic Versus Idiographic Methods

One of the most important goals in scientific research is prediction. Whether it is the prediction that a drug will cause certain beneficial effects in the body or that a surgical operation will improve the functioning of a bodily organ, the scientific investigator seeks to discover relationships that may be universally true. The search for general laws in nature is defined as a *nomothetic approach to science*. However, the individual is affected by numerous idiosyncratic factors, such as physiological, emotional, and social influences, that are complex, unique, and sometimes unpredictable. The *idiographic approach to science* pertains to the intensive study of individuals within their own particular genetic milieu and environment. The nomothetic approach tends to be quantitative research, while qualitative research is generally used with idiographic approaches.

2.5.1 Nomothetic Approach to Science

In nomothetic research, large groups are studied to find general laws and principles that apply to a specific population (Babbie, 2010). Therefore, a certain level of probability is assumed, in that any given individual's behavior or response to an independent variable can be predicted only with a certain level of confidence. Behavior modification and operant conditioning assume that individuals are operating under general laws of nature, especially defined as reward and punishment (Skinner, 1953). The precursors of behaviorism were the logical positivists who theorized that all meaningful scientific propositions are derived from experience and can be expressed in quantifiable physicalistic language (Spence, 1948). This concept of physicalism has tried to incorporate empirical methods of collecting data into the social sciences. The technology of the logical positivists in social science is based on empirical methods of experimental control and objective observation.

The major limitation of a nomothetic approach to social science is in the inability to operationally define and measure social variables, such as motivation, interests, attitudes, emotions, and thinking, and their interactions with one another. Another limitation of the nomothetic approach is that the naming of the disability or disease (e.g., autism, depression) can appear to the patient as a cure. For example the naming of the disease or disability does not necessarily lead to successful treatment, such as when a patient is diagnosed with bipolar depression. He may believe that his problem has been solved by naming the disease (Babbie, 2010).

Behaviorism and scientific empiricism apply a psychophysiological model; historically, the major contributions of behaviorism to social science have been by pioneers such as Pavlov (1927) in classical conditioning, Wolpe (1969) in desensitization experiments, and Miller (1969) in biofeedback and conditioning experiments of the autonomic nervous systems of the body.

2.5.2 Idiographic Approach to Science

Examples of idiographic approaches used in the social sciences include psychoanalysis (Tyson, 2009), phenomenology (Van Boven, Kane, McGraw, & Dale, 2010), Gestalt psychology (Ventegodt, Clausen, & Merrick, 2006), and the humanistic movement (Videler, van Royen, & van Alphen, 2010). The subjective nature of experience and the uniqueness of the individual are, in these approaches, the vantage points for investigations. Social scientists use the case study approach in trying to understand the dynamic forces that influence an individual's behavior. The individual is perceived as an active agent interacting with the world continuously and always in the process of change. Gestalt investigations are concerned with the perceptual processes and individual differences among people and within a humanistic framework (Perls, 1969). These idiographic approaches to scientific knowledge assume that prediction in human beings is limited to the single individual, as no two individuals share the same genetic background, physiological makeup, or psychological experiences.

How does an understanding of these two approaches, nomothetic and idiographic, affect our understanding of research in occupational therapy? In the nomothetic approach, we assume that general laws control human behavior and physiological responses. For example, in medicine, when an individual is treated with a drug for a specific illness, the physician assumes this patient will react as other individuals do to the same drug. Treatment is presented in relation to the illness, not in relation to the specific individual. Researchers investigating cause-effect relationships frequently assume a nomothetic approach. By contrast, with the idiographic approach, the clinician evaluates the patient by considering individual differences and idiosyncratic traits and treats by prescribing a specific regimen. Case studies, single-subject design, and naturalistic observations are the methods used in idiographic approaches. The history of medicine, occupational therapy, rehabilitation, and special education contains many examples of both approaches. In analyzing a research study or designing an experiment, either a nomothetic (quantitative) or idiographic (qualitative) approach may be appropriate.

2.6 Types of Inquiry

There are two categories of scientific inquiry: retrospective and prospective. Each has its own advantages and disadvantages (Hill, 1971).

Retrospective research examines data or events from a historical viewpoint. For example, the investigator may be interested in the causes of multiple sclerosis or the evolution of multisensory teaching. In both cases, the investigation includes the analysis of sequential events leading to the current understanding of disease, events, or methodology. In correlational research, the investigator examines the relationship between two variables or two groups. For example, one might examine the relationship between perceptual abilities and intelligence. In retrospective designs, the findings can only hint at a cause-effect relationship.

Prospective research, on the other hand, directly seeks to predict the effect of the independent variable on the dependent variable, thereby establishing a cause-effect relationship. In experimental prospective designs, the researcher manipulates the independent variable and observes its effect on the dependent variable. For example, in a study examining the effects of aquatic therapy on the reduction of symptoms in individuals with multiple sclerosis, the researcher provides aquatic therapy to an experimental group and compares it to a control group in which no aquatic therapy is provided.

The prospective design is also used in longitudinal research where a researcher examines the effects of a variable over time. For example, longitudinal research would be used in studies of the effects of prenatal exposure to cocaine on academic success are underway (Richardson & Day, 2018).

According to Hill (1971), the following are the advantages and disadvantages of the two approaches:

- In a prospective method, the sample is more easily defined and may be more representative of a target population than in the retrospective design.
- Extraneous variables are more easily controlled in an experimental prospective design.
- In a longitudinal prospective design, such as in the Framingham Heart Study (Dawber & Kannel, 1958), individuals can be followed up with over a long period of time to determine the impact of risk factors.
- In a retrospective design, the subjects can be identified as a convenient sample, and events or variables contributing to the condition can be studied.
- One disadvantage of a retrospective design is that cause-and-effect cannot be determined by the results of the research; rather, a statistical or correlational relationship can be established and used as the basis for a prospective experimental design.

TABLE 2-2

STEPS IN FORMULATING A FEASIBLE QUESTION IN QUALITATIVE, QUANTITATIVE, AND ACTION RESEARCH

STEP TASKS	RATIONALE	EXAMPLE
1. List numerous questions about topics in which the clinician, teacher, or student is interested.	Allows the investigator to select areas of interest and locate relevant studies.	What are the most effective treatment methods for treating spasticity?
2. Locate a secondary source, such as a text or review article.	Enables the researcher to have an overview of the topic and provides a means for locating research articles.	A recent (within the past 5 years) textbook or review article on cerebral palsy.
3. Do a mini-literature review using primary sources (e.g., research articles).	Investigator becomes familiar with the current research in the area of interest.	A current (within the last 3 years) research article on treatment of spasticity
4. Identify an expert in the field.	This expert can serve as an informal consultant for locating resources, identifying additional aspects, and narrowing the research.	A clinician or special educator who has worked with children with cerebral palsy.
5. Narrow the research topic.	When a research topic is too broad, the researcher has difficulty operationally defining the variables or generalizing the results.	Is neurodevelopmental treatment more effective than sensory integration therapy in reducing spasticity in children with cerebral palsy?
6. Determine the feasibility of the research question.	The ability to do the research is dependent on several factors, such as the availability of participants, time elements, costs of the study, or the ability to control extraneous variables.	Neurodevelopmental treatment and sensory integration are used with children with cerebral palsy in a children's care facility.

2.7 MODELS OF RESEARCH

Research is defined as objective, systematic investigation. The process of designing a research study is one of the most creative acts in science. In this process, the researcher can generate new knowledge, synthesize findings from different studies, and develop new theories by being innovative. The research design is an outline of the systematic plan for collecting data. From this outline, the investigator develops a plan of action. Table 2-2 describes the steps involved in designing a research study, and Figure 2-6 gives an example.

The diversity of research designs in occupational therapy is characterized by problem-based research. These studies might include the following: (a) evaluating the efficacy of a treatment method in occupational therapy; (b) surveying the attitudes of a population of individuals with spinal cord injury; (c) carrying out an organizational case study of a sheltered workshop for adults; (d) constructing a rating scale to evaluate student-teachers or interns; or (e) correlating a relationship between perceptual skills and academic

ability. In each of these research examples, a method of data collection serves as the skeleton for the study. The research approach chosen is a decision based on the purposes of the study and the data collection methods available to the investigator. Approaches to research may include qualitative or quantitative analysis, action research, or a combination of any of these. Table 2-3 describes these approaches.

Research models appropriate to problems in occupational therapy, rehabilitation, and habilitation are summarized in Table 2-4 and described in Chapters 3 and 4. These models were identified by analyzing the methods used in the important landmark studies in the biological and social sciences and in the allied health and rehabilitation literature.

Research is not limited to one method. Investigators who carry out an unbiased research plan and collect objective data are engaging in research whether they wear a white coat in a laboratory or do historical research in a library. In practice, some investigators combine both qualitative and quantitative research models. For example, the same study may involve constructing an instrument for measuring

Figure 2-6. Relationship among scientific inquiry, theory, research, and clinical practice. This relationship is pictured using an example of research in TBI.

clinical effectiveness and then carrying out an experimental design. Another frequently used research method is to survey two populations (survey research models) and then compare the responses between the two samples (correlational research model).

The diversity of research models available for the multiple problems of a disability is illustrated by the varied approaches in investigating the aging process. For example, amyloid has been identified hypothetically as a protein that, when accumulating in the body, may be a factor in accelerating the general process of aging. The relationship between amyloid and aging can be analyzed from many perspectives by using more than one research model. For instance, an experimental design using animal research is one possibility (Flood & Morley, 1998). Here, the investigator can form two animal groups, one receiving amyloid injections and the other as a control. The results of this hypothetical design could yield empirical data regarding the direct relationship between amyloid and aging in mammals.

Another design applying a correlational model could be created by retrospectively testing the relationship between the explicit memory of an individual with Alzheimer's disease and that of control subjects without impairment (Fleischman & Gabrieli, 1998). A methodologist may be interested in devising an instrument for detecting the presence of amyloid in the bloodstream ("Consensus Report of the Working Group on ...", 1998). A retrospective clinical case study of Alzheimer's and the examination

of neurological changes is another research possibility (Fukutani et al., 1997). An examination of the relationship between diet and the precursors to amyloid would add another dimension to data collection (Howland et al., 1998).

The research models employed by investigators imply certain hypotheses in generating data collection procedures. Research investigations into specific problems can take place from many perspectives. Knowledge of specific research models enables the investigator to attack problems from more than one dimension. Table 2-5 demonstrates how several research models can be applied to a multifaceted investigation of the aging process.

2.7.1 Action Research

Another application to the scientific method is action research. Action research developed out of Dewey's (1933) concept of learning by doing through creative problem solving. Lewin's (1939) field theory in which he examined the forces in the environment that impacted the individual is the theoretical foundation for action research. *Action research* is defined as a problem-oriented investigation that is applied in site-specific environments, such as an industry, school, classroom, hospital, clinic, community, or home setting. In action research, the teacher or clinician, as the researcher, applies quantitative and qualitative research methods to specific problems originating out of a curriculum, treatment program, or ergonomic situation.

TABLE 2-3

COMPARISON OF QUANTITATIVE AND QUALITATIVE RESEARCH METHODS

	QUANTITATIVE	QUALITATIVE
DEFINITION	• Empirical method that is based on hypothesis testing and control and measurement of variables within a value-free framework	• Study of people and events in a natural setting to make sense of and obtain meaning from the phenomena observed and experienced, emphasizing a value-laden nature of inquiry (Denzin & Lincoln, 1994a)
UNDERLYING ASSUMPTIONS	• Reality is based on natural laws that predict outcome (nomothetic). • Variables are operationalized and the relationships between the variables can be measured. • The hypothesis is stated before data collection occurs. • In experimental design, the investigator manipulates the independent variable(s) and measures the dependent variable(s). • Standardized tests or procedures are used to collect data. • The researcher assumes an objective, unbiased attitude toward participants. • Representative samples of a target population are obtained through random sampling.	• Reality is based on the subjective interpretation of the study (idiographic approach). • Variables are difficult to measure because of the complexity and interconnectedness. • Analysis of data collection is heuristic and ends with grounded theory. • Variables emerge as the researcher collects and analyzes subjective data. • Researcher as an interviewer serves as the instrument for collecting data. • The researcher interacts on a personal, subjective level with the participants. • A snowballing effect is used to obtain a convenience sample of the target population.
MODELS FOR CONDUCTING RESEARCH	• Experimental • Correlational • Methodological • Evaluation • Heuristic • Case study (prospective) • Survey (assessment)	• Case study (retrospective or prospective) • Phenomenology • Biographical or historiography • Ethnography • Grounded theory or heuristic • Survey (interview)
TECHNIQUES OF DATA COLLECTION	• Structured forced-choice questionnaire and surveys • Standardized tests or procedures (performance or paper-and-pencil) • Frequency count or interval recording • Rate of response • Triangulation	• Structured and unstructured interviews • Case studies • Observation • Diaries, journals, and personal experiences • Introspection • Interactional and visual texts • Archival records • Field notes • Triangulation
ANALYSIS OF DATA	• Application of descriptive and inferential statistics to test hypothesis or guiding question	• Content analysis to develop naturalistic generalizations (e.g., themes, meanings, theories)

Adapted from Clifford, C. (1990). *Nursing and health care research: A skills-based introduction.* Englewood Cliffs, NJ: Prentice Hall; Creswell, J. W. (1998). *Qualitative inquiry and research design: Choosing among five traditions.* Thousand Oaks, CA: Sage; Denzin, N. K., & Lincoln, Y. S. (Eds.). 1994. Introduction: Entering the field of qualitative research. In *Handbook of qualitative research* (pp. 1-17). Thousand Oaks, CA: Sage; and Glesne, C., & Peshkin, A. (1992). *Becoming qualitative researchers: An introduction.* New York, NY: Longman.

TABLE 2-4
RESEARCH MODELS

RESEARCH MODEL	TASKS OF RESEARCHER	SIGNIFICANCE
Quantitative		
Experimental (group or case study)	Direct manipulation of independent variables and examination of effects in highly controlled settings	Determine empirically the effectiveness of treatment or classroom procedures
Methodological	Construction of a measuring instrument, curriculum, or therapeutic procedures/approaches	Innovative methods or procedures, including technology
Correlational (retrospective design)	Test of the relationships between non-manipulated variables	Identifying factors that are presumed to have an associational relationship
Qualitative		
Observation (child development, ethnography, descriptive case study)	In-depth study of individuals, groups, or systems	Identify underlying dynamics in individuals or groups or organizational models of practice to affect change
Historical	Investigation of past events through primary sources (e.g., interviews, documents)	Reconstruction of past events to understand contemporary problems
Either Quantitative or Qualitative		
Evaluation	Critical analysis of health care delivery systems and educational programs	Objective and/or qualitative assessment of the effectiveness of systems and treatment programs
Heuristic and operations	Discovery of possible causative factors in chronic disabilities, analysis of time, space, and cost factors	Generate further research by identifying significant variables
Longitudinal (prospective studies)	Follow-up studies to determine the effectiveness of a treatment technique or the effects of variable on maturation	Determine long-term effects of variables (e.g., genetic, environment, and intervention)
Survey	Study of the characteristics of homogeneous populations	Description of general factors that characterize a group

2.7.1.1 Where Can Action Research Be Applied?

Action research can be applied in the following ways:

- Within the school setting, when there is concern about overall achievement, teachers or occupational therapists may use action research to develop ways of changing or modifying the curriculum to allow all students to benefit from instruction.

- When occupational therapists and special education teachers work collaboratively to develop methods for students with developmental disabilities to become more functionally independent in self-care tasks, they may use action research. For example, they examine the effectiveness of teaching work adjustment skills

to a student who has a goal of local employment. The success of the student may possibly enable this method to be applied to another student in the same school or may lead to a revision of the method.

- An occupational therapist fabricates a splint in a hand therapy clinic for patients who have had carpel tunnel release surgery. Using action research, the occupational therapist seeks to devise a splint that keeps the wrist in a neutral position and facilities the healing process.

- In a psychosocial setting, the occupational therapist designs strategies to help patients with a diagnosis of depression to be self-motivated and to self-regulate their symptoms. Action research is used to enable the therapist to select the most effective strategies.

TABLE 2-5	
RELATIONSHIP BETWEEN RESEARCH MODELS: AGING EXAMPLE	
EXPERIMENTAL OR PROSPECTIVE	Use of laboratory animals (induce aging or retard aging) and study of physiological variables (Okuma & Nomura, 1998).
METHODOLOGICAL	Construct tests and instruments to measure neuropsychological aspects of aging (Schinka et al., 2010).
EVALUATION	Evaluate the effectiveness of an independent living facility for individuals who are elderly to increase quality of life (Wang, Kane, Eberly, Virnig, & Chang, 2009).
HEURISTIC	Discover the underlying factors related to premature aging, such as in progeria (Domínguez-Gerpe & Araújo-Vilar, 2008).
CORRELATIONAL OR RETROSPECTIVE	Compare individuals who have retired and who are active in the community with comparable individuals who are inactive (Remsburg, Bennett, Wendel, & Durso, 2002).
QUALITATIVE CASE STUDY	Use a case study analysis of an individual who is older expressing feelings of hopelessness (Markowitz, 2007).
SURVEY	Identify the attitudes of young people regarding Alzheimer's disease (Lundquist & Ready, 2008).
HISTORICAL	Document through a study of federal legislation a society's changing attitudes toward individuals who have Alzheimer's disease (Ahmed, 2001).

- Within the home, an occupational therapist uses action research to modify the home environment so that an individual with a stroke is able to be independent. The occupational therapist considers accessibility, kitchen adaptations, placement for furniture, and electronic equipment to enable an individual to be functional.

Characteristics of action research include:

- Action research occurs in a local, naturalistic setting, sometimes referred to as *site-based*.
- Research may be applied to a setting (e.g., school, organization, hospital, home), a classroom or clinic, or a single individual (e.g., single-subject design).
- The results of the research are usually not generalized outside of the specific setting.
- Quantitative and qualitative research methods can be applied to the investigation. For example, use of standardized tests, observational methods, and statistical analysis may be used to examine the effectiveness of the program.
- Occupational therapists and teachers act as the participant-observer by planning the research, collecting data, and analyzing and interpreting the results. The research is designed and conducted in the teachers' or therapists' own setting as a means of improving one's teaching, therapy, or ergonomic adaptations.

- Problem-solving methods are used to generate possible solutions. For example, a therapist working in a long-term care facility may be looking for ways to increase the morale among staff, or a teacher may be looking for better ways to teach students with ADHD.

2.7.1.2. Possible Outcomes of Action Research for Occupational Therapists

- Students in special education who are receiving services either in a pull-out program (i.e., where students leave the general education classroom to go into a special classroom) or in the general education program will benefit as changes are made in their individualized program because of the outcome of the action research.
- Occupational therapists and special educators work together to modify the program for a student who is having difficulty with handwriting. The special educator and the therapist will look at building up the size of the pencil to make it easier to grasp, use of a neutral position and pincer grip for handwriting, perceptual motor activities to increase performance, methods for improving posture, or changes of furniture to improve ergonomic adaptations.
- Students with developmental disabilities will be taught how to be more independent in activities of daily living within the community.

TABLE 2-6
EXAMPLES OF TYPES OF SCHOLARLY MANUSCRIPTS

SCHOLARLY MANUSCRIPTS	TASKS OF WRITER	SIGNIFICANCE
Position paper	Advocate reforms of health care or educational systems, legislation, ethics of research, standards of practice	Presentation of policy statements and editorials
Theoretical exposition	Explain relationships between variables and predict outcomes	Logical explanation in natural or social science using deductive reasoning
Case study presentation[a]	Present chronological history of an individual, such as one's course of illness or treatment effectiveness	Sequential description of disease process or treatment in an individual
Review paper	Integrate and synthesize published research	Exploration of current state of knowledge in specified field
[a]A case study can be used as a research model in both qualitative and quantitative research.		

- Within occupational therapy, results of action research will enable individuals with spinal cord injuries to become employable in a local community.
- The occupational therapist will devise methods to decrease carpel tunnel syndrome in individuals working in a meatpacking plant.
- Occupational therapists working with an individual with depression will develop strategies for sleep hygiene to enable him or her to sleep better.

2.7.2 Scholarly Models Not Based on the Scientific Method

These research models are not the only methods of organizing knowledge. A theoretical paper in which a scientist integrates and synthesizes knowledge by creating a conceptual model and a position paper in which a health practitioner advocates a governmental policy, such as National Health Insurance, are both examples of nonresearch that are scholarly and original. The important difference between research and a scholarly essay or exposition is that in research the investigator formulates a problem first and then objectively collects empirical data related to the problem. In a nonresearch scholarly article, the investigator presents a position or theory and then cites evidence in its support. Another scholarly model is a case study in which a clinician describes a disease process or a treatment technique with a specific individual. Because this model is case-specific, the author does not usually attempt to control variables or generalize the information to another situation. A review paper can also be a model of scholarly work. In this paper, the author integrates studies to generate a body of knowledge. A summary of scholarly manuscripts are described in Table 2-6.

For the past 100 years, the scientific method has generated many research models. Although for many years research generally was limited to those who did not teach or conduct therapy, there is a need for clinicians and teachers to apply evidence-based practice in their everyday work. Qualitative and quantitative methods can be applied within one's own setting through action research, while scholarly papers can be written through a review of articles in the literature. It is incumbent on those of us in the clinical and teaching fields to use an evidence-based practice model to establish the efficacy of our practices.

3

Quantitative Research Models

The clinical trial is a carefully, and ethically, designed experiment with the aim of answering some precisely framed question. In its most rigorous form it demands equivalent groups of patients concurrently treated in different ways.

—Hill (1971, p. 273)

OPERATIONAL LEARNING OBJECTIVES

By the end of this chapter the learner will be able to:

- Define *quantitative research*.
- Define key terms in quantitative research methods.
- Identify types of quantitative research.
- Critically analyze examples of research from the occupational therapy and special education literature.

Rice, M. S., Stein, F., & Tomlin, G.
Clinical Research in Occupational Therapy, Sixth Edition (pp. 55-104).
© 2019 Taylor & Francis Group.

Quantitative research involves the systematic use of empirical methods to test relationships between variables. Quantitative research is often employed to investigate whether there are statistically significant differences in dependent variables under the influence of an independent variable. The research hypothesis usually describes the research question and establishes the anticipated relationships between the dependent and independent variables.

Empiricism is defined as gaining data through the senses from phenomena that are observable, objective, and verifiable. An example of empirical data is measuring hand strength with a dynamometer. Another example is measuring the rate of words per minute that a student reads. Empirical data must be operationally defined so that they can be reproduced by another investigator. In quantitative research, the investigator begins with a hypothesis that predicts the results of the investigation. While this chapter focuses specifically on quantitative research models, the concepts of research design and methodology (Chapter 7) are closely related to many of the concepts introduced in this chapter. Indeed, successful research amalgamates the concepts from this current chapter with concepts found in Chapter 7. Some key terms used in quantitative research are described in Table 3-1.

3.1 FACTORS IN QUANTITATIVE RESEARCH MODELS

The following factors are the *sine qua non* (i.e., the essential ingredients) of quantitative research models.

- *A justification and rationale for the research*: This includes a justification for the research that is based on the significance of the research. For example, a researcher justifies the need for research in spinal cord injury by describing the number of individuals who incur such an injury and by the cost of the injury. In special education, a teacher may justify the examination of different ways to work with students with autism based on the increasing incidence of this diagnosis.
- *An extensive review of literature*: The researcher identifies and analyzes previous research related to the topic of study. For example, a researcher examining animal-assisted therapy would search databases for previously published studies.
- *Operational definitions of research variables*: The researcher must operationally define each of the variables being examined. These variables include the participants, the setting where the experiment takes place, the intervention, and the outcome measures.

- *Identification of extraneous variables that could confound the results*: The investigator tries to control the static variables, such as gender, age, socioeconomic status, ethnicity, and handedness. The researcher also seeks to control all environmental conditions for the various sub-groups of people studied.
- *Statement of hypothesis or guiding question*: Prior to collecting data, the researcher predicts or hypothesizes about the results of the study.
- *An objective, unbiased method for collecting data*: A research design that can be replicated is developed by the investigator.
- *Separate sections for results and discussion*: After the data are collected, the investigator designs tables, figures, and graphs to depict the results in an objective manner. A discussion of the results is more subjective and allows the investigator to speculate on the implications of the study.
- *Limitations of the study and recommendations for further research*: The researcher acknowledges limitations in the methodology or uncontrolled variables that could have affected the results and makes recommendations that could improve future studies. For example, one limitation might be the limited number of subjects or a less reliable outcome measure.

3.2 EXPERIMENTAL RESEARCH

3.2.1 Purposes of Experimental Research

The researcher uses experimental methods to collect empirical data by manipulating independent variables and observing their effects, seeking maximum control of the data collection procedure and environmental conditions. An experimenter achieves *internal validity* when he or she is able to control extraneous variables that could affect the results (Table 3-2). The degree of experimental rigor depends on these controls.

Figure 3-1 shows the relationship between experimental research and clinical practice. Working together, their purposes are to:

- Compare the effectiveness of clinical intervention methods.
- Observe cause-effect relationships established in a laboratory.
- Examine biopsychosocial factors underlying human responses.

TABLE 3-1
KEY DEFINITIONS IN QUANTITATIVE RESEARCH

CONTROL GROUP	A group selected to compare with the experimental group. This group may be a non-intervention group with no treatment or it may be a group that receives a different treatment method. For example, the researcher may wish to determine the effects of splinting on reducing carpal tunnel syndrome and may introduce exercise in the control group.
DEPENDENT VARIABLE	In clinical research, the treatment effect or outcome resulting from the intervention of the independent variable. For example, the dependent variable in a study of sensory integration therapy could be a reduction of tactile defensiveness in children.
EMPIRICAL DATA	Data based on controlled observation that is observable, measured, verified, and replicated.
EVIDENCE-BASED PRACTICE	Use of contemporary research findings as the basis for clinical reasoning in selecting the most effective treatment method.
EXPERIMENTAL GROUP	A group that is manipulated by the researcher. For example, the experimental group could receive heart rate biofeedback or relaxation therapy or handwriting instruction. The treatment represents the independent variable in experimental research.
EXTERNAL VALIDITY	The degree to which results can be generalized to a target population. External validity depends on the representativeness of a sample and the rigor of the experiment. Replication of a study producing consistent results increases the external validity.
EXTRANEOUS VARIABLE	A variable not manipulated by the researcher but that can potentially affect the results of a study. Extraneous variables can include factors such as gender, intelligence, severity of disability, or socioeconomic status. These variables, if they are uncontrolled, can threaten the internal validity of a study.
HYPOTHESIS	A statement that predicts results and is testable by a systematic methodology. A hypothesis can be either null or stated. (See the following for an example of a null hypothesis.) A stated hypothesis can be either directional or non-directional. An example in the directional form is: "Children will demonstrate greater reading achievement when using a phonetic method when compared to when using a whole language method." An example of a non-directional hypothesis is: "There is a statistically significant difference in reading achievement when using a phonetic method when compared to whole language."
INDEPENDENT VARIABLE	A variable manipulated by the researcher. In clinical research, it represents the treatment method, such as aquatic therapy, progressive relaxation, or phonemic awareness.
INTERNAL VALIDITY	The degree of rigor in an experiment in controlling for extraneous variables and error variance. Potential threats to internal validity have been identified as extraneous historical factors, maturation, instrumentation, and lack of random sampling. Internal validity is an indication of the trustworthiness of the results. Well-designed studies with good control of variables that can potentially distort the results have high internal validity. The quality of a research study is increased by eliminating the threats to internal validity.
NULL HYPOTHESIS	A statement by the researcher that predicts no statistically significant difference or relationship between variables. For example, a clinical researcher states, "There is no statistically significant difference between a prescriptive aerobic exercise and Prozac in reducing clinical depression."

(continued)

TABLE 3-1 (CONTINUED)
KEY DEFINITIONS IN QUANTITATIVE RESEARCH

OPERATIONAL DEFINITION OF A VARIABLE	Specific measure, observation, or criteria that defines a variable. For example, activities of daily living (ADL) skills may be defined as the score obtained on the Barthel Index. An operational definition is important in replicating a study or in evaluating a group of studies using a method, such as through a meta-analysis.
PRE-POST GROUP DESIGN WITH CONTROL GROUP	Classical experimental design where the investigator compares both the within (pre- and post-testing) and the between (experimental and control groups) factors the results obtained by both groups.
RANDOM SAMPLING	An unbiased portion of a target population selected by chance, such as through random numbers.
RELIABILITY	A measure of the consistency of a test instrument. For example, on a test with high reliability, one would expect approximately the same results on two different administrations when there is no change in subject.
REPLICABILITY	The ability to repeat an experiment or scientific procedure. The purpose is to strengthen generalizability of the findings and to ensure external validity.
INTERVENTION PROTOCOL	The operational definition of the independent variable or intervention method. The intervention protocol should have enough detail so that it can be replicated. One purpose of designing a treatment protocol is to evaluate its effectiveness.
VALIDITY	As pertaining to measurement, the degree to which a test or measuring instrument actually measures what it purports to measure.

TABLE 3-2
CONTROL OF EXTRANEOUS VARIABLES

POSSIBLE CONFOUNDING EXTRANEOUS VARIABLES	METHODS TO CONTROL EXTRANEOUS VARIABLES
Demographic variables (e.g., age, socioeconomic status, gender, ethnicity, first language, handedness)	Establish screening criteria that includes range of ages, gender, ethnic groups, home language, or hand dominance.
Cognitive variables (e.g., intelligence, academic achievement, processing abilities)	Administer a screening test to ensure equivalent groups.
Test anxiety	Establish rapport, answer questions, and set the participant at ease prior to any data collection.
Low motivation	Screen out individuals who show reluctance to participate in the study.
Hawthorne effect	Establish a control group and ensure that each group within the study has equal attention.
Test conditions	Ensure that environmental conditions (e.g., lighting, noise, temperature, presence of other people, distractions) do not interfere with data collection.
Reliability and validity of procedure	Use a double-blind control in which the data collector is not aware of the participant's group.

(continued)

TABLE 3-2 (CONTINUED)	
CONTROL OF EXTRANEOUS VARIABLES	
POSSIBLE CONFOUNDING EXTRANEOUS VARIABLES	METHODS TO CONTROL EXTRANEOUS VARIABLES
Experimental bias	Ensure that all individuals collecting data have been trained on the protocol and that inter-rater reliability is high.
Data collection methods	Do a pilot study to examine the reliability and validity of the procedure, or use tests and procedures that have established high validity and reliability.

Figure 3-1. Purposes of experimental research. Note that there are three purposes for research, all of which lead to implications for intervention.

3.2.2 Comparison of Intervention Methods

Is intervention method A more effective than intervention method B? This question is a clinical problem affecting every individual treated by an occupational therapist in a hospital, home, or school setting. Nonetheless, the application of published clinical research remains limited. Many occupational therapists continue to use traditional methods of intervention without searching the literature to determine whether their effectiveness has been established through research. The classical research design employed in testing the relative effectiveness of clinical intervention methods is the paradigm (Figure 3-2).

In this example, the experimental intervention represents the independent or manipulated variable, whereas the degree of improvement represents the dependent variable.

A cause-effect relationship is inferred directly by the experimenter.

Traditionally, the control group has been a non-intervention group or a comparative intervention group. In a nonintervention group, there is a possibility of a Hawthorne effect in which each group does not get equal attention, and the results may be attributable to the attention of the experimental group rather than to the intervention effect. In their classical work on experimental design, Campbell and Stanley (1963) used the term *quasiexperimental* to indicate experimental designs in which there is no comparative control group. For example, in a pilot study, a researcher may want to examine the effects of a stress management program on the reduction of depression by using an experimental group without a control group (Nowak, Preson, & Horoszewski, 2015). This would be considered a quasiexperimental design.

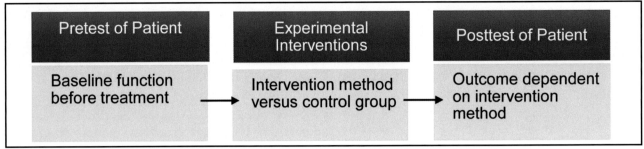

Figure 3-2. Classical clinical treatment paradigm.

An example of a clinical research design using a control condition is a study by Bellows, Gavin, Johnson, Boles, and Davies (2015). In this study, the researchers compared performance on the Bruininks-Oserestsky Test of Motor Proficiency in children from Head Start centers who received the Mighty Moves program to children who did not receive the Mighty Moves program.

Table 3-3 compares the features of two studies: Nowak, Preston, and Horoszewski (2015) and Bellow, Gavin, Johnson, Boles and Davies (2015). Although the basic design is similar, the former study has no control group and uses a smaller sample.

3.2.3 Clinical Research

The clinician's major concern is the effectiveness of a specific intervention method for a specific client. The clinician evaluates the client, establishes intervention goals using RUMBA (i.e., *R*elevant, *U*nderstandable, *M*easurable, *B*ehavioral, and *A*chievable), applies appropriate intervention methods, reevaluates the client's improvement made prior to discharge, and concludes that if the client improved, then the treatment intervention was probably effective. If the intervention method is effective, can the clinician assume that it could be applied to similar clients (i.e., external validity)? Before one can confidently generalize the results, further data must be obtained to validate the results. Using an evidence-based intervention is one way the clinician may validate intervention (Burke & Gitlin, 2012). He or she may also postulate that the selected intervention method is better than other comparable methods. Again, this must be confirmed by comparing the effectiveness of various intervention methods. Another assumption is that the evaluation of intervention outcome is objective. The technique of measuring the effectiveness of an intervention method can make the difference between labeling it successful or ineffective. The test for an adequate outcome measure or evaluation of intervention effectiveness is its reproducibility by other clinicians. General application to other clients, relative effectiveness compared with other methods of intervention, and objective measurement of improvement are factors that clinicians must examine if their results are to be considered valid and generalizable.

Experimental research enables clinicians to compare the relative effectiveness of intervention methods. In clinical research, the occupational therapist carefully documents the effects of intervention over time. The therapist can carry out the research in a group experiment or single-subject design. (See Boxes 3-1 and 3-2 for examples of research studies using experimental design with a single subject or with groups.) In a group experiment, the researcher compares intervention methods with groups of clients. Intervention groups are set up ahead of time, and clients are randomly assigned to each group. Analysis of results is by group statistics. In a single-subject design, the therapist may alternate different intervention methods with the same client (alternating interventions) who may act as his or her own control.

For example, in a group design, clients with arthritis are referred to occupational therapy for intervention. The clinician can employ physical agent modalities, exercise, purposeful activity, and hydrotherapy methods randomly. Functional skills, range of motion (ROM), and self-evaluation of pain in the shoulder joint can be used as measures of improvement. Each intervention group is charted, and statistical analysis can be used to make an inferred probability statement about the relative effectiveness of each intervention method. On the other hand, with a single-subject design, the effect of using upper extremity inhibitive casting to reduce spasticity is studied in a single child with cerebral palsy (Tona & Schneck, 1993). In this case, the investigators measured pre-post performance using the Modified Ashworth Scale, a clinical measure of spasticity. Without further replication, however, the results could not be generalized with confidence to other such clients. Figure 3-3 illustrates how a clinical researcher could chart progress by using a graph.

Other variables that can potentially affect the results should be recorded for each client. In this way, systematic patterns can be noted. A data collection sheet containing information can be statistically analyzed later to compare the relative effectiveness of intervention methods and the systematic influence of extraneous variables. An example of a data collection sheet is illustrated in Figure 3-4.

TABLE 3-3		
COMPARISON OF QUASIEXPERIMENTAL AND EXPERIMENTAL DESIGNS		
	QUASIEXPERIMENTAL	EXPERIMENTAL WITH CONTROL
CITATION	Nowak, M., Preston, H., & Horoszewski, K. (2015). Validity and reliability of an iPod Forearm Goniometer App. *American Journal of Occupational Therapy, 69,* 6911500107p1-6911500107p1.	Bellows, L. L., Gavin, W. J., Johnson, S. L., Boles, R. E., & Davies, P. (2015). Obesity prevention study: A physical activity program improved gross motor skills in preschool children. *American Journal of Occupational Therapy, 69,* 6911515228p1.
SUBJECTS	100 students from Keuka College	218 children from rural Head Start centers.
EXPERIMENTAL GROUP	100 students from Keuka College	126 students from 5 Head Start centers
CONTROL GROUP	None	92 students from 3 Head Start centers
DESIGN	Repeated measures with no control group	Repeated measures design (pre- and post-test) with a control group
TREATMENT PROGRAM	Participants measured four angles of forearm supination and pronation. Two angles were predetermined and the other two were at full ROM.	The experimental group received the Mighty Moves program while the control group did not.
ASSESSMENT OF OUTCOME	Forearm Goniometer App	Bruininks-Oseretsky Test of Motor Proficiency (2nd edition) subtests and body mass index.
RESULTS AND CONCLUSIONS	"The analysis revealed that the app did not accurately measure the predetermined angles. . . . The app did have high reliability between trials, with an overall correlation coefficient of .91." (p. 6911500107p1).	"A significant Group × Time interaction was found for balance ($P < .05$) and speed/agility ($P < .05$), indicating that the intervention group demonstrated a significant increase in these skills compared to the control group." (p. 6911515228p1).

BOX 3-1. EXAMPLE OF AN EXPERIMENTAL CASE STUDY (PROSPECTIVE DESIGN)

1. Bibliographical Notation

Hoffman, H. G., Meyer, W. J. III, Ramirez, M., Roberts, L., Seibel, E. J., Atzori, B., ... & Patterson, D. R. (2014). Feasibility of articulated arm mounted Oculus Rift Virtual Reality goggles for adjunctive pain control during occupational therapy in pediatric burn patients. *Cyberpsychology, Behavior, and Social Networking, 17,* 397-401.

2. Abstract

"For daily burn wound care and therapeutic physical therapy skin stretching procedures, powerful pain medications alone are often inadequate. This feasibility study provides the first evidence that entering an immersive virtual environment using very inexpensive (~$400) wide field of view Oculus Rift Virtual Reality (VR) goggles can elicit a strong illusion of presence and reduce pain during VR. The patient was an 11-year-old male with severe electrical and flash burns on his head, shoulders, arms, and feet (36 percent total body surface area (TBSA), 27 percent TBSA were third-degree burns). He spent one 20-minute occupational therapy session with no VR, one with VR on day 2, and a final session with no VR on day 3. His rating of pain intensity during therapy dropped from severely painful during no VR to moderately painful during VR. Pain unpleasantness dropped from moderately unpleasant during no VR to mildly unpleasant during VR. He reported going "completely inside the computer generated world", and had more fun during VR."

(continued)

Box 3-1. Example of an Experimental Case Study (Prospective Design) (continued)

Results are consistent with a growing literature showing reductions in pain during VR. Although case studies are scientifically inconclusive by nature, these preliminary results suggest that the Oculus Rift VR goggles merit more attention as a potential treatment for acute procedural pain of burn patients. Availability of inexpensive but highly immersive VR goggles would significantly improve cost effectiveness and increase dissemination of VR pain distraction, making VR available to many more patients, potentially even at home, for pain control as well as a wide range of other VR therapy applications. This is the first clinical data on PubMed to show the use of Oculus Rift for any medical application.

3. Justification and Need

The authors detail the primary medical strategy for dealing with pain, namely the heavy reliance on opioid narcotic pain medication. As such, the argument is made that non-narcotic augmentative strategies to relieve pain, particularly during occupational therapy sessions with burn victims, is a worthy pursuit. Thus, the manuscript introduces the concept of immersive VR pain distraction. Although the study cites previous research in this area, the purpose of this study is to determine the feasibility of using newly developed technology that is intended to be even more effective at ameliorating pain through VR.

4. Literature Review

Twenty-five references from a wide variety of sources were used. Cited journals included but were not limited to the following: *Annals of Behavioral Medicine, Archives of Physical Medicine and Rehabilitation, Healthy Psychology, Clinical Journal of Pain,* and *Clinical Psychology.* The years of cited publications ranged from 1963 through 2011.

5. Research Hypothesis or Guiding Question

The guiding question for this research was to "… explore the feasibility of using the Oculus Rift goggles to distract burn patients during occupational therapy and other painful medical procedures" (p. 400).

6. Methods

The participant was an 11-year-old boy who experienced severe electrical and flash burns involving his head, upper extremities, and feet. These burn injuries involved second-degree burns over 36% of his body and third-degree burns over 27% of his body. The intervention involved 3 days.

The participant received the same level of medication on each of the days. The first day, baseline date for two 1-hour sessions dispersed across 6 weeks with 3 sessions/week. The outcome measures included active range of motion (AROM) measurements, the Fugl-Meyer, the Graded Wolf Motor Function Test, the Motor Activities Log, and the Canadian Occupational Performance Measure. This study used a pre-test/post-test/follow-up single experimental case design that employed descriptive statistics to compare performances across time. The timeline involved 6 weeks between the pre- and post-tests and 3 months between the post-test and the follow-up.

7. Results

Improvements on the Graded Wolf Motor Function Test, and the Fugl-Meyer were the most dramatic between the pre- and post-tests; additionally, performance on these two measures showed little decline at the follow-up time period. The variation in performance on the Motor Activities Log varied very little between the three testing periods. The same was largely true for the Canadian Occupational Performance Measure measures of satisfaction and performance. AROM improvements were seen in "shoulder abduction, external rotation, elbow extension and wrist flexion and extension. Of these, some of the shoulder external rotation and elbow extension AROM gains were not maintained at the time of the follow-up testing. The participant also reported decreases in pain, and stiffness over the course of the study" (p. 239).

(continued)

Box 3-1. Example of an Experimental Case Study (Prospective Design) (continued)

8. Conclusions

Hoffman et al. concluded that:

- "Robotic therapy was successful in gaining active movement in the involved UE [upper extremity] ..." (p. 242)

- "The participant also made small gains in functional use" (p. 242)

- "... improvement in motor function does not necessarily translate to functional use" (p. 242)

9. Limitations

As this is a single-case clinical experimental study, generalization of these results is very limiting. Future research is needed using a larger population to increase the external validity of this line of research.

10. Major References Cited

Fasoli, S. E., Krebs, H. I., Stein, J., Frontera, W. R., & Hogan, N. (2003). Effects of robotic therapy on motor impairments and recovery in chronic stroke. *Archives of Physical Medicine and Rehabilitation, 84*, 477-482.

Fugl-Meyer, A. R., Jaasko, L., Leyman, I. Olsson, S., & Steglind, S. (1975). The post-stroke hemiplegic patient: A method for evaluation of physical performance. *Scandinavian Journal of Rehabilitation Medicine, 7*, 13-31.

Law, M., Baptiste, S. Carswell, A. McColl, M. A., Polatajko, H., & Pollock, N. (1998). *The Canadian Occupational Performance Measure* (3rd ed.). Ottawa, Ontario, Canada: Canadian Association of Occupational Therapists Publications.

Taub, E., Uswatte, G., & Pidikiti, R. (1999). Constraint-induced movement therapy: A new family of techniques with broad application to physical rehabilitation—A clinical review. *Journal of Rehabilitation Research and Development, 36*, 1-17.

Box 3-2. Example of an Experimental Research Group Study

1. Bibliographical Notation

Kehoe, R., & Rice, M. (2016). Reality, virtual reality, and imagery: Quality of movement in novice dart players. *British Journal of Occupational Therapy, 79*, 244-251.

2. Abstract

"*Introduction*: Meaning and purpose have been tenets of occupational therapy since the profession's inception. Therefore, it is important to understand how to best employ these central concepts in practice. One way to do this is to study the 'same' task under materials-based, imagery-based, and virtual reality conditions. *Methods*: Participants included 34 adult novice dart players, each of whom experienced all three conditions in a randomized order. Motion capture technology was used to evaluate the quality of motion during the three conditions. *Results*: Similarities between the materials-based and imagery-based condition ($P > 0.0167$) suggest participants utilized preconceived concepts of throwing real darts during these two conditions. Differences between the virtual reality and imagery-based conditions ($P < 0.0167$) suggest that the virtual reality condition utilized a different motor performance, focusing less on perceptions of throwing darts and more on achieving successes within the virtual environment. *Conclusions*: Implications are that utilizing materials-based occupations may be more efficient than imagery-based to enhance development of a skill; imagery-based performance is more similar to the materials-based performance than the virtual reality performance. Virtual reality occupations can be utilized should the patient find meaning and purpose in virtual reality occupations or if the patient cannot engage in a materials-based counterpart."

(continued)

Box 3-2. Example of an Experimental Research Group Study (continued)

3. Justification and Need

There is a growing body of evidence supporting the inclusion of meaningful and purposeful activities as a part of occupational therapy sessions results in enhanced therapeutic outcomes. However, little research within occupational therapy has been done to investigate using video games or VR as a therapeutic strategy. This study used a VR version of the game of darts, which the authors argued does not require actual darts or a dart board and is ubiquitous and culturally relevant within many societies.

4. Literature Review

Twenty-five references from a variety of sources were identified. Cited journals included but were not limited to *American Journal of Physical Medicine and Rehabilitation*, *American Journal of Occupational Therapy*, *Archives of Physical Medicine and Rehabilitation*, *British Journal of Occupational Therapy*, *Canadian Journal of Occupational Therapy*, and *OTJR: Occupation, Participation and Health*. The years of publications cited in this article ranged from 1922 through 2013.

5. Research Hypothesis or Guiding Question

"It was hypothesized that specific kinematic differences between the three conditions would be found. Specifically, it was expected that the material-based condition would elicit a better quality of motor performance than the imagery-based and virtual conditions. It is also hypothesized that the virtual reality-based condition will elicit a better quality motor performance than the imagery condition" (p. 447).

6. Methods

For the study, participants included 34 healthy adults aged 18 to 53 years from the Toledo, Ohio, area. To be included in the study, participants needed to have no or negligible experience playing darts, be fluent in the English language, and be able to stand. Exclusion criteria included having no orthopedic or neurological pathology or condition that would interfere with the ability to play darts. This was a repeated measures design where participants were randomly assigned to one of three orders of presentation involving the three conditions: *real*, *virtual*, and *imagery*. The task involved throwing three darts within the context of each condition. In the real condition, participants were asked to throw three tangible darts at a regulation dart board; in the virtual condition, participants were asked to throw three virtual darts at a virtual dartboard displayed on a television display via an Xbox 360 (Microsoft) and Kinect sensor; and in the imagery condition, participants were asked to throw three imaginary darts at an imaginary dart board. Movement kinetics and kinematics were recorded using a three-dimensional motion capture system. Focused contrasts were used to analyze the differences between the real and the virtual conditions, the real and imagery conditions, and the virtual and the imagery conditions. The alpha was set at .0167. Dependent variables included displacement, peak velocity, movement time, percentage of movement time to peak velocity, movement units, and maximum aperture of the index and thumb.

7. Results

- In general, the imagery and real conditions were more efficient than the virtual conditions, with statistically significantly differences with displacement, movement time, and maximum aperture.

- Exceptions to this trend was that there was a significant difference in peak velocity, with the real condition being more efficient than the imagery condition and the virtual condition being more efficient than the imagery condition.

- There was a significant difference in maximum aperture, with the real condition being more efficient than the imagery condition.

(continued)

Box 3-2. Example of an Experimental Research Group Study (continued)

8. Conclusions

Kehoe and Rice concluded that:

- "... this study partially supports its first hypothesis, as the materials-based condition elicited better motor performances in terms of peak velocity and maximum aperture when compared with the imagery and the virtual reality conditions" (p. 249).

- "This study's second hypothesis was also partially supported. The virtual reality-based condition was found to elicit significantly better motor performances in terms of displacement, peak velocity, and movement time when compared with the imagery condition" (p. 249).

- The real and imagery conditions were largely similar in their kinetic and kinematic performances, whereas these two conditions were largely different than what was observed in the virtual condition. It was surmised that the internal concept of throwing darts during the imagery condition was based upon throwing a real dart.

- "The parameters set by the Kinect sensor as to what is an appropriate movement to elicit a response within the virtual environment may have been the major influence on how the participants planned and executed their motor performances, and not upon the intricacies required for throwing an actual dart" (p. 249).

- "While a VR-based dart throwing intervention may not be effective in eliciting the same motor skills associated with materials- or imagery-based throwing, it is possible to achieve client goals that are biomechanical in nature, such as increasing gross motor ROM of the upper extremity and increasing muscle strength and endurance. Additionally, for those clients who ascribe a large amount of meaning and purpose to playing darts but are not able to participate in the materials-based form of the occupation due to some form of physical limitation, a virtual reality environment may be an appropriate alternative for providing a meaningful and therapeutic occupation" (p. 249).

9. Limitations

The sample size was relatively small, with only 34 participants. There is a possibility of a Type II error. Additionally, it is not possible to guarantee that participants actually imagined throwing darts during the imagery condition. Generalization to special populations served by occupational therapy practitioners is limited and must be done with caution. Finally, the study was conducted in a non-naturalistic lab environment.

10. Major References Cited

DeKuiper, W. P., Nelson, D. L., & White, B. E. (1993). Materials-based occupation versus imagery-based occupation versus rote exercise: A replication and extension. *OTJR: Occupation, Participation and Health, 13*, 183-197.

Harris, K., & Reid, D. (2005). The influence of virtual reality play on children's motivation. *Canadian Journal of Occupational Therapy, 72*, 21-29.

He´tu, S., & Mercier, C. (2012). Using purposeful tasks to improve motor performance: Does object affordance matter? *British Journal of Occupational Therapy, 75*, 367-376.

Hoffman, H. G., Patterson, D. R., & Carrougher, G. J. (2000). Use of virtual reality for adjunctive treatment of adult burn pain during physical therapy: A controlled study. *Clinical Journal of Pain, 16*, 244-250.

Sackaloo, K., Strouse, E., & Rice, M. S. (2015). Degree of preference and its influence on motor control when reaching for most preferred, neutrally preferred, and least preferred candy. *OTJR: Occupation Participation and Health, 35*, 81-88.

3.2.4 Designing Experimental Groups

The advantage of using clinical research is that the experimenter does not need large numbers of subjects to initiate research. The major disadvantage is the experimenter's lack of control in matching the groups on specific variables. For example, there will always be demographic and biopsychosocial differences between two intervention groups.

Experimental research with matched groups increases the internal validity or rigor of the experiment.

In clinical research with groups, the investigator compares the effects of two or more independent variables in a patient population. If the clinical researcher wants to compare intervention method A with intervention method B, he or she must create relatively equal groups and employ reliable and valid measures to test outcomes. The design is illustrated in Figure 3-5.

Figure 3-3. Example of progress chart. On the horizontal axis (X) are the testing days, and on the vertical axis (Y) is the passive resistance to spasticity for each day. (Adapted from Tona, J. L., & Schneck, C. M. (1993). The efficacy of upper extremity inhibitive casting: A single-subject pilot study. *American Journal of Occupational Therapy, 47,* 901-910.)

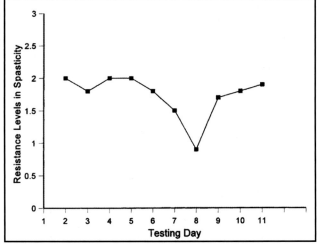

Figure 3-4. Example of a data collection sheet. The information contained on the sheet will change according to the needs of the researcher.

Data Collection Sheet		
Background Data		
1 Patient code number (based on intervention group)		
2 Gender	3 Date of Birth	4 Handedness
5 Diagnosis		
6 Date of onset of illness		
7 Occupation		
8 Years of formal education		
9 Date of data collection		
Test Data		
10 Pretest Scores on dependent variable		

11   Post –test scores
      a 1 week _____
      b 2 weeks _____
      c 3 weeks _____
		d 4 weeks _____
		e 3 months _____

12 Intervention		
13 Other test data, including psychological tests, physiological measures, and self-report		

Experimental research with two or more groups can potentially eliminate the Hawthorne effect. Each group is given equal time and attention to control the effect. The procedure for guarding against the Hawthorne effect is described in Figure 3-6.

The foregoing sequential analysis illustrates the many controls necessary in isolating the experimental or intervention effect and in controlling for extraneous variables. In designing experimental research with a control group, it is important for the researcher to match the groups on variables that could potentially affect the results of the study, such as age, gender, socioeconomic status, intelligence, and education. For instance, how can an investigator design an experiment applying biofeedback techniques in reducing hypertension in patients with post-cardiac disease? The first step in this hypothetical design is to select a population of clients with cardiovascular disease by establishing screening criteria for inclusion based on age, gender, diagnosis, length of hospitalization, and vital capacities. The number of subjects to be included in the study is determined by statistical and practical considerations. (See Chapter 7 for a discussion of these considerations.) Participants are then randomly assigned to an experimental group (e.g., biofeedback) and a control group (e.g., medication). The

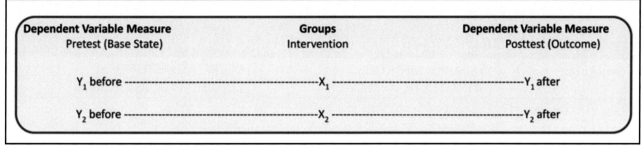

Dependent Variable Measure	Groups	Dependent Variable Measure
Pretest (Base State)	Intervention	Posttest (Outcome)

Y_1 before ---------------------------------X_1---------------------------------------Y_1 after

Y_2 before ---------------------------------X_2---------------------------------------Y_2 after

Figure 3-5. Sequential analysis of control factors in experimental research. Controlling for each of these factors helps prevent possible error due to the Hawthorne effect.

Figure 3-6. Potential factors affecting change in a patient. Each of these factors (i.e., intervention method, patient, intervention setting, and therapist) is multifaceted.

investigator should review the participants' backgrounds to determine if the groups are evenly matched on the relevant variables that are being considered. After two essentially equivalent groups have been established, diastolic and systolic blood pressure are taken in various conditions (e.g., at rest and at several stages of exertion) to establish a baseline. Then the investigator checks to determine if both groups have approximately equal mean blood pressure scores. If not, the groups are reformed until the researcher is satisfied that the two groups are comparable. The two groups then undergo the experiment within a specified time period (e.g., two 2-hour sessions per week over a 3-month period). To avoid researcher bias, the test administrator would not

know whether a subject was in the biofeedback group or the medication group. Research assistants, who would not be told the purpose of the study, would be responsible for implementing the design. This method, called *double-blind control*, eliminates experimenter bias. In a double-blind study, neither the investigator nor the subject participant is made aware of the subject's experimental condition assignment.

Subject motivation, fatigue, anxiety, and distractibility or lack of cooperation are major factors that increase the error variance in experimental research and should be carefully monitored because these variables could affect the results. After the 3-month period, a post-test of blood

		TABLE 3-4	

RESEARCHER-CLINICIAN COMPARISON FOR EVALUATING INTERVENTION OUTCOME

VARIABLE	RESEARCH METHODS (NOMOTHETIC APPROACH)	CLINICIAN METHODS (IDIOGRAPHIC APPROACH)
Intervention method	Experimental variable that is independent, mutually exclusive, and can be replicated in other studies	Clinical method that is modifiable and dependent on the observed needs of the patient and the experiences of the clinician
Other factors affecting intervention	Systematic extraneous variables that must be controlled (e.g., by matching, random assignment, or narrowing the scope of the study)	Individual factors in the patient that account for some patients improving while other patients remain the same or regress
Assessing improvement	Operational definition of measurement instruments for improvement and control for the Hawthorne effect	Clinical impression of patient's progress based on the clinician's initial evaluation and subsequent observed changes at discharge

pressures would be obtained from both groups. It is possible that a training or Hawthorne effect would lower blood pressure in both groups; however, a null hypothesis would be proposed stating that there would be no statistically significant difference between the experimental and control groups. Statistical analysis would be performed to determine whether there is, in fact, a significant difference. A conclusion based on statistical analysis of the data could then be proposed by the researcher. Additionally, the researcher would examine the literature for similar studies to determine if the current results corroborate or contradict these findings. There are many variations of experimental research. One example of a factorial design is examining a possible interactional effect between medication and relaxation therapy in children with attention-deficit/hyperactivity disorder (ADHD).

Before undertaking experimental research with human subjects, ethical and human rights factors must also be considered. Every subject should be informed of the experimental procedures and potential risks involved. (Further discussion regarding this topic along with the human subjects review process is found in Chapter 7.)

3.2.5 Experimental Research Methods and the Effects of Clinical Intervention

Researchers and clinicians have various definitions of improvement. For researchers, improvement is operationally defined and measurable, and the variables that caused the improvement are clearly identified. Clinicians, who work with clients every day, use individual goals and, many times, subjective criteria for evaluating a patient's progress. In addition, clinicians draw upon individual cases from their clinical practice to support or to negate a method of intervention. Table 3-4 summarizes the differences between researchers and clinicians in evaluating intervention outcome.

The problem of investigating the effectiveness of an intervention method is a complex issue. What criteria are used in evaluating improvement? How can other variables in a patient's life space, such as family, friends, diet, activities, and work, be separated from the intervention procedure in the evaluation of improvement? How can the therapeutic relationship be separated from the intervention method in determining its effect on intervention outcome? The interactional effects between the therapist and client, intervention method and client, and external environment and client make it difficult for the experimenter to isolate the specific variables causing specific results. These interrelationships are schematically shown in Figure 3-7.

Before it is possible to determine if one intervention method is more effective than another, the clinical researcher must identify and control possible extraneous variables that could influence the results. Four areas of influence, as shown in Figure 3-7, include variables within the client, therapist, and environment, as well as within the intervention method. All of these factors potentially can affect outcome. Knowing this, the researcher must ask: What specific *intervention* method by what specific *therapist* for what specific *patient* in what specific *environment*

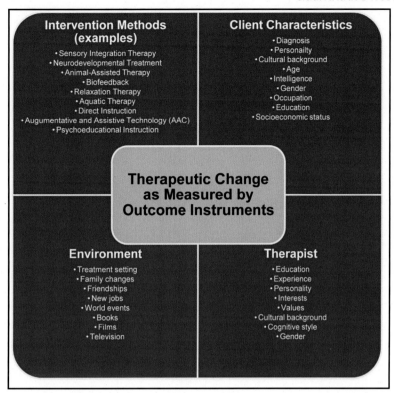

Figure 3-7. Interactional effects of intervention, therapist, patient, and intervention setting. Although the operational definition remains the same, the results obtained on the outcome measures are dependent on the interactional effects of method, therapist, patient, and setting.

is effective as measured by what specific *outcome instruments*? The interactional effects of these variables are shown in Figure 3-8.

3.2.6 Control of Factors Affecting Patient Improvement

When controlling for factors that may account for patient improvement, the researcher considers the following questions within each of the variables listed.

3.2.6.1 Therapist Variables

- Is the therapist's age or gender significant in affecting outcome?
- Is cognitive style (i.e., the characteristic way that the individual perceives the world) a factor?
- How does the therapist's personality affect change?
- Is the therapist's level of education or expertise a factor in improvement?
- What part does the experience of the therapist play in client improvement?
- Are there cultural or ethnic factors in the therapist that facilitate or retard client progress?

- What other qualities of the therapist can potentially affect patient improvement?

3.2.6.2. Client Variables

- Do specific demographic factors (e.g., age, gender, ethnicity, marital status) affect intervention outcome?
- What are the effects of severity of illness and comorbidities on intervention?
- How do the client's intelligence, education, occupation, and social class affect the intervention process?
- Does the congruence or conflict between the personality of the patient and therapist affect outcome?
- Is the patient's home environment a factor?

3.2.6.3 Intervention Method Variables

- Does the therapist need special training to apply the intervention method?
- Is the intervention method reliable (i.e., does it allow the therapist to apply a standard operational procedure or protocol to clients)?
- Is there an underlying theoretical explanation for treatment intervention effect on patient improvement?

Figure 3-8. Interactional effects of intervention (treatment) method, therapist, patient, and intervention (treatment) setting. Although the operational definition remains the same, the results obtained on the outcome measures are dependent on the interactional effects of method, therapist, patient, and setting.

3.2.6.4 Intervention Environmental Variables

- Does the setting where intervention takes place affect outcome (e.g., hospital, clinic, patient's home, classroom, special school, transitional housing, supported employment)?
- How does the timing (the length of individual intervention sessions and frequency of interventions during a week) affect outcome?
- Does group vs. individual intervention affect outcome?
- What are the effects of interactions of co-therapists who are simultaneously treating the same patients?
- Do physical variables in the intervention setting (e.g., lighting, background, sound, color, temperature, atmospheric pressure, visual distractions) affect intervention outcome?

In addition to these four variables (i.e., therapist, patient, intervention method, environment), the researcher must pose the following questions regarding the measurement of outcome.

3.2.6.5 Measurement of Intervention

What criteria are used for measuring outcome? These criteria include the following:

- Change in physical capacity, such as grip strength, spasticity, fine motor dexterity, heart rate, upper extremity strength, and gross motor abilities
- Increase in psychosocial functioning, such as the ability to work, improved self-esteem, improved interpersonal relationships (e.g., with family, peers, authority figures), and the ability to cope with stress
- Cognitive functioning, such as alertness, attention span, memory or information processing, problem solving, and organization
- Improved behavioral performance regarding insomnia, eating disorders, smoking, substance abuse, or sexual dysfunction
- Increase in health-related knowledge, such as nutrition, stress management techniques, the use of activity or exercise, family relationships, and use of and compliance with pharmaceutical drugs
- Occupational habits
- Occupational routines
- Social participation

Figure 3-9. Interaction between intervention methods and therapist characteristics in treating clients with ADHD.

3.2.6.6 Interactional Effects on Intervention Outcome

- The researcher must also account for interactional effects among variables. For example, a therapist with a penchant for order may be more effective using a behavioral modification intervention method than a therapist who has a personality characterized by a strong need for nurturing others. An intervention method that is effectively employed with one therapist may not be as effective with another therapist. The therapist's personality, values, and characteristics impact their ability to work with specific clients and may affect the outcome. Therapists' preferences for working with specific patients are usually indicative of personality variables, although the self-selecting process of the therapists' preference for a specific intervention method, in a specific intervention setting with a designated diagnostic group, may be limited by the therapist's education and experience. As therapists gain insight into their own skills and perceived effectiveness in working with patients, they develop specified preferences. For the researcher evaluating the effectiveness of an intervention procedure, a sensitivity to and awareness of the interactional effects of variables on intervention outcome is a necessity.

- An example of a hypothetical research study examining the interaction between intervention methods in occupational therapy and therapists' characteristics is shown in Figure 3-9. In this example, four methods for treating ADHD in children are compared: behavior therapy, stress management, group psychodynamic, and psychoeducational. The therapists' characteristics in working with clients are typified as the following:

  - *Laissez-faire*: The therapist is permissive in approaching the client
  - *Authoritarian*: The therapist is directive in working with the client
  - *Democratic*: The therapist allows the clients' input into developing interventions

The hypothetical results may show that behavior therapy is most effective with therapists who are authoritarian and that a group psychodynamic approach may be most effective with a therapist who is laissez-faire. The stress management or psychoeducational approaches may be most effective with therapists who use a democratic approach.

3.2.7 Analysis of Human Processes in Typical Subjects

Experimental research models have been used to investigate physiological, psychological, and sociological responses to various stimuli with typical human subjects. In general, experimental research with typical subjects tends to be *nomothetic* in that the researcher seeks general laws of nature that govern kinesthetic, physiological, neurological, sociological, or psychological processes. For example, the researcher might investigate the most effective means to encourage typical child development. Such a study could involve selection of toys, specific teaching methods, nutrition, sensory motor stimulation, or physical activity. In all of these examples, the investigator can use experimental research to compare the different methods.

Potential relationships that can be studied with experimental research are the following:

- Exercise and mood in typical participants
- Cooperative learning groups and achievement
- Cognitive style and choice of leisure activities
- Body alignment and mechanical stress on joints
- Dichotic listening and organization of auditory stimuli into meaningful patterns
- Movement patterns and sport skills
- Verbal reinforcement and learning
- Language stimulation and reading achievement
- Activity and normal aging

3.2.8 Operational Definitions of Normality

When defining normality and selecting typical participants, the investigator should be guided by an a priori screening criterion setting forth attributes in the continuous range of typical functioning. Each screening criterion (e.g., intelligence, muscle strength, ROM, blood pressure, heart rate, reading achievement) must be operationally defined and the range of scores determined to be typical or normal before the study begins. If this guideline is followed, the researcher is more justified in generalizing the results from the data to all typical individuals, within the age ranges represented, who make up the population from which the sample was selected.

In some experiments, *normality* is defined as an ideal state of health without the presence of a disability or disease. In other cases, normality refers to a statistical average of a population where disease and disability are evenly distributed. The following example illustrates the fallacy of rigid criteria for defining normality: A physician evaluating an older individual's blood pressure would take into consideration the age of the individual in concluding that the blood pressure is normal. An individual who is obese would be expected to have a higher blood pressure than an individual who is not, and so forth. The concept of normal blood pressure is dependent on age, gender, and weight as is indicated.

Relative normality needs to be considered when a researcher reports data for typical subjects. Many researchers assume that normality exists as an absolute and that the healthiest age is young adulthood. Concluding that young adults are usually healthy, the researcher often is tempted to select young college students as representative samples of normally healthy individuals. However, the data derived from such a study would be representative only of a young adult population of college students. Whatever group is selected, the researcher must also demonstrate that the subjects had no physiological differences that could influence results. In short, a research subject is considered typical only when compared to a priori screening criteria.

3.3. METHODOLOGICAL RESEARCH

3.3.1 Purposes of Methodological Research

Methodological research involves the objective and systematic investigation for designing instruments, tests, procedures, curriculum, software programs, and intervention programs. Figure 3-10 outlines specific areas of applying methodological research to rehabilitation, occupational therapy, and habilitation.

As seen in Chapter 1, significant advances in medicine and rehabilitation occurred because of technological advances via microscopes, x-ray machines, electrocardiograms, augmentative communication, computer software, computed tomography scans, and the numerous diagnostic scopes, all of which are results of methodological research. The introduction of psychophysiological measures and functional capacity evaluations are examples of the ongoing importance of methodological research and its relationship to clinical practice.

3.3.2 Strategies

In selecting an assessment tool, intervention protocol, or assistive device, the researcher poses the question: What are the relevant factors that must be considered in choosing a test instrument, intervention method, or self-care device? Factors to consider include developmental age, cognitive functioning, sensory-motor abilities, and educational level. The content and format of the instrument or test should be determined after a systematic review of related literature.

An example of a methodological research study is developing a feasible method of independent self-feeding for a group of individuals with severe disabilities. The researcher needs to consider several aspects of feeding, including positioning, utensils, eye-hand coordination, motivational factors, instructional methods, and attention level of the clients. Another example is a researcher interested in devising therapeutic toys for children with cerebral palsy. In this case, factors relating to sensorimotor, cognition, psychosocial aspects, and language should be considered. The sequential analysis shown in Figure 3-11 describes the steps involved in designing a therapeutic toy for children with cerebral palsy.

3.3.3 Designing Intervention Protocol

The *intervention protocol* is an operational definition of an intervention method. It includes all the details in the prescription, preparation, initiation, implementation, documentation, and evaluation. The number of interventions per day or week and the length of the sessions are also included. The intervention protocol should be modified or adjusted to meet the individual needs of the client.

What if an occupational therapist is interested in designing a new intervention protocol for cognitive retraining in adult patients who have sustained a traumatic brain injury (TBI)? How can the clinical researcher assist the occupational therapist in this investigation?

The overall design of the research is organized into five phases:
- *Phase I* is an examination of the need for developing a new cognitive retraining protocol that takes into consideration the incidence of TBI in the population as well as the family, social, and economic costs of TBI. The importance of the study is documented.

Figure 3-10. Methodological research: purposes and content. This figure illustrates the application of methodological research to occupational therapy, rehabilitation, and habilitation. (IADL = instrumental ADL.)

- *Phase II* includes a search of the literature reviewing the etiology, incidence and prevalence rates, and current intervention methods for cognitive retraining. As part of the literature review, the researcher would ideally complete a descriptive meta-analysis that evaluates and compares the research on cognitive retraining methods.

- *Phase III* considers the variables that enter into the design of a specific intervention protocol. The variables considered in devising the protocol are described in Table 3-5. In this phase, the clinical researcher's goal is to design the intervention method so that it can be used by trained occupational therapists to work with individuals with TBI.

- *Phase IV* includes the pilot testing of the intervention protocol. During this phase, the researcher is concerned with the refinement of the procedure and initial evaluation by occupational therapists working with TBI. A rating scale for assessing the clarity and relevancy of the intervention method is developed by the researcher and completed by clinicians. The actual testing of the effectiveness of the intervention protocol cannot be accomplished until the protocol has been operationally defined and then tested for its feasibility. The following issues must also be considered:

  ◦ Are the instructions presented clearly to the client?

  ◦ Are all theoretical assumptions considered when developing the method? For example, when developing a cognitive retraining protocol, the researcher must consider the encoding, storage, and retrieval aspects of information processing.

  ◦ Should the intervention be shortened or lengthened in time?

  ◦ Are there limitations to the intervention procedure? For example, clients with limited cognitive abilities may not benefit from a cognitive retraining protocol.

- *Phase V* includes the evaluation of the intervention protocol, its applicability to individuals with TBI, and the level of skill necessary to administer the intervention. The potential effectiveness of the intervention method compared with other procedures as identified in the literature review should also be considered.

Figure 3-11. Methodological research: construction of a therapeutic toy. Note that the construction includes a literature review, operationalized goals, pilot testing on students with and without disabilities, and evaluation of effectiveness.

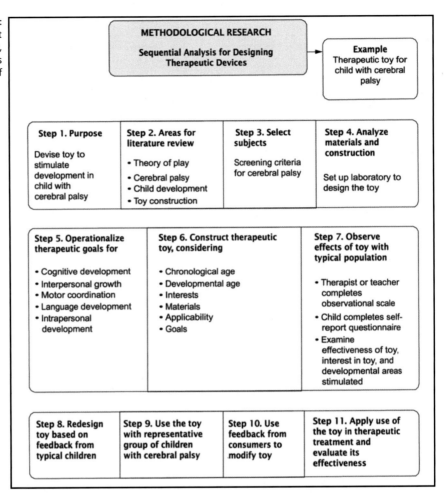

TABLE 3-5
VARIABLES IN DEVISING AN INTERVENTION PROTOCOL

PATIENT	THERAPIST	METHOD
• Diagnosis • Severity of illness • Gender • Intelligence • Education • Socioeconomic status	• Educational level • Experience • Specific training • Cognitive style	• Operationalized intervention goals • Time factors • Manual of directions • Individual vs. group factors

3.3.4 Assessment Instruments

The design of assessment instruments was a traditional role for psychologists who were trained in measurement theory and test construction. Recently, practitioners from diverse disciplines in rehabilitation and education have also become involved in developing new assessment measures that are directly related to professional evaluation.

For example, interest among occupational therapists in perceptual-motor functions and child development has led to the construction of new tests designed for specific populations (Miller, 1988). Application and use of standardized tests are becoming an increasingly important task of the clinician who routinely evaluates the level of patient function. The construction of reliable and valid instruments for measuring human capacities is a relatively fertile area of methodological research in the allied health professions. A more in-depth discussion of testing and measurement is in Chapter 10. Figure 3-12 analyzes the steps involved in test construction.

Figure 3-12. Methodological research: test construction, including rating scales and questionnaires. Note that there is a sequential order to the construction, with many validity checks while the task is being completed.

3.3.5 Questionnaires and Interviews

The need to gather information regarding the characteristics and attitudes of populations has led to the wide abuse of interviews and questionnaires, especially in marketing research. Individuals are deluged by interviews and questionnaires asking whether they use a certain brand of toothpaste or deodorant, ad infinitum. Despite abuses, they can be useful tools in obtaining information about a target population. In constructing interviews or questionnaires, the researcher must resolve the following questions:

- Was there an overall theoretical framework or rationale for selecting the items?
- Do the items measure accurately what the researcher purports to measure? (Validity)
- Are the items clear, unambiguous, and consistent? (Reliability)
- Were the items tested on a representative pilot sample for clarity, reliability, and validity?

For a further discussion of interviews and questionnaires, see Chapter 10.

3.3.5.1 Rating Scales

Rating scales are a type of questionnaire that can be used to quantify information. Rating scales are employed most frequently in evaluating the performance of students, clients, and staff. Typically, the evaluator checks off the description most indicative of performance from a list of adjective phrases. Rating scales are usually of three types: numerical, dichotomous, and descriptive. In a numerical scale, often called a *Likert scale*, ratings are distributed along a continuum, such as in the following example:

Rate each of the following items by circling the number that corresponds to your opinion. (Likert Scale)

Strongly agree   1

Agree   2

Neutral   3

Disagree   4

Strongly disagree   5

a. The United States should adopt a universal health plan for all residents.

1   2   3   4   5

b. Medicare and Medicaid should be combined into one health care system.

1   2   3   4   5

In a dichotomous scale, the extremes are identified, and the rater chooses the extreme that indicates the client's performance. For example:

Circle yes or no.

The patient's ability to assemble small parts is adequate.

Yes   No

In a descriptive scale, the rater chooses a phrase from a presented list. For example:

Circle the descriptive phrase that is most accurate.

1. On a specific task (e.g., addressing envelopes), the worker in a supported employment needs supervision.

- All of the time

- Some of the time

- Once in a while

- Rarely

- None of the time

3.3.6 Treatment Facilities

How can a clinical researcher contribute to the design of an effective intervention environment for clients with disabilities? The tasks of designing sheltered workshops, adult day care, outpatient clinics, and halfway houses are a joint effort by architects, administrators, therapists, and other rehabilitation personnel. The researcher applying methodological research to the construction of an intervention environment should first pose the question: What factors must be considered in designing a therapeutic environment for clients? Using answers to this question, the researcher can generate a plan that considers several variables. A tentative outline for research follows.

3.3.7 Methodological Review: Treatment Facilities

1. Formulating the purposes for the treatment facility:
    a. Disabilities served (e.g., individuals with mental illness, intellectual disabilities, or physical impairments)
    b. Intervention goals (e.g., cognitive and physical enhancement, functional skills, independent living, social participation)
    c. Demographic considerations for screening clients (e.g., age, gender, level of care)
    d. Location of treatment facility (e.g., urban, suburban, rural) and impact on neighborhood
2. Surveying need for intervention facility by documenting:
    a. Number of potential clients to be serviced
    b. Number of other intervention facilities in service area

    c. Attitudes toward facility's location by potential clients, community residents, and health care providers
3. Reviewing literature describing similar programs:
    a. Identifying model programs
    b. Architectural descriptions of physical layouts
    c. Analysis of staff functions and patient ratios
    d. Policies regarding patient admissions, discharges, and follow-up
    e. Evaluation research of intervention effectiveness
    f. Administrative considerations (e.g., budgeting, departmental responsibilities)
4. Stating guiding assumptions and rationale for:
    a. Setting screening criteria for client admission and discharges
    b. Designing physical layout and geographical location
    c. Proposing staff positions
    d. Setting criteria for evaluating effectiveness
5. Surveying resources of community for:
    a. Potential source of staff
    b. Transportation facilities
    c. Consultative services
    d. Community support
6. Survey cost-effectiveness factors:
    a. Construction cost
    b. Cost of providing patient care and intervention
    c. Cost of providing supportive and maintenance services
    d. Sources of potential income
        i. Private pay
        ii. Insurance and any third-party payments
        iii. Government entitlements (i.e., Medicaid and Medicare)
        iv. State and federal grants
        v. Private foundations

3.3.8 Designing Education Curricula

The training of occupational therapists, dietitians, rehabilitation counselors, speech-language pathologists, audiologists, physical therapists, special educators, school psychologists, and other related professional groups involves interdisciplinary approaches. What knowledge in the areas of physiology, anatomy, psychology, and sociology are necessary? What interpersonal skills in working with clients with disabilities must be developed? What evaluation and intervention procedures should be taught? These questions regarding the content of educational curricula are continually reevaluated considering the rapid growth of the occupational therapy profession. Parallel to the growth of the curricula content areas is the interest in designing methods for effectively communicating knowledge to occupational therapy students. How do students learn most effectively? What should be the role of problem-based learning, computer-assisted instruction, distance learning, technology, preceptor and intern supervision, and lecture in the educational curricula? These questions lend themselves to methodological research. The researcher methodically designs a curriculum after identifying the relevant factors from an extensive review of the literature.

3.3.9 Physical Evaluation Techniques and Intervention Hardware

Another area of methodological research that is appropriate to the allied health professions pertains to the use of machines and hardware for evaluating a patient's functional capacity. Electromyography, electrodiagnostic recording, perceptual-motor tests, visual, auditory and kinesthesis testing, and manual muscle testing are examples of the broad areas for potential research.

Occupational therapists may use physical agent modalities, often in conjunction with physical therapists. Physical agent modalities include ultrasound, diathermy, infrared light, ultraviolet rays, hydrotherapy, electrical stimulation, hot packs, acupuncture, TENS (transcutaneous electrical nerve stimulation), biofeedback, and paraffin. New methods of intervention, especially in muscle retraining, are now relying on electrophysiological methods involving oscilloscopes, telemetry, and computers. The growth in the prosthetics field has been the result of the combined talents of researchers coming from backgrounds in engineering, neurophysiology, and occupational therapy. Orthotics, the development of splints and braces for individuals with physical disabilities, is another area for research in occupational therapy.

In Box 3-3, the investigators examine the Useful Field of View and the Stroke Drivers' Screening Assessment to determine which is the most useful to guide clinical practitioners in evaluating the skill of driving after a stroke.

3.4 EVALUATION RESEARCH

3.4.1 Purposes of Evaluation Research

Evaluation research examines the effectiveness of programs that provide direct health care, prepare health personnel, and administer services for private and governmental agencies. When engaged in evaluation research, the investigator considers a total organizational unit and the components that comprise it. Program effectiveness, quality of service, productivity, organizational communication, cost-effectiveness, stated objectives, and personnel practices are areas considered in evaluation research. Evaluation research is commonly applied in the following programs, services, and agencies:

- Certification of hospitals (e.g., Joint Commission on Accreditation of Hospital Organization)
- Accreditation of college or educational program (e.g., the National College Accreditation of Teacher Education or the Accreditation Commission of Occupational Therapy Education)
- Rehabilitation agency evaluation (e.g., The Rehabilitation Accreditation Commission)
- Analysis of cost-per-patient intervention (e.g., Medicare guidelines, Diagnostic Related Groups)
- Outcome studies of patients or clients
- Needs assessment (e.g., community's health needs, available resources)
- Evaluation of program effectiveness using a priori criteria

A historical example of the impact of evaluation research on changing an institution was the report *Medical Education in the United States and Canada* by Flexner, Pritchett, and Henry (1910), which was made into the Carnegie Foundation for the Advancement of Training. Flexner personally toured the 155 medical schools that existed in the United States and Canada at that time. Although he did not use a standardized questionnaire or test instrument for evaluation, he did apply specific criteria in evaluating the quality and effectiveness of medical schools in preparing physicians. These criteria were the following:

- The entrance requirements for gaining admission to the medical school (e.g., minimal standards, high school graduation or equivalent, college education).
- The number of students in full- or part-time attendance.
- The size of the faculty, including the number of full-time professors and part-time instructors.
- The financial resources available to the college from endowments, student tuition, and clinical fees.
- The quality and adequacy of the physical plant, including laboratory classrooms, lecture halls, medical and laboratory equipment, refrigerator plants, amphitheater for observation of surgery and clinical interviews, and medical library.
- Professional supervision available to the students in the laboratories.
- The opportunities for student practice in clinics and availability of hospital patients.

Based on these criteria, Flexner found a wide discrepancy in standards of medical education in the schools he visited. Based on his observations, he concluded that many medical schools were doing a disservice to the public by preparing poorly educated physicians. He recommended that there be fewer medical schools.

Flexner's evaluations of the 155 medical schools led to dramatic changes in medical education that occurred between 1910 and 1925. He recommended (a) that medical schools and hospitals enter into teaching relationships, (b) state boards reject applicants for medical degrees who graduate from medical schools that were inadequate, and (c) examinations for state licensure be rigorous. He hoped that "perhaps the entire country may some day be covered by a health organization engaged in protecting the

Box 3-3. Example of Methodological Research

1. Bibliographical Notation

Rodger, S., Chien, C. W., Turpin, M., Copley, J., Coleman, A., Brown, T., & Caine, A. M. (2016). Establishing the validity and reliability of the Student Practice Evaluation Form-Revised (SPEF-R) in occupational therapy practice education: A Rasch analysis. *Evaluation & the Health Professions, 39,* 33-48.

2. Abstract

"This study investigated construct validity and internal consistency of the Student Practice Evaluation Form-Revised Edition Package (SPEF-R) which evaluates students' performance on practice education placements. The SPEF-R has 38 items covering eight domains, and each item is rated on a 5-point rating scale. Data from 125 students' final placement evaluations in their final year study were analyzed using the Rasch measurement model. The SPEF-R exhibited satisfactory rating scale performance and unidimensionality across the eight domains, providing construct validity evidence. Only 2 items misfit Rasch model's expectations (both related to students' performance with client groups, which were often rated as not observed). Additionally, the internal consistency of each SPEF-R domain was found to be excellent (Cronbach's α = .86 to .91) and all individual items had reasonable to excellent item-total correlation coefficients. The study results indicate that the SPEF-R can be used with confidence to evaluate students' performance during placements, but continued validation and refinement are required."

3. Justification and Need

The SPEF-R is the primary tool for evaluating occupational therapy student performance during clinical/practical fieldwork placement in Australia. Although content and face validity have been established for the SPEF-R, its construct validity and reliability have yet to be established.

4. Literature Review

Twenty-five references from a wide variety of sources were cited. The cited journals included but were not limited to *Australian Occupational Therapy Journal, Applied Psychological Measurement, American Journal of Occupational Therapy, Hong Kong Journal of Occupational Therapy, Archives of Physical Medicine and Rehabilitation,* and *Journal of Outcome Measurement.* The years of the cited publications ranged from 1978 to 2011.

5. Research Hypothesis or Guiding Question

The perspective of the study was to determine the construct validity and reliability of the SPEF-R. No hypotheses or guiding questions were explicitly stated.

6. Methods

This study utilized a secondary analysis approach incorporating existing data from clinical educator ratings on student performance at the end of 10-week placement. Data from 125 students were included in the analyses. Construct validity was determined on the 38-item SPEF-R using the Rasch Measurement Model. More specifically, internal consistency was ascertained using rating scale analysis, test unidimensionality, and test targeting. Internal consistency was measured using the Cronbach's α coefficient.

7. Results

The analyses revealed that the SPEF-R was found to have satisfactory construct validity in that the rating scale performance and unidimentionality were acceptable. Additionally, the Cronbach's α coefficient was in the excellent range and therefore can be considered to have excellent reliability.

(continued)

Box 3-3. Example of Methodological Research (continued)

8. Conclusions

Rodger et al. concluded that:

- "… the 5-point rating scale worked appropriately to differentiate students' level of placement performance" (p. 43).

- "… the unidimensionality of the SPEF-R was investigated and found to demonstrate with distinct constructs (as per the eight domains)" (p. 43).

- "… the ceiling effects and poor targeting for more skilled students are not considered problematic for the SPEF-R" (p. 44).

- "… the SPEF-R was found to have excellent reliability" (p. 44).

9. Limitations

While Rasch analyses are versatile in analyzing instrumental validity and reliability, there are other methods that can be incorporated to provide an even more comprehensive and definitive determination of construct validity.

10. Major References Cited

Allison, H., & Turpin, M. (2004). Development of the student placement evaluation form: A tool for assessing student fieldwork performance. *Australian Occupational Therapy Journal, 51*, 125-132.

Duncan, P. W., Bode, R. K., Lai, S. M., & Perera, S. (2003). Rasch analysis of a new stroke-specific outcome scale: The Stroke Impact Scale. *Archives of Physical Medicine and Rehabilitation, 84*, 950-963.

Lim, S. M., Rodger, S., & Brown, T. (2009). Using the Rasch analysis to establish the construct validity of rehabilitation assessment tools. *International Journal of Therapy and Rehabilitation, 16*, 251-260.

Thompson, M. M., & Ryan, A. G. (1996). The influence of fieldwork on the professional socialisation of occupational therapy students. *British Journal of Occupational Therapy, 59*, 95-104.

World Federation of Occupational Therapists. (2002). *Revised minimum standards for the education of occupational therapists.* Forrestfield, Australia: Author.

public health against the formidable combination made by ignorance, incompetency, commercialism, and disease" (Flexner et al., 1910, p. 173). All of these recommendations were eventually implemented and led to the founding of the American Medical Association. Evaluation research as used by Flexner was directed toward the improvement of an institution, specifically the medical profession.

When properly used, evaluation research can be useful (Weiss, 1972) in deciding whether to:

- Continue or discontinue a program.
- Improve an agency's practices and procedures.
- Add or drop specific program strategies and techniques.
- Use a program as a model for new agencies.
- Utilize more fully the services of a program on a geographical basis.
- Accept or reject theoretical approaches underlining an agency's program.

These purposes are achieved only after the investigator has collected objective and valid data. The research steps include (a) the stated need for evaluation research; (b) a review of the literature, comprising a description of programs and criteria used; (c) an objective research design for

collecting data through interviews, questionnaires, attitude scales, and clinical observation; (d) statistical analysis of records and examination of the physical plant; (e) comparisons of program with objective criteria; (f) separate sections on results and discussion of findings; and (g) the evaluation team's recommendation for reaccreditation, probation, or closing of the program. Figure 3-13 identifies examples of potential areas for evaluation research in occupational therapy, rehabilitation, and habilitation.

3.4.2 Strategies of Evaluation Research

The issue of researcher bias is of prime consideration in evaluation research. The underlying purpose of evaluation research is to apply objective assessment to a facility, agency, or intervention program. How does a researcher objectively evaluate an organization? How are criteria established for measuring the effectiveness of a program? Are criteria established by the evaluation research team based on ideal theoretical considerations or by the intervention agency that is being evaluated? What expertise in research is needed in evaluating the competence and abilities of health professionals? What controls should be established in the research methods to reduce investigator bias?

Figure 3-13. Four examples of the application of heuristic research.

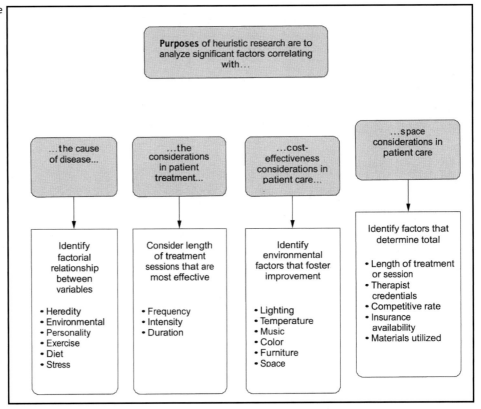

The following hypothetical example explores the process of evaluation research as applied to a residential school for adolescents with severe behavior disorders:

1. Stated purposes of evaluation are set forth, such as:
   a. Continued school certification or accreditation
   b. Evaluation of intervention effectiveness
   c. Direct and indirect costs per student intervention
   d. Widening of services to include more diverse client groups
   e. Change in delivery of services to reduce residential population and to include more day care or community-based intervention
   f. The overall decision to cease operation before evaluation research is undertaken must involve a mutual understanding of the purpose between the evaluators and those being evaluated. If the purposes are unclear or if there is a hidden agenda, then the research objectivity could become undermined and the evaluation could serve more as a political maneuver than as a means to collect objective data. For example, if the evaluators seek to close a program by collecting negative or damaging information and by omitting any positive attributes, then the evaluation's integrity is compromised.

2. The formation of a research team of evaluators is dependent on the stated purposes of the evaluation and the specific areas considered. Expertise and experience in program administration, budgeting, intervention techniques, special education, vocational rehabilitation, research methodology, interviewing techniques, and familiarity with educational requirements and job descriptions of professional and nonprofessional staff members are necessary to provide appropriate expertise and knowledge levels for the members of an evaluation research team. Evaluation research demands a sophisticated level of expertise that is essential in the research process. The responsibility of judging the effectiveness of the program is delegated to the research team. As the level of effectiveness is a relative judgment, it is important that each member of the evaluation team understand and accept the criteria being used as the measuring sticks. Experience of the members of the team in working in other intervention agencies and familiarity with the evaluation process, either as a supervisor in a clinic or in an educational environment, are necessary requisites for doing evaluation research. The size of the research team, responsibility based on the areas of expertise and experience represented, and the availability of consultants are considered in forming an effective evaluation research team.

3. The descriptive data will include:
   a. History of the organization, including why it was established and names and backgrounds of founders
   b. Flow chart of administration, including lines of responsibility, and departmental components
   c. Description of the physical plant, including a detailed layout of the facilities

TABLE 3-6

HYPOTHETICAL RESULTS OF A RESIDENTIAL TREATMENT PROGRAM

VARIABLE	NUMBER	PERCENT
Capacity of program	55	100
Average daily attendance of residents during last 6 months	50	90
Average length of residence for each individual discharged in last 6 months	3 months	N/A
Number of individuals in residence for over 1 year	15	30
Number of direct care workers (treatment personnel)	10	N/A
Number of full-time professional staff, excluding administrators	6	N/A
Number of part-time consultants	3	N/A
Number of full-time teachers	5	N/A

d. Staff resumes, including education and experience of administrators, intervention staff, and supporting personnel

e. Job descriptions of work responsibilities

f. Rehabilitation and intervention services offered, including but not limited to medical, psychological, educational, child care, and prevocational

g. Formal and informal meetings, conferences, and patient staffings

h. Intake policies, orientation, and discharge procedures

i. Follow-up care and evaluation of discharges

j. Relationships with community and outside agencies

k. Numerical data regarding maximum client capacity of facility, present number of clients, average length of residence, number of referrals, and discharges over time

4. Criteria of effectiveness are established by the research team. The criteria are based on a priori standards or objectives furnished by the administrator of the program. Areas for criteria include:

   a. *Intervention effect*: Percentage of clients who have made successful and unsuccessful adjustments after discharge. Definition of successful and unsuccessful outcome should be operationally defined.

   b. *Physical plant*: Safety, health, and accessibility for those individuals with mobility impairment meeting the Americans with Disability Act (1990) requirements; fire requirements

   c. *Professional staff*: Percentage of staff having professional educational backgrounds (resumes, number of years at facility, reasons for leaving previous position)

   d. *Staff ratio*: Number of clients per intervention staff

   e. *Staff salaries*: Average salaries as compared with national average or salaries in comparable agencies

   f. *Continuing education*: Opportunities for staff to attend conferences, workshops, or inservices

g. *Discharges*: Number over time and reasons for client discharge

5. Criteria can also be established by selecting characteristic patterns from programs considered to be successful models, although flexibility in employing these models is necessary when applying criteria. The severity of the disability in clients serviced and the financial resources available to an agency are factors that must be considered when analyzing outside criteria.

6. Interviews with staff and residents are necessary to transform the highly subjective process of discerning salient information from the complexities of social data. The limitations of the interview process should be recognized by the researcher. The very nature of communicating feelings and attitudes is limited by the natural suspiciousness of the interviewee and his or her reliance on memory to provide information. It is not the authors' intent to discuss interviewing techniques in detail, but it shall be sufficient to note that researchers utilizing interview information must be certain that the interviewers have had training. Leading questions, long and complicated questions, and rambling and unrelated items, which untrained interviewers often use, provide data that subsequently bias the results (see Jensen [2013] for further information).

7. The next process in evaluation research is the synthesis of objective descriptive data and objective interview material. The Results section of the report should be separated from the Discussion and Conclusions. Results are raw data that are objective findings. Results should not be flavored" by subjective analysis or undone by interpretations. The results should remain separate from critical analysis. Table 3-6 lists hypothetical data that would be included in a Results section.

8. The interpretative summary consists of a qualitative discussion of the results apart from the quantitative results. For example, qualitative or naturalistic information could include staff opportunities to innovate

new programs, the informality of the communication process, the accessibility of administrators, the feelings of hope and optimism generated by the staff, the willingness of the agency to change the consumer with disabilities' involvement in intervention planning, the use of community resources, the integration of new technology with present methods, and the facilitation of professional growth through supervision.

9. The conclusions and recommendations of evaluation research are a vital part of the report. How does the research team decide that an intervention program is effective and should have continued support by the community or that an intervention program is ineffective, not responsive to the needs of a community, and should be terminated?

Over the last 50 years, we have seen the decline and closing of large, isolated institutions that served individuals with physical and psychiatric disabilities who mainly came from poor backgrounds. These institutions were closed because they had become custodial warehouses without providing for the needs of the individuals. Nevertheless, when the institutions were supported by governmental agencies in the United States in the 1920s up until the 1960s, there were few alternatives for community-based intervention. Did evaluation research play a role in the closing of institutions during the 1960s and 1970s?

The criteria identified in evaluative research must be consistent with the needs of the target population. These needs relate to values in human society, such as economic independence, social relationships, educational development, self-esteem, and whatever else the research team or agency sets forth as the goals and objectives. It should be clear that if an agency is not meeting "stated needs" of those individuals who are treated, educated, or serviced and alternative agencies or facilities are available, then the community should not continue to support an institution's existence.

The following research models are ex post facto in nature: heuristic, correlational, clinical observation, survey, and historical. Clinical observation is unique in that it can be either ex post facto (retrospective) or prospective. The data collection procedure in ex post facto research is retrospective because the presumed independent variable has already occurred. Kerlinger (1986) differentiated experimental research and ex post facto research on the basis of the lack of direct control by the researcher in ex post facto designs. For example, in experimental research, the investigator hypothesizes "if X then Y" and manipulates the X. In ex post facto research, the investigator observes Y (the dependent variable) and hypothesizes X (the independent variable). The researcher in ex post facto designs can only presume a past cause-effect relationship. In many ex post facto designs, the investigator seeks historically to reconstruct cause-effect relationships.

Suchman (1967) identified several areas of potential abuse as follows:

- *Eyewash*: An attempt to justify an ineffective program by deliberately selecting only those aspects that appear successful and overlooking important parts of the program.
- *Whitewash*: An effort whereby the evaluators try to cover up program failure and inadequacies by avoiding these areas when evaluating the program. The evaluators may solicit testimonials to divert attention from the general failure of the program.
- *Submarine* or *torpedo*: A device to destroy a program regardless of its worth or usefulness in delivering health services. This often occurs in administrative power struggles when opponents and their programs are attacked.
- *Posture*: Used by evaluators when they want to appear scientific and objective when, in fact, they carry out a superficial and incomplete evaluation.
- *Postponement*: A tactic of using evaluation research, for example, to answer public reaction to scandalous conditions in an institution. The real purpose of this ploy is to defuse public outrage by substituting research for action.
- *Substitution*: An attempt to hide an essential part of a program that is an obvious failure and to shift emphasis to areas that are controversial.

From the foregoing examples, it is evident that evaluation research can serve not only to provide objective data, but also as a tactic to keep an inadequate program operative or to discredit an effective program.

An example of evaluation research in occupational therapy is found in Box 3-4. The authors of this research study evaluated the effectiveness of an occupational therapy program with older adults who were living in independent housing.

3.5 Heuristic Research

3.5.1 Purposes of Heuristic Research

Kerlinger (1986) described a heuristic view of science as that which "emphasizes theory and interconnected conceptual schemata that are fruitful for further research" (p. 8). The main purpose of heuristic research is to discover relationships between variables as a means of generating further investigations. In heuristic research, the researcher fishes for correlational relationships as a means to build a theory and design further research.

The researcher engaged in heuristic research seeks to discover significant relationships by correlating variables with a specific disease or factors affecting intervention. Research in cardiovascular diseases, learning disorders, mental illness, arthritis, multiple sclerosis, cancer, and AIDS are appropriate areas for heuristic research, as well as investigations of space, time, and cost factors in the intervention environment.

Box 3-4. Example of Evaluation Research

1. Bibliographical Notation

Clark, F., Azen, S. P., Zemke R., Jackson, J., Carlson, M., Mandel, D., … Lipson, L. (1997). Occupational therapy for independent-living older adults. A randomized controlled trial. *Journal of American Medical Association, 278,* 1321-1326.

2. Abstract

"*Context*: Preventive health programs may mitigate against the health risks of older adulthood. *Objective*: To evaluate the effectiveness of preventive occupational therapy (OT) services specifically tailored for multiethnic, independent-living older adults. *Design*: A randomized controlled trial. *Setting*: Two government subsidized apartment complexes for independent-living older adults. *Subjects*: A total of 361 culturally diverse volunteers aged 60 years or older. *Intervention*: An OT group, a social activity control group, and a non-treatment control group. The period of treatment was 9 months. *Main Outcome Measures*: A battery of self-administered questionnaires designed to measure physical and social function, self-rated health, life satisfaction, and depressive symptoms. *Results*: Benefit attributable to OT treatment was found for the quality of interaction scale on the Functional Status Questionnaire ($P=.03$), Life Satisfaction Index-Z ($P=.03$), Medical Outcomes Study Health Perception Survey ($P=.05$), and for 7 of 8 scales on the RAND 36-Item Health Status Survey, Short Form: bodily pain ($P=.03$), physical functioning ($P=.008$), role limitations attributable to health problems ($P=.02$), vitality ($P=.004$), social functioning ($P=.05$), role limitations attributable to emotional problems ($P=.05$), and general mental health ($P=.02$). *Conclusions*: Significant benefits for the OT preventive treatment group were found across various health, function, and quality-of-life domains. Because the control groups tended to decline over the study interval, our results suggest that preventive health programs based on OT may mitigate against the health risks of older adulthood."

3. Justification and Need

Findings from the literature suggest that effective activity-based intervention can enhance the lives of elderly individuals. "In response to this need, we conducted between 1994 and 1996 a randomized controlled trial, the Well Elderly Study, to evaluate the effectiveness of preventative OT specifically targeted for urban, multiethnic, independent-living older adults" (p. 1321).

4. Literature Review

The authors examined the literature on normative aging, activity-theory and aging, quality-of-life issues in aging, and the role of occupational therapy with the elderly. Forty-three references were used, selected from the following journals: *Social Indicators Research, Social Science in Medicine, American Journal of Occupational Therapy, International Journal of Aging and Human Development, Journal of Gerontology and Psychological Science, Journal of Gerontology, Journal of Clinical Psychology, Journal of the American Medical Association,* and *Research in Nursing Health*.

5. Research Hypothesis or Guiding Question

"We hypothesized that mere participation in a social activity program does not affect the physical health, daily functioning, or psychosocial well-being of well elderly individuals; and compared with participation in a social activity program or an absence of any treatment, preventative OT positively affects the physical health, daily function, and psychosocial well-being of well elderly individuals (1-sided alternative)" (p. 1322).

6. Methods

Three-hundred sixty-one elderly adults, aged 60 and older, were randomly assigned to one of three groups: an occupational therapy group, a social activity group, and a no treatment group. Participants came from government subsidized housing for independent living, private homes, and other facilities in the community. In the occupational therapy group, participants were exposed to didactic teaching of community living and use of adapted equipment, and performed activities emphasizing grooming, nutrition, exercising, and shopping. Those in the social activities group were involved in "community outings, craft projects, films, played games, and attended dances" (p. 1322). Five questionnaires were used to measure outcome.

(continued)

Box 3-4. Example of Evaluation Research (continued)

7. Operational Definition of Variables

Functional status, life satisfaction, depression, perceptions of health, and physical and mental health status were evaluated through self-report.

8. Conclusions

The occupational therapy program in general was more effective than the other two groups. "The OT program enabled subjects to construct daily routines that were health promoting and meaningful given the context of their lives" (p. 1325).

9. Limitations

"The results may not generalize to older adults in different living situations (e.g., single-family dwellers, nursing home residents) or of different socioeconomic status" (p. 1326).

10. Major References Cited

Fisher, B. J. (1995). Successful aging, life satisfaction and generativity in later life. *International Journal of Aging and Human Development, 41,*230-250.

Carlson, M., Fanchiang, S.-R., Zemke, R., & Clark, F. (1996). A meta-analysis of the effectiveness of occupational therapy for older persons. *American Journal of Occupational Therapy, 50,* 89-98.

Larson, K. O., Stevens-Ratchford, R. G., Pedretti, L. W., & Crabtree, J. L. (1996). *ROTE: The role of occupational therapy with the elderly.* Bethesda, MD: American Occupational Therapy Association.

Levine, R. E., & Gitlan, L. N. (1992). A model to promote activity competence in elders. *American Journal of Occupational Therapy, 47,*147-153.

3.5.2 Application of Pilot Studies in Heuristic Research

Pilot studies are innovative studies that examine a problem or question to determine if the research is viable. These studies often have a small number of participants and the investigator does not control all of the extraneous variables. Limitations of the research methodology are identified. While pilot studies are carried out in other research designs, pilot studies in heuristic research require both an exploration of a theoretical basis and recommendations for further research.

The following is a relatively recent list of pilot study examples from occupational therapy that are heuristic:

- Arthanat, S., Curtin, C., & Kontak, D. (2015). An evaluation protocol for selection of educational technologies for students with developmental disabilities: A demonstration study using iPad apps. *Journal of Occupational Therapy, Schools, & Early Intervention, 8*(3), 236-255.
- Bone, C., Cheung, G., & Wade, B. (2010). Evaluating person-centred care and dementia care mapping in a psychogeriatric hospital in New Zealand: A pilot study. *New Zealand Journal of Occupational Therapy, 57,* 35-40.
- Chang, Y. J., Chen, S. F., & Huang, J. D. (2011). A Kinect-based system for physical rehabilitation: A pilot study for young adults with motor disabilities. *Research in Developmental Disabilities, 32*(6), 2566-2570.
- Crowe, T., Sanchez, V., Weber, A., & Murtagh, A. (2016). The influence of a Mexican cultural immersion experience on personal and professional healthcare practices. *Occupational Therapy International, 23*(4), 318-327.
- Doyle, S., Bennett, S., & Gustafsson, L. (2013). Clinical decision making when addressing upper limb post-stroke sensory impairments. *British Journal of Occupational Therapy, 76,* 254-263.

3.5.3 Assumptions Underlying Heuristic Research

In engaging in heuristic research, the investigator:
- Seeks to discover statistically significant relationships between variables
- Seeks data for theory building; the result of research provides the basis for theoretical formulations
- Uses deductive methods to analyze a research problem.
- Analyzes a research problem retrospectively; that is, the researcher starts with the presumed effect (dependent variable) and works back to the presumed causative factors (independent variables)

- Understands that results derived from heuristic research are not conclusive, implying that further investigation using prospective research is needed to substantiate cause-effect relationships

3.5.4 Method of Heuristic Research

Factor analysis enables an investigator to correlate many variables and to systematically analyze interactional patterns. This method is especially appropriate in analyzing biopsychosocial illnesses where there are a combination of presumed causative factors rather than a single etiological factor. Weaver (1947) characterized research in the 17th, 18th, and 19th centuries as typifying the era of the two-variable problems in simplicity. In medicine during the early part of the 20th century, a single etiological factor was correlated with the effects of disease (two-variable research). Today, however, both modern medical research and social sciences research are engaged in investigating complex health problems that involve multiple causes. For example, drug addiction, intellectual disability, arteriosclerosis, Alzheimer's disease, and dyslexia have multiple causes. An application of a two-variable model, where the investigator searches for the single cause of the disease, is inadequate in biopsychosocial research. On the other hand, heuristic research lends itself to the study of multiple factors that are interactive in nature. The Framingham Study of heart disease (Dawber, Meadors, & Moore, 1951) is an example of heuristic research. The strategy involved in these studies was to identify numerous risk factors that are significantly more frequent in patients with heart disease than in the normal population. The purposes of heuristic research are diagramed in Figure 3-13.

3.5.5 Identification of Correlating Factors

In heuristic research, the investigator seeks to derive the major factors that correlate significantly to assess their relative importance. Descriptive and inferential statistics, as well as multiple regression, factor analysis, and path analysis, are appropriate for analyzing the relative significance of factors that may be important in generating further research.

A major problem in this research model is in the selection of a diagnostic group. It is critical that screening criteria be used in selecting a research sample. The researcher cannot assume that a patient's diagnosis is accurate. There is much controversy in the diagnosis of chronic illnesses, such as asthma, schizophrenia, arthritis, fetal alcohol syndrome, and failure to thrive, that requires the investigator to use rigorous methods for operationalizing diagnostic categories. After the investigator has developed and refined the screening criteria for subject selection, the next problem is to select a population of subjects that will be the source for a representative sample.

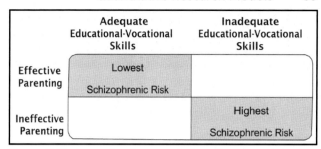

Figure 3-14. Interaction between independent and dependent variables in the risk of developing schizophrenia. An explanation of the development of schizophrenia must take into account all major variables, not just a single variable.

Parallel to the process of subject selection is the compiling of investigative variables. These variables are derived by analyzing the following areas:

- *Demographic*: Age, gender, occupation, educational level, marital status, income
- *Psychosocial*: Personality, intelligence, attitude, lifestyle
- *Biochemical*: Physiological, somatotype, nutritional, genetic

3.5.6 Interactional Effects in Heuristic Research

Heuristic research requires the investigator to make an exhaustive search for variables that can potentially contribute to the onset of a disease. It is necessary for the investigator to take a holistic view of the problem of etiology to avoid the trap of two-variable research that lacks an analysis of interactional effects. For example, let us suppose hypothetically that schizophrenia is a result of the interactional effects of genetics, child development, and lack of skills in educational, vocational, or social arenas. In studying the exclusive relationship between genetics and schizophrenia, a researcher will have mixed results because other major factors have not been considered. Results cannot be generalized to all patients with schizophrenia. Figure 3-14 illustrates hypothetically the interaction between the three independent variables (i.e., genetics, child development, and competence) and the dependent variable (diagnosis of schizophrenia).

The diagram shows that those individuals who have effective parenting and educational and vocational competence are the least likely to develop schizophrenia, even if they have a genetic vulnerability factor. Schizophrenia results only through the interaction of three variables: genetic, parental, and educational-vocational competence.

This hypothetical example shows the complexity of factorial designs that test the interactional effects of multiple causes. It is highly probable that many chronic illnesses result from this type of interactional pattern. Nonetheless, only through rigorous, painstaking research will it be possible to identify interactional effects. Heuristic research

TABLE 3-7	
ANALYSIS OF TIME FACTORS IN INTERVENTION	
IDEAL	PRAGMATIC
• Time needed for application of intervention method; dependent on the client's treatment goals • Time needed to meet short-term objectives or goals • Time needed for preparation and progress notes	• Number of patients under care in proportion to the number of hours allocated for intervention (client load) • Traditional practices (therapy schedules) • Third-party reimbursement for service (insurance)

provides the framework to investigate multiple factors in the development of a disease process.

3.5.7 Analysis of Time Factors in Client Intervention

What are the determining factors in planning intervention time for patients? Why is 1 hour/week sufficient for some clients while 2 hours/week are prescribed for others? What proportion of intervention time is a function of pragmatic issues, such as the availability of a therapist? What consideration for time is given to the physical and emotional needs of the client? How is intervention time planned for client groups? All of these questions are suitable for research analysis. In general, only a few studies have analyzed time factors in patient care (Atwal et al., 2014; Baillargeon-Normand, Rochette, Gaulin, 2016). Yet time is one of the most basic factors in clinical intervention. An analysis of the factors considered in determining the length of time for interventions should consider both the ideal factors and pragmatic issues (Table 3-7).

3.5.8 Analysis of Cost-Effectiveness Factors in Client Intervention

What are the real economic costs for intervention? What does it cost to treat a patient in a hospital compared with the intervention in an outpatient clinic? What are the costs for direct patient care by professionals as compared with non-professional health technicians trained for specific health purposes? What is the cost of a massive public health prevention program compared with existing costs for treating a specific disability group? What factors are considered in determining fees for health services? How are salaries for health workers determined? What is the economic worth of a health professional? These questions are typical of the pressing economic problems facing industrialized and developing countries where the demand for health care far outreaches the resources that countries can allocate for prevention and intervention. If a society is to determine rationally how its economic resources can be used most

effectively for implementation, then it must examine objectively the underlying factors affecting the costs of health care (Ke et al., 2013).

3.5.9 Analysis of Space Factors in Patient Care

As with time and cost, space has received little attention from clinical researchers. Ethnologists and social anthropologists analyzed the effect of space in animal behavior and health (Baratchi, Meratnia, Havinga, Skidmore, & Toxopeus, 2013; Johnson, 2015). There are a few studies that suggest a direct relationship between life space and psychological reactions (Mey & Gunther, 2015; Polku et al., 2015).

In psychiatry, it has been evident that space affects a client's emotions and behavioral patterns. Goffman (1961) described the syndrome of passivity and depersonalization as being the result of institutionalization. A contemporary definition of space is not limited to the traditional 19th century view that space represents area. Since Einstein's theory of relativity, space has taken on new meaning, implying in conceptual terms that space is the distance between two events. Space involves events, occurrences, or movement. An individual's space represents the potential area for movement. In this concept of space, factors related to increasing or diminishing space are appropriate. Hospitalization, imprisonment, and institutionalization are situations in which the patient, prisoner, or inmate are deprived of space and consequently has fewer opportunities for movements and events. In treating a patient, what considerations are given to space? Are wards or private rooms considered on any other basis than economic? Do groups occupying space limit the number of events or increase the movement of patients? Questions involving space are invariably linked to issues of group vs. individual intervention. What is the relationship between the number of clients in a group, the area of movement, and the events taking place in a group? What is the meaning of differently sized and configured spaces to the client—favorable or unfavorable for comfort, participation, and health? Issues related to the size of client groups in occupational therapy clinics involve space factors.

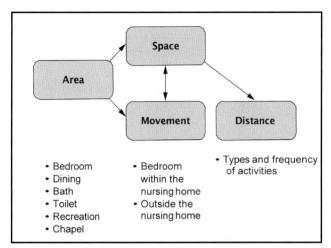

Figure 3-15. Analysis of space factors in a nursing home.

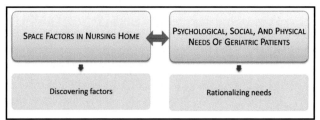

Figure 3-16. Integration of data with need theory. In this example, the data obtained from analyzing space factors in the nursing home with the needs of elderly patients (obtained through a literature review) is integrated.

A researcher employing a heuristic research model seeks to discover underlying factors affecting space. For example, how would a researcher analyze the problem of determining the space needs of elderly clients in a nursing home? Figure 3-15 illustrates this example.

The first step is to define operationally the space of elderly clients. The next step is to discover the physical, psychological, and social needs of elderly clients. A review of the literature and a survey of existing programs would provide the data. Maslow's (1954) theory of a hierarchy of needs and Havighurst's (1952) activity theory could be applied to an analysis of psychological and emotional needs. Theories of aging and health could provide the framework for setting physical and health goals. The third step in the research process is to integrate the data derived from analyzing space factors in a nursing home with biopsychosocial needs. This is illustrated in Figure 3-16.

The goals of heuristic research in this example are to:
- Discover the factors comprising space in a nursing home
- Analyze the effects of these factors in psychological adjustment, social relationships, and physical health maintenance
- Identify in the literature the needs of the elderly.
- Integrate space factors with need theory
- The reader may be puzzled with the example in Figure 3-16. How, the reader may ask, does the heuristic researcher know that he or she has identified all the factors related to space and all the needs of elderly clients? The answer is that researchers cannot conclude that the data collection is complete. Heuristic research is a method of discovery, and research in general is an ongoing process that functions as a feedback loop. As

more information is gathered, analyzed, and integrated with previous data, the researcher comes closer to solving questions. Box 3-5 gives an example of heuristic research.

3.6 CORRELATIONAL RESEARCH

3.6.1 Purposes of Correlational Research

Many studies published in occupational therapy are primarily correlational and retrospective. This research is analogous to experimental research in that the investigator tests a hypothesis. Unlike the experimental researcher, however, the investigator does not manipulate independent variables, nor does he or she investigate a cause-effect relationship. In correlational research, the investigator compares the relationships between variables by measuring the extent to which the variables co-vary. It is applied frequently to questions in the social sciences because the very nature of the problem limits the experimenter from inducing causal effects. If, for example, a researcher's purpose is to correlate characteristics in an individual suffering from alcoholism with causative factors, then he or she is limited to an ex post facto design where it is not possible to induce experimentally the onset of alcoholism. The researcher in this example is limited to a retrospective analysis of the assumed causes of alcoholism. Kerlinger (1986), in discussing the value of nonexperimental research, concluded that "social, scientific, and educational problems do not lend themselves to experimentation, although many of them do lend themselves to controlled inquiry of the nonexperimental kind" (p. 359)

A sequential analysis of correlational research is diagramed in Figure 3-17. These steps are reviewed in the following section.

Box 3-5. Example of Heuristic Research

1. Bibliographical Notation

Rabadi, M., Galgano, M., Lynch, D., Akerman, M., Lesser, M., & Volpe, B. (2008). A pilot study of activity-based therapy in the arm motor recovery post stroke: A randomized controlled trial. *Clinical Rehabilitation, 22*, 1071-1082.

2. Abstract

"To determine the efficacy of activity-based therapies using arm ergometer or robotic or group occupational therapy for motor recovery of the paretic arm in patients with an acute stroke (< or = 4 weeks) admitted to an inpatient rehabilitation facility, and to obtain information to plan a large randomized controlled trial. Prospective, randomized controlled study. The setting was a stroke unit in a rehabilitation hospital. Thirty patients with an acute stroke (< or = 4 weeks) who had arm weakness (Medical Research Council grade 2 or less at the shoulder joint). Occupational therapy (OT) group (control) (n = 10), arm ergometer (n = 10) or robotic (n = 10) therapy group. All patients received standard, inpatient, post-stroke rehabilitation training for 3 hours a day, plus 12 additional 40-minute sessions of the activity-based therapy. The primary outcome measures were discharge scores in the Fugl-Meyer Assessment Scale for upper limb impairment, Motor Status Scale, total Functional Independence Measure (FIM) and FIM-motor and FIM-cognition subscores. The three groups (OT group versus arm ergometer versus robotic) were comparable on clinical demographic measures except the robotic group was significantly older and there were more haemorrhagic stroke patients in the arm ergometer group. After adjusting for age, stroke type and outcome measures at baseline, a similar degree of improvement in the discharge scores was found in all of the primary outcome measures. This study suggests that activity-based therapies using an arm ergometer or robot when used over shortened training periods have the same effect as OT group therapy in decreasing impairment and improving disability in the paretic arm of severely affected stroke patients in the subacute phase."

3. Justification and Need

This study lists multiple novel rehabilitation techniques, such as constraint-induced therapy, robotic training, and other intensive activity tasks, like bilateral arm training with rhythmic cueing to increase functional motor recovery. Recently there has been a reduction in the amount of time of hospitalization in the inpatient rehabilitation as a cost-containment measure, which has motivated the evaluation of techniques that complement conventional therapies to enhance potential post-stroke motor recovery. This researchers in this study decided to investigate whether an activity-based programme (of bilateral arm training using the ergometer or unilateral arm training with a robot) would be more effective than occupational group therapy for the same amount of intensity and duration of treatment in decreasing arm motor impairment and improving disability in moderately sever stroke patients during their acute rehabilitation hospital stay. This study also hopes to use the findings to design a larger randomized controlled trial study.

4. Literature Review

This study had 51 references from a wide variety of sources. Cited journals included, but were not limited to, *Archives of Physical Medical Rehabilitation, Neurology, Stroke, Neurorehabilitation and Neural Repair, Behavior Brain Science, Scandinavian Journal of Rehabilitation Medicine, Physical Therapy*, and *American Journal of Physical Medicine Rehabilitation*. The years of cited publications ranged from 1951 to 2008.

5. Research Hypothesis or Guiding Question

No hypotheses or questions were stated in the article.

6. Methods

Thirty-three participants were recruited with an acute stroke (less than or at 4 weeks) who had arm weakness (Medical Research Council grade two or less at the shoulder joint). Each patient received standard occupational and physical therapy by their assigned therapist for 3 hours/day. Each participant also received 12 additional sessions of 40 minutes/day, 5 days/week, consisting of arm ergometer, robot, or occupational therapy alone based on randomization.

(continued)

Box 3-5. Example of Heuristic Research (continued)

The Monark arm ergometer is a bidirectional hand cycle that is used for upper body aerobic exercise. It uses all muscle groups of the upper limb. The intensity to which the paretic arm was subjected was a count of the number of movements completed at 1 minute and over the 40 minute session. Each participant exercised for 20 minutes of continuous cycling at zero resistance, had a 5 minute break, and then again cycled for 20 minutes. The unaffected arm helped move the paretic arm

The robot-aided therapy consisted of goal-directed, robot-assisted arm movement, and a customized interactive computer-generated video program provides visual feedback to the participant about the accuracy and speed of reaching a given target. The participants paralyzed arm initially receives passive movement, but as the voluntary movement returns the robot assists the participant to initiate, guide, and complete the motor activity required for point-to-point movements. Each participant completed two 20 minute programs with a 5 minute break between each session. The intensity of this treatment is displayed electronically by the robot.

The control occupational therapy group received 40 minutes of group therapy led by a certified occupational therapist assigned to that specific stroke unit who is competent in the group therapy protocol. Therapy focused on self-range of motion exercises focusing on patient-directed movements at the affected shoulder, elbow and hand when able. Each participant was encouraged to use his or her unaffected arm in actively assisting the paretic arm movement. The participants in this group had moved his or her arm an average of 16 to 18 times/minute either by the participant themselves supporting or assisting the paretic arm, or helped by the therapist. The primary outcomes measured arm motor weakness by a variety of tests that are commonly implemented in rehabilitation settings and whose change scores have been correlated with functional motor improvement. The assessments used include the discharge scores in the Fugl-Meyer Assessment Scale for upper limb motor impairments, the FIM, the FIM-motor, and the FIM-cognition subscores for disability. The secondary outcome measures were discharge scores on the following assessments: Motor Power Scale for muscle strength, Action Research Arm Test for arm-hand function, Modified Ashworth Scale for muscle tone, and the Fugl-Meyer Assessment Scale for arm pain and ROM.

7. Results

All three of the groups had demonstrated improvements in both motor impairment and functional scores. Among the three groups, there were no differences in the discharge Fugl-Meyer Assessment Scale upper extremity impairment score, the Motor Status Scale, FIM-total, FIM-motor subscore, and FIM-cognition subscore. The ergometer group had performed better than the occupational therapy group on the Fugl-Meyer Assessment Scale wrist-hand score, and the robot group had performed better on the Motor Status Scale shoulder-elbow score than the occupational therapy group. The robot group had performed better on the Motor Power Scale, Modified Ashworth Scale, and the pain score than the occupational therapy group. The ergometer group had performed better on the Modified Ashworth Scale and the pain score than the occupational therapy group did. The degree in these impairment and functional scores overall favored the occupational therapy group compared to the robot group or the arm ergometer group.

8. Conclusions

Rabadi et al. (2008) concluded that the activity-based therapies, which include the arm ergometer and robot, were no more effective in improving disability and decreasing impairment than occupational therapy during the subacute phase of stroke.

9. Limitations

The first limitation is that this study was a single-center study. Secondly, there was a small sample size. Thirdly, the treatment plan is debatable whether the 12 sessions of 40 minutes/day 5 days/week is sufficient to induce cerebral reorganization to supplement a change. Finally, these techniques do require supervision.

(continued)

Box 3-5. Example of Heuristic Research (continued)

10. Major References Cited

Broeks, J. G., Lankhorst, G. J., Rumping, K., & Prevo, A. J. (1999). The long-term outcome of arm function after stroke: Results of a follow-up study. *Disability Rehabilitation, 21*, 357-364.

Kunkel, A., Kopp, B., Muller, G. Villringer, K., Villringer, A., Taub, E., & Flor, H. (1999). Constraint-induced movement therapy for motor recovery in chronic stroke patients. Archive*s of Physical and Medicine and Rehabilitation, 80*, 624-628.

Nakayama, H., Jorgensen, H. S., Raaschou, H. O., & Olsen, T. S. (1994). Recovery of upper extremity function in stroke patients: The Copenhagen Stroke Study. *Archives of Physical and Medicine and Rehabilitation, 75*, 394-398.

Taub, E., Miller, N. E., Novack, T. A. Cook, E. W., Fleming, W. C., Nepomuceno, C. S., … Crago, J.E. (1993). Technique to improve chronic motor deficit after stroke. *Archives of Physical and Medicine and Rehabilitation, 74*, 347-354.

Taub, E., Unswatte, G., & Pidikiti, R. (1999). Constraint induced movement therapy: A new family of techniques with broad application to physical rehabilitation—A clinical review. *Journal of Rehabilitation Research and Development, 36*, 237-251.

Figure 3-17. The sequential analysis of correlational research.

3.6.2 Identification of Research Variables

As clinicians in the health fields, we are all concerned with the question of etiology. Why did this patient become schizophrenic? Why did this individual develop learning problems? What factors led to arthritis? What environmental factors contributed to juvenile delinquency? These questions regarding etiology and relationships between variables are amenable to investigation through correlational research, even though the causative aspect of the question cannot be answered definitely.

The first step in correlational research is to identify the variables in a target population to be studied. These variables are presumed causative factors and may be genetic, neurophysiological, psychosocial, or cultural. The variables are identified from clinical observations, by examining previous studies or theoretical papers, or through deductive reasoning. The presumed independent and dependent variables are identified. Because the researcher does not actively induce the levels of the independent variables, only an associational or statistical relationship can be assumed.

3.6.3 Formulating Hypotheses in Correlational Research

The researcher formulates a hypothesis after reviewing the related literature. The hypothesis can be a *directional hypothesis*, that is, predicting a significant positive or negative relationship between two variables. For example, the researcher predicts that there is an increase of abnormal reflexes in children with cerebral palsy compared with typical children. A hypothesis stated in a null form predicts

TABLE 3-8	
ASSOCIATIONAL RELATIONSHIPS BETWEEN VARIABLES	
VARIABLES	**POPULATIONS COMPARED**
Kinesthetic ability	• Blind • Normal vision
Self-concept	• Children with intellectual disabilities in inclusive settings • Children with intellectual disabilities in self-contained settings
Carpal tunnel syndrome	• Computer operators using the computer 6 or more hours a day • Clerical workers using the computer less than 4 hours a day
Visual-motor perception	• Children from dysfunctional families • Children with mental health disorders
Auditory processing	• Individuals with autism • Individuals with learning disabilities
Cancer	• Asbestos workers • Typical individuals

no significant relationship. For example, the *null hypothesis* can be stated as, "There is no difference between the presence of abnormal reflexes in children with cerebral palsy compared with typical children." The decision whether to formulate a directional hypothesis or a null hypothesis is based on direct or implied evidence from previous research.

Other examples of directional hypotheses in correlational research are as follows:

- Individuals who are blind have a significantly greater kinesthetic ability than individuals with normal vision.
- Individuals with intellectual disabilities educated in an inclusive setting will show higher self-concept than those educated in a self-contained program.
- Carpal tunnel syndrome occurs more frequently among individuals using a computer for 6 or more hours daily when compared with individuals using a computer for less than 4 hours daily.
- Children from dysfunctional, low-income families have better visual perceptual abilities than auditory processing abilities.
- There is a higher percentage of cancer among asbestos workers than in the population at large.

In all of the foregoing examples of directional hypotheses, the variables are associated with a target population. Analyzing the hypotheses one by one, we find the relationships shown in Table 3-8.

In the foregoing hypotheses, variables and populations are compared. Hypotheses can test the effects of multiple variables in one population or, conversely, the differences among multiple populations on one variable. A researcher cannot test multiple variables in multiple populations in one hypothesis. For example, it is fallacious to offer a hypothesis such as the following: High cholesterol level and hypertension are more prevalent among cardiac patients than among a normal population. Each variable (i.e., high cholesterol level, hypertension) should be stated in a separate hypothesis.

The null hypothesis posits that there will be no relationship between two variables; for example, there is no relationship between smoking and heart disease. The decision whether to state a hypothesis in a directional form or as a null hypothesis should be an outcome of the literature review. If previous studies indicate directionality, then the researcher should state a directional hypothesis. Moreover, a one-tailed test should only be used if the relationship in the other direction is of no research or clinical interest. On the other hand, if the researcher finds no evidence for a directional hypothesis in a review of the literature or if the research or clinical interest exists in either direction, then a bi-directional hypothesis should be stated. The form in which the hypothesis is stated has implications when analyzing the data statistically. For those readers without statistical background, it will suffice to say that when a researcher is comparing statistically significant differences between two variables with a *t*-test, a null hypothesis usually indicates a two-tail test of significance, and a directional hypothesis usually indicates a one-tail test of significance.

3.6.4 Operational Definitions of Variables

Before a hypothesis can be tested, the investigator must operationally define the variables stated in the hypothesis. The operational definition includes the specific test or procedure used in measuring a variable. If an investigator is measuring mild cognitive deficits, then the procedure given by Geslani, Tierney, Herrmann, and Szalai (2005) might be indicated as the operational measure.

3.6.5 Selection of Sample

Screening criteria are necessary when selecting a sample. It is not enough simply to state that patients with diabetes or epilepsy will be compared with a typical population. The investigator must indicate how the patients have been diagnosed, the severity of the illness considered, and other demographics identifying the population such as age, gender, occupation, socioeconomic status, education, and geographical area. The screening criteria devised by the investigator serve as a reference point in generalizing the results to a population. Universality and external validity depend on the screening criteria devised for subject selection.

3.6.6 Data Collection Procedure

Can the test procedure be replicated? Has the investigator tried to reduce factors such as subject fatigue, anxiety, extraneous distractions, lack of cooperation, and any other factors that threaten the internal validity of the investigation? The test procedure should be described in detail by the investigator, including the time of day when the subjects are tested, the number in the group, the environmental conditions, the length of time for testing each subject, and the sequence in presenting the operational measures.

3.6.7 Interpretation of Results

In general, research has a cumulative effect. Usually, the results of one study are not enough to be conclusive. Many factors affect the results in correlational research that are not directly controlled by the investigator. These limitations affecting internal validity do not negate correlational research. The advantages of correlational research are that investigations can be easily replicated and that large data sets can easily be mined. Before an investigator proposes a conclusion based on the results of one study, he or she should cross-validate the correlational results with another sample. Furthermore, he or she must integrate the results with previous research. If the results are contradictory, then further research is indicated. If the results are cross-validated and are consistent with previous literature, then it may be justified to suggest that adequate evidence has been found. There is a need in research to be conservative rather than premature. An example of correlational research is found in Box 3-6.

3.7 SURVEY RESEARCH

3.7.1 Definition of Survey Research

Survey research, as defined in this text, is the descriptive study of populations. The main purpose of survey research is to obtain accurate objective descriptions about a specific universe of people or entities, such as a group of individuals with disabilities or the curriculum requirements in occupational therapy. The major task of the survey researcher is to obtain reliable and valid data from a representative sample of a population. In some cases, the researcher will be able to survey the total population or universe without relying on a representative sample.

3.7.2 Purposes of Survey Research

Health, social, and educational planners use descriptive survey research as the basis for needs assessment for developing health strategies, programs, and physical plants. The changing needs of populations as derived from surveys can contribute to the planning of health centers, inclusion practices for individuals with disabilities, allied health training programs, community mental health centers, and adult day care centers. Survey research should play an essential part in assessing the needs of a population where the planning of services is involved.

Along with community planning, survey research is an important tool for learning about the general attitudes of people. Many studies are sponsored by governmental agencies and legislators to solicit general opinion on topics such as national health insurance, malpractice in health, legalization of abortion, ethics in research, inclusion of individuals with disabilities in educational and community settings, and other controversial issues where majority opinion is often considered in the formulation of national policy and to guide the enactment of laws.

Survey research need not be limited to questioning individuals. Methodologies in survey research assessing the physical characteristics of groups are also applicable. Recently, governmental grants in health research have funded studies that screen a population for the presence of a disability. School populations are screened for deficits in hearing and vision acuity. Diabetes tests, chest X-rays to detect lung cancer, cardiovascular screening utilizing blood cholesterol counts, blood pressure measurements, and testing for HIV are some of the examples of survey research utilizing physical measurements to screen for health defects in large populations. Public health agencies use survey research as a means of identifying trends in the incidence

Box 3-6. Example of Correlational Research

1. Bibliographical Notation

Chae, G. S., & Chang, M. (2016). The correlation between occupational performance and well-being in stroke patients. *Journal of Physical Therapy Science, 28*, 1712-1715.

2. Abstract

"[Purpose] This study was performed to evaluate the occupational performance of stroke patients and their environment by occupational self-assessment and to investigate the relationship between occupational performance and well-being. [Subjects and Methods] This study enrolled ninety-two stroke patients who were receiving occupational therapy at a general hospital, a rehabilitation hospital, or a community welfare center in the cities of Busan and Gimhae, Republic of Korea. Occupational performance and well-being were investigated with Occupational Self-Assessment Version 2.2 and the Personal Well-being Index-Adult. [Results] Analysis of the correlation between occupational performance as assessed by the 'Myself' and 'My Environment' sections of Occupational Self-Assessment Version 2.2 and well-being revealed moderate positive correlation for both sections. [Conclusion] The relationship between occupational performance and well-being was identified. Further studies are needed to reveal whether improvement of occupational performance could affect well-being in various dimensions."

3. Justification and Need

The authors note that a focus of occupational therapy is occupational performance, particularly when treating individuals with stroke. Occupational therapy often involves occupational performance associated with the fulfillment of life roles, employment, and leisure activities. Many of these can be categorized as being either ADLs or IADLs. The authors also explore the concept of well-being and describe it as a "state of recognizing harmony in all aspects of life: satisfaction, pleasure, spiritual experience, and happiness" (p. 1712). The purpose of the study is to explore the relationship between occupational performance and well-being.

4. Literature Review

This study had 19 references from a variety of sources. Cited journals included but were not limited to *American Journal of Occupational Therapy, BioMedCentral Neurology, Journal of Affective Disorders, British Journal of Occupational Therapy, Canadian Journal of Occupational Therapy, Scandinavian Journal of Occupational Therapy,* and *Stroke.* The years of cited publications ranged from 1988 through 2015.

5. Research Hypothesis or Guiding Question

No specific hypothesis was offered; however, the purpose of the study was to "evaluate the occupational performance of stroke patients and their environment by occupational self-assessment and to investigate the relationship between occupational performance and well-being" (p. 1712).

6. Methods

Ninety-two stroke survivors aged 40 to 63 years participated in this research, with 61 male and 31 female. Inclusion criteria involved participants scoring at least 24 on the Mini-Mental State Examination-Korean version. The Occupational Self-Assessment and the Personal Well-Being Index-Adult were used as the data collection tools. The Occupational Self-Assessment has two portions, the first being "Myself" (21 questions) and the second being "My Environment" (8 questions). The Personal Well-Being Index contained 8 quality of life items. One hundred and one surveys were delivered with 92 being returned.

7. Results

There was a statistically significant correlation of .432 between Occupational Performance (Myself) and Well-Being. Similarly, there was a statistically significant correlation of .427 between Occupational Performance (My Environment) and Well-Being.

(continued)

BOX 3-6. EXAMPLE OF CORRELATIONAL RESEARCH (CONTINUED)

8. Conclusions

Chae and Chang concluded that:

- There was a "significant positive relationship between occupational performance and well-being was indicated based on analysis of the questionnaires" (p. 1714).

- "The occupational performance of 'getting along with others' was relatively well performed, but that of 'taking care of others for whom I am responsible' was not" (p. 1714).

- "Among the 'My Environment' items for occupational performances, 'people who do things with me' and 'people who support and encourage me' were scored highest, which suggested that the stroke patients needed help from family and other people and were relatively well supported" (p. 1714).

9. Limitations

The sample of convenience was limited to two cities. Because of the nature of correlations, it is not known if there is a causative effect between occupational performance and well-being, only that there is a positive relationship.

10. Major References Cited

Baron, K., Kielhofner, G., Iyenger, A., Goldhammer, V., & Wolenski, J. (2006). *The Occupational Self-Assessment* (version 2.2). Chicago, IL: Model of Human Occupation Clearinghouse.

Baum, C. M., & Law, M. (1997). Occupational therapy practice: Focusing on occupational performance. *American Journal of Occupational Therapy, 51,* 277-288.

Law, M., Cooper, B., Strong, S., Stewart, D., Rigby, P., & Letts, L. (1996). The person-environment-occupation model: A transactive approach to occupational performance. *Canadian Journal of Occupational Therapy, 63,* 9-23.

Wilcock, A. (1993). A theory of the human need for occupation. *Journal of Occupational Science, 1,* 17-24.

---

of diseases and health problems. The information comprising the survey data is obtained from physicians, hospitals, clinics, and other health agencies that compile disease statistics. Table 3-9 from the *Morbidity and Mortality Weekly Report* is an example of epidemiological statistics, that is, data showing cases of specified reportable diseases in the United States.

3.7.3 Statement of Problem in Survey Research

The first step in survey research is to state the problem in question form. The problem should be researchable, requiring measurable data that can be collected and analyzed. In stating a problem in survey research, the investigator must operationally define the population to be surveyed in terms of geographical area and demographic characteristics, such as age, gender, socioeconomic status, education, and marital status. The identified population must be rigorously defined, otherwise there can be confusion in the *external validity* or in generalizing the results from the representative sample to the larger population. This, of course, is not an issue when the total population is surveyed. The following are hypothetical questions related to survey research:

- What is the present occupational status of clients who have been discharged from a supported employment program where they had been for at least 1 year?

- What are the minimal competencies required in different programs for teacher preparation in special education?

- What rehabilitation services do individuals with spinal cord injuries perceive as the most important?

- What are the socioeconomic characteristics of individuals using community mental health centers?

- What are the cholesterol levels of sedentary office workers?

- How are service dogs used by occupational therapists as adjunctive therapy?

- What are the specific intervention techniques that occupational therapists use in working with clients with AIDS?

- What methods are used for teaching reading in resource rooms?

3.7.4 Survey Research Methodology

After identifying a researchable problem, the target population, and the variables to be measured in the sample, the

TABLE 3-9

PROVISIONAL CASES OF INFREQUENTLY REPORTED NOTIFIABLE DISEASES (<1000 CASES REPORTED DURING THE PRECEDING YEAR) IN THE UNITED STATES

WEEK ENDING JULY 3, 2010

Disease	*Cumulative Number (Through 7/3/2010)*
Botulism, total	35
Foodborne	4
Infant	23
Other (wound & unspecified)	8
Brucellosis	53
Chancroid	27
Cholera	2
Cyclosporiasis	54
Hansen disease	18
Hanta virus pulmonary syndrome	4
Hemolytic uremic syndrome, post-diarrheal	70
Influenza-associated pediatric mortality	54
Listeriosis	283
Measles	28
A, C, Y, and W-135	132
Serogroup b	62
Other serogroup	6
Unknown serogroup	206
Mumps	2,064
Novel influenza A infection virus	1
Psittacosis	4
Q fever total	47
Acute	36
Chronic	11
Rabies, human	1
Rubella	4
Streptococcal toxic-shock syndrome	91
Syphilis, congenital (age < 1 year)	80
Tetanus	1
Toxic-shock syndrome (staphylococcal)	45
Trichinellosis	1
Tularemia	22
Typhoid fever	164
	(continued)

TABLE 3-9 (CONTINUED)	
PROVISIONAL CASES OF INFREQUENTLY REPORTED NOTIFIABLE DISEASES (<1000 CASES REPORTED DURING THE PRECEDING YEAR) IN THE UNITED STATES	
Disease	*Cumulative Number (Through 7/3/2010)*
Vancomycin-intermediate *Staphylococcus aureus*	50
Vancomycin-resistant *Staphylococcus aureus*	1
Vibriosis (non-cholera Vibrio species infections)	162
Viral hemorrhagic fever	1

Note: Table adapted from TABLE I of the Morbidity and Mortality Weekly Report, 59(26), pp 820-833 by the Centers for Disease Control and Prevention, National Center for Health Statistics, 7/9/2010. Data are cumulative through the week ending 7/3/2010. Retrieved from http://wonder.cdc.gov/mmwr/mmwr_reps.asp?mmwr_year=2010&mmwr_week=26&mmwr_table=1

investigator formulates the procedure for collecting data and the measuring instruments. Sampling procedures (discussed in more detail in Chapter 7) should be objective and unbiased and provide an accurate as possible description of the population. Random sampling, where the investigator selects a sample from the total population, is the best method to achieve an unbiased, representative sample. The external validity of the results is, of course, increased as the percentage of the population sampled increases. For example, a random sample of 50% of the population will be more accurate than a random sample of 30% of the population. Use of stratified samples can increase the accuracy of a survey if there are real strata in the population. In a stratified sample, the sample is divided into groups based on strata such as gender, age, diagnostic, or socioeconomic status. Of course, the determination of how large a sample to include in a survey is often based on practical considerations, such as the cost of the survey and the time allocated to the research project.

The principle methods for collecting data in survey research are the personal interview, mail (regular or e-mail), online, and telephone. Table 3-10 lists the relative merits of these four procedures.

3.7.5 Selection of Questionnaire

In selecting a measuring instrument for data collection, the survey researcher often is in the position of devising a self-made questionnaire. Whether the questionnaire is custom-designed for a study or has already been published, the researcher must account for the reliability and validity of the instrument. Before the investigator devises the instrument, a thorough search of published questionnaires should be undertaken. The latest edition of the Buros Mental Measurement Yearbook (Carlson, Geisinger, & Jonson, 2014) and other compendiums of tests and questionnaires, as well as abstracting journals are excellent sources for locating specific instruments for a study.

Surveys involving the measurement of physical variables in human research are also dependent on the reliability and validity of the instruments used. Procedures are employed

for increasing the validity of a subject's response, such as taking three blood pressure readings or three grip strength readings. Usually, the instruments used in collecting data are reliable and valid, such as the x-ray, electrocardiogram, and blood typing, but sometimes, because of subject anxiety or variability caused by external circumstances, one test result can be inaccurate. Figure 3-18 describes the sequential steps in undertaking survey research.

3.7.6 Constructing a Questionnaire in Survey Research

The questionnaire is the most commonly used and most frequently self-devised measuring instrument. Simply defined, a questionnaire is a standardized list of objective questions or statements to elicit personal opinions. The purpose of a questionnaire is to obtain information directly from a sample. Ultimately, the goal may be to generalize to a larger population. The format of a questionnaire is designed in accordance with the following:

- Content (e.g., demographic variables, personality characteristics, behavioral patterns, health history)
- Form of question (e.g., forced-choice or open-ended)
- Level of data collected (e.g., objective or attitudinal)

The steps in devising a questionnaire are listed in Table 3-11.

3.7.7 Item Construction

In constructing items, the researcher should be aware of the following:

- The choices available to the subjects should be exhaustive. On some items, a place for "other, please specify" should be provided.
- The choices should be mutually exclusive.
- The items presented should be unambiguous and precise. A pilot study testing the reliability of items is essential.

TABLE 3-10

RELATIVE MERITS OF THE PRINCIPLE SURVEY METHODS

PERSONAL INTERVIEW	MAIL	TELEPHONE	EMAIL/INTERNET-BASED
Advantages			
• Most flexible means of obtaining data because questions can be elaborated on or revised during the interview • Open-ended questions are possible • Accountability of the respondent is increased • Nonverbal cues can be observed • Lack of response generally very low • Equalize the types of subjects (e.g., men vs. women) • Establishment of rapport may increase validity and reliability of the response • Likely to be most expensive of all methods • Training the interviewer is required • Dangers of interviewer bias that may result in skewed results (halo or devil effect) • Scheduling • Time required for obtaining data	• Wider and more representative distribution of sample possible • No field staff • Cost per questionnaire relatively low • People may be more frank on certain issues (e.g., sex) • No interviewer bias; answers in respondent's own words • Respondent can answer at leisure; has time to think things over • Certain segments of population more easily approachable • Bias due to poor response rate (e.g., <30%) • Control over who answers the questionnaire may be lost • Interpretation of omissions to questions may be difficult • Cost per return may be high if the response rate is poor • Open-ended questions may result in poorer response rate or difficulty interpreting • Only those interested in subject may reply • Likely to be slowest response time of all	• Cost per response relatively low • Control over interviewer bias easier; supervisor can be present at interview • Quick way of obtaining data • Flexibility possible by elaborating or revising questions • Current lists of telephone numbers easily obtained • Shortened interviews because of time • Questions must be short and to the point • Open-ended questions usually avoided because of possibility of misinterpretation • Certain types of questions cannot be used (e.g., visual material) • Certain segments of population are not available (e.g., those without telephones)	• Wide and large representative distribution of sample possible • Cost per response is low or minimal • Quick way of obtaining data • Email addresses readily available • Respondent can answer at leisure • Certain segments of population more easily approachable • Enhanced ability to automate and tabulate responses • Bias due to poor response rate (e.g., <30%) • Control over who answers the questionnaire may be lost • Interpretation of omissions to questions may be difficult • Certain segments of population are not available (e.g., those without email) • Open-ended questions may result in poorer response rate or difficulty interpreting • Only those interested in subject may reply • Ambiguities in questions • Technology may hinder responses

Adapted from Ferber, R., & Verdoom, P. J. (1962). *Research methods in economics and business* (p. 210). New York, NY: Macmillan.

Figure 3-18. The sequential steps in survey research.

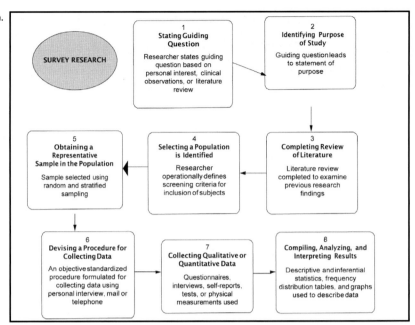

TABLE 3-11	
AN EXAMPLE OF THE STEPS IN CREATING A MAIL QUESTIONNAIRE	
STATE RESEARCH QUESTION	• What are the role functions of a public school occupational therapist?
CARRY OUT LITERATURE REVIEW	• Locate studies on public school occupational therapists.
IDENTIFY KEY AREAS FOR ITEMS IN THE QUESTIONNAIRE	• Description of school environment, faculty, and staff • Description of occupational therapists • Occupational therapy facilities and space • Student demographics • Classification of students treated by occupational therapist • Treatment techniques employed by occupational therapists • Occupational therapy treatment goals for diagnostic groups • Treatment modalities used by occupational therapists • Outcome measures for diagnostic groups • Quality assurance through progress monitoring of individual students
DEVISE SURVEY FORMAT	• Forced choice check off • Ranking priorities • Avoiding open-ended questions • Allowing opportunity for comment
EXPERT EVALUATION	• Send questionnaire to three public school occupational therapists asking them to evaluate each item using a specified form and make suggestions for improvement • Send questionnaire to research design expert
REVISE QUESTIONNAIRE	• Base revisions on expert recommendations • Limit time for completion to 10 to 15 minutes
FINAL DRAFT	• Have local public school occupational therapist complete questionnaire before mailing to participants • Work out final bugs and consider aesthetics of format

- Items should ask only one question. Avoid double-barreled questions.
- The respondent should have enough information to answer the item.
- The researcher should have a rationale for each item asked. The questionnaire should not be padded with irrelevant items.
- Negative questions should be avoided.
- Leading questions that force a response should be omitted. The respondents should not be able to give expected answers or opinions.

Examples of questionnaire items using various formats follow:

- *Likert-type scales* rate subjects by their agreement or disagreement with a statement on a scale usually of 1 to 5 or 1 to 7. For example, if an investigator is interested in surveying the attitudes of the general public with respect to research on children, an item such as the following could be considered for inclusion in the study:

All experimental research with children is unethical.

1	2	3		4	5	6	7
Disagree Very Strongly	Disagree Strongly	Disagree		No Opinion	Agree	Agree Strongly	Agree Very Strongly

- *Multiple-choice questions* can be used to elicit opinions or attitudes. Suppose a researcher is interested in surveying a group of patients with post–myocardial infarction on their attitudes toward the disability. The following multiple-choice question is one example:

If I had a severe pain in my chest, I would first do the following:

1. Call my private physician.

2. Call an ambulance.

3. Call the emergency rescue unit of the police.

4. Lie down and rest.

5. Other, please specify.

- *Rank order items* are used by researchers as a way of determining priorities. For example, a survey soliciting perceptions of intervention from former patients with psychiatric problems could include the following item:

From the list below of mental health workers, rank in order the most important persons who helped you improve in the hospital. Start numbering with 1 as the person who helped you most; 2, the second most helpful person; and so on:

Mental Health Worker Rank

Attendant _____

Nurse _____

Occupational therapist _____

Psychiatrist _____

Psychologist _____

Social worker _____

Other: Please specify occupation: _____

- *Incomplete sentences* are used in questionnaires to measure informational level, personality traits, and attitudes. For example:

Children with intellectual disabilities are different from normal children in …

- *Multiple adjective checklists* can be used to elicit perceptions, such as in the following example:

Circle the appropriate adjectives.

In general, older patients in nursing homes are:

independent	dependent
happy	sad
well-nourished	poorly fed
active	passive
neglected	supervised
healthy	sick

Please read the survey.

1. For each question on the survey, indicate whether the question is stated clearly or if it should be restated or eliminated.
2. Add additional questions that you feel would improve the validity of the questionnaire.

Answer the following questions.

3. Do you feel the survey is too lengthy? _____ Yes _____ No
   If you feel the questionnaire is too long, please place a line through the questions you would omit.
4. Do you find the questionnaire interesting? _____ Yes _____ No
   If you answered no, please tell us what you found uninteresting or irrelevant.
   _____
   _____
5. Were the questions arranged in a logical sequence? _____ Yes _____ No
   If you answered no, please indicate how you would rearrange the questions.
   _____
   _____
6. List further comments and include suggestions for decreasing research bias when administering questionnaire.
   _____
   _____

Thank you for your time. Any feedback you can give us will greatly enhance our study.

Figure 3-19. Evaluation form for survey questionnaires.

- *Open-ended questions* are used in the interviews when the researcher wants the subject to discuss an issue in detail. Examples of such questions are:

  - What is your opinion of including students with disabilities in the general education program?
  - What do you think the purpose(s) of prisons are?
  - What type of policy should the United States adopt for health insurance?

Depending on the ingenuity and creativeness of the researcher, other types of questionnaire items can be constructed, such as true-false questions, analogies, and rating scales. As with constructing any test instrument, it is critical that the investigator check the reliability and validity of the questionnaire before collecting data.

3.7.8 Evaluation of Survey

Once the survey has been developed, it will be important to have experts in the field evaluate it. This will improve reliability and validity and eliminate ambiguous questions. An example of an evaluation form is found in Figure 3-19. This form can be adapted as necessary.

3.7.9 Application of Survey Research to Occupational Therapy

In recent years, occupational therapists have expanded their role functions to include health planning and research. The future role of occupational therapists in planning community health services and health programs in schools is related to needs assessment research (Söderback & Paulsson, 1997). Figure 3-20 gives examples of the application of survey research and needs assessment.

3.7.9.1 Distribution of Health Care

One of the essential purposes of survey research is to guide the direction and planning of health services in a community. Health planners need hard data before they can recommend the construction of a health facility or hospital or the allocation of additional financial resources to a community health agency. Community health planning, therefore, is vitally linked to survey research. Legislators and developers who are persuaded by community pressures for new facilities need data to justify their positions. Survey research has taken on new importance in the current debate on whether the federal government should be responsible for the total health needs of the population. The data provided by survey research, such as the distribution of health personnel, the proportion of hospital beds for a designated population, and the number of various services provided in defined health catchment areas, can enable legislators to decide whether the present system of delivering health services is adequate for the country or whether a national system for health care would meet the needs of the population more equitably. Survey research can be combined with evaluation research in examining the effectiveness of a health delivery system.

3.7.9.2 Planning Therapeutic Services

Community organization of health services is a good example of the applicability of survey research to the needs of a population. Questions such as "What are the health needs of a community?" and "What are the health resources available?" are areas that occupational therapy researchers can directly examine through survey research. Survey research in health is comparable to market research in advertising. In market research, the individuals in a business collect data regarding the need for a product in the community and the community's attitude toward the introduction of new merchandise. Health planners have sometimes failed miserably in surveying a community before introducing a halfway house, a clinic for treating individuals with addictions, or a child health center. The failure usually has been the result of unexpected resistance from the community to the apparent visibility of individuals with social or physical disabilities in a neighborhood. Survey research can be used to anticipate a community's negative attitudes or even to expose the unrealistic fears that are attached to individuals with disabilities, and thus provide the means for counteracting the effects of social stigma.

3.7.9.3 Educational Planning

Educational planners and administrators often are asked by deans and presidents of colleges to determine if there is a need for a specific allied health training program (e.g., occupational therapy). Are there positions in schools, hospitals, or community agencies for occupational therapists when they graduate from a new program? Do vacancies in occupational therapy exist in hospitals and community clinics at present? Will there be an increased demand for occupational therapists in the future? In what geographic areas are the needs most pressing? These questions are directly assessable through survey research. Questions regarding level of training (i.e., associate, bachelor's, graduate, postgraduate, and continuing education) can be answered through a survey methodology.

Other important concerns that health educators should consider in designing curriculums are course content, clinical reasoning, and skill knowledge. What theoretical content and level of training should the occupational therapy program provide? In designing curriculums, health educators must be aware of the expectations of administrators. Have graduates of an occupational therapy program been adequately prepared to provide services needed by individuals with disabilities? On what basis does the educator determine the content of a training program? The need for continual feedback and interaction between educators and health administrators is necessary to create meaningful development of the occupational therapy profession. The occupational therapy educator must decide whether the education provided is directly or indirectly related to the needs of the individual with disabilities. If the education of the occupational therapists is directed toward clinical practice and specialization, then occupational therapist educators must be responsive to the community's needs. Survey research can provide the data gathered from the community to answer many questions in educational planning in occupational therapy.

3.7.9.4. Occupational Health Planning

There is an increasing need to investigate the prevention of occupational injuries through ergonomics. Other areas include the relationship between mental health and job satisfaction, and the study of environmental conditions, such as noise, ventilation, chemical contamination, and radiation. The distribution of accidents and the statistical relationship between occupation and disease are related to the application of survey research to occupational health. Occupational therapists, in consultation with industrial researchers, can provide information about workers' occupation patterns, nutritional needs, and protective equipment. Occupational health planning should not be done in a vacuum. There are obvious needs for descriptive data regarding frequency of diseases or accidents and the attitudes of workers toward using ergonomic methods before preventive programs can be implemented.

Research in occupational health must also consider psychosocial factors, such as the relationship between personality and accident-proneness; the effects of boredom, low morale, and poor motivation on job satisfaction and mental health; and the effects of job modification on productivity and injury prevention.

3.7.9.5 Preventive Programs in Schools and Communities

For the child from a low-income or socially disadvantaged family, school represents the greatest potential escape from a life of deprivation and misery. The school is one of the few institutions that can help the child overcome parental neglect or other disadvantages. It was not by happenstance but through careful research that during the 1960s social reformers saw the need to incorporate Head Start programs, work-study curriculums, nutritional programs, and vocational education into schools located in inner-city neighborhoods and poor rural regions. Survey research has been used in the past as a means to justify the existence of new programs in the schools, but there has been a backlash to the abuse of survey research in areas where data have been gathered and the needs of a community identified without any program implementation. Community leaders may be rightly suspicious of researchers who come into

a neighborhood or community to determine the need for services and making a promise to start new programs, only to leave without any follow-up.

Occupational therapists, in conjunction with allied health professionals and educators, have much to contribute in the areas of nutrition, health education, career planning, recreation, and developmental screening in schools and community centers. Survey research can provide the data for planning these services. Nonetheless, community support and follow-up are necessary if survey research is to have any impact on planning preventive programs. Box 3-7 gives an example of survey research.

3.8 Summary

Quantitative research offers occupational therapy clinicians the means to demonstrate the effectiveness of their intervention protocols. The importance of evidence-based practice is established primarily through the results of quantitative research. The various quantitative research models described in this chapter can assist clinicians in developing new ways to evaluate outcome, design intervention methods, and implement a needs assessment. Action research provides the occupational therapist with data to solve occupational problems at the local level. Qualitative research, as described in the Chapter 4, can be integrated with quantitative research to investigate research questions more thoroughly and can even address new types of questions pertaining to human beings.

BOX 3-7. EXAMPLE OF SURVEY RESEARCH

1. Bibliographical Notation

Cahill, S. M., McGuire, B., Krumdick, N. D., & Lee, M. M. (2014). National survey of occupational therapy practitioners' involvement in response to intervention. *American Journal of Occupational Therapy, 68*, e234-e240.

2. Abstract

"*Objective*: We sought to describe occupational therapy practitioners' perceived levels of preparedness for and involvement in school-based Response to Intervention (RtI) initiatives. *Methods*: We mailed a survey to a random sample of 1,000 practitioners from the American Occupational Therapy Association's [AOTA] Early Intervention and School Systems Special Interest Section. *Results*: Of 295 returned surveys (29.9% response rate), 19 were excluded because of missing or incomplete data. Three-quarters of respondents (77.6%) reported that their districts implemented RtI. Two-thirds of respondents (66.3%) indicated that lack of resources limited their involvement in RtI; two-thirds (67%) said that district guidelines that describe expectations for practitioners' involvement would help increase their participation. Many respondents cited the need for continuing education and supported moving from a caseload to a workload model. *Conclusion*: Occupational therapy practitioners would benefit from specific district guidelines outlining the services they are able to provide within the context of RtI."

3. Justification and Need

The authors define RtI as a "team-based, multitiered problem-solving framework that relies on data-based decision making to support students who are at risk for academic failure because of learning or behavioral difficulties" (p. e234). The authors also note that there is little research investigating how school-based occupational therapists collaborate with educators to facilitate students' general educational goals. They also go on to state that more research is needed to understand the various ways occupational therapy practitioners can contribute and how they would be perceived by their fellow teammates within the schools.

4. Literature Review

This study had 25 references from a variety of sources. Cited journals included but were not limited to *American Journal of Occupational Therapy, Journal of Learning Disabilities, Journal of Occupational Therapy in Schools and Early Intervention, Journal of Psychoeducational Assessment, Physical and Occupational Therapy in Pediatrics*, and *Learning Disabilities Research and Practice*. The years of cited publications ranged from 1993 through 2011.

5. Research Hypothesis or Guiding Question

No hypotheses or guiding questions were stated; however, the authors stated that the purpose of the study was to "describe how occupational therapy practitioners across the United States are involved in RtI and their attitudes toward being involved in such initiatives. Specifically, we describe four areas: current involvement of occupational therapy practitioners in RtI, beliefs of practitioners in relation to their participation, perceived barriers to practitioners' involvement, and factors perceived as facilitating practitioners' involvement in RtI" (p. e237).

6. Methods

Survey research was conducted and distributed to 1000 occupational therapists who were among the 4354 subscribing members of AOTA's Early Intervention and School Systems Special Interest Section. The investigators developed a 15-item questionnaire that ascertained respondents' RtI involvement and attitudes in being involved in RtI activities, as well as respondents' demographic information. The surveys were sent through the U.S. postal service with a stamped envelope with a return address.

(continued)

Box 3-7. Example of Survey Research (continued)

7. Results

With a 29% response rate, 295 surveys were mailed back to the investigators. Of these, 276 surveys were included in the data analysis (17 surveys were excluded due to improper and incomplete respondent actions). The researchers found that more than 77% of the respondents reported that their school district was engaged in RtI, with 44% indicating that their school districts fully implemented RtI. Although 69% of respondents believed RtI was beneficial, only 60% believed that the school employees did not have an awareness of all that occupational therapy could contribute. Given that, 53% of the respondents believed that school personnel would like to see occupational therapy be more involved with RtI initiatives.

8. Conclusions

The authors concluded that:

- "Occupational therapy practitioners working in RtI participate on school-based problem-solving teams, coach teachers, and provide one-to-one interventions to students in general education." (p. e240)

- Lack of resources for RtI implementation limits practitioners' involvement in such initiatives.

- School district guidelines that describe the roles and expectations of practitioners are needed.

- Moving from a caseload model to a workload model may support increased participation by practitioners in RtI initiatives.

9. Limitations

The study was limited to occupational therapy practitioners who subscribed to the AOTA's Early Intervention and School Special Interest Section. By its design, survey research relies on those individuals who are willing to return the questionnaire and therefore may have inherent bias in the responses.

10. Major References Cited

Burns, M., Appleton, J., & Stehouwer, J. (2005). Meta-analytic review of responsiveness-to-intervention research: Examining field-based and research-implemented models. *Journal of Psychoeducational Assessment, 23*, 381-394.

Cahill, S. (2010). Contributions made by occupational therapists in RtI: A pilot study. *Journal of Occupational Therapy in Schools and Early Intervention, 3*, 3-10.

Fuchs, D., Mock, D., Morgan, P., & Young, C. (2003). Responsiveness-to-intervention: Definitions, evidence, and implications for the learning disability construct. *Learning Disabilities Research and Practice, 18*, 157-171.

Reeder, D. L., Arnold, S. H., Jeffries, L. M., & McEwen, I. R. (2011). The role of occupational therapists and physical therapists in elementary school system early intervening services and Response to Intervention: A case report. *Physical and Occupational Therapy in Pediatrics, 31*, 44-57.

Telzrow, C., McNamara, K., & Hollinger, C. (2000). Fidelity of problem-solving implementation and relationship to student performance. *School Psychology Review, 29*, 443-461.

4

Qualitative Research Models

Qualitative methods can inform the understanding of a problem, the development of an intervention, and the understanding of how an intervention is delivered by agencies and received by participants. In process evaluations, qualitative data can contribute insights into how interventions operate and how outcomes are reached, although in practice, qualitative research is not always used to inform the trials in which they are a part.

—Cooper et al. (2014, p. xx)

OPERATIONAL LEARNING OBJECTIVES

By the end of this chapter the learner will:
- Define *qualitative research*.
- Describe the qualitative research process.
- Recognize the difference between quantitative and qualitative research designs.
- Enhance rigor in qualitative designs.
- Identify qualitative data collection methods.
- Identify the principles of qualitative data analysis.
- Critically analyze examples of qualitative research from the health literature.

Rice, M. S., Stein, F., & Tomlin, G.
Clinical Research in Occupational Therapy, Sixth Edition (pp. 105-140).
© 2019 Taylor & Francis Group.

4.1 DEFINING QUALITATIVE RESEARCH

Qualitative research is defined as the study of people and events in their natural setting.

Qualitative research is multi-method in focus, involving an interpretive naturalistic approach to its subject matter. This means that qualitative researchers study things in their natural settings, attempting to make sense of or interpret phenomena in terms of the meanings people bring to them. Qualitative research involves the studied use and collection of a variety of empirical materials—case study, personal experience, introspective, life story, interview, observational, historical, interactive, and visual texts—that describe routine and problematic moments and meaning in individuals' lives (Denzin & Lincoln, 1994b, p. 2).

In this method, researchers use multiple and interconnected methods, seeking to explore perceptions and experiences to understand phenomena in terms of the meanings that experiences have for people. These phenomena are examined in context and from the individual's point of view. In rehabilitation settings, the phenomena investigated include the experience of disability or a chronic medical condition, or of rehabilitation itself. The people involved may be clients, their family members, or occupational therapists.

Among health and rehabilitation personnel, there is a rapidly growing interest in exploring the views of clients and their families (Bamm, Rosenbaum, Wilkins, Stratford, & Mahlberg, 2015; Ferguson, Ferguson, & Taylor, 1992; Llewellyn, 1995; Morse, 1994; Westby & Backman, 2010). This interest is being shaped by two forces. The first is the disability movement. Consumers of health and related services are actively campaigning for a less medical approach to disability and a more positive acceptance of people with disabilities' place in society (French, 1994; Pazzaglia, Haggard, Scivoletto, Molinari, & Lenggenhager, 2016). The second is the coming together of researchers in medical and social science disciplines. This has led to the demise of the traditional illness-based view of disability. In its place, disability is regarded as a social construction. This view considers the ways in which particular societies regard impairments and the influence of situational factors, such as poor socioeconomic conditions, on the incidence of disability (Oliver, 1991; Plantinga, Johansen, Schillinger, & Powe, 2012). Another trend in patient-physician relationships is the sharing of medical records with patients. In a study in the United Kingdom, Fisher, Bhavnani, and Winfield (2009) described how patients' electronic access to medical records helped patients to make more informed decisions and reinforced trust and confidence in their doctors.

Exploring the viewpoint of the client or patient requires different research designs from those usually employed in the medical and health sciences. Allied health researchers are turning to sociology (the study of groups) and to anthropology (the study of cultures) for more appropriate research models. Investigators in these disciplines have been unraveling the complex interactions between individuals since the end of the 19th century (Weber, Parsons, & Weber, 1964).

Qualitative research models differ from those in the positivist quantitative tradition in three fundamental ways. First, qualitative researchers are interested in "participatory and holistic knowing" (Reason, 1998, p. 12). This contrasts with the distance and objectivity found particularly in experimental research designs. Second, there is a focus on critical subjectivity in qualitative research. This involves researchers acknowledging their primary subjective experience or bias. The researcher becomes his or her own "research instrument." This is in direct contrast to the notion of the objective researcher in experimental research designs. Third, researchers working in the qualitative tradition hold the view "that knowledge is formed in and for action" (Reason, 1998, p. 12). Action, as it naturally occurs, is viewed as the appropriate context for the development of knowledge.

4.2 CHARACTERISTICS OF QUALITATIVE RESEARCH

There are four fundamental characteristics of qualitative research:

1. Phenomena are investigated and interpreted in their natural settings, considering the sociocultural-historical context.

2. Multiple methods are used to understand and offer interpretations of the meanings held by participants about these phenomena.

3. The researcher, along with the informant, occupies a central place in the qualitative research process.

4. An inductive process is used to develop general principles from the study of specific instances.

Phenomena are investigated and interpreted in their natural settings, considering the sociocultural-historical context. Qualitative research often takes place in the field. Qualitative researchers get involved in the natural setting to understand the meanings held by participants about the phenomena under investigation. From this involvement and understanding, qualitative researchers develop insight and knowledge. This knowledge may be in the form of patterns or themes or a fully developed theory about the phenomena studied. Whatever the case, the resulting knowledge is grounded in direct field research experience rather than imposed a priori through hypotheses or deductive propositions (Glaser & Strauss, 1967).

Multiple methods are used to understand and offer inter-pretations of the meanings held by participants about these phenomena. Qualitative researchers use an array of methods to collect information about, describe, and interpret events and meanings in individuals' lives. The basic methods used for gathering data are interviewing, observation, and documentary analysis. The strategies most commonly used to analyze data include content or theme analysis, grounded theory procedures, and story analysis. These strategies are employed in the search for regularities in the meanings that participants hold about the phenomena under investigation. For some researchers, these regularities are viewed as a form of conceptual order; for others, their interest lies in the repetition of patterns across the data.

The researcher, along with the informant, occupies a central place in the qualitative research process. In qualitative research, the researcher is acknowledged as an individual located within a historical context and within a research tradition or traditions. Researchers bring to the research process particular sets of beliefs about the world that guide their actions. In contrast to experimentally based research designs, qualitative researchers attempt not to impose preexisting expectations on the phenomena or setting under study. Rather, the researchers' set of beliefs functions as an interpretive framework (Guba, 1990). This interpretive framework guides the research purpose and shapes the research questions and the methods employed to address these questions. In addition to an interpretive framework, qualitative researchers become familiar with the literature and develop guiding questions to focus on the purposes of the research.

An inductive process is used to develop general principles from the study of specific instances. In qualitative research, the analysis begins with specific instances of data and builds toward general principles. This contrasts with the deductive process employed in the quantitative tradition in which hypotheses are constructed prior to data collection and then tested. In qualitative research, preparing the research text is the final stage of the inductive analysis process. The research text is a construction that integrates and interprets data and the researcher's understanding of the area of study. The completed product is the public text, which may be delivered either as a research report, journal article, book, or seminar paper.

4.3 TYPES OF QUALITATIVE RESEARCH

Qualitative research is a term widely used to indicate methods that subscribe to the characteristics described previously. For example, Tesch (1990) listed 46 different research approaches under the rubric of qualitative research. Some research methods more closely fit the characteristics described; others are less closely associated. Historically, several qualitative methods have become standard in the medical and health literature (Morse, 1994). These include case study, field study, focus group research, ethnography, and oral history (Table 4-1). Other methods, such as ethnoscience, discourse analysis, transformative research, and hermeneutics, are not as familiar.

Discourse analysis and ethnoscience are concerned with the study of the characteristics of language as a communication tool and as culture, respectively. Transformative research involves the research subjects as active participants in developing and implementing the research project to overcome the usually passive nature of the research process by turning this into a transforming activity. Researchers employing hermeneutics take as their central theme, the understanding of events in relation to the context of which these are part, with special reference to the historical context.

Another approach to classifying qualitative research is by the research purpose. Some approaches are ideal for identifying regularities, patterns, or themes. Others are better suited to generating and refining tentative theoretical propositions. Still others are more useful for intense, intimate study of a phenomenon using personal reflection. There is ongoing debate in the qualitative research literature about this diversity of approaches and associated methodological issues (Denzin & Lincoln, 1994a; Higgs, 1997). Each approach has adherents in the core disciplines of psychology, psychiatry, sociology, and anthropology.

It is not by chance that many of the important contributions in the social sciences have emerged from clinical observation and case study methods (Dukes, 1965). Freud in his search for an understanding of the psychodynamics of mental illness, Gesell's (1928) rigorous observation of child development, Piaget's (1926) conceptualization of cognitive development through detailed analysis of clinical responses, and Henry's (1971) naturalistic observation of families of children with emotional disturbance all made a significant impact on understanding human behavior through qualitative research. Clinical observation as a research method has the potential to contribute greatly to the fields of occupational therapy. Table 4-2 lists some of the major studies in the social sciences based on clinical observation research methods.

Clinical observation research employs four methods: individual case study, child development studies, field observation (ethnography), and operations research. The definition, purposes, procedure, and application to occupational therapy and special education are listed in Table 4-3.

TABLE 4-1

FIVE APPROACHES TO QUALITATIVE RESEARCH

	CASE STUDY (RETROSPECTIVE OR PROSPECTIVE)	GROUNDED THEORY OR HEURISTIC STUDY	PHENOMENOLOGICAL	ETHNOGRAPHY OR FIELD STUDY	BIOGRAPHICAL
DEFINED	Exploration of an individual, organization, program, or event through an in-depth data collection using multiple sources of information (Creswell, 1998)	General method for generating or discovering theory during the data collection (Strauss & Corbin, 1998)	"From the individual descriptions, general or universal meanings are derived, in other words, the essences of structures of the experience" (Moustakas, 1994, p. 13)	Examination of a cultural or social group through extended participant observations to determine the meanings of behavior, language, and interactions of the group (Creswell, 1998; Vidich & Lyman, 2003)	Study of an individual; this study may be through "portrayals, portraits, profiles, memoirs, life stories, life histories, case studies, autobiographies, journals, diaries, and on and on—each suggesting a slightly different perspective under consideration" (Smith, 1994, p. 278)
EXAMPLE OF STUDY	Emerson, H., Cook, J., Polatajko, H., & Segal, R. (1998). Enjoyment experiences as described by persons with schizophrenia: A qualitative study. *Canadian Journal of Occupational Therapy, 65,* 183-192.	Creighton, C., Dijkers, M., Bennett, N., & Brown, K. (1995). Reasoning and the art of therapy for spinal cord injury. *American Journal of Occupational Therapy, 49,* 311-317.	Hasselkus, B. R., & Dickie, V. A. (1993). Doing occupational therapy: Dimensions of satisfaction and dissatisfaction. *American Journal of Occupational Therapy, 48,* 145-154.	Frank, G., Bernardo, C. S., Tropper, S., Noguchi, F., Lipman, C., Maulhardt, B., & Weitze, L. (1997). Jewish spirituality through actions in time: Daily occupations of young orthodox Jewish couples in Los Angeles. *American Journal of Occupational Therapy, 51,* 199-206	Frank, G. (1996). Life histories in occupational therapy clinical practice. *American Journal of Occupational Therapy, 50,* 251-264.
METHODS OF DATA COLLECTION	• Interviewing • Naturalistic observational techniques		• Mute evidence • Personal experience		

TABLE 4-2
MAJOR CONTRIBUTIONS FROM CLINICAL OBSERVATION METHODOLOGIES IN THE SOCIAL SCIENCES

SOCIAL SCIENTISTS	MAJOR WORK	METHOD	PUBLICATION DATE	FIELD OF INVESTIGATION
Sigmund Freud and Josef Breuer	*Studies in Hysteria*	Case study	1895	Psychiatry
Margaret Mead	*Coming of Age in Samoa*	Field observation	1928	Cultural anthropology
Arnold Gesell	*Infancy and Human Growth*	Developmental observation	1929	Child development
Jean Piaget	*The Psychology of Intelligence*	Developmental observation	1947	Cognitive development
Alfred Stanton, M. S. Schwartz, and Morris Schwartz	*The Mental Hospital*	Operations research	1950	Psychiatry
Robert White	*Lives in Progress*	Case study	1952	Personality
Jules Henry	*Pathways to Madness*	Field observation	1965	Family casework
Rene A. Spitz	*The First Year of Life: A Psychoanalytic Study of Normal and Deviant Development of Object Relations*	Developmental observation	1965	Child psychiatry
Joseph Church	*Three Babies: Biographies of Cognitive Development*	Case study	1966	Cognition
Oscar Lewis	*La Vida*	Field observation	1966	Cultural anthropology
Bruno Bettelheim	*The Empty Fortress*	Case study	1967	Child psychiatry
Robert Coles	*Children of Crisis*	Field observation	1967	Social psychiatry
Eric Berman	*Scapegoat*	Field observation	1973	Family casework
Mary D. Salter Ainsworth, Mary C. Blehar, Everett Waters, and Sally N. Wall	*Patterns of Attachment*	Clinical observation	1978	Social psychology
Jack Fadely and Virginia Hosier	*Case Studies in Left and Right Hemispheric Functioning*	Case study	1983	Perception
Stephen Marks	*Three Corners: Exploring Marriage and the Self*	Case study	1986	Family relationships
Sylvia Kenig (Ed.)	*Who Plays? Who Pays? Who Cares? A Case Study in Applied Sociology, Political Economy and the Community Mental Health Centers Movement*	Case Study	1992	Community mental health

(continued)

TABLE 4-2 (CONTINUED)				
MAJOR CONTRIBUTIONS FROM CLINICAL OBSERVATION METHODOLOGIES IN THE SOCIAL SCIENCES				
SOCIAL SCIENTISTS	MAJOR WORK	METHOD	PUBLICATION DATE	FIELD OF INVESTIGATION
Kelley Johnson	*Deinstitutionalizing Women: An Ethnographic Study of Institutional Closure*	Case study	1998	Deinstitutionalization
Steven Pinker	*The Blank Slate*	Clinical observation	2002	Psychology
Jonathan Kozol	*The Shame of the Nation: The Restoration of Apartheid Schooling in America*	Field observation	2005	Educational philosophy
Oliver Sacks	*Musicophilia: Tales of Music and the Brain*	Case study	2007	Neuropsychology
Temple Grandin	*The Way I See It: A Personal Look at Autism and Asperger's*	Case study	2008	Autism

TABLE 4-3			
APPLICATION OF CLINICAL OBSERVATION METHODS			
METHOD	PURPOSE	PROCEDURES FOR COLLECTING DATA	APPLICATION TO FIELDS
Individual case study	Understanding of underlying dynamics of illness	• Interviewing • Testing • Examination of personal documents • Case research	• Investigation of health problems, chronic diseases, and individual factors
Child development studies	Description of the sequential, hierarchical processes in human development	• Objective observation in a controlled setting • Mechanical audiovisual recordings	• Examination of normal and abnormal patterns in development

Field observations (ethnography)	Examination of the interaction between members of a social group, educational group, or family	• Naturalistic observation
		• Process recordings of interactions
		• Unobtrusive measurement
			• Description of group interaction in:
			  ○ Dysfunctional families
			  ○ Halfway houses
			  ○ Residential treatment programs
			  ○ Education classrooms
			  ○ Socioeconomic units
			(continued)

TABLE 4-3 (CONTINUED)			
APPLICATION OF CLINICAL OBSERVATION METHODS			
METHODS	**PURPOSES**	**PROCEDURES FOR COLLECTING DATA**	**APPLICATION TO FIELDS**

Operations research	Analysis of administrative problems in organization systems	• Flow charts of organizational structure
		• Job descriptions
		• Communication patterns
		• Decision-making process
			• Examination of interrelationships among systems
			  ∘ Political
			  ∘ Economic
			  ∘ Health care
			  ∘ Educational

4.3.1 Case Study

There is much criticism by experimentalists of the case study approach as a model for research, primarily directed toward the subjectivity of the researcher and the inability to generalize to a population based on one subject. The most important purpose of the case study is in the intensive investigation of one individual. Through a thorough study the researcher can examine factors that ordinarily would be difficult either in an experimental study involving a group of subjects or in a correlational study.

To illustrate, let us suppose an investigator is interested in learning why patients who are older and living in a nursing home develop feelings of hopelessness and disengage from the mainstream of society. The researcher poses the question: What factors in an older person's life contribute to feelings of hopelessness and disengagement? In this study, the investigator is limited to an ex post facto research model. It would be possible to answer this question by comparing a group of older individuals who display feelings of hopelessness with another group of older individuals who are actively engaged in independent activities. In this hypothetical study, the researcher could test whether individuals who have personalities characterized by an external locus of control feel more hopeless than a similar geriatric sample who characteristically have a more internal locus of control and feel less hopeless.

The reader will recognize this research model as correlational. In a correlational model, the researcher is restricted by the test instruments used in measuring the variables of locus of control and hopelessness and by the limitations in controlling for the individual differences among participants. For example Singh and Misra (2009) conducted a study of loneliness, depression, and sociability in old age.

On the other hand, a case study approach would allow the investigator the freedom to search for individual factors that could easily be overlooked in a correlational study, but on closer investigation prove to be a critical variable in generating dependency and hopelessness. The flexibility of a case study and the creativity afforded to the researcher

compensate for the apparent lack of external validity or the ability to generalize to a larger population.

The general outline of case study research is like all aspects of research in that the researcher justifies the need for investigation, reviews previous literature, states guiding questions for data collection, and obtains data through observation and measurement. In contrast to a random controlled trial and correlational research, in the case study the researcher is limited in generalizing the results. The main purpose of a case study is to explore relationships that can generate further research or case study replications. The general format of a case study follows.

4.3.1.1 Need for the Study

In this section of the study, the investigator explores the significance of the study and the multiple effects of a problem on family, educational and health institutions, and society in general. The investigator examines the prevalence of the problem and its relationship to occupational therapy. The investigator should also discuss the appropriateness of using a qualitative case study model. If a case study is used as a pilot study, such as to collect data about a problem before undertaking a larger study, then it should also be stated. A case study should not be used in place of an experimental or correlational study. For example, a case study may be more appropriate than an experimental or correlational methods in an in-depth study of a complex chronic disability such as drug addiction (van Emmerik-van Oortmerssen, Vedel, van den Brink, & Schoevers, 2015).

Potential issues for justifying the need for a case study may include the number and percentage of a population affected by a disability regarding its incidence and prevalence in relation to mortality rates and the number of hospitalization admissions and physician visits. Other items to consider may include exploring the evaluation tests and treatment methods are currently provided by occupational therapists. The investigator should also discuss in this section what the possible implications of the results from a case study could provide. Investigations into the dynamic factors affecting the etiology and pilot interventions in

TABLE 4-4	
EXAMPLE OF SCREENING CRITERIA (DELINQUENT YOUTH)	
AGE	16 years old
GENDER	Male
SOCIOECONOMIC FACTOR	Working-class family
INTELLIGENCE	Average nonverbal IQ
FAMILY	Dysfunctional, non-intact due to divorce, separation, or parent desertion
SCHOOL STATUS	Special education setting
GEOGRAPHIC AREA	Urban
BEHAVIOR	Delinquent, with vandalism, truancy, and deviant behavior that results in adjudication, probation, or referral to residential treatment setting

individuals diagnosed with arthritis, schizophrenia, clinical depression, autism, dementia, drug and alcohol addictions, and attention-deficit/hyperactivity (ADHD) disorders are particularly appropriate for case study research.

4.3.1.2 Review of Literature

The investigator should do an extensive review of the literature on the question and critically examine the variables in the case study. Research related to etiology and treatment is particularly important in a case study. The literature review should provide the investigator with a general overview of the current state of knowledge. Research journals, textbooks, conference proceedings, electronic databases, and other sources of information should be reviewed. An outline should guide the investigator in deciding what aspects of the research problem to include, the extensiveness of the review, and the sources used to obtain information. (For a more detailed discussion on reviewing literature, see Chapter 6.)

The literature review should also include an examination of case study methods for collecting and reporting data, such as video recording, interviewing, reliability of case records, medical history recording, and psychological testing. These areas are especially important to the investigator who is unfamiliar with the case study methods.

4.3.1.3 Research Methodology

In this section, critical variables are operationally defined, a screening criteria for subject selection is delineated, a procedure for interviewing and testing the subject is stated, test instruments are identified, and reliability and validity data are reported. A screening criteria should be based on a rationale considering representative statistical data for a target population. For example, if an investigator is interested in doing a case study of a youth who is delinquent, he or she would consider gender, age when most delinquency occurs, socioeconomic group factors, school status, cognitive level, family, and delinquent acts committed. The variables identified should be obtained from a review of the literature, statistical abstracts, and clinical observations. From these sources the researcher operationalizes the screening criteria as outlined in Table 4-4.

The investigator should also consider exclusionary criteria, that is, factors that potentially affect the results. These variables may include brain damage, mental illness, or language difficulty. After the researcher has determined inclusion and exclusion criteria, the next task is to plan a procedure for selecting a participant for the case study. This may entail contacting a juvenile facility, a court, or an agency working with delinquent youth. The cooperation of the agency is crucial to the research. The participant and the parent or guardian must be told of the purposes of the study through informed consent. The plan for collecting data is another important part of the research methodology. This includes the following questions:

- At what setting will the study take place?
- What psychological tests, evaluation instruments, questionnaires, and interview schedules will be employed?
- During what time period will the study take place (e.g., hours of day, school time or evening, time of year)?

4.3.1.4 Results

The data gathered for a case study include the subject's history, informal and formal assessments, collateral information from case records, interviews with the individual and family members, and clinical reports. Difficulties can arise in a case study that threatens the researcher's objectivity White (1952) believed that "It is impossible to study another person without making evaluations, and it is hard to keep the evaluations from being seriously distorted by one's personal reactions to the subject" (p. 99). The investigator must acknowledge this limitation of a case study. One way to do this is to have more than one interviewer obtain an independent history on the same individual. In this way, investigator bias and personal views can be isolated. Another method is to make the investigators aware of their own rigidities, assumptions, and prejudices "through increased familiarity with their own personalities" (White, 1952, p. 100). However, most important is the need to acknowledge that there will always be investigator subjectivity in the conduct and reporting of any study, particularly in an intensive case study. The preferred way to demonstrate that the reported results accurately reflect the individual's responses and the investigator's neutrality is to ensure that the investigator is aware of bias and presumptions that may affect the results of the case study. Investigators often keep a reflective journal in which these themes of possible bias are explored and documented.

Most investigators, in reporting a case study, use a chronological outline starting from the subject's early childhood and continuing through his or her current age. A topical biography is another way to organize data. For example, in a case study of a subject with osteoarthritis, the investigator may want to report data under subject headings, such as possible etiological factors (e.g., genetic vulnerabilities, joint injuries, allergies, emotional disturbances, endocrine disorders) or interventions (e.g., occupational therapy, physical therapy, chemotherapy, psychological counseling). An interpretive summary and a recommendation for further research follow the reporting of results.

In short, case study research is a viable method for obtaining credible data pertaining to the life of an individual with disabilities. It is an idiographic approach to research that considers individual differences in etiology of disease and specific adaptations in coping with a disability. Box 4-1 gives an example of a qualitative case study.

4.3.2 Operations Research

Ackoff and Rivett (1963) described the three essential characteristics of operations research: "(1) systems orientation, (2) the use of interdisciplinary teams, and (3) the adaptation of scientific method" (p. 10). Operations research was developed in Great Britain during World War II, mainly for the purpose of using radar effectively to combat German air attacks (Crowther & Whiddington, 1948). Subsequently, during the 1950s, large corporations employed operations research teams to analyze production methods as a way of increasing efficiency. Wiener's (1948) contributions in cybernetics and in the application of the feedback principle expanded systems theory to biological, sociological, and psychological dimensions. For example, using the technology of cybernetics, the methodology of operations research, and systems theory, researchers have examined the processes used to implement evidence-based care in a primary care practice (Huebsch et al., 2015), physiology of respiration (Pribram, 1958), equipment design and human engineering (Shrader, 2006; U.S. Department of Defense, Joint Services Steering Committee, 1963), political life (Easton, 1961), the city as a system (Blumberg, 1971), clinical rotation (Reid, Seavor, & Taylor, 1991), higher education (Cheng, 1993), family planning (Huezo, 1997), obstetric care (Sibley & Armbruster, 1997), and rehabilitation (Doarn, McVeigh, & Poropatich, 2010).

Efficiency in industrial production has been one of the areas in which operations research has been widely applied.

Feigin, An, Connors, and Crawford (1996) applied operations research to restructure IBM's manufacturing strategy. The goal of the efficiency expert in a factory is to minimize expenditures and maximize production. By analyzing the industrial system of production, the operations researcher can determine where costs can be reduced and production increased. Factors such as competitive costs of raw materials and plant machinery, redeployment of labor, employee morale, and distribution of goods are all considered in operations research. Essentially, operations research analyzes a system by identifying all those factors that affect input or raw materials and output or finished product. The feedback in this system represents the critical analysis of input and output and the resultant changes in the total system of production (Figure 4-1).

The concept of operations research and systems theory have also been applied to research problems in health care (Dickinson et al., 2010; Jacob & Shapira, 2010; Uomoto & Williams, 2009). For example, hospital management provides an excellent area for operations research. For hospital administrators, the problems of expanding costs and depersonalized care for health consumers have become increasingly more aggravated during recent decades. Although society seeks improved, expanded health care for larger portions of the population, hospitals have to find more efficient methods to service more clients and to provide them with sophisticated diagnostic methods for detecting and treating illnesses with the most advanced technology. Specifically, these problems include (a) architectural design, (b) medical equipment, (c) hospital staffing, including availability of consultants, (d) cost sharing for using expensive machinery, and (e) issues such as managed care. Operations research as applied to the fields of allied health and rehabilitation uses observational data and systems analysis to identify critical issues and solve problems. Health problems appropriate for operations research include the following:

- Zika virus and epidemiology (Nunes et al., 2016)
- Depersonalization of clients in long-term care (Kliebsch, Stürmer, Siebert, & Brenner, 1998)
- Effect of tele-emergency services on recruitment and retention of rural physicians in the United States (Potter, Mueller, Mackinney, & Ward, 2014)
- Inadequate funding for long-term care (Xakellis, Frantz, Lewis, & Harvey, 1998)
- Recurrence of chronic disease among vulnerable populations (Woods et al., 1997)
- Lack of rehabilitation services in forensic psychiatry (Muñoz, Moreton, & Sitterly, 2016)
- Inefficient emergency care in urban hospitals (Ernst, Houry, & Weiss, 1997)
- Day care for elderly or adults with severe disabilities (Macdonald, Epstein, & Vastano, 1986)
- Quality of life for patients with post-polio syndrome (Jacob & Shapira, 2010)

Box 4-1. Example of a Qualitative Case Study

1. Bibliographical Notation

Chan, A. S., Tsang, H. W., & Li, S. M. (2009). Case report of integrated supported employment for a person with severe mental illness. *American Journal of Occupational Therapy*, 63, 238-244.

2. Abstract

"*Objective*: We illustrate the implementation of an integrated supported employment (ISE) program that augments the individual placement and support model with social skills training in helping people with severe mental illness (SMI) achieve and maintain employment. *Method*: A case illustration demonstrates how ISE helped a 41-year-old woman with SMI to get and keep a job with support from an employment specialist. An independent, blinded assessor conducted data collection of employment information, including self-efficacy and quality of life, at pretreatment and at 3-month, 7-month, 11-month, and 15-month follow-up assessments. *Results*: The participant eventually stayed in a job for 8 months and reported improved self-efficacy and quality of life. *Conclusion*: The case report suggests that ISE could improve the employment outcomes of people with SMI. Moreover, changes in the participant's self-efficacy and quality of life were shown to be driven by the successful employment experience."

3. Justification and Need

The authors documented the need for individuals with SMI to obtain and maintain competitive employment as only 15% to 30% are employed. A protocol for the integrated supported employment program was tested and evaluated, with one individual diagnosed with depression.

4. Literature Review

Twenty-nine references were cited in the study. Cited journals included but were not limited to *Community Mental Health Journal, American Journal of Occupational Therapy, Psychiatric Rehabilitation Journal, American Journal of Psychiatry, Schizophrenia Bulletin, British Journal of Medical Psychology, Psychiatric Services, Psychiatric Quarterly, Archives of General Psychiatry, Social Indicators Research, Psychiatry, Social Psychiatry and Psychiatric Epidemiology, Journal of Nervous and Mental Disease, Journal of Behavior Therapy and Experimental Psychiatry, International Journal of Psychosocial Rehabilitation, Psychologia,* and *American Journal of Rehabilitation.*

5. Research Hypothesis or Guiding Question

The authors assessed how integrated supported employment can improve the employment outcome of an adult with chronic depression.

6. Methods

The integrated supported employment program was operationally defined applying vocational assessment, individual employment plan, social skills training, vocational placement, and follow-along support. The program was in place for 7 months.

7. Results

The individual stayed in her job for 8 months. She expressed that she was satisfied in her job and was able to maintain a good relationship with her supervisor and coworkers.

8. Conclusions

The authors felt that the program supported the application of integrated supported employment program and was developing an e-learning package for clinicians.

(continued)

Box 4-1. Example of a Qualitative Case Study (continued)

9. Limitations

As this was a qualitative study without a control group, more research is needed to validate the conclusions. The protocol developed in the study needs to be replicated to assess its applicability in a wide range of vocational rehabilitation programs.

10. Major References Cited

Bond, G. R. (2004). Supported employment: Evidence for an evidence-based practice. *Psychiatric Rehabilitation Journal, 27,* 345-359.

Drake, R. E., McHugo, G. J., Bebout, R. R., Becker, D. R., Becker, D. R., Harris, M., … Quimby, E. (1999). A randomized clinical trial of supported employment for inner-city patients with severe mental illness. *Archives of General Psychiatry, 56,* 627-633.

McGurk, S. R, Mueser, K. T., & Pascaris, A. (2005). Cognitive training and supported employment of persons with severe mental illness: One-year results from a randomized controlled trial. *Schizophrenia Bulletin, 31,* 898-909.

Figure 4-1. Simple feedback model.

- Integrated care for returning veterans (Uomoto & Williams, 2009)
- Computer-based cognitive remediation for schizophrenia (Dickinson et al., 2010)
- Learning difficulties in children with ADHD (Bennett, Power, Eiraldi, Leff, & Blum, 2009)
- Characteristics of traumatic brain injury (TBI) assessed in the workplace (Bootes & Chapparo, 2002)
- Waiting time for total hip replacement (Hajat et al., 2002)
- Computerized contingency management in a drug addiction treatment program (Vahabzadeh, Lin, Mezghanni, Epstein, & Preston, 2009)
- Roles of nonmedical health care workers (Mitchell, 2009)
- Challenges in occupational therapy (Gewurtz, Stergiou-Kita, Shaw, Kirsh, & Rappolt, 2008)

In all of the foregoing problems, the underlying assumption is that a system—a unified interconnected whole—exists. The systems researcher analyzes the specific components of the system and their interrelationships. In these examples, the systems are identified as rural health, long-term care, legislation process, general hospitals, chronic illness, emergency care, and adult day care. Box 4-2 provides an example of an operational research study.

4.3.3 Developmental Observations

"Experimental observation, with conditions so clearly defined that they can be duplicated and so delimited that only a single variable remains for study is scientifically a goal to work toward" (Gesell, 1928, p. 23). This description, stated almost one century ago, remains the benchmark for research on child development. Developmental observation research is concerned with the rigorous investigations into the processes, stages, and hierarchical steps in human development. How does speech develop? What are the sequential stages in the areas of language, ambulation, psychosocial development, and cognition? These and other questions are examples of research problems that lend themselves to developmental observation methods. The investigator seeks to identify the processes involved in development, the approximate ages when landmarks are reached, and the biopsychosocial factors that shape development.

A key assumption in developmental research is that human behavior unfolds at critical stages. In Table 4-5, some examples of approximate ages are given for achieving

Box 4-2. Example of Operations Research

1. Bibliographical Notation

Bennett, A. E., Power, T. J., Eiraldi, R. B., Leff, S. S., & Blum, N. J. (2009). Identifying learning problems in children evaluated for ADHD: The Academic Performance Questionnaire. *Pediatrics, 124,* e633-e639.

2. Abstract

"*Objective*: The objective of this study was to assess the usefulness of the Academic Performance Questionnaire (APQ) to identify low reading and math achievement in children who are being evaluated for attention-deficit/hyperactivity disorder (ADHD). *Methods*: Charts of 997 patients who were seen in a multidisciplinary ADHD evaluation program were reviewed. Patients who were in first-through sixth-grade and had complete APQ and Wechsler Individual Achievement Test II Basic Reading and Numerical Operations subtests were enrolled in this study. The 271 eligible patients were randomly assigned to a score-development group (n = 215) and a validation group (n = 56). By using data from the score-development sample, APQ questions that predicted low academic achievement were identified and the scores for these questions were entered into a logistic regression to identify the APQ questions that independently predicted low achievement. *Results*: Only 2 APQ questions, 1 about reading and 1 about math, independently predicted low achievement. By using these 2 questions, the area under the receiver operating characteristic curve was 0.834, and the optimal combination of sensitivity and specificity occurred when the total score for the 2 items was >4. This cutoff had a sensitivity of 0.86 and a specificity of 0.63 in the score-development group and a sensitivity of 1.0 and a specificity of 0.53 in the validation sample. *Conclusions*: The APQ may be a useful screening tool to identify children being evaluated for ADHD who need additional testing for learning problems. Although the predictive value of a negative screen on the APQ is good, the predictive value of a positive test is relatively low."

3. Justification and Need

The authors stated that learning disorders co-occur with ADHD in 20% to 30% of children and are typically identified by a psychoeducational assessment. Primary care physicians who evaluate children for ADHD often find it difficult to identify which children they should refer for additional assessment of academic skills. The purposes of this study were to (a) examine the test-retest reliability of the APQ and (b) evaluate the validity of the APQ with regard to predicting low achievement in reading and/or math.

4. Literature Review

The authors cited 17 references. Cited journals included but were not limited to *Pediatrics, Journal of Pediatric Psychology, Journal of Learning Disabilities, School Psychology Review,* and the *Journal of Developmental Behavior Pediatrics.*

5. Research Hypothesis or Guiding Question

Is the APQ helpful in identifying those students with ADHD who will have difficulty in reading and math achievement?

6. Methods

The charts of 997 students who were seen in a multidisciplinary ADHD evaluation program were reviewed. Students who were in first through sixth grade and had complete APQ and Weschler Individual Achievement Test-II (WIAT-II) Basic Reading and Numerical Operations subtests were enrolled in this study. The 271 eligible students were randomly assigned to a score-development group (n = 215) and a validation group (n = 56). By using data from the score-development group, APQ questions that predicted low academic achievement were identified and the scores for these questions were entered into a logistic regression to identify the APQ questions that independently predicted low achievement.

(continued)

BOX 4-2. EXAMPLE OF OPERATIONS RESEARCH (CONTINUED)

7. Results

Results of this study demonstrate that using only two questions from the APQ, one about math and one about reading, as a screen produces a test with acceptable test-retest reliability and sensitivity.

8. Conclusion

The APQ may be a useful initial screening tool for assessing learning problems among children who present with symptoms of ADHD or other school problems. Before the APQ can be implemented as a primary care screening tool, additional research is needed to confirm its predictive validity in a primary care setting assessing children with a diverse range of demographic characteristics.

9. Limitations

"This study was a retrospective chart analysis of children with ADHD who attended a multi-disciplinary center. The results of this study should be considered in the context of the following limitation: the children in this study did not have a full psychoeducational assessment. For clinical efficiency, only the two subtests of the WIAT-II that best correlate with overall reading and math scores were selected. A more complete academic assessment may have changed the classification of some children who scored near the cutoff. In addition, we did not assess other important skills, such as writing, spelling, and phonics. Thus, the ability of the APQ questions to detect children with low achievement in these areas could not be assessed."

10. Major References Cited

Glascoe, F. P. (2001). Can teachers' global ratings identify children with academic problems? *Journal of Developmental and Behavioral Pediatrics, 22*, 163-168.

Gresham, F. M., & MacMillan, D. L. (1997). Teachers as "tests": Differential validity of teacher judgments in identifying students at-risk for learning difficulties. *School Psychology Review, 26*, 47-60.

Leslie, L. K., Weckerly, J., Plemmons, D., Landsverk, J., & Eastman, S. (2004). Implementing the American Academy of Pediatrics attention-deficit/hyperactivity disorder diagnostic guidelines in primary care settings. *Pediatrics, 114*, 129-140.

Polaha, J., Cooper, S., Meadows, T., & Kratochvil, C. J. (2005). The assessment of attention-deficit/hyperactivity disorder in rural primary care: The portability of the American Academy of Pediatrics guidelines to the "real world." *Pediatrics, 115*, e120-e126.

TABLE 4-5	
DENVER DEVELOPMENTAL SCREENING TEST-II	
DEVELOPMENTAL SKILLS	**HIERARCHICAL SEQUENTIAL ACTIVITIES FROM BIRTH TO 6 YEARS**
Gross motor	Lifts head at age 2 months to walks backward (heel-to-toe) at age 6 years
Fine motor	Visually tracks objects to midline at age 2 months to draws a man with 6 distinct parts at age 6 years
Language	Responds to bell at age 2 months to defines 6 words at age 6 years
Personal-social	Regards face at age 2 months to dresses without supervision at age 5 years

Note: From normative data, age levels were established as to when children develop individual skills. Normal limits (upper and lower) were validated for each hierarchical activity.

Adapted from Frankenburg, W. R., Dodds, J. B., Archer, P., Shapiro, H., & Bresnick, B. (1990). *The Denver Developmental Screening Test-II (DDST-II)*. Denver, CO: Denver Developmental Materials.

TABLE 4-6	
SUGGESTED AREAS FOR RESEARCH QUESTIONS	
AREAS OF DEVELOPMENT	**EXAMPLES OF RESEARCH QUESTIONS**
Social	What are the sequential stages that lead to cooperative play in children?
Emotional	What are the origins of anxiety?
Cognitive	What types of logic are used by 3-year-old children?
Language	What is the most favorable age for learning a second language?
Academic	What cognitive processes are related to reading?
Moral	What factors facilitate moral learning in 8-year-old children?
Motor	What are the sequential stages of development in eye-hand coordination?
Feeding	What is the relationship between obesity in infancy and obesity in adolescence?

a developmental landmark. The typical child is expected to pass a test item related to chronological age. The child's rate of development is relative to the norm response for specific chronological age groups. For example, the Denver Developmental Screening Test (Frankenburg et al., 1990) makes the assumption that human development progresses in a linear direction influenced by genetically based parameters. In this model, the child is ready at specific ages to learn to walk, play games cooperatively with other children, write, speak, or perform any number of other developmental tasks. Environmental experiences provide the opportunities for development to occur.

4.3.3.1 Stating the Guiding Question

The first task of the researcher is to state a research question that focuses and guides the generation of data. Piaget (1926), in the first sentence of his book, *The Language and Thought of the Child*, wrote: "The question which we shall attempt to answer in this book may be stated as follows: What are the needs which a child tends to satisfy when he talks?" (p. 1). Gesell and Thompson (1923), in their research on infant behavior, also began with a guiding question: "When does this orthogenetic patterning of the human individual begin?" (p. 9).

The potential areas for research using developmental observation are considerable. An outline of the broad scope of development and specific research questions, listed in Table 4-6, demonstrates the wide spectrum of developmental research.

The questions listed in Table 4-6 represent only a fraction of the potential research appropriate for developmental observation. The aspect of development selected by a researcher and the research questions generated provide the engine for the study. The justification and need for the study are based on practical and clinical issues.

4.3.3.2 Need for Study in Developmental Observation

For the occupational therapist, developmental research provides an interpretive bedrock for evaluating clients or students. Is this individual functioning within normal limits? To answer this question, norms pertaining to development are needed. Developmental studies therefore provide benchmarks for interpreting the developmental level and constructing sequential intervention programs. In children with developmental disabilities, such as cerebral palsy, intellectual disability, autism, or severe social deprivation, data from developmental observations are used by therapists to monitor progress in response to the intervention. The rationale behind this approach is that development progresses sequentially and in a hierarchal fashion in the typical child but can be delayed, incomplete, or impaired in the child with a developmental disability. The developmental therapist reconstructs the sequential stages in an area of development and facilitates the child's progress through each stage. Steps along a linear developmental progression are programmed for the individual child starting at his or her current level of performance.

The results of developmental observation research have a direct effect on evaluating and treating children with developmental disabilities. After delineating the need for

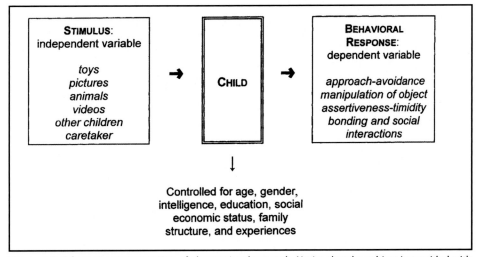

Figure 4-2. Schematic representation of observational research. Notice that the subject is provided with stimuli so as to elicit a response. The data collected are the behaviors elicited by the stimuli.

the study, the researcher designs an observational method for collecting data.

4.3.3.3 Observational Methods for Collecting Data

The technique of observation of infant behavior is not a subject that lends itself to free and easy generalization. Nor does the question "What is the best technique?" permit a simple answer. Observation methods must vary considerably with the age of the infant and with the objectives in view (Gesell, 1928).

The observational method that the developmental researcher selects should provide objective descriptive data that are representative of the child's repertoire of behavior. This is accomplished by providing the child with a stimulus that will elicit the desired behavior, schematically represented in Figure 4-2.

The researcher selects the stimulus after operationally defining the area of development in terms of the behavioral response. Tests for assessing a child's level of development such as the Bayley Scales of Infant Development-3 (Anderson & Burnett, 2017; Bayley, 2005), the Mullen Scales of Early Learning (Mullen, 1995), the Miller Function and Participation Scales (Miller, 2006), and the Goal-Oriented Assessment of Lifeskills (Miller & Oakland, 2013) are examples of this method. In the Bayley Scales of Infant Development-3, cognitive abilities are operationally defined by the following tasks:

6 months	Plays with single object (e.g., banging it)
9 months	Relational acts emerge (e.g., placing spoon in cup; placing lid on pot)
24 months	Symbolic play (e.g., pretend to drink from a cup)
36 months	Symbolic play becomes more complex (e.g., pretend to call someone on make-believe phone)

Developmental Factors	Operational Definition
Object permanence	An object is wrapped in a sheet of paper while the child is watching. The child is asked to find the object.
Manual dexterity	Child puts pegs into a peg board in a timed or untimed condition. The time taken to complete the task is age-specific.

Questions arise in this context. How does the researcher know that all aspects of a developmental factor are being considered and that the operational definition of a developmental factor is valid? These questions are pertinent in developmental research, and they demand a rationale from the investigator.

Figure 4-3. Position of the camera and baby when taking observational data.

Figure 4-4. Illustration of a photographic dome used by Gesell (1928) in observational research.

In reporting developmental data, the researcher should describe factors in the child that affect the results. These factors include age, gender, intelligence, education, socioeconomic status, family structure, and experiences. The identification and control of these factors by inclusion in the research reduces ambiguity in interpreting the results.

In addition to operationally defining the developmental factors and identifying variables within the child, the researcher must construct an objective environment for collecting valid data. Examples of study environments in developmental research are shown in Figures 4-3 and 4-4. Arrangements for observation are part of a standard procedure. Adaptations in this method include the use of a photographic dome as developed by Gesell (1928) or the use of study rooms with one-way mirrors, where the observer is not seen by the subject. Box 4-3 gives an example of a study using developmental research.

4.3.4 Longitudinal Research (Prospective Designs)

Are there developmental factors that over a time period cause changes in a person's anatomical and physiological processes, predisposing him or her to illness? Does prolonged exposure to smog cause lung cancer? Do obese adults develop heart disease when they are middle-aged at a higher rate than non-obese adults? Do children who have high IQs become leaders in the society when they are adults? What is the prognosis for high-risk children who come from socially disadvantaged environments? What is the relationship between occupational hazards and the later onset of disease? These problems are all affected by time factors.

Longitudinal research is a method used in observing the effects of independent variables on dependent variables over a prolonged period of time. The investigator uses longitudinal research to predict an outcome based on the presence of causative factors. For example, a team of researchers may study groups of individuals over a period of 20 years (from young adult to middle age) and observe whether certain groups are more vulnerable to heart attacks than others. In occupational therapy, a researcher may examine the long-term effects of sensory integration therapy on academic achievement in children with learning disabilities. Box 4-4 provides an example of longitudinal research relating cholesterol to coronary heart disease.

4.3.5 Field Observation (Ethnography)

About the same time that Gesell (1928) was experimenting with his photographic dome, cultural anthropologists developed scientific methods for collecting data describing the everyday lives of aboriginal people. Franz Boas, the noted anthropologist, wrote in the foreword to Margaret Mead's classic study *Coming of Age in Samoa* (1928) the following, which summarized field research:

> Through a comparative study of these data and through information that tells us of their growth and development, we endeavor to reconstruct, as well as may be, the history of each particular culture. Some anthropologists even hope that the comparative study will reveal some tendencies of development that recur so often that significant generalizations regarding the processes of cultural growth will be discovered. (p. xiii)

Box 4-3. Example of Developmental Observation

1. Bibliographic Notation

Kawaguchi, H., Murakami, B., & Kawai, M. (2010) Behavioral characteristics of children with high functioning pervasive developmental disorders during a game. *Journal of Epidemiology, 20*(Suppl. 2), S490-S497.

2. Abstract

"Background: To evaluate children's sociability through their behavior, we compared the motion features of children with high functioning pervasive developmental disorders (HFPDD) and typical development (TD) during a game. We selected 'Jenga' as the game because this is an interactive game played by two people. *Methods*: We observed the behavior of 7 children with HFPDD and 10 children with TD. An optical motion capture system was used to follow the movement of 3-dimensional position markers attached to caps worn by the players. *Results*: The range of head motion of the children with HFPDD was narrower than that of the control group, especially in the X-axis direction (perpendicular to the line connecting the two players). In each game, we calculated the range of motion in the X-axis of each child and divided that figure by the matched adult player's range. The average ratios of children with HFPDD and TD were 0.64 and 0.89 (number of games are 61 and 18), and the difference of these two ratios is significant ($P < 0.001$). *Conclusions*: This ratio has sensitivity to identify HFPDD children and could be useful in their child care."

3. Justification and Need

"We attempted to derive a behavioral indicator connected to sociability based on comparing the behavioral characteristics of two groups of children, children who are socially challenged (with high functioning pervasive developmental disorders (HFPDD) and those who are not (children with [TD])" (p. S491).

4. Literature Review

The authors cited 45 references from the literature. Cited journals included but were not limited to *Journal of Epidemiology, Trends in Cognitive Science, Brain Imaging Behavior, Child Development, Science, Journal of Child Psychiatry and Psychology, Developmental Psychology, Perceptual and Motor Skills, Japanese Journal of Child Adolescent Psychiatry*, and *Early Development and Parent*. The majority were published in the last 10 years.

5. Research Hypothesis or Guiding Question

The authors sought evidence to demonstrate that children with HFPDD as compared to a normal typical group of children responded differently in their social behavior as observed in playing a Japanese game.

6. Methods

Six video cameras, two microphones, and an optical motion capture system set up inside an observation room recorded the social interaction of the participants.

7. Results

The results of the observations indicated that HFPDD children have problems conveying their interests through movement and seemed to have difficulty in nonverbal communication.

8. Conclusions

"Making the assumption that children with developmental disorders are creating communicative signals, if we make efforts to pick up those signals, and educate widely with this objective, we may be able to create a society where children with developmental disorders can live comfortably" (p. S497).

(continued)

Box 4-3. Example of Developmental Observation (continued)

9. Limitations

Further research is needed to replicate the study with another group of children with HFPDD to determine if the methodology is reliable and valid in observing children at play.

10. Major References Cited

Frith, C. D., & Frith, U. (2006). The neuron basis of mentalizing. *Neuron, 50*, 531-534.

Ozonoff, S., & Miller, J. N. (1995) Teaching theory of mind: A new approach to social skills training for individuals with autism. *Journal of Autism and Developmental Disorders, 25*, 415-433.

Rogers, S. J., Hepburn, S. L., Stackhouse, T., & Wehner, E. (2003). Imitation performance in toddlers with autism and those with other developmental disorders. *Journal of Child Psychiatry and Psychology, 44*, 763-781.

Sallows, G. O., & Graupner, T. D. (2005). Intensive behavioral treatment for children with autism: Four-year outcome and predictors. *American Journal of Mental Retardation, 110*, 417-438.

Yamamoto, J., Kakutani, A., & Terada, M. (2001). Establishing joint visual attention and pointing in autistic children with no functional language. *Perceptual Motor Skills, 92*, 755-770.

Box 4-4. Example of a Longitudinal Study

1. Bibliographic Notation

Sendroy-Terrill, M., Whiteneck, G. G., & Brooks, C. A. (2010). Aging with traumatic brain injury: Cross-sectional follow-up of people receiving inpatient rehabilitation over more than 3 decades. *Archives of Physical Medicine and Rehabilitation, 91*,489-497.

2. Abstract

"*Objective*: To investigate aging with [TBI] by determining if long-term outcomes after TBI are predicted by years postinjury and age at injury after controlling for the severity of the injury and sex. *Design*: Cross-sectional follow-up telephone survey. *Setting*: Community residents who had received initial treatment in a comprehensive inpatient rehabilitation hospital. *Participants*: Survivors of TBI (N = 243) stratified by years postinjury (in seven 5-year cohorts ranging from 1 to over 30 years postinjury) and by age at injury (in 2 cohorts of people injured before or after age 30). *Interventions*: None. *Main Outcome Measures*: Measures of postconcussive symptoms, major secondary conditions including fatigue (Modified Fatigue Impact Scale), physical and cognitive activity limitations (FIM [Functional Independence Measure], Alertness Behavior Subscale of the Sickness Impact Profile, Medical Outcomes Study 12-Item Health Status Survey Short Form), societal participation restrictions (Craig Handicap Assessment and Reporting Technique), environmental barriers (Craig Hospital Inventory of Environmental Factors), and perceived quality of life (Satisfaction with Life Scale). *Results*: Most problems identified by the outcome measures were reported by one fourth to one half of the study participants. Increasing decade's postinjury predicted declines in physical and cognitive functioning, declines in societal participation, and increases in contractures. Increasing age at injury predicted declines in functional independence, increases in fatigue, declines in societal participation, and declines in perceived environmental barriers. *Conclusions*: This investigation has increased our understanding of the aging process after TBI by demonstrating that both components of aging (years postinjury and age at injury) are predictive of several outcomes after TBI."

3. Justification and Need

The purpose of this descriptive exploratory study was to determine whether age at injury is associated with progressive functional decline. This hypothesis has important intervention implications, particularly because the advent of neuroprotective therapies for dementia will make it important to identify people at risk for cognitive decline in late life.

(continued)

Box 4-4. Example of a Longitudinal Study (continued)

4. Literature Review

The authors did an extensive review of the literature with 54 references cited. Cited journals included but were not limited to *Archives of Physical Medicine and Rehabilitation, Brain Injury, Annals of Neurology, Journal of Head Rehabilitation Trauma, Archives in Neurology, Neurorehabilitation, Journal of Neurology, Journal of Trauma*, and *Journal of the American Medical Association*.

5. Research Hypothesis or Guiding Question

The primary hypothesis stated that older patients show greater decline in neurological function over the first 5 years after TBI than younger patients.

6. Methods

The study was identified as a longitudinal cohort study. It included participants who met the following criteria: (a) age of 16 years or older at the time of TBI, (b) arrival at a hospital emergency department within 8 hours after injury, (c) receipt of acute and rehabilitation treatment at a traumatic brain injury model system affiliated hospitals, (d) complete Disability Rating Scale (DRS) 25 scores taken at 1- and 5-year follow-up evaluations, and (e) provision of informed consent directly or by proxy. At the time of this investigation, 1127 patients were eligible to receive a 5-year post-TBI DRS evaluation specified in the traumatic brain injury model system protocol, and 624 (55%) patients had complete DRS data 5 years post-TBI. Four hundred twenty-eight patients had complete DRS outcome data at both year 1 and year 5 (38 %) and constituted the cohort analyzed here.

7. Results

All three age groups improved between admission and rehabilitation through year 5, and the magnitude (or slope) of improvement among the three age groups was similar through the first year post-injury. Paired-sample *t*-test results show significant improvement in functioning as measured by the four outcome measures (i.e., DRS, FIM, cognitive domain of the FIM, Extended Glasgow Outcome Scale) over time among the youngest group. In addition, the intermediate group showed significant improvement on the DRS, and the oldest did not show significant improvement on any of the outcome measures. Change scores for the outcome measures were examined as a marker of the magnitude of improvement between year 1 and year 5. The two younger groups showed greater change in DRS than the oldest group, and there were no differences in magnitude of change among the other outcome measures.

8. Conclusions

The study supported the primary hypothesis that older survivors of TBI show greater functional decline than younger survivors. Results from this study show that younger survivors of TBI showed significant improvement in disability ratings between the year 1 and year 5 post-injury, whereas older counterparts did not show significant improvement in outcome measures over the same time period. Furthermore, the results suggest older survivors have a higher risk of functional decline than younger survivors because patients aged 26 years or younger showed a lower rate of decline over a 4-year span than older patients.

9. Limitations

One limitation of the study was the potential for systematic bias created by subjects lost to follow-up. Employment could be overestimated because of the loss of subjects with prior histories of substance abuse. Another limitation of the present investigation is that it is difficult to determine whether the decline in disability rating over time experienced by the oldest group is attributed to disabling effects of brain injury or simply decline associated with normative aging. Future studies may need to incorporate an orthopedic control group separated into age groups.

(continued)

Box 4-4. Example of a Longitudinal Study (continued)

10. Major References Cited

Consensus Conference. Rehabilitation of persons with traumatic brain injury (NIH Consensus Development Panel on Rehabilitation of Persons with Traumatic Brain Injury). (1999). *Journal of the American Medical Association, 282,* 974-983.

Flanagan, S. R., Hibbard, M. R., & Gordon, W. A. (2005). The impact of age on traumatic brain injury. *Physical Medicine and Rehabilitation Clinics of North America, 16,* 163-177.

Thurman, D. J., Alverson, C., Dunn, K. A., Guerrero, J., & Sniezek, J. E. (1999). Traumatic brain injury in the United States: A public health perspective. *Journal of Head Trauma Rehabilitation, 14,* 602-615.

Whitnall, L., McMillan, T. M., Murray, G. D., &Teasdale, G. M. (2006). Disability in young people and adults after head injury: 5–7 year follow up of a prospective cohort study. *Journal of Neurology, Neurosurgery, and Psychiatry, 77,* 640-645.

Mead (1928) attempted to answer the question "Are the disturbances which vex our adolescents due to the nature of adolescence itself or to the civilization?" (pp. 6-7). She lived in Samoa for 6 months, and there she analyzed the life and development of 68 girls between the ages of 8 and 20 years. She was particularly concerned with three villages on the island of Tau.

In her field study, Mead (1928) painted a vivid and complete picture of the island life of adolescent girls. She felt that certain characteristics, basically Samoan, enable adolescent girls to pass through puberty without the storms and crises that are part of living in Western society. Chiefly, a Samoan girl may leave her immediate household and go to live with another family at any time, especially if she feels put upon. Other characteristics concern life roles, absence of double standards, familiarity with disasters such as death, casual family relationships as opposed to intense ones, and a specific place in society for each member. Further, the author pointed to a tolerance for sexually diverse behavior and concomitant lack of guilty feelings about such behavior, absence of extreme poverty, and a less stressful environment as reasons for a more serene adolescence than that found elsewhere in the world.

Mead's pioneering research led to the field of ethnography: to reconstruct accurately a particular culture and to search for patterns that can be generalized to a specific population or provide theoretical insights into the human condition. The observations occur in a natural setting, such as in a village, an urban neighborhood, a family home, a playground, a street corner, an Israeli kibbutz, or a family coping with severe socioeconomic challenges in New York City (see also Hall, 1966; Jessor, Colby, & Shweder, 1996).

Henry's (1971) in-depth study of five families in which a child with psychosis was present is a bleak and brilliant example of field observation. He proposes that the main difference between "them and us" is "that they [families with a child with psychosis] seem to go to extremes and do too many things that are upsetting" (p. xx). Henry detailed communication patterns, physical interaction, and positions of power in each of the five families. He

faithfully recorded the emotional content of the parents' communication patterns and the effects on their children. To record accurately, he lived with four of the five families for a short time and relied on a trained observer to supply similar observations about the fifth family. The five studies involved field visits to each family once per week. Rapport was established when the investigator informed each family that this kind of observation would perhaps aid other children with psychosis. He maintained confidentiality in the study by altering some of the details of family life and all of the names of the families.

4.3.5.1 The Application of Field Observation (Ethnography) to Occupational Therapy

What research problems are appropriate to field observations? Some possibilities are as follows:

- Research involving the culture of individuals with disabilities living in specialized environments, such as halfway houses, forensic units, adult day care, psychiatric hospitals, communities for individuals with physical disabilities, and residential institutions for the individuals with profound intellectual disabilities (Gleason, 1990; McColl & Paterson, 1997)
- Client advocacy (Sachs & Linn, 1997)
- Occupational therapy practice (Fitzgerald, Mullavey-O'Byrne, & Clemson, 1997)
- Meaning of play (Gleason, 1990)
- Mental health day programs (Townsend, 1996)
- Inclusionary settings for individuals with special needs (Falk-Ross, 1996; Miller, 1990)
- Daily occupations of Orthodox Jewish couples (Frank et al., 1997)
- Cultural diversity (Adger, 1994; Klimidis, Minas, & Kokanovic, 2006; Luera, 1994; Malave & Duquette, 1991; Whiteford, 1995)
- Cultural competency of health care professionals (Noble, Noble, & Hand, 2009)
- Ethnogeriatric studies (McBride & Lewis, 2004)

- Aging adult children with disabilities and their families (Barnhart, 2001)

4.3.5.2 Advantages of Field Observation

The main purpose of field observation or ethnography is to describe accurately the social structure and social processes engaged in by a group of people. The investigator observes the interactions between members of a group, records their responses, and describes their formal codes for communications and the unwritten rules that guide their behaviors (Frederic, 1928; Mead, 1928). In the field study, the investigator may attempt to become a participant observer, performing the occupational roles and enacting the forms of activities of the people studied, in order to gain deeper insight into their meanings. One major advantage of the field observation is that data obtained from this method are not affected by artificial laboratory conditions. Another advantage is that the investigator observes behavior directly rather than eliciting verbal responses, such as through group personality tests. A third advantage is that the observer, who is not an indigenous member of the culture, will interpret patterns and behaviors differently from the way that these are acknowledged by those within the culture. Indeed, the "outsider" assists in bringing to the forefront patterns that, being embedded in "insider" behavior, are sometimes not readily described or easily recognized by members of the group.

Which research method would be appropriate for examining the interactions in a residential school for individuals with profound developmental delays? It is not possible to construct experimental conditions or control for all of the possible variables that could affect the dependent variable, which is, in this example, the rate of development in the child. The most appropriate method would be qualitative research, where the investigator observes, like an ethnographer in a natural setting, the structures and processes of the institution and the transactions and interactions between all the participants in the institutional setting.

4.3.5.3 Methods of Field Observation

The investigator using field observation research is initially guided by research questions that focus on the important issues in social structures and social processes, such as education, vocational preparation, health care, child-rearing practices, sexual expression, ethical standards, peer relationships, leisure patterns, and recreation (Box 4-5). Broad areas selected for field observation are decided before the investigator collects data. The preparation for field observation is detailed in the Research Design section. Here the investigator decides:

- The total time period for field observation
- The methods used in establishing rapport with the group
- The broad areas in a social structure to be investigated

- The observational recording devices to be used (e.g., audio or video recorders)
- Methods for obtaining informed consent and preserving the confidentiality of group
- Interview protocols for collecting data (e.g., rating scales, questionnaires, attitude surveys)

4.3.6 Historical Research

4.3.6.1 Definition

Historical research is a systematic method for reconstructing events that happened in the past to describe and understand them. As applied to occupational therapy, historical research pertains to (a) the chronology of events in occupational therapy, (b) the interrelationship between these events, and (c) the critical factors influencing them. For example, one might want to describe the events and identify the individuals that led to the formation of the discipline of occupational therapy in 1917. In studying historical data in occupational therapy, the investigator examines the individuals who were significant in shaping events and creating change, as well as the institutions or organizations that were part of the historical process. The scientific approach to collecting historical data is similar to all methods of research in that the investigator proposes a research problem, states guiding questions, collects data, interprets the results, and arrives at conclusions and implications. The main differences between historical research and other types of research models are in the format of guiding questions and in the use of related literature. In historical research the guiding questions serve as the rationale for collecting data and the literature review and examination of artifacts provide the data, while the literature review generates guiding questions in other qualitative methods.

4.3.6.2 Purposes

Fraenkel and Wallen (1990) suggested five purposes for historical research:

1. "To make people aware of what has happened in the past so they may learn from past failures and successes" (p. 411): For example, cone stacking has been used rather than craft activities to increase fine motor coordination. The craft activity is client centered and increases motivation, whereas the cone stacking is a non-meaningful repetitive activity.

2. "To learn how things were done in the past to see if they might be applicable to the present day problems and concerns" (p. 411): The model used in adult day centers from the 1950s and 1960s was successful in treating individuals with psychosocial illnesses. Adult day care centers now use this model in caring for individuals with Alzheimer's disease.

3. "To assist in prediction" (p. 412). Special education has alternated between placing students with special needs into self-contained classrooms and into the general

BOX 4-5. EXAMPLE OF ETHNOGRAPHIC RESEARCH

1. Bibliographic Notation

Berinstein, S., & Magalhaes, L. (2009). A study of the essence of play experience to children living in Zanzibar, Tanzania. *Occupational Therapy International*, 16, 89-106.

2. Abstract

"This study aimed to gain an understanding of the essence of play experience to children in Zanzibar, Tanzania. A phenomenological approach using the photovoice method was adopted. The study was carried out over 4 weeks, with 12 boys and 4 girls. Four key themes emerged from the analysis of 116 photographs: creative play, physical play/games, football and equipment play. The findings suggest that play experience in Zanzibar has aspects of creativity and resourcefulness, and influences from tradition, culture and poverty. Furthermore, that opportunity for play may differ for children in Tanzania, compared with children in Western countries. Unequal boy and girl participants, and the lack of representation of children with a disability were some limitations of this study. The occupational therapy profession may want to further investigate the opportunities for play for children living in developing countries. Additionally, it may be valuable to look at different aspects of play, such as its meaning to children from different cultures and its potential restorative value for children who have experienced traumatic events."

3. Justification and Need

Play is recognized to be universal in nature but is influenced by its cultural context. The context and culture of Tanzania will influence how children living in poverty experience play. This study aimed to gain an understanding of the essence of play experience to children living in Zanzibar, Tanzania.

4. Literature Review

Forty-two references were cited in this study. Cited journals included but were not limited to *American Journal of Occupational Therapy, Australian Journal of Occupational Therapy, Child: Care, Health and Development, Canadian Journal of Occupational Therapy, Archives of Pediatrics and Adolescent Medicine, Pediatrics, Journal of Children and Poverty, Journal of Community Practice, Health, Education and Behavior,* and *Journal of Advanced Nursing*.

5. Research Hypothesis or Guiding Question

Does the opportunity for play, as well as the meaning of play, differ in Tanzania as compared to Western countries?

6. Methods

A phenomenological approach using the photovoice method was used to explore the essence of play experience to children living in Zanzibar. The participants were students, ranging from ages 10 to 13 years old, from a school in Zanzibar. This school has students from varying socioeconomic backgrounds who are predominantly of the Muslim religion and speak Swahili as their first language.

7. Results

Four categories emerged from the photovoice process that included creative play, physical play/games, football, and equipment play. Children seemed to view play as about just having fun, about getting fit, about strengthening the body, and for social interaction. In Zanzibar, play seems to have aspects of creativity, resourcefulness, differences between boys and girls, and influences from tradition and culture.

(continued)

Box 4-5. Example of Ethnographic Research (continued)

8. Conclusions

Play seems to be self-driven, outside the relationship of the family, a social endeavour, and about waking the body up and occupying free time, as opposed to being about developing social, physical, and cognitive skills. Furthermore, despite the lack of adult encouragement and available resources to play, children find ways to engage in play together.

9. Limitations

The available time to carry out this research was limited first to the duration of the first author's (researcher) occupational therapy placement in Zanzibar. Second, assistance was limited to the researcher's supervisor in Canada. Third, financial assistance was limited to what the researcher could afford. More support may have allowed for the opportunity to work more closely with the participants. Moreover, financial support would have allowed the researcher to hire a translator for the duration of the 4 weeks and purchase more disposable cameras to permit more opportunity to practice. Other factors limiting this study were the researcher's lack of previous experience in carrying out photovoice and the language barrier that existed.

10. Major References Cited

Burdette, H. L., & Whitaker, R. C. (2005). Resurrecting free play in young children. *Archives of Pediatrics & Adolescent Medicine, 159,* 46-50.

Ginsburg, K. R. (2007). The importance of play in promoting healthy child development and maintaining strong parent-child bonds. *Pediatrics, 119,* 182-191.

McArdle, P. (2001). Children's play. *Child: Care, Health and Development, 27,* 509-514.

Simo-Algado, S., Mehta, N., Kronenberg, F., Cockburn, L., & Kirsh, B. (2002). Occupational therapy intervention with children survivors of war. *Canadian Journal of Occupational Therapy, 69,* 205-217.

---

education program. Examination of mainstreaming in the 1980s demonstrated that these students would not succeed in the general education program without support from special educators, occupational therapists, and other allied health personnel.

4. "To test hypotheses concerning relationships or trends" (p. 412). Over the last 80 years, an examination of trends of employment settings has shown a change for occupational therapists from hospital-based settings to schools, home health care, and other community-based settings.

5. "To understand present educational practices and policies more fully" (p. 412). To understand Medicare reimbursement, occupational therapists study previous legislation and litigation leading to the present policies.

4.3.6.3 Historical Research Related to Occupational Therapy

The following are some examples of historical research related to occupational therapy:

- Bockoven, J. S. (1971). Occupational therapy—A historical perspective. Legacy of moral treatment—1800s to 1910. *American Journal of Occupational Therapy, 25,* 223-225.

- Cockburn, L. (2005) . Canadian occupational therapists' contributions to prisoners of war in World War II. *Canadian Journal of Occupational Therapy, 72,* 183-188.

- Frank, G. (1992). Opening feminist histories of occupational therapy. *American Journal of Occupational Therapy, 46,* 989-999.

- Friedland, J., & Silva, J. (2008). Evolving identities: Thomas Bessell Kidner and occupational therapy in the United States. *American Journal of Occupational Therapy, 62,* 349-360.

- Gutman, S. A. (1995). Influence of the U.S. military and occupational therapy reconstruction aides in World War I on the development of occupational therapy. *American Journal of Occupational Therapy, 49,* 256-262.

- Hamlin, R. B. (1992). Embracing our past, informing our future: A feminist revision of health care. *American Journal of Occupational Therapy, 46,* 1028-1035.

- Horghagen, S., Josephsson, S., & Alsaker, S. (2007). The use of craft activities as an occupational therapy treatment modality in Norway during 1952-1960. *Occupational Therapy International, 14,* 42-56.

- Newton, S. (2007). The growth of the profession of occupational therapy. *U.S. Army Medical Department Journal, Jan-Mar,* 51-58.
- Peloquin, S. M. (1991). Occupational therapy service: Individual and collective understandings of the founders, Part 2. *American Journal of Occupational Therapy, 45,* 733-744.
- Reitz, S. M. (1992). A historical review of occupational therapy's role in preventive health and wellness. *American Journal of Occupational Therapy, 46,* 50-55.
- Stecco, C., & Aldegheri, R. (2008). Historical review of carpal tunnel syndrome. *La Chirurgia degli Organi di Movimento. 92,* 7-10.
- Woodside, H. H. (1971). Occupational therapy—A historical perspective. The development of occupational therapy 1910-1929. *American Journal of Occupational Therapy, 25,* 226-230.

4.3.6.4 Hypothetical Historical Questions in Occupational Therapy

- How did occupational therapists treat individuals with polio during the 1950s?
- What treatment techniques were used by occupational therapists in large mental hospitals during the 1930s?
- What were some of the experiences and education of noted individuals in occupational therapy?
- How is occupational therapy treated in the literature by individuals who write about their disability experiences?
- How have different philosophical viewpoints in occupational therapy influenced intervention in the schools?
- What is the history of the use of arts and crafts in occupational therapy?
- What are the major theories that have influenced clinical treatment trends through time?

4.3.6.5 Format of Historical Research

The outline of historical research is as follows:
- *Part I*: The statement of problem and significance of the study (e.g., how the study impacts on occupational therapy)
- *Part II*: Guiding questions and methods for collecting data
- *Part III*: The results, including the collection of data from primary and secondary sources
- *Part IV*: A discussion of the results based on previous data from other studies
- *Part V*: Conclusions, implications of results, and recommendations for further study

4.3.6.5.1 Part I: The Statement of Problem and Significance of the Study.

What are potential areas for historical research in occupational therapy? How does one determine its significance?

These are issues of concern for the historical researcher or historiographer planning a study. Barzun (1974), in a discussion of psychohistory, stated that the primary purpose of the new history is explanation, and the ulterior motive is action. He wrote, "The type of explanation sought is the scientific; that is, showing a connection ('durable link') between the facts and a definable cause. Classification, then analysis, then prediction is the sequence that leads naturally to action" (Barzun, 1974, p. 60). Barzun (1974) suggested that the historiographer's main motive is to obtain evidence in support of a cause. In effect, the historical researcher is a tool for change. This approach to medicine and health care can lead to research supporting causes that advocate change in the delivery of health care, public health education, and the training and preparation of health professionals. The vulnerability of this approach is that the researcher could subjectively determine what evidence to cite. The historiographer should start with a relevant problem and objectively collect data. Table 4-7 outlines the relationship between the researcher's motive and the problem being investigated using the historical research model.

4.3.6.5.2 Part II: Guiding Questions and Methods for Collecting Data

After narrowing the area of investigation to a researchable question, the researcher states any assumptions underlying the study. These assumptions are the researcher's preliminary opinions, attitudes, and knowledge in the area. For example, if a researcher is interested in what factors led to the development of the rehabilitation movement in the 20th century, tentative assumptions could be proposed. These are:

- The rehabilitation movement developed in response to the health needs of the chronically disabled individual.
- The rehabilitation movement was facilitated by governmental legislation related to social security.
- The industrialized countries were first to educate specialized rehabilitation workers.
- World War I and World War II generated the need for developing a technology for restoring function in soldiers who were severely wounded.
- The first leaders in the rehabilitation movement were social reformers.

Continuing with these examples, the researcher generates the following questions:
- What was the historical chronology of the rehabilitation movement?
- How did social welfare programs influence rehabilitation legislation?
- How did advances in medical treatment influence rehabilitation of individuals with chronic disabilities?
- When did the allied health professions emerge and affect the rehabilitation movement?
- What scientific technology facilitated advances in rehabilitation medicine?

TABLE 4-7	
RELATIONSHIPS BETWEEN RESEARCHER'S MOTIVE AND INVESTIGATED PROBLEM	
MOTIVE OF RESEARCHER	**STATEMENT OF PROBLEM**
Establishing the occupational therapist as an independent practitioner	How did the independent health practitioner evolve historically?
Integrating the individual with intellectual disability into the community	What factors led to the institutionalization of individuals with mental retardation from 1900 to 1950?
Incorporating wellness in health education of public schools	What is the history of health education in public schools?
Ensuring the right of access to primary health for every individual	Historically what are the determining factors regarding access to health care?
Gaining parity in health insurance coverage for psychosocial disabilities	Why have insurance companies typically restricted reimbursement for psychosocial disabilities?

- Who are the leaders and supporters of the rehabilitation movement?

These guiding questions provide the content areas for the literature search and collection of data. The plan for collecting the data should be carefully formulated. The *research plan* is the outline of primary and secondary sources to be used in the data collection procedure. These sources include the following:

- Published books, periodicals, newspapers, and pamphlets
- Unpublished conference proceedings and minutes of meetings
- Official records and vital statistics
- Governmental documents, archives, and publications
- Personal letters, diaries, and memoirs
- Collateral interviews of eyewitnesses
- Audio recordings and films

4.3.6.5.3 Part III: The Results

The essential task of the historical researcher is to collect data and evaluate it for reliability and validity. By obtaining various sources of information, the researcher can cross-check the data, thereby substantiating conclusions. This procedure is called *triangulation*. *Primary sources* that represent first-hand data, such as eyewitnesses and contemporary documents, are the best evidence for the historical researcher. In comparison, *secondary sources* are the interpretations and critiques of historical evidence based on primary data. Primary sources are the raw data for historical research, while secondary sources serve as supportive evidence. In researching a problem, the investigator should seek evidence that is direct, objective, and verifiable. It should be clear that one unit of datum is not conclusive. The *personal equation*, which is the observer's effect on what is being observed and measured, must be controlled by the investigator's substantiating evidence from more than one primary source in eyewitness accounts.

Secondary sources such as encyclopedias, textbooks, and critical essays are useful in initially obtaining an overview of an historical problem. These sources represent the generally accepted versions of historical events that have been retold in a reductive manner. The critical historiographer need not accept any evidence until primary data can substantiate the facts.

4.3.6.5.4 Part IV: Discussion of Results and Part V: Conclusions and Recommendations

The raw data of a historical study must be critically analyzed by the investigator for its validity before any conclusions or generalizations can be made. The historical researcher must examine every document and piece of evidence with a skeptical eye, seeking substantiating proof for the authorship and the accuracy of its contents. *External criticism* of a document is a testimony of its authenticity. The Hippocratic writings are an example of unknown authorship and unknown copyright date. It is important for the historical researcher to substantiate the author of every document, the date it was written, and the place of origination or presentation, as evidence for external validity. Indirect means for collecting evidence are frequently used by historians. These methods include archeology and paleography (e.g., study of ancient manuscripts and examination of art objects). Ancient medical instruments used in surgery were discovered through archeological evidence. Questions that might be asked when examining external validity include the following (Fraenkel & Wallen, 1990):

- Did the purported author actually write the document or report the event?
- Do we know the exact date that the document was written?
- Do we know where the document was written or where the observation took place?

TABLE 4-8

HISTORY OF POLIO RESEARCH IN THE UNITED STATES

TIME	EVENT	SETTING	CONTRIBUTORS
1884	Polio epidemics identified	United States	
1907	Initial research in polio	Rockefeller Institute	Flexner
1910–1913	Poliovirus implicated	Rockefeller Institute	Flexner
1920–1930	Transmission of polio	Rockefeller Institute	Olitsky
1938	Warm Springs Foundation	Georgia	Roosevelt
1938	Electron microscope	Germany	Borries
1946	Immunization of monkeys	Johns Hopkins	Morgan
1948–1951	Identification of poliovirus	University of California Johns Hopkins University of Pittsburgh	Kessel Bodian Salk
1949	Cultivation of poliovirus	Harvard	Enders
1952	Salk vaccine (dead intramuscular vaccine)	University of Pittsburgh	Salk
1954	Mass vaccinations	University of Michigan	Francis
1958	Sabin Vaccine (oral live vaccine)	University of Cincinnati	Sabin

Adapted from Benison, S. (1972). In G. Holton (Ed.). *The twentieth-century sciences: Studies in the biography of ideas* (pp. 308-343). New York, NY: W.W. Norton & Company.

- Are we sure that the writing of the document and the observation were not influenced by external events or individuals?
- Are we sure the document is genuine?

The next step of the historical researcher is to establish the validity or truth contained in a document. This process is called *internal criticism*. The purpose of this process is to establish as near as possible the actuality of an event. Fraenkel and Wallen (1990) suggested the following types of questions:

- Was the author an eyewitness to the event?
- Did the author participate in the event?
- What expertise did the author have to discuss or report the event?
- Was the author biased or subjective in the observation, or did the author have a vested interest in the event's interpretation?

Historical surveys of medical progress are frequently filled with interpretative statements that go beyond the evidence and selective omissions that fail to give a true perspective of events or individuals who had an impact on treatment. It is left to the historical researcher in occupational therapy to carefully evaluate the biases of the authors when interpreting evidence. Generalizations and synthesizing statements should be carefully documented. In examining the causes of events, the historiographer takes a multidimensional point of view when examining the influences of contemporary practices of treatment, discoveries, patterns of dysfunction, governmental and community intervention, war, and natural disasters. One variable rarely changes the course of history.

A good example of historical research is a scholarly manuscript by Saul Benison (1972), "The History of Polio Research in the United States: Appraisal and Lessons." In this article, Benison documented the chronological events that led to a safe and effective vaccine for preventing polio. He analyzed the problem from three perspectives: (a) time of events, (b) settings where research took place, and (c) individuals and scientists who had an impact on the problem and facilitated progress in the development of a vaccine. These three factors are detailed in Table 4-8.

In documenting the chronology of events and the individuals who made important contributions to the development of a successful polio vaccine, Benison (1972) used the following primary sources:

- Contemporary accounts of the early polio epidemics from 1894 to 1910
- Autobiographical notes
- History of the Rockefeller Institute
- Foreign journals
- Scholarly articles by Flexner, Pritchett, & Henry (1910)
- Conference proceedings

- Research articles
- *Bulletin of the History of Medicine*
- National Foundation Archives
- History of Warm Springs
- Private communication
- Minutes of committees
- Files from the National Foundation
- Biographical essays
- Final reports of research grants
- Congressional hearings

In total, Benison (1972) used 117 citations to document his article. He concluded that the development of a successful polio vaccine was a cooperative effort by researchers in major universities funded by two private organizations—the Rockefeller Foundation and the National Foundation—with external support from the U. S. Public Health Service. Benison's lesson in the article was that modern medical progress is a cooperative effort where researchers from diverse settings are supported by the federal government, private foundations, and voluntary health agencies.

The historical research article by Benison (1972) is an example of rigorous documentation providing strong external validity. Benison's article should serve as a model for research in occupational therapy. See Box 4-6 for another example of historical research.

Potential areas for historical research in occupational therapy include the following:

- Biographies of founders of the discipline of occupational therapy
- Development of innovative assistive technology
- Development of social attitude toward psychosocial illness
- Chronological analysis of the treatment of a disability
- History of the occupational therapy discipline
- History of a hospital, health facility, organization, or institution
- History of reimbursement practices
- History of movements in occupational therapy (e.g., rehabilitation, normalization)

4.4 COLLECTING QUALITATIVE DATA

There are many ways to collect qualitative data. Table 4-9 gives some examples. These are more fully explained in the following paragraphs.

4.4.1 Interviewing

The most common data collection method in qualitative research is interviewing. Using interviews as a research method rests on the assumption that "the perspective of others is meaningful, knowable, and able to be made explicit" (Patton, 1990, p. 270). In short, researchers conduct interviews to find out about things that cannot be directly observed. Everyday familiarity with conversational or therapeutic interviews can lead novice researchers to regard interviewing for research purposes as quite straightforward; however, to effectively use interviewing as a research method requires knowledge of, and practice with, available techniques.

Research interviews take several forms. Interviews can be done face-to-face, over the telephone, or in a group. The format may be structured, semi-structured, or open-ended. Interviewing may be used to collect personal experiences, to understand a particular phenomenon, or to identify the perspective of a particular group of people. Interviews may be brief or lengthy, they may be one-off, or part of a series.

Oftentimes, investigators will employ a combination of interviewing approaches if this suits the purpose of the research and the research questions. For example, an interview may begin with a standardized, structured format, followed by sections made up of semi-structured questions. Alternatively, the interview may begin with an unstructured, open-ended format and conclude with a set of standardized questions. The type of interview that will best suit the research purpose needs particular care and thought.

4.4.1.1 Structured Interviewing

In this type of interview, the interviewer uses a preestablished set of questions in a uniform manner. Although the questions may be open-ended, the interviewer cannot alter the predetermined format. The aim of this structured approach is to achieve as close as possible a standard format across interviewers and respondents. One disadvantage of this approach is that the interviewer is not able to pursue topics of interest that arise during the interview.

4.4.1.2 Semi-Structured Interviewing

This type of interviewing utilizes a general interview guide. The issues to be covered in the interview are predetermined; however, question format and exact content are not prespecified. Rather, the interviewer uses a guide that can be adapted, as necessary, during the interview. Semi-structured interviewing is an effective use of time while still allowing the interviewer to build up rapport and conduct the interview in a flexible way. This approach is particularly appropriate for group interviews where it can be used to encourage all participants to contribute to the topic under discussion.

Box 4-6. Example of Historical Research

1. Bibliographical Notation

Sachs, D., & Sussman, N. (1995). Historical research: The first decade of occupational therapy in Israel: 1946-1956. *Occupational Therapy International, 2,* 241-256.

2. Abstract

"The present study examined the first decade of the development of occupational therapy in Israel: 1946-1956. The structural-functional approach to the study of professions, which provided the theoretical framework for this study, identifies three formal organizations in the professions: the practice, the educational system, and the association. The purpose of this article was to follow the development of occupational therapy and to examine the interrelations of the profession's three formal organizations in the reviewed period. The methodology of the study was based on qualitative historical methods. Data collection included oral histories, and published and unpublished written material. Data organization and analysis were within the framework of the structural-functional approach. Data analysis indicated that 'expansion' was a major theme affecting the development of occupational therapy, the reason for which lies within the historical background of the period under investigation. In addition, data indicated that the practice was the strongest and most active organization in occupational therapy and that expansion in practice was beyond the capacity of both the educational system and the professional association. The interrelations of the three formal organizations, and the rapid expansion of occupational therapy practice, had a lasting effect on the development of occupational therapy in Israel."

3. Justification and Need

Because "historical research sheds light on present behaviors and practices" (p. 242), this study was completed to "understand current theories and practices more accurately, and to plan intelligently for the future" (p. 242).

4. Literature Review

Forty-two references were cited in the study. Articles came from a wide variety of sources, including files at the Occupational Therapy School at the Hebrew University from 1947 to 1954; archives of Hadassah 1941-1949; *Israeli Journal of Occupational Therapy; Health Services in Israel: A Ten Year Survey 1948-1958*; and Trade Unions in Israel.

5. Research Hypothesis or Guiding Question

The guiding questions explicitly stated were (a) "How did the practice [in occupational therapy] develop and how did it adapt itself to the growing needs of the healthcare services?" (b) "How did the educational system cope with practice needs?" and (c) "How did the association [Israeli Occupational Therapy Association] meet the needs of the profession?" (p. 244)

6. Methods

Interviews were held with nine female occupational therapists who had been practicing between 1946 and 1956 and who were considered prominent leaders in the development of occupational therapy in Israel. Primary documents including memoirs and archived materials were accessed by the investigators. These materials were analyzed using the structural-functional approach (Parsons, 1939). The credibility of the data was obtained by validating oral testimonies with contemporary documents.

7. Results

The historical development was organized into three periods, each covering the practice, the education system, and the professional association: (a) Preliminary Period, 1941-1945; (b) The Formative Years, 1946-1948; and (c) Expansion: 1949-1956.

(continued)

Box 4-6. Example of Historical Research (continued)

8. Conclusions

"Analysis of the data indicates that the practice was the strongest and most active organization [as compared with education and professional association] in the function of occupational therapy. Expansion in the practice was beyond the capacity of the education and the association…. By employing historical research methods and a conceptual framework to the study of professions, this study exposed the origin of some of the problems faced by occupational therapy in Israel" (pp. 254-255).

9. Limitations

The study only interviewed nine individuals when collecting the bulk of the data. In addition, some contemporary documents were not available and presumed to have been lost due to war conditions.

10. Major References Cited

Archives of Hadassah. (1941–1949). *Occupational therapy correspondence services*. New York: Hadassah.

Files at the Occupational Therapy School, 1st Class. (1947–1949). Jerusalem, Israel: Hebrew University.

Files at the Occupational Therapy School, 2nd Class. (1949–1951). Jerusalem, Israel: Hebrew University.

Files at the Occupational Therapy School, 3rd Class. (1952–1954). Jerusalem, Israel: Hebrew University.

Grushka, T. (1959). *Health services in Israel: A ten year survey 1948–1958*. Jerusalem, Israel: Ministry of Health.

Grushka, T. (1968). *Health services in Israel*. Jerusalem, Israel: Ministry of Health.

Sussman, N. (1989). *The history of occupational therapy in Israel: The first decade—1946-1956*. Unpublished master's thesis. New York, NY: New York University.

4.4.1.3 Unstructured Interviewing

Unstructured interviews are sometimes referred to as *informal conversational interviews* or *in-depth interviews*. The purpose of this approach is to interview respondents without imposing any a priori categories on the content or format of the interview. The emphasis is on listening and on understanding each interviewee's individual point of view, not on explaining interviewees' perspectives within a predetermined interpretive framework (Holstein & Gubrium, 1995).

Unstructured interviews often occur as part of observation in field research. They may also be used with a specific purpose in mind, such as exploring one or more issues in depth. In unstructured interviewing, most of the questions flow from the immediate interview context. Specific questioning techniques are used to elicit, as clearly as possible, the way that each interviewee constructs meaning. For example, Spradley (1979) suggested three types of questions: descriptive, contrast, and structural. Patton (1990) also listed several alternative questioning formats. Whichever techniques are used, the researcher's primary task is to understand as fully as possible the interviewee's point of view.

Unstructured interviews are particularly useful for interviewing individuals over a period of time. Later interviews can be used to elaborate information gathered in earlier interviews to help build a comprehensive picture of the topic being investigated. One disadvantage of unstructured interviewing is the time involved. Another is the resources needed to analyze the quantity and variety of information gained.

4.4.1.4 Group Interviews

Interviewing people in groups is gaining popularity in allied health research. Group interviews are commonly called *focus groups*. Focus groups may be structured, semistructured, or unstructured. Group interviews are a cost-effective and efficient way to gather information. However, interviewers need to be experienced in managing group processes. For example, aspects of group interaction, such as the tendency of one or more members to dominate the group or the group members sliding into group think, may impede the interview process (Frey & Fontana, 1995).

4.4.1.5 Attentive Listening

The role of self is critical in interviewing. Interviewing requires a commitment to, and an interest in, understanding another's point of view. Developing skills as an attentive listener are as important, if not more so, than becoming a skilled questioner. To resist the temptation to fit individuals into predetermined response categories requires careful listening and skillful questioning. Questions need to be as unambiguous, focused, and value-free as is humanly

	TABLE 4-9	
METHODS OF COLLECTING DATA IN QUALITATIVE RESEARCH		
TYPE	**DEFINITION**	**RESEARCH EXAMPLE**
Interviewing	• Data collection method for obtaining information through face-to-face verbal exchange, through mail, or through telephone surveys. Interviews can occur in a single session or over multiple sessions. Interviews can be group or individually obtained and can be structured, semi-structured, or unstructured. Structured interviews have specific questions that are answered by the interviewee, whereas unstructured interviews have no specific questions but may have general areas of discussion. Semi-structured interviews are a combination of both (Fontana & Frey, 1994).	Focus groups: Semi-structured group interview • Lau, A., Chi, I., & McKenna, K. (1998). Self-perceived quality of life of Chinese elderly people in Hong Kong. *Occupational Therapy International, 5,* 118-139.
Naturalistic observational techniques	• "The act of noting a phenomenon, often with instruments, and recording it for scientific or other purposes" (Morris, 1973, p. 906). Qualitative observation occurs in the natural setting among the targeted population without intervention by the observer. The focus of naturalistic observation is to examine "trends, patterns, and styles of behavior" (Adler & Adler, 1994, p. 378). • Naturalistic observation occurs through videotaping, audiotaping, photography, or through participant observation.	Observational case study • Henry, J. (1971). *Pathways to madness.* New York, NY: Random House.
Mute evidence	• Primary sources, such as field notes, diaries, memos, letters, and official records (e.g., marriage licenses, banking statements, driving records), but not audio tapes or videotapes that can be heard or viewed.	Historiography • Benison, S. (1972). The history of polio research in the United States: Appraisal and lessons. In G. Holton (Ed.), *The twentieth-century sciences: Studies in the biography of ideas* (pp. 308-343). New York, NY: W.W. Norton & Company. • Jonsson, H. (1998). Ernst Westerlund—A Swedish doctor of occupation. *Occupational Therapy International, 5,* 155-171.
Personal experience	• Understanding of someone's life story through questioning who we are through the narrator, through our relationship to the text, and the way we interpret the text (Clandinin & Connelly, 1994). The life stories told by an individual become a means of educating oneself and others. Autobiography, case histories, and life stories are all part of personal experience.	Personal journals • Jung, B., & Tryssenaar, J. (1998). Supervising students: Exploring the experience through reflective journals. *Occupational Therapy International, 5,* 35-48.

possible. Compiling such questions and learning how to create a context in which interviewees are willing to answer openly and honestly require effort and practice. The rewards are well worth the time spent.

4.4.1.6 Using an Audio Recorder

Using an audio recorder is an efficient and accurate method to record an interview, although this needs to be done unobtrusively so as not to inhibit interviewees' responses. Researchers can easily become dependent on using an audio recorder, and disaster strikes if for any reason a recorded account is not possible. Not using an audio recorder requires a methodical approach and self-discipline to make sure that the researcher's notes are adequate. This is essential if the researcher is to gather the richest possible information in as many situations as possible.

There are instances in which audio recording is not a suitable means of documenting information. Using an audio recorder may invade the privacy of the participant by drawing attention to the interviewee. Circumstances may mitigate against adequate sound recording, particularly in open and crowded public places, such as a shopping center. Audio recording may be inappropriate when the aim is to keep interviews as informal as possible.

Experience suggests that interviewees frequently share valuable information when audio recording is not possible (e.g., on the sidewalk, just after the machine is turned off). No matter how relaxed interviewees become with an audio recorder, occasions still occur when information is withheld for privacy reasons or because of personal embarrassment. It is, therefore, unwise to rely only on recorded interviews. Alternative procedures are described in Section 4.4.3 on field notes

4.4.2 Observation

Observation is essential to understanding human and natural phenomena. As Adler and Adler (1994) noted, "as long as people have been interested in studying the social and natural world around them, observation has served as the bedrock source of human knowledge" (p. 377). Observation in qualitative inquiry goes by several terms: *participant observation, direct observation, field research,* or *qualitative observation.* Whatever the term employed, the essence of observation "lies in the prolonged and unobtrusive presence of a *sensitive* and *trained* observer among the people being studied" (Edgerton & Langness, 1978, p. 339, italics added). All observational methods require disciplined training and rigorous preparation.

The primary purpose of observation in qualitative research is to describe. Description includes the setting, the activities taking place, the participants, and the meaning of the setting and its activities from the perspective of the participants. Observing activities as they take place provides the researcher with direct first-hand experience. This is essential to a full understanding of the phenomena

under investigation. There are several sources of data in fieldwork settings. These include the physical setting, social interactions and activities (both planned and informal), the language used, nonverbal communication, unobtrusive indicators, program documents, and "notable non-occurrences" (Patton, 1990). In any setting, however, there is far more happening than can be accurately observed and documented. Therefore, qualitative researchers usually employ a framework to guide their fieldwork observations.

Several dimensions to observing need careful consideration in the research design phase. These are the role of the observer, portrayal of role and purpose, and duration and focus of observation.

4.4.2.1 Role of the Observer

The first dimension relates to the extent to which the observer not only observes but also participates in the setting. There are several typologies of observer involvement in research settings. For example, Gold (1958) outlined four modes: the complete participant, the participant-as-observer, the observer-as-participant, and the complete observer. The latter is rarely used now owing to the ethical concerns about covert observation.

Adler and Adler (1994) suggested three roles for researchers as observers: the complete member-researcher, the active member-researcher, and the peripheral member-researcher. These roles fall along a continuum. The role chosen will depend on the purpose and nature of the research study. The peripheral member-researcher is part of a setting while remaining removed from the core activities. The active member-researcher participates in the core activities of the setting. The complete member-researcher is one who already has full membership in the setting or converts to genuine membership during the study.

4.4.2.2 Portrayal of Role and Purpose

Researchers may explicitly explain their observer role and purpose, may choose not to disclose any information about their observational role, or may portray their role somewhere in between these two extremes. The nature of the research questions and the access the researcher has to the setting and his or her position within that setting will influence how much others are told about the researcher role. For example, in primarily evaluative research, there will usually be full and complete explanation of the observational component. As Patton (1990) succinctly noted, "People are seldom deceived or reassured by false or partial explanations—at least not for long" (p. 212). By contrast, in research of a more public nature, there may be little need to describe exactly what will be observed, or when, how, and why it will be observed.

4.4.2.3 Duration and Focus of Observation

Observation may only occur once, happen for a limited period, or be of varying duration carried out multiple times over an extended period. The duration of the observational period relies heavily on the purpose of the research. For example, research investigating complex processes that change over time, such as adaptation to acquired disability, require prolonged observation. In contrast, the timeliness and resources available for evaluation research often determine how much—or how little—observation occurs.

Not everything in a single research project warrants observation. The focus and scope of the observation needs to be considered when framing the research question. For example, decisions will need to be made about whether to observe a small number of occasions in great depth or many occasions in less depth.

4.4.3 Field Notes

Field notes are the basic tool of the qualitative researcher. As Patton (1990) noted, "There are many options in the mechanics of taking field notes.... *What is not optional is the taking of field notes*" (p. 239). Taking field notes can be used to substitute for audio recording interviews. Note taking can also be used to expand the recorded account to include enriching descriptions of visual pictures of participants' facial expressions, gestures, and other nonverbal behaviors. Taking notes also expands the opportunities to collect data. For example, taking notes can provide a documented account of participants' reactions and interactions.

As noted previously, researchers need to learn to observe methodically. Similarly, learning to systematically document observations requires the researcher to develop disciplined methods. The first step in this process is to decide on a format. Field notes can be in a notebook or composed into a computer or tablet. The second step is to organize the different types of field notes according to their content, which will vary according to their purpose. The purposes of field notes include maintaining a transcript file, a personal log, or an analytical log (Minichiello, Aroni, Timewell, & Alexander, 1995).

The transcript file contains descriptive data about the observation or interview setting. This includes where the observation took place, who was present, and what social interactions and activities took place. This file may also contain a diagram of the setting. The transcript file also contains either a transcription of the interview or a written account of the observation. The secret of making good field notes for the transcript file is to be descriptive, concrete, and detailed. The researcher needs to avoid interpretation or judgment, loosely defined comparisons, and abbreviations that, although making sense at the time of documenting, may mean nothing at all when reviewing the file. This file should also contain direct quotations of what the research participants say. The quotations may be documented in the actual transcript of a recorded interview. If not, it is critical that the researcher record relevant information in the participants' own words. Participants' words can

be differentiated from the researcher's descriptions by using quotation marks.

The personal log is the repository for the researcher's thoughts on the field research. This log includes personal feelings, reactions to the fieldwork experience, and personal and methodological reflections during the study. Writing this log needs to be done as soon as possible after each encounter in the field. It is not possible at the end of a study to go back and capture the feelings, reactions, and reflections that occurred during fieldwork. Keeping the personal log in the form of a journal may be helpful. Using headings and subheadings will help to organize the material and make it easier to review the contents in the analysis stage. The headings will vary according to research focus. For example, headings can be used to organize the material according to the sequence of events.

The analytical log contains the researcher's insights and reflections on data collection and analysis in the context of the theoretical framework of the study. Minichiello et al. (1995) suggested that this is where the researcher asks and answers questions such as: What is it that I know so far? What do I not know? What do I need to know? How do I collect this information? This log also provides a record or audit trail of the analysis and theoretical propositions as these develop throughout the study.

4.4.4 Political and Ethical Context for Research

The political context sets the background for any research project. This context ranges from the micropolitical of personal relationships to the macropolitical of government sponsorship of research. Feminist research and research about race and ethnicity have highlighted the potential nature of research as a political activity. Grappling with the political context may seem overwhelmingly daunting to the beginning researcher. This is more so because little is written about how experienced researchers understand and deal with the political dimensions of the contexts in which they are working (Shaffir & Stebbins, 1991). Consideration of the political context is crucial in the research design phase.

Much has been written about the stages of fieldwork, particularly strategies for entering and leaving the field (see Schatzman & Strauss, 1973; Shaffir & Stebbins, 1991). Personal factors such as age, race, and gender of both the researcher and the participants affect fieldwork. Other influences on fieldwork include the nature and status of the researcher's institution and the institution where the research occurs (e.g., a prestigious teaching hospital compared to a community health center). *Gatekeeping*—the term used to describe institutional power holders blocking access to people served by their institution—does occur in the health and welfare fields. For example, family workers may be unwilling to inform client families about a proposed research project or may tell only some families and not others. This may be done on the grounds that some families are more likely to be willing to participate, are more articulate, or are more able to withstand yet another intrusion into their lives. Frequently, however, those families not informed are less well-educated, from minority ethnic groups, or are disadvantaged parents. Professional gatekeeping applied to these families may result in biased participant selection for the research.

Professional associations, academic institutions, funding bodies, and medical facilities have ethical standards and convene human ethics committees. These have a mandate to permit or disallow proposed research according to federal and state regulations. Traditionally, the ethical precepts of biomedical research have been applied to social science research, although this research is more likely to be of a qualitative nature. These regulations, although providing a useful framework, may offer little guidance for the proper and ethical conduct of research in the field. Of primary interest to field researchers are issues of consent, privacy, confidentiality, trust, and betrayal (Bulmer, 1982).

Gaining the informed consent of research participants is essential to the ethical conduct of any research; however, informed consent is not as straightforward as it first appears. For example, what happens to individual behaviors if they are informed a priori that they will be observed? What constitutes informed consent under circumstances such as mental illness, cognitive limitations, extreme youth, and extreme age? Research in the medical, rehabilitation, and allied health fields is often carried out with individuals identified as vulnerable subjects on ethics clearance forms. Obtaining informed consent from research participants in these groups may require special procedures (Booth & Booth, 1994; Llewellyn, 1995).

A major aim for ethical researchers is to protect the privacy and confidentiality of research participants. Typical ways that this is done include keeping data in locked storage, destroying identifying material, and using pseudonyms in research reports. Safeguards also need to be in place against less obvious intrusions on participant privacy and confidentiality. For example, the researcher's institutional affiliation, the description of the research context, or the bibliography of the research report may give away the research location and the likely participants.

Finishing a field research study presents a further ethical concern. At the beginning of a research study, intense effort (possibly over weeks, months, or even years) will have gone into building trust with the research participants. At the end of the study, the researcher leaves while the participants remain. After a period of engagement, the participants may feel betrayed or, at the very least, let down. There are no simple rules to deal with this possibility. Each researcher must find a way to leave the field in an acceptably ethical manner. Fontana and Frey (1994) suggested a three-point guide to exercising moral responsibility toward research participants: "to our subjects first, to the study next and to ourselves last" (p. 373).

4.5 ANALYZING QUALITATIVE DATA

There is a diverse variety of methods for analyzing qualitative data (see Bryman & Burgess, 1994; Miles & Huberman, 1994; Strauss & Corbin, 1998; van Manen, 1990). Qualitative data analysis methods are based on the following general principles.

4.5.1 Principles

The first principle is that the analysis is conducted concurrently with data collection. This means that as analysis occurs, the researcher develops further questions that guide ongoing data collection. The researcher analyzes the data, proposes new questions or tentative propositions, and then checks these out by returning to the data. This proposing and verifying process illustrates the movement between inductive and deductive procedures typical of qualitative analysis procedures.

The second principle is that the analysis process is systematic. Methods vary according to schools of thought and the researcher's interpretive framework. All methods make use of systems that involve reflection, are open to examination, and can be applied to more than one researcher. Miles and Huberman (1994) described their system as follows: "Margin notes are made on the field notes, more reflective passages are reviewed carefully, and some kind of summary sheet is drafted. At the next level are coding and memo writing" (p. 432). These memos are analytic in nature and result from reflection on the data. Memos help the process of generating an increasingly more abstract conceptualization from the concrete field data (Miles & Huberman, 1994).

The third principle is that, during the analytic process, the data are divided into segments; however, these segments of data remain part of the whole. Dividing the data into segments is carried out by using content analysis procedures. The researcher reviews the data from transcribed interviews or questionnaire responses or field notes and gives a name or code to each unit of meaning. This process is called *open coding* (Strauss & Corbin, 1998). The names or codes given to these units of meaning are developed directly from the text data or are generated from previous studies, from the relevant literature, or from a combination of all of these sources.

The fourth principle is that comparison is the main intellectual tool employed by the researcher in doing the analysis. Comparison is used to "discern conceptual similarities, to refine the discriminative power of categories, and to discover patterns" (Tesch, 1990, p. 96). Glaser and Strauss (1967) developed the term *constant comparative analysis* to describe the process whereby the researcher compares and contrasts elements of data in a search for recurring regularities. These regularities are further compared and contrasted to develop concepts. These concepts

---

Table 4-10

What to Store, Retrieve From, and Retain

- Raw material: Field notes, tapes, site documents
- Partially processed data: Write-ups, transcriptions. Initial version and subsequent corrected, cleaned, commented-on versions
- Coded data: Write-ups with specific codes attached
- The coding scheme or thesaurus, in its successive iterations
- Memos or other analytic material: The researcher's reflections on the conceptual meaning of the data
- Search and retrieval records: information showing which coded chunks or data segments the researcher looked for during analysis and the retrieved material; records of links made among segments
- Data displays: Matrices or networks used to display retrieved information, along with the associated analytic text; revised versions of these
- Analysis episodes: Documenting of what was done, step by step, to assemble the displays and write the analytic text
- Report text: Successive drafts of what is written on the design, methods, and findings of the study
- General chronological log or documentation of data collection and analytic work
- Index of all the above material

Adapted from Miles, M. B., & Huberman, A. M. (1994). *Qualitative Data Analysis. An Expanded Sourcebook* (2nd ed.). Thousand Oaks, CA: Sage.

---

are then compared and contrasted to form internally consistent and mutually exclusive categories.

The fifth principle is that the researcher refines the category organizing system as familiarity with the data develops. Using the comparative process, the researcher clusters together categories that are alike. The organizing system remains flexible, becoming more conceptually sound and parsimonious as the researcher develops a deeper understanding of the phenomena under study. This occurs as the categories are expanded and elaborated, which occurs by building on existing information, making links between items of information, and proposing and verifying new information. Category organization is continually refined until *theoretical saturation* is reached (Glaser & Strauss, 1967). Theoretical saturation is said to occur when new data lead to redundancy and the categories appear to be conceptually sound.

The sixth and final principle is that the goal of qualitative analysis is synthesis of the data into a higher level of conceptualization. In this process, a qualitative researcher has dual roles. The first is to describe phenomena as they exist—the what, how, when, and where. The second is to interpret and explain these phenomena as concepts. Patton (1990) suggested that this involves *discovering* and *uncovering*.

- Discovering involves elaborating concepts that are obvious to participant and researcher alike.
- Uncovering requires clarifying or elaborating already existing sociological concepts or building new concepts from the research setting.

In summary, the aim in qualitative research designs is not casual determination, prediction, or generalization as in quantitative research. Rather, qualitative researchers aim to elucidate relationships, investigate and interpret connections, and, by doing so, develop an understanding about particular phenomenon and their place within existing theoretical knowledge about the social world.

4.5.2 Practice

Qualitative data is, most frequently, text derived from interview transcripts, questionnaire responses, field notes, and documents such as case records. The researcher may also use photographs and video (Harper, 1989). The volume of text data gathered can create a data management challenge. Miles and Huberman (1994) provided a useful summary of storage and retrieval requirements (Table 4-10).

Qualitative researchers need to develop a data management system that suits their own style or that of the research team and the purpose of the research. Traditional methods for organizing data include using notebooks, file folders, card systems, and filing cabinets. Newer methods include word-processing programs, databases, spreadsheets, and other computer-based programs. Storage and retrieval of data can be done quickly and efficiently by computer.

Recent developments in computer software mean that researchers can also get help with data analysis. Several computer-based text analysis programs, known as *Computer Assisted/Aided Qualitative Data Analysis* (CAQDAS), aids in qualitative analysis, such as transcription analysis, coding and text interpretation, recursive abstraction, content analysis, discourse analysis, and grounded theory methodology. When choosing a software package, the researcher needs to be aware of the assumptions underlying the design of the software and to decide whether such assumptions are congruent with the research purpose and design. For example, a common assumption is that concepts are of a hierarchical nature (such that A is an instance of a higher order concept B, and so on). Three widely known qualitative data analysis programs are Nvivo (http://www.qsrinternational.com/), Ethnograph (http://www.qualisresearch.com/), and ATLAS/ti (http://atlasti.com/). Reviews of available programs and their functions, advantages, and shortcomings are available at the CAQDAS Networking Project (http://caqdas.soc.surrey.ac.uk/) and Qual Page (http://www.qualitativeresearch.uga.edu/QualPage/).

4.6 CREDIBILITY IN QUALITATIVE RESEARCH

In qualitative research designs, the aim is to make sense of the meanings that people apply to phenomena in the social world. Therefore, qualitative researchers want to make sure that their research findings are credible in the everyday sense of being plausible, believable, and trustworthy, as well as being reliable and valid (Leung, Bo, Hsiao, Wang, & Chi, 2014; Morse, 1994). Researchers using experimental designs and quantitative methods for collecting and analyzing data use constructs of reliability and validity. Many investigators have written about ways to address credibility in qualitative research. These range from applying of the experimental concepts of reliability and validity to suggesting alternative concepts better suited to qualitative designs (see Kirk & Miller, 1986; Lincoln & Guba, 1985). Among these writers, there is general agreement that three elements of the inquiry process must be addressed. These are the research techniques used, the researcher's credibility, and the assumptions underpinning the study.

Credibility of the research techniques can be checked by testing rival explanations, searching for negative cases, and triangulation. The first, testing rival explanations, requires the researcher to consider and test out alternative explanations to the one proposed and then to report the results. Searching for negative cases is a related process. In this instance, the researcher searches for cases that do not fit the proposed patterns or themes identified from the data. Identifying negative or outlier cases increases understanding of the commonly occurring cases and, therefore, the totality of the phenomenon under investigation. The last way to check credibility is by a process called triangulation.

Triangulation has come to mean the use of multiple methods, sources, analysts, or theoretical perspectives to verify the information gained in different arenas (Carter, Bryant-Lukosius, DiCenso, Blythe, & Neville, 2014). The aim of triangulation is "to guard against the accusation that a study's findings are simply an artifact of a single method, a single source, or a single investigator's bias" (Patton, 1990, p. 470). Triangulation of methods may involve collecting both quantitative and qualitative data for comparison and potential reconciliation. This helps to expand and elaborate the quality of information gained by one method alone.

Triangulation of sources involves comparing the consistency of information derived from varying sources, such as comparing the data gathered from interviews and observations, from public and private documents, or from informants making the same claim independently. Triangulation across analysts is becoming more common. For example, this can take the form of agreement between the field notes of one observer and the observations made by another. Lastly, some investigators have suggested triangulation of theoretical perspectives. This means applying more than one theoretical perspective to the research findings to reveal any differences and similarities (Patton, 1990).

As mentioned at the beginning of this chapter, the researcher is an integral part of the qualitative research process. Concern for researcher credibility is therefore an inherent part of the verification process. Researcher credibility is dependent on training, experience, and acknowledgment of the researcher role in the research process. Most of all, credibility requires a clear and concise explanation of the researcher role and contribution to the study findings. It is the researcher's responsibility to explain the extent of possible researcher effect on the study and whether changes in perceptions or responses occurred during the study or whether any predispositions or biases influenced the study findings. A description of the researcher's interpretive framework allows the reader to understand exactly how the researcher framed the research question and collected and analyzed the data.

The final element is the need for concise clarification by the researcher of the philosophical orientation underpinning the study. For example, there is continuing debate about the place of objectivity in scientific inquiry. This often takes the form of competition between the two paradigms of quantitative and qualitative research (Guba, 1990). Clear explanation by the researcher of the philosophical orientation of the study helps to place the study findings within a particular interpretive framework and allows readers to judge the authenticity of the study results for themselves. Frank and open explanation in reporting research enhances credibility (Linkov, Loney, Cormier, Satterstrom, & Bridges, 2009).

Readers of qualitative research need a method to evaluate study credibility and the contribution to knowledge of the study findings. Frost, Reeve, Liepa, Stauffer, and Hays (2007) concluded that "Various qualitative (e.g., focus groups, behavioral coding, cognitive interviews) and quantitative approaches (e.g., differential item functioning testing) are useful in evaluating the reliability and validity of PRO [patient reported outcomes] instruments" (p. s94).

Some tests deal specifically with evaluating qualitative studies (e.g., Higgs, 1998). The following questions proposed by Schwandt and Halpern (1988; as cited in Miles & Huberman, 1994, p. 439) provide useful criteria for readers in the medical and rehabilitation research literature:

- Are findings grounded in the data? (Is sampling appropriate? Are data weighted correctly?)
- Are inferences logical? (Are analytic strategies applied correctly? Are alternative explanations accounted for?)
- Is the category structure appropriate?
- Can inquiry decisions and methodological shifts be justified? Were sampling decisions linked to working hypotheses?

- What is the degree of researcher bias (e.g., premature disclosure, unexplored data in field notes, lack of search for negative cases, feelings of empathy)?
- What strategies were used for increasing credibility (e.g., second readers, feedback to informants, peer review, adequate time in the field)?

In summary, qualitative research offers a diversity of methods well-suited to the interests of researchers in occupational therapy. The increasing popularity of these methods is evident in the growing number of qualitative studies reported in the occupational therapy literature and in the appearance of journals devoted specifically to qualitative research studies.

5

The Research Problem

The great working hypotheses in the past have often originated in the minds of the pioneers as a result of mental processes which can best be described by such words as "inspired guess," "intuitive hunch," or "brilliant flash of imagination."

—Conant (1951, p. 48)

OPERATIONAL LEARNING OBJECTIVES

By the end of this chapter the learner will:
- Identity a feasible research topic in an area of clinical practice, administration, or education.
- Write a paragraph justifying the need for a research study.
- Identity a feasible research problem.
- Formulate relevant questions pertaining to a research problem.
- Identify possible psychological blocks in the investigator and flaws in research designs that could potentially deter the research.
- Outline a general plan for data collection.

Rice, M. S., Stein, F., & Tomlin, G.
Clinical Research in Occupational Therapy, Sixth Edition (pp. 141-154).
© 2019 Taylor & Francis Group.

5.1 THE NEED FOR PROBLEM-ORIENTED RESEARCH IN THE HEALTH PROFESSIONS

Since the middle of the 20th century, health research in the United States has multiplied beyond the volume that could have been predicted one century earlier. During the 19th century, a medical scientist could easily have read most of the published research in a wide range of health specialties. A scholar in the sciences in the 19th century would also be familiar with the literary and artistic worlds. Today that is impossible. Snow (1964) in his discussion of the two worlds of science and humanities was one of the first to recognize the isolating effect of specialization in the 20th century. Scientists and humanists now live in two cultures, deprived of the sharing and communication that existed in the 18th and 19th centuries. Specialization and the narrowing of interest in scientific topics have led to a multiplicity of professional associations and published journals.

Currently, there are thousands of scientific journals published monthly, semimonthly, and quarterly. Many of these are accessible electronically where scholars can read articles directly from the internet. A gap exists between the methods used in social science research and research in the biological and physical sciences. Quantitative research is more prevalent in the biological and physical sciences, whereas the social sciences apply more qualitative research methods for collecting data. Research in the social sciences is most vulnerable to criticism because of the subjective nature of qualitative research. On the other hand, there is a pressing need for social progress (e.g., the reduction of alcoholism, drug addiction, juvenile crime, and mental illness). The gap between research in the social sciences and its impact on social problems has led to criticism of applied research. However, one need only examine the history of medical progress to realize the tremendous gains science has made through applied research, such as in the reduction of heart disease, the increase in survival rates for patients with cancer, and advances in surgical techniques for cataracts. There is also a strong need for basic research in areas that may not seem relevant at the moment, as with cellular research and microbiology, where theory and basic research performed 50 years ago have led to practical results, such as in the understanding of the immune system and how it impacts individuals with AIDS. There is a need for basic research into life processes, such as in DNA expression, muscle metabolism, and neurological and cognitive areas of human development. The need exists for problem-oriented research that can be applied to topics in health, medicine, occupational therapy, and special education. A research study begins with establishing the need, significance, and implications of the results.

5.2 SELECTING A SIGNIFICANT RESEARCH PROBLEM

How does a researcher select a significant area for investigation? What factors in an individual's personal life, education, or clinical experience generate a research interest? In the introduction of his book *On the Motion of the Heart and Blood in Animals*, William Harvey (1628/1938) described his purpose in investigating the problem of circulation of blood:

Since, therefore, from the foregoing considerations and many others to the same effect, it is plain that what has ... been said concerning the motion and function of the heart and arteries must appear obscure, inconsistent, or even impossible to him who carefully considers the entire subject, it would be proper to look more narrowly into the matter to contemplate the motion of the heart and arteries, not only in man, but in all animals that have hearts; and also by frequent appeals to vivisection, and much ocular inspection, to investigate and discuss the truth. (p. 73)

Harvey selected the problem of investigating the circulatory system after he evaluated the previous studies as contradictory and inconclusive. His motivation to study the problem was based on his desire to bring clarity to an area of medicine that is vital to human survival. This desire to clarify is an important motivating force in the researcher. There are numerous examples in the history of scientific research of individuals seeking to understand the basic anatomic and physiologic processes of human beings.

Other motivating forces can also generate research. Individuals can pursue a research area because they seek insight into a disease or disability that has touched their own life or the life of a family member or close friend. In 1847, Ignaz Semmelweis, a relentless investigator, pursued the causes of puerperal fever (i.e., blood poisoning associated with childbirth) after the death of a friend. Louis Braille, blinded at the age of 4, became a teacher of the blind and in 1824 devised a reading method for the blind. Some situations that may motivate an individual to pursue an area of research include the following:

- A clinician becomes a researcher after becoming aware of the need for more effective treatment methods or diagnostic instruments. There are many instances in the history of medicine where practitioners became part-time researchers and made notable contributions through their efforts. For instance, A. R. Luria, a Russian neuroscientist, became interested in the way the brain worked after evaluating neurological injuries occurring in soldiers. He used case study research to explore neurological disorders and from this developed a concept of how an undamaged brain works.

- A dramatic increase in the incidence of a disease produces national priorities for research. In the United States during the last 50 years, there has been a significant amount of research effort directed at cancer, cardiovascular disease, and AIDS. These areas have received added attention from researchers partially because of the dramatic increases in the incidence of these illnesses and partially because of the availability of federal grant support. It is no secret that a research investigator's career can become determined by national politics and priorities. On the other hand, the abuse of federal grant support in the opportunism of research can also become an overriding problem in neglecting research areas that are significant but receive little interest from the granting foundations and governmental agencies.

- An interest in a content area is generated by an inspiring teacher. There is no doubt that universities are an ideal place for research because they can play an active yet neutral role in facilitating research efforts. Universities need not be caught in political decisions.

- A student develops an interest on a research topic through intellectual curiosity spurred by intense reading and study. As the student gains more understanding in a specific area, more questions are raised, which motivate research.

From these motivating forces and others, the researcher selects an area of investigation. From this point, how does one maintain momentum and nurture research interests sometimes in the face of insignificant results and tedious, laborious work? The story of Fleming's discovery of penicillin in 1929 is an example of persistence. The impetus for Fleming's investigation was the catastrophic rate of death that occurred during World War I from infected wounds. Fleming sought a chemical substance that would destroy the pathogenic germs entering the body from an open flesh wound. After 10 years of painstaking laboratory work that involved growing bacterial colonies and observing the reactions of chemicals, he was successful in discovering a powerful therapeutic agent that would eventually change the course of medical practice. There were two landmark events in his work. The first occurred in 1922 when he noticed that a foreign chemical substance prevented a bacterial colony from growing. At this point in his work, he was unable to isolate or identify the chemical substance. In 1928, he noticed that a bacterial culture of staphylococci had accidentally become contaminated by mold. He found that the mold produced a substance that retarded the growth of the bacteria. The chemical substance was later identified by an American mycologist, Thom, as *Penicillium notatum*. After the substance was identified, Fleming was able to produce penicillin in the laboratory and experiment with its effect on bacteria and on normal human tissues. It was not until 1943, about 20 years after Fleming's original investigations, that penicillin was mass produced in Great Britain and the United States. In analyzing Fleming's discovery, a combination of persistence and responsiveness to accidental discovery was the key factor. Fleming first asked a researchable question: Is there a chemical substance that can stop the growth of harmful bacteria in the bloodstream without destroying normal human tissue? He persisted in his efforts to solve the problem over a period of 25 years until his successful discovery of penicillin.

Compared to medicine, research originating from occupational therapy fields is in earlier stages of development. Potential directions for research abound in the areas of evaluation and treatment, as well as professional education and administration. Research originates out of the relationship between the evaluation and treatment of a specific disability. By analyzing a disability, the clinical researcher tries to determine where the major gaps in knowledge exist. For instance, in evaluating and treating the client with arthritis, are there effective evaluative instruments? What treatment methods have been demonstrated to be effective? What factors in the client's life affect the course of the illness? From this analysis, the researcher can identify a research problem. This same process of generating research also is evident in analyzing the educational and administrative aspects of occupational therapy in addressing questions such as whether to admit students into a program, how to provide effective supervision and evaluation of staff, how to maintain morale in job satisfaction, and how to design the curriculum. The need for research is justified when a researcher can establish the significance of the results. For example, the researcher should ask, "If I collect this data, what impact will the results have on intervention, education, or administration?" A researcher should clearly state the implications of the study, relating it to the evaluation or treatment of a specified disability or the educational or administrative practices that could be affected by the results. Before data are collected, the researcher should be able to think through the impact of the results. An *if* (results positive or negative) … *then* (recommendations and options taken) contingency is the initial strategy proposed by the researcher.

5.3 IDENTIFYING PROBLEMS RESULTING FROM A DISABILITY

In selecting a disability area for research, investigators can be guided by their own clinical experience in an area of specialization. For example, the significance of a problem can be gauged by the leading causes of death and the leading causes of hospitalization. The 15 leading causes of death in the United States in 2007 are shown in Table 5-1.

For the researcher, these disabilities and diseases represent significant health problems. Evaluation and diagnosis are ongoing concerns for the therapist. Methodological research, such as in diagnostic hardware, clinical observational methods, screening procedures, and objective

TABLE 5-1
FIFTEEN LEADING CAUSES OF DEATH FOR 2014

CAUSE	
All causes	2,626,418
Diseases of heart	614,348
Malignant neoplasms	591,699
Chronic lower respiratory diseases	147,101
Accidents (unintentional injuries)	136,053
Cerebrovascular diseases	133,103
Alzheimer's disease	95,541
Diabetes mellitus	76,488
Influenza and pneumonia	55,227
Nephritis, nephrotic syndrome and nephrosis	48,146
Intentional self-harm (suicide)	42,773
Septicemia	38,940
Chronic liver disease and cirrhosis	38,170
Essential hypertension and renal disease	30,221
Parkinson's disease	26,150
Pneumonitis due to solids and liquids	18,792
All other causes	535,666

Note: The table shows the number and rank for the top causes of death in the United States in 2014. The data include all races and were obtained from page 5 of the *National Vital Statistics Report,* 65(4), June 30, 2016, published by the Centers for Disease Control and Prevention. Retrieved from https://www.cdc.gov/nchs/data/nvsr/nvsr65/nvsr65_04.pdf

tests, can become the focal point of an investigation. The development of specific treatment techniques or protocols that can be generalized to a population with disabilities represents another fertile direction for researchers. Treatment techniques such as sensory-integration therapy, constraint-induced movement therapy, neurodevelopmental therapy, aquatic therapy, hippotherapy, stress management, and biofeedback are a few examples of research areas generated from examining the needs of people with disabilities.

5.4 IDENTIFYING SIGNIFICANT ISSUES IN PROFESSIONAL EDUCATION

Who should become occupational therapists? Are there specific abilities, personalities, intellectual potentials, or academic achievements necessary before entering a professional preparatory program? What is the rationale for each characteristic? How are admission requirements for entrance to an occupational therapy program determined? Who among the faculty and staff in the occupational therapy departments determines policy for admission? These questions examine the assumptions underlying the education of occupational therapists. The recruitment, screening, and selection of students pose realistic problems to the occupational therapy educator that should provide significant areas for investigation.

Along with the admission process, the curriculum is a potential area for research. The educational curriculum includes the traditional and flipped classroom teaching methods, online teaching environment, curricular content, audiovisual aids, clinical education, problem-based learning, experiential learning, service learning, and student evaluation. Examples of these potential areas of research in educating occupational therapy students are listed in Table 5-2.

Administration of clinical programs, personnel policies, budgetary planning, physical plant layouts, and job satisfaction are often neglected areas of research, although the effect of administrative policies sometimes have more impact on the course of a client's disability than the direct effects of treatment. Public health policies to mass vaccinate a population, the access to health care, and the staff morale are all critical areas of concern that have important implications in the total health needs. These are all potential areas for research.

5.5 JUSTIFYING THE RESEARCH PROBLEM

Once a research area is identified by the investigator, statistical data should be cited that indicate the extent of the problem. See Table 5-3 as an example of statistical data. A problem involving one of the 15 leading causes of death or hospitalization is obviously significant. Nonetheless, how does one justify investigating a rare disease, such as amyotrophic lateral sclerosis, that affects proportionately fewer people? On the other hand, should the freedom of an investigator be restricted by governmental agencies deciding which areas to fund research? The question of research significance does touch on societal values. Priorities are established by nations in areas of health that realistically affect research efforts. It is assumed that the individual scientist should have the freedom to pursue any area of investigation as long as it does not endanger the lives or well-being of the subjects. However, research should not be isolated from the pressing needs of a society. If, for example, osteoarthritis becomes a problem of epidemic proportions in the United States in the early 21st century, then society should justly allocate a larger percentage of its health resources to those researchers seeking means to reduce the incidence of osteoarthritis. Establishing research priorities

TABLE 5-2
METHODOLOGY AND CONTENT OF PROFESSIONAL PROGRAMS IN OCCUPATIONAL THERAPY

CLASSROOM TEACHING METHODS	CURRICULA CONTENT	PRESENTATION METHODS	CLINICAL EDUCATION	STUDENT EVALUATION

• Case studies
• Laboratory experiences (e.g., testing or treatment)
• Lecture
• Problem-based learning
• Role playing
• Seminar
• Student-oriented group projects
• Flipped classroom
• Online teaching
	• Basic sciences
	• Dynamics of interactions
	• Evaluation and treatment techniques
	• Practice areas (e.g., geriatrics, mental health, pediatrics, physical disabilities)
	• Research design
	• Supervision and administration
		• Audiovisual methods
		• Computer-assisted instruction
		• Distance learning
		• Internet
		• Presentation software (e.g., PowerPoint)
		• Videos
		• Video conferencing
		• Online learning environments/tools
			• Level 1: Short-term experiences with or without supervision
			  ○ Observations (single day)
			  ○ Clerkships (weekly)
			• Level 2: Two 3-month affiliations with supervision
			  ○ Internships or affiliations
			  ○ Optional affiliations in a specialty area
				• Grades: Number and letter grades
				• Grades: Pass/fail
				• Individual counseling
				• Observation of students in clinical settings
				• Competency-based evaluation

TABLE 5-3
PREVALENCE OF SELECTED CHRONIC CONDITIONS IN ADULTS IN UNITED STATES, 2015

CHRONIC CONDITION	PERCENT OF ADULTS OVER 18
Arthritis	21.0
Chronic joint symptoms	28.4
Diabetes	8.9
Low back pain	29.1
Physical function difficulties (e.g., very difficult to or cannot grasp or handle small objects)	1.8
Vision	9.0
Hearing	14.4
Adapted from the Centers for Disease Control and Prevention, National Center for Health Statistics. (2015). Tables of summary health statistics. Retrieved from https://www.cdc.gov/nchs/nhis/SHS/tables.htm	

in a democratic society involves the participation of a broad spectrum of groups who represent the policy makers, clinicians, consumers, and researchers. Governmental agencies, universities, pharmaceutical companies, and private foundations are the primary sources for the financial support of research, and thus, are the policy makers for research. The recipients of research grants are those clinical practitioners, students, educators, and administrators who have convinced policy makers of the significance and validity of their research proposals.

In summary, the researcher justifies an investigation by establishing the need for a study based on an analysis of a health problem and the implications of the results. The need for an investigation is documented by the following statistical data:

- The incidence (initial occurrences) and prevalence (existing cases in the population) of a disability, derived from primary statistical data.
- The leading causes of death (mortality) as reported by national and international centers for health statistics (e.g., World Health Organization).
- The number of first admissions and readmissions to a hospital caused by a disability, obtained from national and state public health agencies.
- The number of physicians and outpatient visits reported as the result of a disability.
- The days lost at work because of specific health problems, compiled from Department of Labor Statistics and Workers Compensation.
- The incidence of social disabilities (i.e., alcoholism, drug addiction, adult crime, juvenile delinquency, and child abuse), available through the national and state public health agencies and the state attorney general's office.
- The number of occupational therapists employed in the United States as provided by professional organizations, the *Occupational Outlook Handbook* (published by the U.S. Department of Labor), and state employment agencies.
- Statistics on the number of hospitals, outpatient clinics, state institutions for individuals with intellectual disabilities and mental illness, rehabilitation centers, and other patient care facilities, usually available from public health agencies or through directories published by municipal and state organizations and private social service agencies.

5.6 NARROWING THE INVESTIGATION

Problem-oriented research is a process of asking questions and gathering data. The investigator generates a question and intellectually ponders the possible outcomes. This ability to formulate research questions and to predict outcomes is an essential part of the research process. The Socratic method of teaching is based on this principle of questions and answers that invariably lead to other questions and answers until a topic is exhausted. This method is also used in problem-based learning where students examine a case study by asking relevant questions and developing hypotheses.

Brainstorming a problem is another method for generating questions by creative free association. The researcher must be able to freely generate questions that on initial examination may seem unrelated or unfeasible. Many great discoveries, when they were first reported publicly, seemed like "hair-brained" ideas that would never work. Roentgen, a physicist, accidentally discovered x-rays when examining the results of passing electricity through a vacuum tube. He then proceeded to ask himself questions regarding its applicability to medical diagnosis. On hearing of Roentgen's discovery in 1895, people in the streets were incredulous. Many felt that x-rays would be used like a camera to spy on people or to expose them. Later medical scientists raised questions regarding the potential of x-ray in diagnosis and in the treatment of cancerous growths.

This process of asking questions and observing the outcome is the essential part of research. At first, the question may be general, ill-conceived, unclear, and incongruous. As the researcher explores and defines what is actually being asked, the research question becomes sharper until, as Wallas (1926) stated:

> Our mind is not likely to give us a clear answer to any particular problem unless we set it a clear question, and we are more likely to notice the significance of any new piece of evidence, or new association of ideas, if we have formed a definite conception of a case to be proved or disproved. (p. 84)

The persistent effort on the part of the researcher to brainstorm a problem, to think it through, to ponder silently, or to discuss it with a colleague brings the researcher closer to a solution. For some investigators, the problem incubates, while for others the problem stirs. Whatever the style is, the researcher must be able to stay with a problem while trying to overcome the apparent pitfalls and culs-de-sac that are created. Many a researcher is stymied by the assumption of others that the problem is too complex or impossible to solve or by the knowledge that others have failed. The investigator must persist in working through the problem. For example, low back pain is a significant health problem that affects a large number of sedentary and manual workers. It directly affects economic productivity, psychological well-being, and participation in sports and leisure activities. Although it is widespread in the population and it has significant implications, practitioners have been only partially successful in treating this disability. Experienced occupational therapists observe that low back pain is an elusive syndrome that is difficult to diagnose and sometimes difficult to separate from symptom magnification or psychosomatic effects. Other clinicians are hesitant to investigate the problem because of the subjective nature of measuring pain. Others state that the neurophysiology is too complex to investigate. These reactions to low back pain should not deter research. Investigators entering into an area of research can become overwhelmed by the immensity of a problem, but they need not try to solve all aspects of the problem, including objective diagnosis and successful treatment. Researchers should instead attempt to focus on a portion of a research problem that is feasible

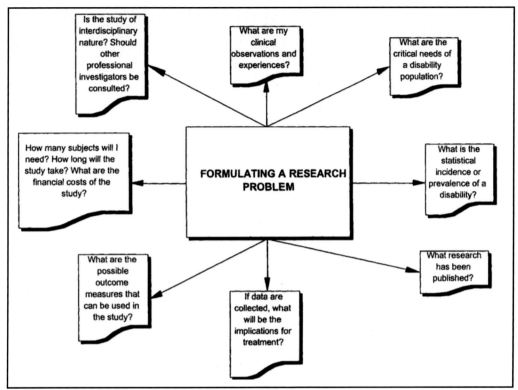

Figure 5-1. Clinical formulation of a research problem.

within the limitations of time and resources available. The process of formulating a research problem by a clinician is summarized in Figure 5-1.

Let us examine hypothetical examples of research questions originating in significant health problems (Table 5-4). These research questions are derived directly from an analysis of a health problem. The specificity of the question depends on the uniqueness of the investigator's interests. After researchers identify an area of investigation and document the significance of the study, they are faced with the task of narrowing the area of investigation into a feasible chunk within a designated time span. Some researchers devote their entire professional life to a specific area of research; others drastically change their research areas as they broaden their interests.

5.6.1 Determining Feasibility

In the process of narrowing the investigation to a feasible study, the investigator should, as a preliminary procedure, carefully examine the following questions:
- How long will data collection take?
  - *Laboratory experiments*: The length of time required for preparing and collecting data for each participant
  - *Travel time*: The length of time required to get to and from the data collection site

- *Interview time*: Time for each subject multiplied by total number of subjects equals total interview time
- *Mail survey*: Researcher must account for response time and possibly a second mailing
- *Correlational study*: Individual or group testing time periods
- *Methodological*: Consideration of time for constructing instrument and obtaining reliability and validity data
- What measuring instruments are available for testing constructs and variables?
  - *Cost*: Expenses incurred to obtain test instruments
  - *Expertise*: Level of competency or experience needed to administer and interpret test results
- Are participants readily available? Where can participants be obtained?
  - *Screening criteria*: Used to determine participant inclusion
  - *Incentives for the participants*: Will payment or some other incentive be given to the participants?
- What expertise is needed to carry out the treatment procedure?
  - What are the total financial costs of the research, and who will finance them?
  - How long will it take for approval by the institutional review board (IRB) of ethical standards?

TABLE 5-4
HYPOTHETICAL RESEARCH QUESTIONS RELATED TO DISABILITY

DISABILITY	RESEARCH QUESTION
AIDS	How can prescriptive exercise help in reducing symptoms?
Cerebral palsy	Is development sequential and hierarchical in children with motor lesions in the cerebral cortex?
Depression	What is the role of exercise in increasing serotonin?
Hypertension	Can blood pressure rates be self-regulated through biofeedback techniques?
Learning disability	What are significant factors in facilitating handwriting?
Mental retardation	How does the environment facilitate or restrict learning?
Multiple sclerosis	What are the effects of stress on triggering episodes?
Schizophrenia	Can relaxation therapy help the individual to manage stress?

5.7 PSYCHOLOGICAL BLOCKS IN SELECTION OF A RESEARCH PROBLEM

Many times, graduate students confronted with the task of completing a thesis, dissertation, or study that involves collecting primary data are stymied in selecting a researchable topic. Students often belabor the process and frequently change their research area. In the process of selecting a feasible research problem, the student can become frustrated and blocked. In overcoming these psychological blocks, the student should examine the consequences of a research study and its potential significance. The following examples are typical of the psychological blocks that interfere with selecting a research problem.

- A research topic is dropped prematurely because the investigator fails to locate enough published studies related to the topic.
- The investigator is overwhelmed by the multiplicity of studies published in an area and concludes that further research is not necessary because the area has already been researched sufficiently. The investigator drops the topic without rigorously evaluating the validity and conclusiveness of results.

- The research topic selected is too broad, considering the time constraints of an investigator. Instead of narrowing the research topic to a feasible study the investigation is terminated.
- A preliminary investigation of a research area reveals difficulty in measuring an outcome variable. The investigator drops the study without seeking to construct an instrument that could reliably and validly measure the outcome.
- An investigator is motivated to explore a research area with the goal of making an important and original contribution to the body of knowledge. The investigator refuses to delimit a study after realizing the amount of time necessary to complete the study and subsequently terminates the investigation.

Selecting a researchable problem should be an ongoing process where the investigator explores the relevance, feasibility, applicability, and significance of a study. The worksheet guide in Box 5-1 lists the areas that a researcher should be aware of in the process of selecting and narrowing a researchable problem.

5.7.1 Worksheet Guide for Selecting a Research Problem

Box 5-1 provides a worksheet that can be used to select a research problem.

Box 5-1. Worksheet Guide for Selecting a Research Problem

1. What is the target population? (e.g., group with disabilities, student or clinician from the allied health profession)

2. What are the perceived needs of the population (e.g., investigating causes of disability, evaluation and diagnostic methods, student performance, evaluation of therapists' effectiveness, investigation of treatment techniques, evaluation of personal factors)?

3. What are the primary and secondary sources relevant to responses 1 and 2?

Journal articles	1.
	2.
	3.
Annual reviews	1.
	2.
	3.
Textbooks	1.
	2.
	3.
Statistical compendiums	1.
	2.
	3.

4. Are independent and dependent variables identifiable?

Independent variables (presumed cause):	1.
	2.
	3.
Dependent variables (presumed effects):	1.
	2.
	3.

5. How can the research impact …

- Treatment:

- Education:

- Administration:

(continued)

Box 5-1. Worksheet Guide for Selecting a Research Problem (continued)

6. Can research variables be operationally defined?

7. What explanation or theory accounts for the presumed relationship between variables?

8. What research model's are relevant to the study? Identify model and state research question relative to research model.

Qualitative

- Experimental (pre-test/post-test):

- Methodological (construction of instrument):

- Evaluation (evaluation of health care system):

- Correlation (relationship between variables):

Quantitative

- Survey (description of population):

- Historical (reconstruction of events):

- Clinical or naturalistic observation (dynamic analysis of subject):

- Heuristic (discovery of relationships):

9. Research problem/question

- State the research problem:

- State the hypothesis in null or directional form:

- State the guiding question:

10. To which groups are the research findings directed? (e.g., clinicians, individuals with disabilities, students, academicians, program administrators)

Feasibility Check

- Where can participants be obtained?

- How many participants are necessary?

- What tests, instruments, or apparatuses will be necessary to measure outcome?

(continued)

BOX 5-1. WORKSHEET GUIDE FOR SELECTING A RESEARCH PROBLEM (CONTINUED)

11. What are financial costs?

• Travel:

• Mailings:

• Tests:

• Protocols:

• Clinical time:

• Apparatus:

• Computer analysis:

• Books and duplicating:

• Clerical and typing:

• Laboratory analysis of findings:

12. Analysis of time (list the projected time sequence or dates for completion of research phases)

Initiation of study	Review of literature	Preparation for data collection	Approval from IRB	Collection of results	Writing discussion chapter	Completion of study

5.8 WHY RESEARCH PROPOSALS ARE NOT APPROVED

The following list of major reasons for the disapproval of research proposals is based on the authors' experiences as raters on governmental and university committees. The list is summarized in Table 5-5.

• *The research problem is insignificant, and the results will have little impact on clinical practice currently or in the future.* An example of an insignificant problem is an investigation of the relationship of low birth weight with the incidence of cerebral palsy. A literature search in this area already confirms that low birth weight is one among many risk factors for cerebral palsy. Nonetheless, not all infants with cerebral palsy are born prematurely nor are all infants with low birth weight destined to have cerebral palsy. This study will have little impact on our understanding of the causes of cerebral palsy and will not provide insight into its prevention and treatment. The projected results from this type of study would have a splintering effect where one variable is linked to a disability that has already been found to have multiple causes. A better study in a related area would be to examine the effects of low birth weight on one area of development, such as motor function. In this way, the investigator can narrow the research and control for extraneous variables that could have a potential effect on the results.

• *The hypothesis presented is not supported by scientific evidence and seems speculative.* As a hypothetical example, a researcher proposes that a computer application for cognitive rehabilitation is effective in treating individuals with brain injuries. The investigator equates improvement with the client's ability to learn a computer game. The investigator does not demonstrate through a literature review that there is a carryover of this computer skill to the learning of functional skills in independent living. A better study is to investigate the types of skills that are facilitated while learning with a computer.

• *The research problem is more complex than the investigator presents, and it needs to be narrowed down.* For example, a researcher proposes to examine the effects of sensory integration therapy on children with attention-deficit/hyperactivity disorder (ADHD). Both variables are complex and must be operationally defined. Sensory integration therapy includes several components in treatment, whereas ADHD is a complex disorder with multiple causes. A better study is to identify one aspect of sensory integration therapy, such as vestibular stimulation, and evaluate its effectiveness with a measurable variable, such as motor proficiency, as assessed by the Miller Assessment for Preschoolers (Miller, 1988).

TABLE 5-5

REASONS WHY RESEARCH PROPOSALS ARE DENIED

- The research problem is insignificant, and the results will have little impact on clinical practice currently or in the future.
- The hypothesis presented is not supported by scientific evidence and seems speculative.
- The research problem is more complex than the investigator presents, and it needs to be narrowed down.
- The anticipated results from the study will be of only local significance and lacks external validity or generalizability.
- The research proposed has too many uncontrolled elements.
- The research methodology seems overly complex and difficult to replicate.
- The proposed outcome measures are either inappropriate, unstandardized, unreliable, or invalid.
- Extraneous variables are left uncontrolled and may influence the results.
- Overall design of the study seems incomplete and not well-conceived.
- The statistical tests suggested for analyzing the data are not appropriate.
- Selection of subjects for the study is not representative of a target population.
- The treatment procedure under investigation has not been adequately defined in enough detail to replicate.
- The literature review seems outdated and lacks landmark studies in the area of investigation.
- The equipment identified in the study is outmoded or unsuitable.
- The investigator has not proposed adequate time for completion of the study.
- Resources are inadequate to complete the study.
- The setting and environment for the study are unsuitable.
- The investigator has not considered the ethical nature of the study, such as stating the potential physical and psychological risks to subjects in an informed consent form, or has not received approval from an IRB regarding human subjects.

- *The anticipated results from the study will be of only local significance and lacks external validity or generalizability.* An example of a flawed proposal is when a researcher designs a survey of job satisfaction for occupational therapists in a local school district without considering the generalizability to a larger sample or population. The data collected from this study would have only local interest and could not be generalized to teachers in other schools. In a better study of job satisfaction among occupational therapists, the researcher would determine first the demographics of an average occupational therapists, considering age, gender, and educational level. These variables could be used to determine if the occupational therapists are representative of a larger population. The survey would be designed with the intention of applying it to a more general sample. Questions would be generated that examine the broad issues of job satisfaction among occupational therapists in general rather than looking at local issues that affect job satisfaction in that particular school district.
- *The research proposed has too many uncontrolled elements.* For example, a researcher wants to study the effects of in utero exposure to alcohol on children born with fetal alcohol syndrome. The amount of alcohol exposure is unknown and is dependent on the mother's self-report, which is often unreliable. In addition, the home environment and genetic makeup are variables that may play a part in the child's behavior. These variables are difficult to measure and are often neglected by the researcher. A better approach is a retrospective case study analysis of an infant with fetal alcohol syndrome and the child's mother, exploring the dynamics of the case.
- *The research methodology seems overly complex and difficult to replicate.* For example, a researcher wants to examine the relationship between the onset of a depressive episode and an individual who is vulnerable. The interaction between family relationships, work situations, and personal attitudes are complex and make it difficult to identify the interactive factors that result in depression. Because of the individuality of each episode, replication of the study using a group method or survey would be difficult and might distort results. A better study would include a qualitative research method using an in-depth case study approach to identify within each individual the interactive effects that trigger depression.

- *The proposed outcome measures are either inappropriate, unstandardized, unreliable, or invalid.* A researcher investigating the effects of exercise on depression creates a scale for depression without testing for its reliability or validity. A better approach to measurement is to use more than one instrument to measure outcome (i.e., triangulation). For example, the investigator can use a physiological measure, a standardized test, and a client self-report. These three measures will increase the internal validity of the study in assessing outcome.

- *Extraneous variables are left uncontrolled and may influence the results.* For example, a researcher wants to examine the effect of a specific treatment method on improving motor skills. Although the researcher is careful to administer pre- and post-tests, extraneous variables, such as practice at home, additional interventions, or sessions per week, are not included in the analysis. These variables will most certainly affect the results. A better study would be to take frequent measures of performance, perhaps at the beginning and end of each therapy session, to determine changes in skill level. Another possibility is to have the client and researcher keep a log describing motor performance.

- *Overall design of the study seems incomplete and not well-conceived.* In this example, elements of the research proposal are missing, such as controlling for extraneous variables that could possibly influence the results or a large section of the literature review is omitted. It is important for the researcher to work with an outline that lists the essential components of a research proposal.

- *The statistical tests suggested for analyzing the data are not appropriate.* An investigator has collected ordinal data, such as ranking of students on an achievement test. Rather than using a nonparametric test, such as the Spearman Rank Order Correlation used for ordinal type data, the researcher inappropriately applies a parametric test, such as the Pearson correlation coefficient statistical test used for interval scale data. The statistical test applied should be based on the measurement scale of data. The assumptions of parametric statistics, such as normality of data distribution, should be followed. The appropriate statistics are based on the assumptions underlying the statistical tests.

- *Selection of subjects for the study is not representative of a target population.* If it is known that the incidence of traumatic brain injuries (TBIs) is higher for males than females by more than 2 to 1 and that more than 50% of clients with TBIs are between the ages of 15 and 24 years, then the investigator should try to select participants who reflect these statistics. This is especially true for studies where the investigator intends to generalize results to a representative sample. Nonetheless, there are studies in which the investigator is interested in examining a non-representative sample that is a portion of the target population, such as females or children with TBIs. Then the investigator must delineate clearly the target population in the title of the study.

- *The treatment procedure under investigation has not been adequately defined in enough detail to replicate.* An investigator identifies the independent variable as counseling; however, not enough detail is given regarding the type, frequency, and duration of counseling. Therefore, this study cannot be replicated.

- *The literature review seems outdated and lacks landmark studies in the area of investigation.* In reviewing the literature, it is wise to first examine current secondary texts or to survey articles in the area to identify the major landmark studies that are cited frequently. An up-to-date literature review also can be found by scanning the current journals in a subject area and by looking at the journal's yearly index.

- *The equipment identified in the study is outmoded or unsuitable.* For example, a test that has been standardized on adults is used for children. This is inappropriate and unsuitable for the study.

- *The investigator has not proposed adequate time for completion of the study.* In outlining the proposal for a study, the researcher should set up a timeline graph that breaks down the components of the study into time periods (see Box 5-1).

- *Resources are inadequate to complete the study.* For example, a research plan includes a request for funds to pay assistants to collect data. The funds requested for support are insufficient to complete the study.

- *The setting and environment for the study are unsuitable.* In this instance, the investigator attempts to complete a complex study without securing an appropriate environment for the study, such as a fully equipped laboratory or testing area that is free from distracting noise.

- *The investigator has not considered the ethical nature of the study, such as stating the potential physical and psychological risks to subjects in an informed consent form, or has not received approval from an IRB regarding human subjects.* For example, a researcher begins to collect data for a study on apraxia and its relationship to students with learning disabilities before the IRB has approved the research design. This is unethical, and data collected cannot be used in the final analysis.

5.9 SUMMARY

How does one create a research project? Where do research ideas come from? What are the essential variables in formulating a research problem? Occupational therapy is an applied health profession meaning that the focus in the profession is in problem solving and clinical reasoning as applied to helping the client achieve desired social participation in his or her everyday life. Research in occupational therapy is problem oriented and focused on developing the assessments and interventions to assist clients. In this chapter, the emphasis is on helping the researcher to select a significant research project related to occupational therapy practice. Education in the preparation of becoming an occupational therapist, administration related to occupational therapy, and client intervention are the three major areas of research in occupational therapy. This chapter is the transition from formulating a significant research question to implementing the project. In the next chapters, the reader is introduced to the nuts and bolts of research, literature review, methodology, statistics, selecting a test instrument, and scientific writing.

6

Review of the Literature

That "the library" as yet unspecified—is the repository of by far the largest part of our recorded knowledge needs no demonstration. The author of an active article on West Africa who reports that the annual rainfall in Fernando, PA, is 100 inches found this information in the library—in a book. It is most unlikely that he measured the rain himself.

—Barzun & Graff (1970, p. 63)

OPERATIONAL LEARNING OBJECTIVES

By the end of this chapter the learner will:

- Identify the main purpose of a literature review.
- Initiate a computer-based library search, such as PubMed, MEDLINE (Medical Literature Analysis and Retrieval System Online), OT Search, CINAHL (Cumulative Index to Nursing and Allied Health), ERIC (Education and Resources Information Center), PsychINFO, and RehabDATA.
- Compare and contrast referral and primary sources.
- Initiate a search of the literature identifying relevant and up-to-date research articles.
- Critically evaluate the validity of research studies.
- Outline a comprehensive search of the related literature.

Rice, M. S., Stein, F., & Tomlin, G.
Clinical Research in Occupational Therapy, Sixth Edition (pp. 155-179).
© 2019 Taylor & Francis Group.

6.1 THE NEED FOR A LITERATURE REVIEW

What is a good literature review in the age of evidence-based practice? In general, a good literature review cites the relevant studies that have been used to justify research in an objective way. The first task of the researcher is to find the related studies through a search of databases. The second step is to evaluate the reliability and validity of the studies' results. In the 21st century the quality of published research has been put to the test because of the number of predatory journals that publish research without quality review. The Beall's List of Predatory Journals is updated frequently and available online (http://beallslist.weebly.com). Knowledge is part of a cumulative process in which information expands based on the previous work of researchers. Breakthroughs in knowledge do not occur suddenly. The scientist first explores the previous literature to determine (a) what has been accomplished, (b) what questions still remain, and (c) what research is recommended based on the results of the literature.

Scientific research is a force that advances knowledge. For many scientists, discovery of new information or technology is a process of juxtaposing research from diverse fields in relation to an identifiable problem. Wiener (1948), a mathematician who pioneered work on cybernetics (which eventually led to the invention of the computer), attained success by brainstorming with engineers, psychiatrists, educators, and physicists. These specialists were able to share their ideas, and their collaboration stimulated the examination of a problem from many perspectives. From this experience, Wiener developed a theory of thinking based on the integration of physical science theory with behavioral observations. The lesson from Wiener's careful research is that investigators exploring the literature should not only examine studies directly related to a problem, but also try to find studies from other fields that have an indirect or implied relationship to their question.

For example, if a researcher is interested in examining the relationship between staff morale and treatment effectiveness, there may be a need to search the literature in management psychology if a preliminary search reveals a lack of studies in occupational therapy (Osaro & Chima, 2014). The diversity of findings adds strength to a study, especially if corroboration of data appears from different professions. The Hawthorne effect, which was first noted in factory workers (Landsberger, 1958), is now widely accepted as a factor in clinical research. For example, a study by McCarney et al. (2007) found that there was a moderate Hawthorne effect in a study of patients diagnosed with Alzheimer's disease. Spinoffs from research in the space programs (https/spinoff.nasa.gov), such as the advances in nutrition, specialized clothing, computer programming, temperature control, and monitoring of vital bodily functions, are examples of applying data generated from a seemingly unrelated field.

The main goals of the investigator in searching the literature are to:

- Make an exhaustive search of the most up-to-date research
- Identify the landmark studies that have an important impact in the area investigated
- Evaluate the validity of the research findings
- Integrate and synthesize the results into content areas.
- Summarize the findings from previous studies
- Identify limitations of the published findings and recommend further research
- Justify the current research study based on the literature review

These goals are part of the overall preliminary process of research that precedes data collection.

6.2 CONCEPTUAL VIEW OF A LITERATURE SEARCH

The steps involved in a conceptual view of the literature search are shown in Figure 6-1. Each of these steps is described below.

1. The first step in initiating a literature search is to identify the key words in the study. The key words may be identified through (a) reading a secondary source, (b) clinical experience with a particular population, (c) reviewing a journal article, or (d) examining a thesaurus of terms, such as MeSH. The MeSH database can be used to find Medical Subject Heading terms, which are used to build a literature search strategy. ERIC is another database that publishes a thesaurus. These key words can be linked to the independent variable (e.g., intervention technique), dependent variable (e.g., desired outcome), outcome measure or test instrument (e.g., Allen's Cognitive level), target population (e.g., individuals with cognitive difficulties), contextual setting (e.g., assisted living center), age range (e.g., elderly), or frame of reference (e.g., occupational behavior).

2. The next step in a literature search is to locate a recent textbook or review article in which the researcher can obtain an overall summary of the major research in the specific area. For example, a researcher may be interested in the effectiveness of occupational therapy on the achievement of students with learning disabilities. The researcher would examine a recent textbook on pediatric occupational therapy, such as *Occupational Therapy for Children and Adolescents* (7th edition) by Case-Smith and Clifford O'Brien (2015), to gain an overall view of treatment and to identify recent references. The textbook may help identify key words and narrow the focus of the study.

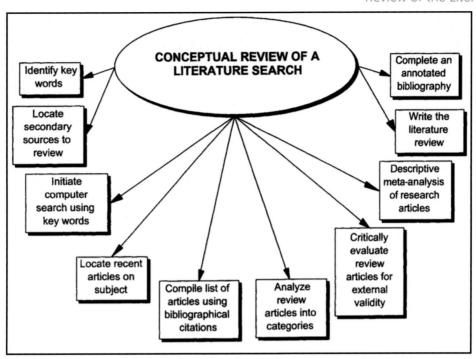

Figure 6-1. Conceptual review of the literature search.

3. Next, the researcher is ready to do an online search of recent articles in the field of study. PubMed, MEDLINE, Embase, Cochrane Library, OTseeker, CINAHL, and ERIC are examples of databases that can be used. Another way to examine recent articles is to look at the article in current issues or review the cumulative yearly index in recent occupational therapy journals. Examining the bibliography in relevant articles may also help to locate other articles. After the researcher has identified relevant articles, it is important to file the bibliographic citations and abstract for later use. (See discussion of occupational therapy databases later in this chapter.)

4. The next step is the categorization of the articles into types of publications, such as review, research, or theoretical papers (Table 6-1). Articles can also be categorized into subject areas for easier review.

5. The researcher must critically evaluate each article for external (i.e., generalization of results) and internal (i.e., rigor of the methodology) validity. The researcher examines how the variables were controlled, the subject selection, the randomness of the selection, the reliability and validity of the outcome measures, and the operational definition of the independent variable.

6. A descriptive tabulation of research studies identified by the literature review is next. The researcher designs a table that includes the title of the study, the date of publication, the authors or researchers, the number of subjects, the treatment methodology, the outcome measures, the statistical results, and conclusions. See the example of exercise and depression in Table 6-2.

7. The researcher is now ready to write the literature review from an outline. The review should include an integrated summary of the various articles.

8. Finally, the researcher should develop an annotated bibliography. Articles should be organized by subject heading, with research articles listed separately from theoretical articles. The annotated bibliography should include the published abstract. The purpose of the abstract is to provide the reader with a quick overview of the problem under investigation, the methods used in data collection, the results reported, and the conclusions. The abstract is an intermediary step between the bibliographical citation and the complete journal article. Because the abstract is a self-contained summary, it can provide the researcher with all of the information desired in a specific research area. The annotated bibliography serves as a primary data source for the research study and it helps the reader gain an overview of the research study.

6.3 LOCATING SOURCES OF RELATED LITERATURE

More than 5000 periodicals are currently published annually in medical and health-related areas that are of interest to occupational therapists. The literature search task would be enormous if the investigator had to review each periodical individually. How can the investigator quickly obtain a list of studies that are relevant to narrow

TABLE 6-1	
CATEGORIZATION OF PUBLICATIONS	
TYPES OF PUBLICATIONS	**EXAMPLES OF PUBLICATIONS**
Primary data research	• Journal articles • Dissertations • Theses • Conference proceedings • Government documents • Statistical surveys
Review articles	• Journal articles • Monographs
Evaluation findings	• Joint Commission on Accreditation results • Special commissions
Conceptual or theoretical papers	• Journal articles • Monographs • Conference proceedings
Position papers	• Journal articles • Associational and organizational statements • Monographs • Editorials
Secondary and tertiary information	• Popular magazines • *Scientific American* • Encyclopedias • College texts
Other publications	• Test manuals • Reference books for test instruments • Book reviews • Software programs and reviews • Manuals for self-help devices
Bibliographic references	• Books in print • Information retrieval system • Directories of reference

the search and reduce the number of hours examining the online catalog and library stacks? For the persevering investigator seeking to identify every study conceivable, the task could be endless. Realistically, the investigator accepts the limitation that some published and unpublished studies will not be located. For example, studies published in foreign journals that have not been translated, recent unpublished papers presented at conferences and institutes, ongoing research where the investigator has not published the findings, and research studies by students presented in unpublished theses, dissertations, or special studies may not be found. These are realistic limitations to every study. Nonetheless, with the availability of computer systems for information retrieval, the present-day investigator can locate a vast portion of the literature.

The literature search is divided into two areas: referral sources and primary sources of data. These two areas are outlined in Table 6-3. The first step in searching the literature is to locate where the relevant studies are reported, that is, in which journal, source book, or dissertation. The referral source supplies bibliographical information locating a specific study. The use of key words allows the researcher to more easily identify those studies that cover a particular topic. Frequently, the key words for a specific article are listed immediately before or after the abstract. This is illustrated in Figure 6-2, in which the key words (e.g., adolescence, learning disabilities, school-based,

TABLE 6-2

EFFECT OF EXERCISE ON DEPRESSION: EXAMPLE OF DESCRIPTIVE TABULATION

STUDY	SUBJECTS	TREATMENT TECHNIQUE[a]	OUTCOME MEASURES	RESULTS
Blue, 1979. Aerobic running as a treatment of moderate depression.	2 adult patients with chronic depression	Aerobic running program 3 times per week for 9 weeks	Zung (1965) SDS	Significant reduction of depression
Bosscher, 1993. Running and mixed physical exercises with depressed psychiatric patients.	24 men and women diagnosed with depression and hospitalized in psychiatric hospital	E: Short-term running therapy 3 times per week for 8 weeks; C: mixed physical and relaxation exercises 3 times per week for 8 weeks	Zung (1965) SDS	Significant improvement for running group; no significant improvement for mixed physical and exercise group
Brollier, Hamrick, & Jackson, 1994. Aerobic exercise: A potential occupational therapy modality for adolescents with depression.	4 adolescent boys from a private psychiatric hospital with diagnosis of depression	Brisk walking and running 3 times per week for 1 hour over a 65-day period	BDI (Beck, Ward, Mendelson, Mock, & Erbaugh, 1961)	Results showed a general decrease in depression scores of all subjects
Doyne, Chamblass, & Beutler, 1983. Aerobic exercise as a treatment of depression in women.	4 women with MDD	Aerobic exercise for 6 weeks	BDI (Beck et al., 1961); DACL (Lubin, 1981)	Significant reduction in depression scores compared with pre-exercise screening phase
Doyne et al., 1987. Running vs. weightlifting in the treatment of depression.	40 women diagnosed with depression	E1: walked/ran on indoor track in 7-minute intervals for 8 weeks; E2: used weightlifting machine for 8 weeks; C: no treatment	BDI (Beck et al., 1961); HRDS (Hamilton, 1960), DACL (Lubin, 1981)	Both aerobic groups and the weightlifting group showed significant improvement in depression; no change was observed in the control group
Greist et al., 1979. Running as a treatment for depression.	13 men, 15 women; aged 18 to 30 years	E: 10 patients ran 3 to 4 times per week; C: 18 in psychotherapy	Response Symptom Checklist (Greist et al., 1979)	Running was as effective as psychotherapy

(continued)

TABLE 6-2 (CONTINUED)
EFFECT OF EXERCISE ON DEPRESSION: EXAMPLE OF DESCRIPTIVE TABULATION

STUDY	SUBJECTS	TREATMENT TECHNIQUE[a]	OUTCOME MEASURES	RESULTS
Kaplan, Mendelsons, & Dubroff, 1983. The effect of a jogging program on psychiatric inpatients with symptoms of depression.	12 women, 6 men; aged 15 to 38 years; patients in acute care psychiatric ward	Warm-up and cool-down exercises; 20 minutes of graded walking/jogging on indoor track; short discussion of exercise and health-related topics	Self-report questionnaire (5-point Likert scale); observation by coleaders	Decreased sleep disturbances and increased self-esteem
Martinsen, Medhus, & Sandvik, 1985. Effects of aerobic exercise on depression: A controlled study.	43 patients with MDD; ages 17 to 60 years	E: 9 patients receiving TCAs and aerobic exercise for 1 hour 3 times per week for 9 weeks; E2: 15 patients receiving aerobic exercise but no TCAs; C1: 14 patients receiving TCAs and occupational therapy 3 times per week for 9 weeks; C2: 5 patients receiving occupational therapy but not TCAs	CPRS (Åsberg, Perris, Schalling, & Sedval 1987); BDI (Beck et al., 1961)	Significantly lower depression scores for those participating in aerobic exercises than others; maximum oxygen uptake noted in aerobic training groups resulted in greater antidepressive effects
Martinsen, Hoffart, & Solberg, 1989. Comparing aerobic with nonaerobic forms of exercise in the treatment of clinical depression: A randomized trial.	90 inpatients of a psychiatric hospital with diagnosis of depression	E: 43 patients participating in brisk walks and jogging 3 times per week for 8 weeks; C: 47 patients participating in muscular strength, flexibility, and relaxation exercises 3 times per week for 8 weeks	BDI (Beck et al., 1961); MADRS (Montgomery & Åsberg, 1979)	Depressed scores in both groups were reduced significantly, but no significant difference was observed between groups
Rape, 1987. Running and depression.	21 White men running 15 or more miles per week; 21 White males, nonexercisers	Matched two-group design comparing runners with nonexercisers	BDI (Beck et al., 1961)	Runners were significantly less depressed than were nonexercisers

[a]E = experimental group. C = control group.

BDI = Beck Depression Inventory; CPRS = Comprehensive Psychopathological Rating Scale; DACL = Depression Adjective Check-Lists; HRDS = Hamilton Rating Scale for Depression; MADRS = Montgomery and Åsberg Depression Rating Scale; MDD = major depressive disorder; SDS = Self-Rating Depression Scale; TCA = tricyclic antidepressant.

TABLE 6-3
THE LITERATURE SEARCH IN OCCUPATIONAL THERAPY

REFERRAL SOURCES	PRIMARY SOURCES OF DATA
• Information retrieval systems • Abstracting periodicals and bibliographic indexes • Directory of references • Annual reviews	• Journals • Theses • Conference proceedings • Government documents • Statistical compendiums • Unpublished studies

Ethical Dilemmas in School Based Therapy: Implications for Occupational Therapy
Josephine Mae Smith
Key Words: Adolescence, learning disabilities, school-based ethics, occupational therapy, decision making
Abstract: An analysis …

Figure 6-2. An example of key words listed before the abstract and journal article. The use of these key words will lead the reader to other related articles.

ethics, occupational therapy, decision making) have been listed before the abstract. A student or researcher looking for related articles would use one or more of these key words in the online search.

Each database has its own thesaurus that contains key words or concepts by using a controlled vocabulary, which provides a structure for classifying articles into given topics. Most databases are accessed online through library websites. Many of these searchable databases have a text box search option to search subject terms. If this option is used, a list of subject terms comes up based on the words entered into the search text box. This list of subject terms can provide a more focused search strategy. For more specialized words, such as the names of tests or the specific intervention theories (e.g., sensory integration, cognitive-behavioral, neurodevelopmental therapy), the exact term will suffice to locate the articles. As noted previously, MEDLINE uses MeSH subject headings.

The Thesaurus (https://www.nlm.nih.gov/mesh): MeSH is the National Library of Medicine's (NLM) controlled vocabulary thesaurus. It consists of sets of terms naming descriptors in a hierarchical structure that permits searching at various levels of specificity.

MeSH descriptors are arranged in both an alphabetic and a hierarchical structure. At the most general level of the hierarchical structure are very broad headings such as "Anatomy" or "Mental Disorders." More specific headings are found at more narrow levels of the 11-level hierarchy, such as "Ankle" and "Conduct Disorder." There are 27,883 descriptors in 2016 MeSH. There are also over 87,000 entry terms that assist in finding the most appropriate MeSH Heading, for example, "Vitamin C" is an entry term to "Ascorbic Acid." In addition to these headings, there are more than 232,000 headings called *Supplementary Concept*

Records (formerly Supplementary Chemical Records) within a separate thesaurus.

MeSH Applications: The MeSH thesaurus is used by NLM for indexing articles from 5600 of the world's leading biomedical journals for the MEDLINE/PubMED database in 2016. It is also used for the NLM-produced database that includes cataloging of books, documents, and audiovisuals acquired by the library. Each bibliographic reference is associated with a set of MeSH terms that describe the content of the item. Similarly, search queries use MeSH vocabulary to find items on a desired topic.

Establishing and Updating MeSH: The MeSH staff continually revises and updates the MeSH vocabulary. Staff subject specialists are responsible for areas of the health sciences in which they have knowledge and expertise. In addition to receiving suggestions from indexers and others, the staff collects new terms as they appear in the scientific literature or in emerging areas of research, define these terms within the context of existing vocabulary, and recommend their addition to MeSH. Professionals in various disciplines are also consulted regarding broad organizational changes and close coordination is maintained with various specialized vocabularies.

MeSH Data: MeSH, in machine-readable form, is provided at no charge via electronic means. The MeSH website (http://www.nlm.nih.gov/mesh) is the central access point for additional information about MeSH and for obtaining MeSH in electronic form. (NLM, 2018, para. 1-5)

Most information retrieval systems use *Boolean logic* as the strategy to build search statements. Boolean logic uses the logical operators *and, or,* and *not* to represent relationships between topics in a symbolic manner (Figure 6-3). Some systems also use the search operators of *with* and in. The use of the term *with* identifies those articles in which the connected terms are used in the same field (e.g., traumatic brain injury (TBI) with cognitive-behavior therapy), whereas the use of the term *in* specifies the particular field

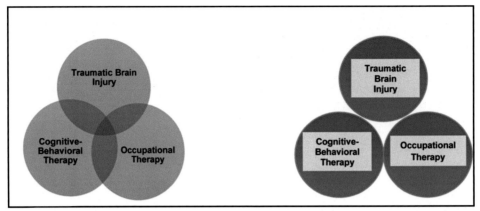

Figure 6-3. An example of Boolean thinking. In the first example, the researcher is interested in information about traumatic brain injury *and* cognitive-behavior therapy *and* occupational therapy. The articles retrieved from the search will be found in the intersection that contains all three terms. In the second example, articles about traumatic brain injury, cognitive-behavior therapy, *or* occupational therapy will be found. The first example is a more specific search that yields a smaller number of articles.

(traumatic brain injury in title). By combing search terms with these logical operators, the researcher can limit or enlarge the search. For example, if a researcher is looking for articles regarding the treatment of TBI using cognitive-behavior therapy in occupational therapy settings, the search term would be written as

> traumatic brain injury and cognitive-behavior therapy and occupational therapy

Use of these terms with the delimiter and would limit the search to only those articles in which both TBI and cognitive-behavior therapy have been discussed. Articles that contain only etiology or only treatment will not be obtained. If, on the other hand, the researcher is interested in articles that describe either TBI or cognitive-behavior therapy, the search statement is written as

> (traumatic brain injury and occupational therapy) or (cognitive-behavior therapy and occupational therapy)

Articles that examine TBI or cognitive-behavior therapy and occupational therapy and those that examine both TBI and cognitive-behavior therapy will be obtained. Thus, this search statement produces a larger list of citations, including the citations from the first search statement. As each system uses a slightly different search technique, it will be necessary to obtain specific information about search strategies for the system used (e.g., OT Search, MEDLINE, or ERIC).

6.3.1 Information Retrieval Systems

Automated systems for storing and retrieving information have revolutionized libraries. Although print-only journals still exist, many journals also include an online

version of the print edition and others are now exclusively online. Through computer and internet technology, persons seeking information have access to an enormous amount of information available through these online journals. Many online journals can be accessed through the journal's publisher for free or through a fee-based system. Many hospital and university libraries subscribe to various searchable database conglomerates and provide access to databases and electronic online journals for clinicians, faculty, staff, and students. The particular type of searchable database(s) offered by any given institution is determined by the type of subscription with which the institution has contracted. The major information retrieval systems relevant to research in medicine, rehabilitation, health care, and education are described in this section. Additionally, there are a few databases that are free to the public and can be accessed through any computer connected to the internet, such as PubMed and Google Scholar.

PubMed (http://www.ncbi.nlm.nih.gov/pubmed/): PubMed comprises more than 19 million citations for biomedical literature from MEDLINE, life science journals, and online books. Citations may include links to full-text content from PubMed Central and publisher websites (http://www.ncbi.nlm.nih.gov/sites/entrez). PubMed is accessible through any computer that is connected to the internet.

MEDLINE (https://www.nlm.nih.gov/bsd/medline.html): MEDLINE is a database focused on biomedical literature. It has a fascinating history as a product of MEDLARS, which was developed during the Cold War as a repository of biomedical information.

MEDLINE is the [NLM] journal citation database. Started in the 1960s, it now provides more than 24 million references to biomedical and life sciences journal articles back to 1946. MEDLINE includes citations from more than 5,600 scholarly journals published around the world. Publishers submit journals to an NIH [National Institutes of

Health]-chartered advisory committee, the Literature Selection Technical Review Committee (LSTRC), which reviews and recommends journals for MEDLINE. The LSTRC considers the quality of the scientific content of a journal, including originality and the importance of the content for the MEDLINE global audience, using the guidelines found on the NLM Fact Sheet MEDLINE Journal Selection. The MEDLINE database is directly searchable from NLM as a subset of the PubMed database as well as through other numerous search services that obtain the data from NLM's Data Distribution program. In addition to the comprehensive journal selection process, what sets MEDLINE apart from the rest of PubMed is the added value of using the NLM controlled vocabulary, Medical Subject Headings (MeSH), to index citations. (U.S. National Library of Medicine., 2018)

The National Network of Libraries of Medicine is composed of eight regional medical libraries in the United States that provide searches for health scientists. These federally designated regional medical libraries also provide consultative services and interlibrary loan privileges to other medical libraries within their region. Contact information for the NLM Regional Offices is available at http:/nnlm.gov. The NLM houses a National Information Center on Health Services Research and Health Care Technology (Box 6-1).

OT Search (http://www1.aota.org/otsearch/index.asp): OT Search (formerly called OT BibSys) is a bibliographic database that requires payment of a yearly fee to access. It was developed and is owned by the American Occupational Therapy Association (AOTA). Many occupational therapy programs pay the site fee so that their students and faculty can have access to the database. The database covers literature in occupational therapy and related subject areas, such as rehabilitation, education, psychiatry and psychology, and health care delivery and administration. On the website, information that identifies the material and the abstract necessary for obtaining the full text of the indexed resources is available.

The repository for the official documents for AOTA is located in the Wilma L. West (WLW) Library.

The collection includes monographs, journals, dissertations, theses, conference proceedings, and audiovisual materials covering the literature of occupational therapy and related subject areas, including rehabilitation, education, psychiatry or psychology, and health care delivery and administration.

The contents of the WLW Library are indexed in OT Search, which is an online bibliographic database with over 41,900 bibliographic records. Drawing from this database, the library operates as a national clearinghouse of occupational therapy information for AOTA members and occupational therapy

professionals. Librarians can assist in performing literature searches, obtain factual information for specific queries, provide guidance on additional sources of information, or send photocopies of documents in compliance with copyright laws (American Occupational Therapy Foundation, n.d.)

The WLW Library also houses a variety of resources related to research, education, and occupational therapy practice. These resources include:

- WLW Library resource notes
- Research competencies for occupational therapy
- Responsible conduct of research
- Research priorities and parameters of practice for occupational therapy
- Research across the curriculum archives of the AOTA, which are housed in the WLW Library (http://www.aotf.org/resourceswlwlibrary)

CINAHL (http://www.cinahl.com): This database, updated monthly, covers English-language journals and literature from 1937 to the present in the disciplines of nursing and allied health, including emergency services, health education, and social services in health care. Publications from the following allied health fields are indexed:

- Athletic training
- Audiology
- Cardiopulmonary technology
- Dental hygiene
- Emergency services
- Health information management
- Medical assisting
- Medical/laboratory technology
- Nutrition and dietetics
- Occupational therapy
- Physical therapy and rehabilitation
- Physician assistants
- Radiologic technology
- Respiratory therapy
- Social service in health care
- Speech-language pathology
- Surgical technology

Selected journals are also indexed in the areas of consumer health, biomedicine, and health sciences librarianship. In total, more than 5400 journals are regularly indexed; of these, more than 600 journals provide full-text articles. CINAHL maintains more than 5.4 million records. The database also provides access to health care books, nursing dissertations, selected conference proceedings, standards of professional practice, educational software, and audiovisual materials in nursing and other health-related fields. CINAHL uses nearly 13,000 subject headings. More information about CINAHL can be found at http://www.ebscohost.com/cinahl

Box 6-1. National Information Center on Health Services Research and Health Care Technology

The 1993 NIH Revitalization Act created the National Information Center on Health Services Research and Health Care Technology (NICHSR) at the NLM to improve "… the collection, storage, analysis, retrieval, and dissemination of information on health services research, clinical practice guidelines, and on health care technology, including the assessment of such technology."

The Center works closely with the Agency for Healthcare Research and Quality, formerly the Agency for Health Care Policy and Research, to improve the dissemination of the results of health services research, with a special emphasis on the growing body of evidence from reports and technology assessments, which provide organizations with comprehensive, science-based information on common, costly medical conditions and new health care technologies.

The overall goals of the NICHSR are to make the results of health services research, including practice guidelines and technology assessments, readily available to health practitioners, health care administrators, health policy makers, payers, and the information professionals who serve these groups; to improve access to data and information needed by the creators of health services research; and to contribute to the information infrastructure needed to foster patient record systems that can produce useful health services research data as a byproduct of providing health care.

Products and Services

The NICHSR coordinates the development of information products and services related to health services research.

- HealthSTAR (Health Services Technology, Administration, and Research) was an online bibliographic information service that resided as a separate database available from the NLM from February 1994 (originally called HSTAR) to December 2000. Materials that comprised HealthSTAR have now migrated to other NLM online web-based environments: (1) journal citations are being added weekly to NLM's PubMed (http://pubmed.gov/); (2) books, book chapters, technical reports, and conference papers are added regularly to NLM's online catalog, LocatorPlus (http://locatorplus.gov); and (3) meeting abstracts from AcademyHealth (formerly Academy for Health Services Research and Health Policy and the Association for Health Services Research), Health Technology Assessment International (formerly International Society of Technology Assessment in Health Care), and the Cochrane Colloquium annual conferences have moved to the NLM Gateway (http://gateway.nlm.nih.gov/). Users can go to these specific environments to search for HSR literature or they can use the NLM Gateway to simultaneously search across all information services.

- HSRProj (http://www.nlm.nih.gov/hsrproj/) and the NLM Gateway (http://gateway.nlm.nih.gov) under the Other Collections category a database of citations to research-in-progress funded by federal and foundation grants and contracts, became available in 1995. HSRProj builds upon a database developed in prototype by staff of AcademyHealth and the Cecil Sheps Center at the University of North Carolina with funding from the Pew Charitable Trust. It includes over 5000 citations to ongoing or recently completed research funded since 2000.

- HSRR (Health Services and Sciences Research Resources; http://www.nlm.nih.gov/nichsr/hsrr_search/) is a free, searchable catalog of research datasets, instruments, and software relevant to health services research, behavioral and social sciences, and public health.

- HSTAT (Health Services/Technology Assessment Text; http://hstat.nlm.nih.gov) is a free, web-based resource of full-text documents that provide health information and support health care decision making. The HSTAT's audience includes health care providers, health service researchers, policy makers, payers, consumers, and the information professionals who serve these groups. It includes Agency for Healthcare Research and Quality evidence reports, guideline documents, and technology assessments, NIH Consensus Development Conference Statements and Technology Assessment Workshop Reports, the U.S. Task Force on Preventive Services' Guide to Clinical Preventive Services, HIV/AIDS Treatment Information Service approved guidelines, and Substance Abuse and Mental Health Services Administration treatment improvement protocols.

- DIRLINE, (available from NLM Gateway http://gateway.nlm.nih.gov under the Consumer Health category) the NLM's Directory of Information Resources onLINE, has a special subfile covering health services research organizations, including those involved in technology assessment and development of practice guidelines.

(continued)

Box 6-1. National Information Center on Health Services Research and Health Care Technology (continued)

In addition to its online databases, NICHSR and other NLM staff develop guides, fact sheets, bibliographies, and other products targeted to health services researchers. To find many of these, go to the Health Services Research and Public Health Information Programs website at http://www.nlm.nih.gov/hsrph.html.

Outreach and Training

The NICHSR collaborates with other NLM components and with members of the NNLM to exhibit NLM products and services and to present specially focused training classes at national meetings of HSR-related organizations. The NICHSR provides training programs for medical librarians to improve their ability to respond to health services research questions and to support the conduct of such research, as well as training activities directed toward producers and users of health services research.

Research and Development

The NICHSR supports several intramural and extramural research and development projects designed to improve access to useful health services research data. Current efforts include the following: expansion of the Unified Medical Language System Metathesaurus to improve its utility in creating and retrieving computer-based patient records; and funding of extramural research and evaluation involving the creation and use of computer-based patient records.

For more information on NICHSR, contact:

National Information Center on Health Services Research and Health Care Technology

National Library of Medicine

8600 Rockville Pike

Building 38A, Room 4S-410, Mail Stop 20

Bethesda, MD 20894

Voice: (301) 496-0176; Fax: (301) 402-3193

email: nichsr@nlm.nih.gov; Internet: http://www.nlm.nih.gov/nichsr/

NLM's home page is http://www.nlm.nih.gov.

For a complete list of NLM Fact Sheets visit http://www.nlm.nih.gov/pubs/factsheets/factsheets.html Or, write to: Office of Communications and Public Liaison, National Library of Medicine, 8600 Rockville Pike, Bethesda, Maryland 20894. Fax: (301) 496-4450: email: publicinfo@nlm.nih.gov

Reprinted with permission from U.S. National Library of Medicine. (2018). About the National Information Center on Health Services Research and Health Care Technology (NICHSR). Retrieved from https://www.nlm.nih.gov/nichsr/about-NICHSR.html

ERIC (http://eric.ed.gov/): ERIC is the world's most widely used index for educational-related literature. Established in 1966, ERIC is supported by the U.S. Department of Education's Office of Educational Research and Improvement and is administered by the U.S. National Library of Education.

ERIC is the largest education database in the world, containing more than 1.5 million records for journal articles, research reports, curriculum and teaching guides, conference papers, dissertations and theses, and books. Currently, more than 650,000 records are from scholarly journals; more than 225,000 records are from reports, conference proceedings, and the like; and more than 14,000 records are from reference works. Many of these records contain links to the full-text documents in ERIC, but the user can also access full-text from the publisher when available or use the library's linked full-text resources when available. Additional full text from ProQuest for many of the journals indexed in ERIC is available through ProQuest Education Journals. The bundle of ERIC Plus Text includes the ERIC index and ProQuest Education Journals, and users can link directly from records in an ERIC search to full text from ProQuest Education Journals (http://proquest.libguides.com/eric).

PsychINFO (apa.org): PsychINFO is an online database with over 4 million records that covers the disciplines of psychology and related fields, including psychiatry, sociology, anthropology, education, pharmacology physiology, linguistics, and psychopharmacology. PsychINFO indexes records published from the 1800s, with some material being originally published in the 17th and 18th centuries. The records include journal articles, books, dissertations, and other secondary publications.

RehabDATA (naric.com): RehabDATA, produced by the National Rehabilitation Information Center (NARIC), is the leading literature database on disability and rehabilitation. The collection spans 1956 to the present. The database describes over 80,000 documents covering physical, mental, and psychiatric disabilities; independent living; vocational rehabilitation; special education; assistive technology; law; employment; and other issues as they relate to people with disabilities. RehabDATA results may also include abstracts from the international research collection, originally developed by CIRRIE. More than 120,000 documents are abstracted in this database. NARIC adds approximately 4000 items to RehabDATA each year, including 1000 international research documents.

Four main categories of documents are included: (a) reports, studies, and papers submitted by projects funded by the National Institute on Disability, Independent Living, and Rehabilitation Research (as featured in the NIDILRR Program Directory); (b) articles published in rehabilitation-related periodicals; (c) international research originally collected by the Center for International Rehabilitation Research (CIRRIE) project; and (d) commercially published books. Some non-print materials are also included (NARIC, 2018).

AbleData (http://www.abledata.com): ABLEDATA, also funded by NIDRR, provides information in the area of assistive technology and rehabilitation equipment.

AbleData's most significant resource is the AbleData database of assistive technology, which contains objective information on more than 35,000 assistive products (over 22,000 of which are currently available). For each product, we provide a detailed description of the product's functions and features, price information (when available), and contact information for the product's manufacturer and/or distributors. We also offer information on non-commercial prototypes, customized and one-of-a-kind products, and do-it-yourself designs.

OTseeker (http://www.otseeker.com): OTseeker is an occupational therapy database

[t]hat contains abstracts of systematic reviews and randomized controlled trials relevant to occupational therapy. Most trials have been critically appraised and rated to assist you to evaluate their validity and interpretability. These ratings will help one to judge the quality and usefulness of trials for informing clinical interventions. In one database, OTseeker provides you with fast and easy access to trials from a wide range of sources in occupational therapy.

Using the search window, users can determine the internal validity and the statistical integrity of the study. The database was initiated in 2003 and is updated on a regular basis.

6.3.1.1 Other Databases and Periodicals for Occupational Therapists

OTDBase (http://www.otdbase.org/) is provided for a fee and contains abstracts from about 20 international occupational therapy journals. The system is user friendly and cross-indexes articles.

Embase, or the Excerpta Medica Database (http://embase.com), is a comprehensive biomedical and pharmacological database produced by Elsevier and includes the following features:

- "Journal coverage from 1947 to the present
- Over 32 million records, including MEDLINE titles
- Over 8,500 journals from over 95 countries, including MEDLINE titles
- Over 2,900 indexed journals unique to Embase
- Over 1.5 million records added yearly, with an average of over 6000 each day
- Over 2.3 million conference abstracts indexed from more than 7000 conferences dating from 2009
- Full-text indexing of drug, disease and medical device data (Elsevier.com, n.d., para. 1)

Internet Mental Health (http://mentalhealth.com/home/introduction.html) is a free online database for professionals and patients that provides information on the 54 most common mental disorders.

Publishing original, refereed papers, *Health Education Research* deals with all the vital issues involved in health education and promotion worldwide—providing a valuable link between the health education research and practice communities.

Health Education Research gives highest priority to original research focused on health education and promotion research, particularly intervention studies with solid research designs. The journal welcomes rigorous qualitative studies or those that concentrate on hard-to-reach populations. Because of the high number of submissions, cross sectional studies, instrument development, psychometric studies, and pilot data are assigned lower priority. Medical or professional health education studies are not within the scope of the journal's themes unless they are directly related to the broad area of changing health behaviors and the conditions that influence health. (Health Education Research, n.d.)

CSA Sociological Abstracts (http://www.proquest.com/products-services/socioabs-set-c.html) indexes the international literature of sociology and related disciplines in the social and behavioral sciences. It includes a companion file, Social Services Abstracts.

Social Services Abstracts (https://www.proquest.com/products-services/ssa-set-c.html) provides bibliographic coverage of current research focused on social work, human services, and related areas, including social welfare, social policy, and community development. The database includes abstracts of journal articles and dissertations, as well as citations to book reviews.

Dissertation Abstracts Online (http://www.proquest.com/products-services/dissertations/find-a-dissertation.html). Virtually every major research library in the world provides access to the ProQuest Dissertations & Theses (PQDT) database through one of several formats.

PQDT Database: With more than 2.3 million entries, the PQDT database is the most comprehensive collection of dissertations and theses in the world. Students, faculty, and other researchers search the database for titles related to their scholarly interests. Of the millions of graduate works listed, we offer over 1.9 million in full text format. PQDT is a subscription database, so consult your library for availability.

Biological Abstracts (http://www.ovid.com/site/catalog/DataBase/24.pdf) report the world's bioscience research. This database contains more than 11.3 million records, with more than 250,000 being added every year. Indexed are journal records in areas of life science, genetics, anatomy, physiology, environmental pollutants, nutrition, psychiatry, and public health, as well as other biology-related records.

Web of Science (https://clarivate.libguides.com/directlinks). Core Collection provides researchers, administrators, faculty, and students with quick, powerful access to the world's leading citation databases. Authoritative, multidisciplinary content covers over 12,000 of the highest impact journals worldwide—including open access journals—and over 160,000 conference proceedings. You'll find current and retrospective coverage in the sciences, social sciences, arts, and humanities, with coverage dating back to 1900. Focus is on the essential data from across more than 250 disciplines.

Current Contents Connect (http://wokinfo.com/products_tools/multidisciplinary/CCC):

[i]s a current awareness database that provides easy web access to complete tables of contents, abstracts, bibliographic information, and abstracts from the most recently published issues of leading scholarly journals, as well as from more than 7000 relevant, evaluated websites.

NIH Office of Extramural Research (http://grants.nih.gov/grants/oer.htm) is an online database that contains information about health research currently supported by various agencies of the NIH, thereby allowing scientists and administrators of science programs to identify current research activities in areas relating to their own endeavors.

Annual Reviews (http://www.annualreviews.org/) "publishes authoritative reviews in 40 focused disciplines within the Biomedical, Life, Physical, and Social Sciences. Among the most highly cited in scientific literature, they are

available online and in print to individuals, institutions, and consortia worldwide" (Annual Reviews, 2018, para. 1).

Google Scholar (https://scholar.google.com/) allows you to search

[f]or scholarly literature. From one place, you can search across many disciplines and sources: articles, theses, books, abstracts and court opinions, from academic publishers, professional societies, online repositories, universities and other websites. Google Scholar helps you find relevant work across the world of scholarly research (Google Scholar, 2018, para. 1).

Similar to the Science Citation Index database, records in Google Scholar are linked to other published work that has cited that record. Google Scholar can be accessed by any computer that has internet access.

The Cochrane Library (http://www.cochranelibrary.com/cochrane-database-of-systematic-reviews/index.html) "is the leading resource for systematic reviews in health care. The CDSR includes Cochrane Reviews (the systematic reviews) and protocols for *Cochrane Reviews*, as well as editorials. The CDSR also has occasional supplements. The CDSR is updated regularly as *Cochrane Reviews* are published 'when ready' and form monthly issues"

Our mission is to promote evidence-informed health decision-making by producing high-quality, relevant, accessible systematic reviews and other synthesized research evidence. (Cochrane Library, 2018)

6.3.3 Sources for Health Statistics

Statistical information is an essential part of the literature search. The incidence of diseases, hospitalization rates, occupational accidents, infant mortality rates, and the leading causes of death are examples of data compiled by government agencies and published in periodicals available to researchers. A common source of primary statistical information is the National Center for Health Statistics (https://www.cdc.gov/nchs/index.htm).

FedStats (https://nces.ed.gov/partners/fedstat.asp) provides additional information.

FedStats, which has been available to the public since 1997, provides access to the full range of official statistical information produced by the Federal Government without having to know in advance which Federal agency produces which particular statistic. With convenient searching and linking capabilities to more than 100 agencies that provide data and trend information on such topics as economic and population trends, crime, education, health care, aviation safety, energy use, farm production and more, FedStats is your one location for access to the full breadth of Federal statistical information.

Statistical reports are issued periodically. The Vital and Health Statistic Series, complied by the National Center for Health Statistics, may be useful to health care researchers. The complete list of this series is available at https://www.cdc.gov/nchs/products/series.htm:

- *Series 1: Programs and collection procedures*: Reports that describe the general programs of the National Center for Health Statistics and its offices and divisions, data collection methods used, definitions, and other material necessary for understanding the data.

- *Series 2: Data evaluation and methods of research*: Studies of new statistical methodology, including experimental tests of new survey methods, studies of vital statistics collection methods, new analytical techniques, objective evaluations of reliability of collected data, and contributions to statistical theory.

- *Series 3: Analytical and epidemiological studies*: Reports presenting analytical or interpretive studies based on vital and health statistics, carrying the analysis further than the expository types of reports in the other series.

- *Series 4: Documents and committee reports*: Final reports of major committees concerned with vital and health statistics and documents, such as recommended model vital registration laws and revised birth and death certificates.

- *Series 5: International vital and health statistics reports*: Analytical and descriptive reports comparing U.S. vital and health statistics with those of other countries.

- *Series 10: Data from the National Health Interview Survey*: Statistics on illness, accidental injury, disability, use of hospital, medical, dental, and other services, and other health-related topics, based on data collected in a continuing national household interview survey.

- *Series 11: Data from the National Health Examination Survey; the National Health and Nutrition Examination Surveys, and the Hispanic Health and Nutrition Examination Survey*: Data from direct examination, testing, and measurement of national samples of the population provide the basis for two types of reports: (a) estimates of the medically defined prevalence of specific diseases in the United States and the distributions of the noninstitutionalized population with respect to physical, physiological, and psychological characteristics; and (b) analysis of relationships among the various measurements without reference to an explicit finite universe of persons.

- *Series 12: Data from the institutional population surveys*: Statistics relating to the health characteristics of persons in institutions and on medical, nursing, and personal care received, based on national samples of establishments providing these services and samples of the residents or patients. This series was discontinued after 1969. Information in this series appears in Series 13.

- *Series 13: Data from the National Health Care Survey*: Statistics on the utilization of health manpower and facilities providing long-term care, ambulatory care, and family planning services.

- *Series 14: Data on health resources, manpower, and facilities*: Statistics on the numbers, geographic distribution, and characteristics of health sources, including physicians, dentists, nurses, other health manpower occupations, hospitals, nursing homes, and outpatient and other inpatient facilities.

- *Series 15: Data from special surveys*: Statistics on health and health-related topics collected in special surveys that are not a part of the continuing data systems of the National Center for Health Statistics.

- *Series 16: Compilations of advance data from vital and health statistics*: These reports provide early release of data from the health and demographic surveys of the National Center for Health Statistics. Many of these releases are followed by detailed reports in the Vital and Health Statistics Series.

- *Series 20: Data on mortality*: Various statistics on mortality other than as included in regular annual or monthly reports. Special analyses by cause of death, age, and other demographic variables; geographic and time series analyses; and statistics on characteristics of death not available from the vital records based on sample surveys of those records.

The Global Health Observatory (http://www.who.int/gho/en/) "is the WHO's [World Health Organization] portal providing access to data and analyses for monitoring the global health situation. It provides critical data and analyses for key health themes, as well as direct access to the full database" (WHO, 2018, para. 1). Data from the WHO programs, including health-related databases, reports, and geographical maps and country profiles from WHO member nations, can be found here.

The *Demographic Yearbook* and other reports are published by the statistical office of the United Nations, Department of Economic and Social Affairs, New York (http://unstats.un.org/unsd/demographic/default.htm). Statistics compiled from 250 countries of the world are included. Topics include population rates, mortality rates by disease, life expectancy tables, and marriage, divorce, and migration statistics.

Other statistical compendiums include the following:
- U.S. Bureau of the Census (http://www.census.gov/)
- U.S. Bureau of Labor Statistics (http://www.bls.gov/)
- U.S. Department of Agriculture (http://www.usda.gov/wps/portal/usda/usdahome)

6.3.4 Directories of References

Directories of references are books that provide a comprehensive source for locating studies in specified fields. They provide lists and short reviews of available textbooks, journals, bibliographies, dictionaries, atlases, databases, and government documents. The following directories are a sample of the many reference resources available to the clinical researcher. The main limitation of directories is the rapidity with which new sources of information are created, which makes it almost impossible for a directory to be up to date. When using a directory, the researcher should be aware of the copyright date.

- Blake, J. B., & Roos, C. (Eds.). (1967). *Medical reference works 1679-1966: A selected bibliography.* Chicago, IL: MLA. The purpose of the publication, as stated by the editors, is "To survey the world's bioscientific, medical, and allied health literature and select and organize from it an annotated list of the major works useful in gaining access to publications or frequently needed data" (p. iii). Indexes and abstracts, bibliographies, proceedings of Congress, dictionaries, periodicals, and directories related to areas such as medicine, anatomy, medical education, hospitals, neurology, psychiatry, nursing, nutrition, pediatrics, physical medicine and rehabilitation, psychology, public health research in progress, and sociology are listed in the publication.
- Bowker Company (http://www.bowker.com/) is a leading source for national and international bibliographic information in both printed and digital material. The company provides information to consumers in areas such as books and serials in print. Typically used by librarians and book sellers, it can be a resource for finding specific books in the health sciences.
- Post, S. G. (Ed.). (2004). *Encyclopedia of bioethics: Volumes 1-5* (3rd ed.). New York, NY: Gale Cengage Learning/Macmillan Reference USA. The text is also available in electronic format. The fifth volume may be of special interest, as it contains the appendices, including primary documents, numerous bibliographies, and a list of additional resources.
- Huber, J. T., Boorkman, J. A., & Blackwell, J. (2014). *Introduction to reference sources in the health sciences* (6th ed.). New York, NY: Neal-Schuman Publishers. The book contains bibliographic and informational sources of monographs, periodicals, abstracting services, databases, U.S. government documents and technical reports, conferences, medical and health statistics, and audiovisual reference sources.
- Walters, L., Kahn, T. J., & Goldstein, D. M. (Eds.). (2009). *Bibliography of bioethics* (Vol. 35). Washington, DC: Georgetown University, Kennedy Institute. (Also available at http://bioethics.georgetown.edu/publications/biobib/index.html.) This bibliography of

Mary Johnson (mjohnson@yahoo.com)
Sent: Friday July 16, 2010 3:20 PM
To: John T. Clark

Dear Mr. Clark,
Please send me a reprint of your article Occupational Therapy for Adults with Alzheimers published in *Occupational Therapy for Adults* (2010), volume 8, pp. 35-40.
If it is in electronic form, please send it to mjohnson@yahoo.com. If it is in print, please send it to Mary Johnson, 1927 Main Street, Anytown, ME 02217.

Thank you very much,
Mary Johnson

Figure 6-4. An example of an email request for an article. Notice that the request includes the author, title of article, date of article, journal, and page numbers. If the article is unpublished, the request should state that.

bioethical topics has been published annually since 1975. It provides a comprehensive cross-disciplinary listing of journals, newspaper articles, monographs, essays, court decisions, and audiovisual materials. The bibliography is designed for anyone concerned with bioethics, including scientists, health professionals, and legal scholars.

6.3.5 Current Research

Current research not included in computer retrieval systems or annual reviews can be found in the most recently published periodicals. Most university and medical libraries have reading rooms where current scientific journals are placed on open shelves or online.

A perusal of newly published articles may be helpful in gaining an overview of a topic and establishing an up-to-date bibliography of related literature. Key words will often be listed under the abstract. Use of these key words to identify additional literature through databases and indexes may result in additional material. Current journals will also be helpful in locating individuals engaged in ongoing research, allowing researchers to request current reprints of articles, unpublished research, and conference papers. In general, most scholars will be flattered to receive requests from individuals genuinely interested in their work, and they will respond readily. The standard format in requesting reprints is to list the bibliographical citation (i.e., journal, volume, date, and title) as in the example in Figure 6-4.

6.3.6 Journals

A list of occupational therapy journals published around the world is supplied in Table 6-4.

TABLE 6-4

COMPENDIUM OF THE MAJOR JOURNALS IN OCCUPATIONAL THERAPY

AMERICAN JOURNAL OF OCCUPATIONAL THERAPY (AJOT)

http://www.aota.org/Publications-News/AmericanJournalOfOccupationalTherapy.aspx

The primary mission of AJOT is to publish peer-reviewed research examining the effectiveness and efficiency of occupational therapy practice so that occupational therapy professionals can make informed, evidence-based decisions about best practices. In addition, the journal aims to publish (a) research documenting the reliability and validity of occupational therapy instruments; (b) studies demonstrating a relationship between occupational engagement and the facilitation of community participation and health; and (c) articles that provide a forum for scholars to debate professional issues that affect education, practice, and research

AMERICAN JOURNAL OF PHYSICAL MEDICINE & REHABILITATION

http://journals.lww.com/ajpmr/Pages/aboutthejournal.aspx

The *American Journal of Physical Medicine & Rehabilitation* focuses on the practice, research, and educational aspects of physical medicine and rehabilitation. Monthly issues keep physiatrists up-to-date on the optimal functional restoration of patients with disabilities, physical treatment of neuromuscular impairments, the development of new rehabilitative technologies, and the use of electrodiagnostic studies. The journal publishes cutting-edge basic and clinical research, clinical case reports, and in-depth topical reviews of interest to rehabilitation professionals.

ANNALS OF INTERNATIONAL OCCUPATIONAL THERAPY

www.routledge.com/9781630915094/OTannals

The *Annals of International Occupational Therapy* is a quarterly peer-reviewed journal that includes original articles that focus on research as related to the clinical practice of occupational therapy worldwide. Manuscripts that are appropriate for the journal include randomized controlled trials, meta-analyses and systematic reviews, and prospective and retrospective case studies and case reports. Also appropriate are conceptual reviews, correlational studies, research on educational issues, and surveys of factors or variables impacting occupational therapy practice.

THE ARCHIVES OF PHYSICAL MEDICINE AND REHABILITATION

http://www.archives-pmr.org/content/about

The *Archives of Physical Medicine and Rehabilitation* is the official journal of the American Congress of Rehabilitation Medicine, an organization focused on the creation and use of knowledge in the rehabilitation process. The *Archives of Physical Medicine and Rehabilitation* publishes original, peer-reviewed research and clinical reports on important trends and developments in medical rehabilitation and related fields.

This international journal brings researchers and clinicians authoritative information on the therapeutic utilization of physical, behavioral, and pharmaceutical agents in providing comprehensive care for individuals with chronic illness and disabilities. The journal's content is relevant to all members of medical rehabilitation teams, including physicians, nurses, counselors, therapists, and case managers.

ASIAN JOURNAL OF OCCUPATIONAL THERAPY (ASIAN JOT)

http://www.jstage.jst.go.jp/browse/asiajot

The Asian JOT, which is published by the Japanese Association of Occupational Therapists, publishes articles to promote occupational therapy in Japan and Asian countries. It is accessible to the public through the internet. This journal is particularly aimed at disseminating the aspects of clinical, research and education of occupational therapy in the Asian region as well as Japan to the rest of the world.

(continued)

Table 6-4 (continued)

Compendium of the Major Journals in Occupational Therapy

AUSTRALIAN OCCUPATIONAL THERAPY JOURNAL (AOTJ)

http://onlinelibrary.wiley.com/journal/10.1111/(ISSN)1440-1630

The AOTJ is the official journal of Occupational Therapy Australia, and welcomes manuscripts relevant to the theory, research, practice, and education of occupational therapy. The journal aims to promote research and interdisciplinary communication, and provide a forum for discussion of issues relevant to occupational therapists. The journal is dedicated to promoting occupational therapy internationally.

BRITISH JOURNAL OF OCCUPATIONAL THERAPY (BJOT)

https://us.sagepub.com/en-us/nam/journal/british-journal-occupational-therapy

BJOT is the official journal of the Royal College of Occupational Therapists and is a monthly peer-reviewed publication. Its purpose is to publish articles with international relevance that advance knowledge in research, practice, education, and management in occupational therapy. BJOT aims to be the publication of choice for people to access, disseminate, and guide the implementation of occupational therapy knowledge and evidence worldwide so that occupational therapists, service users, and key stakeholders can make informed decisions.

CANADIAN JOURNAL OF OCCUPATIONAL THERAPY (CJOT)

http://journals.sagepub.com/home/cjo/

CJOT was first published in September 1933. Since that time, it has fostered advancement and growth in occupational therapy scholarship. The mission of the journal is to provide a forum for leading-edge occupational therapy scholarship that advances theory, practice, research, and policy. The vision is to be a high-quality scholarly journal that is at the forefront of the science of occupational therapy and a destination journal for the top scholars in the field, globally. Consistent with its mission and vision, the principal content of the journal depicts empirical findings and theoretical/conceptual arguments pertaining to occupation-based, client-centred enablement with relevance to Canadian occupational therapy practitioners. The majority of the papers present full-length empirical studies across the full range of methodologies. Registered RCT [randomized controlled trial] protocols and theoretical papers and conceptual reviews that provide a new and critical perspective on a topic of relevance to occupation-based, client-centred practice are also encouraged. The journal also publishes brief reports presenting preliminary empirical findings or theoretical/conceptual arguments that have the potential to inform future research in occupational therapy. Letters to the editor that encourage critical discussions on topics published within, or are of relevance to, CJOT are encouraged. Book reviews and invited commentaries are published on occasion. As CJOT is an English/French bilingual journal, articles are published in the language of submission with the title, key words, and abstract translated into the other language. This journal is a member of the Committee on Publication Ethics and follows its guidelines for ethical publishing.

HONG KONG JOURNAL OF OCCUPATIONAL THERAPY (HKJOT)

https://journals.sagepub.com/home/hjo

HKJOT is the official peer-reviewed publication of the Hong Kong Occupational Therapy Association. It is published twice per year by Elsevier.

The journal's aims are to promote the development of theory and practice in occupational therapy and facilitate documentation and communication among educators, researchers, and practitioners. The journal also works to advance availability, use, support and excellence of occupational therapy on behalf of the Association to the public, and maintain professional standards to promote better understanding of occupational therapy.

(continued)

TABLE 6-4 (CONTINUED)

COMPENDIUM OF THE MAJOR JOURNALS IN OCCUPATIONAL THERAPY

INDIAN JOURNAL OF OCCUPATIONAL THERAPY (IJOT)

http://aiota.org/publications/ljot

IJOT is published three times per year in April, August, and December by the All India Occupational Therapists Association.

The journal publishes original scientific research papers, case reports, preliminary articles, and information on all aspects of occupational therapy. It welcomes articles from all over the world. Letters to the editor are welcome.

The Editorial Board reserves the right to refuse any matter for publication and decision of the board must be accepted as final.

IRISH JOURNAL OF OCCUPATIONAL THERAPY (IJOT)

http://www.emeraldgrouppublishing.com/services/publishing/ijot/index.htm

The aim of IJOT is to contribute and stimulate critical debate and evidence-based practice by disseminating research findings, expert opinion, theoretical arguments, and developments within clinical practice and professional education in Ireland and internationally. The journal will publish original articles that will add to the knowledge base within occupational therapy and further evidence-based practice and critical debate within the profession. The journal contributes to theory, practice, education, research, and professional developments within occupational therapy. Theoretical papers, qualitative, quantitative, and mixed methods research studies and systematic reviews are equally welcome. Practice reports of innovative service developments and short papers appraising the evidence base for specific interventions will also be considered for publication.

ISRAELI JOURNAL OF OCCUPATIONAL THERAPY (IJOT)

http://www.isot.org.il

IJOT was founded and produced by the Israel Society for Occupational Therapy in order to meet the needs of the various professions: collecting, processing, and concentrating knowledge, and imparting knowledge to occupational therapists and other professionals. The journal serves as a platform for professionals to convey their professional outlook and to share their clinical and research work with their colleagues and the community.

JOURNAL OF HAND THERAPY

http://www.jhandtherapy.org/content/aims

The *Journal of Hand Therapy* is designed for hand therapists, occupational and physical therapists, and other hand specialists involved in the rehabilitation of disabling hand problems. The journal functions as a source of education and information by publishing scientific and clinical articles. Regular features include original reports, clinical reviews, case studies, editorials, and book reviews.

JOURNAL OF OCCUPATIONAL SCIENCE (JOS)

http://www.tandfonline.com/action/authorSubmission?journalCode=rocc20&page=instructions

JOS publishes original research and scholarly papers on human occupation, defined here as things people do that have meaning and occupy people's time, with a particular focus on the reciprocal relationship of occupation and health and well-being. Studies of populations, communities, groups and individuals are accepted, as well as explorations of people's development as occupational beings, patterns of occupation, societal structuring of occupation, and differential access to occupation. Humanist, indigenous, population, transactional, evolutionary, biological, ecological, historical, sociopolitical, philosophical, and biographical perspectives of occupation will be considered.

(continued)

TABLE 6-4 (CONTINUED)

COMPENDIUM OF THE MAJOR JOURNALS IN OCCUPATIONAL THERAPY

JOURNAL OF REHABILITATION MEDICINE

https://www.medicaljournals.se/jrm/about/jrm

The *Journal of Rehabilitation Medicine* is an international peer-review journal published in English, with at least 10 issues published per year. Original articles, reviews, case reports, short communications, special reports and letters to the editor are published, as well as editorials and book reviews. The journal strives to provide its readers with a variety of topics, including functional assessment and intervention studies, clinical studies in various patient groups, methodology in physical and rehabilitation medicine, epidemiological studies on disabling conditions, and reports on vocational and sociomedical aspects of rehabilitation. The journal is read by a wide group of health care professionals, including specialists in rehabilitation medicine, neurology, clinical neurophysiology, general medicine, psychologists, physiotherapists, occupational therapists, and social workers. Contributions from all parts of the world and from different professions in rehabilitation are welcome.

NEW ZEALAND JOURNAL OF OCCUPATIONAL THERAPY (NZJOT)

https://www.otnz.co.nz/public/publications/new-zealand-journal-of-occupational-therapy/

NZJOT is a peer-reviewed journal dedicated to the publication of high quality national and international articles that are research based and grounded in occupational therapy practice. It is published twice per year—in April and September.

OCCUPATIONAL THERAPY IN HEALTH CARE

https://www.tandfonline.com/loi/iohc20

Occupational Therapy in Health Care is a journal of contemporary practice in occupational therapy. It provides occupational therapy practitioners with a forum to stay up to date on current methods and theories in the field. Focused on everyday practice, the journal addresses the concerns of new and experienced therapists, presenting innovations in client evaluations and treatments, current research findings, critical reviews of current textbooks, and descriptions of novel programs and of fieldwork innovations.

OCCUPATIONAL THERAPY IN MENTAL HEALTH

https://www.tandfonline.com/loi/womh20

Occupational Therapy in Mental Health provides professionals with a forum in which to discuss today's challenges—identifying the philosophical and conceptual foundations of the practice; sharing innovative evaluation and treatment techniques; learning about and assimilating new methodologies developing in related professions; and communicating information about new practice settings and special problem areas particular to psychiatric occupational therapy.

Authors are strongly encouraged to submit manuscripts electronically. If submitting a disk, it should be prepared using MS Word and should be clearly labeled with the authors' names, file name, and software program used.

OPEN JOURNAL OF OCCUPATIONAL THERAPY (OJOT)

http://scholarworks.wmich.edu/ojot/about.html

OJOT is published through Western Michigan University's Department of Occupational Therapy in the College of Health and Human Services. The mission of OJOT is to publish high-quality articles that focus on applied research, practice, and education in the occupational therapy profession. OJOT is an open-access, peer-reviewed journal with quarterly publications. Peer-review is completed by members of the OJOT Editorial Review Board, who are selected through an application process assessing the individual's experience and areas of specialty in practice, education, and/or research.

(continued)

TABLE 6-4 (CONTINUED)

COMPENDIUM OF THE MAJOR JOURNALS IN OCCUPATIONAL THERAPY

OTJR: OCCUPATION, PARTICIPATION AND HEALTH

https://us.sagepub.com/en-us/nam/otjr-occupation-participation-and-health/journal202285

OTJR is published quarterly by the American Occupational Therapy Foundation, Inc. This international peer-reviewed journal offers empirical, theoretical, and review articles to readers interested in factors of human participation and how such factors influence health and well-being.

PHYSICAL & OCCUPATIONAL THERAPY IN GERIATRICS

https://www.tandfonline.com/loi/ipog20

Physical & Occupational Therapy in Geriatrics has functioned as a forum for allied health professionals, as well as others, with a focus on rehabilitation of the geriatric client to share information, clinical experience, research, and therapeutic practice. Each issue focuses on current practice and emerging issues in the care of the older client, including rehabilitation and long-term care in institutional and community settings, and innovative programming; the entire range of problems experienced by the elderly; and the current skills needed for working with older clients. Contributors consider the current methods of managing older people at home, in assisted living, alone, or with families. Contributors address policy issues that affect the styles of living of older people, and discuss projects relating to research and teaching, as they may affect practice in the field of gerontology.

PHYSICAL & OCCUPATIONAL THERAPY IN PEDIATRICS (POTP)

https://www.tandfonline.com/loi/ipop20

POTP delivers vital information to all therapists involved in developmental and physical rehabilitation of infants, children, and youth. Designed for physical and occupational therapy pediatric professionals in hospitals, rehabilitation centers, schools, and health and human services agencies, the journal provides the latest clinical research and practical applications that no professional will want to miss. Current clinical advances and research findings are important for all therapists, and each issue of this journal brings therapists the latest discoveries in therapy as related to their work with children. With an emphasis on implications and applications for therapy practice, the journal includes case reports, and reviews/critiques of new measures.

This comprehensive journal is recognized for its useful balance of research and clinical practice articles.

REHABILITATION PSYCHOLOGY

https://www.researchgate.net/journal/0090-5550_Rehabilitation_Psychology

Rehabilitation Psychology is a quarterly peer-reviewed journal that publishes articles in furtherance of the mission of Division 22 (Rehabilitation Psychology) of the American Psychological Association and to advance the science and practice of rehabilitation psychology. Rehabilitation psychologists consider the entire network of biological, psychological, social, environmental, and political factors that affect the functioning of persons with disabilities or chronic illness. Given the breadth of rehabilitation psychology, the journal's scope is broadly defined. Suitable submissions include papers describing experimental investigations, survey research, evaluations of specific interventions, outcome studies, historical perspectives, relevant public policy issues, conceptual/theoretical formulations with implications for clinical practice, reviews of empirical research, detailed case studies, and professional issues.

SCANDINAVIAN JOURNAL OF OCCUPATIONAL THERAPY (SJOT)

http://www.tandfonline.com/action/journalInformation?journalCode=iocc20

SJOT is an internationally well-recognized journal that aims to provide a forum for occupational therapy research worldwide, especially the Nordic countries.

(continued)

TABLE 6-4 (CONTINUED)
COMPENDIUM OF THE MAJOR JOURNALS IN OCCUPATIONAL THERAPY
SOUTH AFRICAN JOURNAL OF OCCUPATIONAL THERAPY (SAJOT)
http://www.sajot.co.za/index.php/sajot SAJOT is the official journal of the Occupational Therapy Association of South Africa and is a leading publication for research into occupational therapy in Africa. SAJOT publishes and disseminates research articles that contribute to the scientific knowledge of the profession and its outcomes with particular reference to service delivery in Africa. It provides a platform for debate about issues relevant to occupational therapy in Africa which will also contribute to the development of the profession worldwide.
WORK: A JOURNAL OF PREVENTION, ASSESSMENT & REHABILITATION
http://www.iospress.nl/journal/work/ *Work* is an interdisciplinary, international journal that publishes high-quality peer-reviewed manuscripts covering the entire scope of the occupation of work. The journal's subtitle has been deliberately laid out: The first goal is the prevention of illness, injury, and disability. When this goal is not achievable, the attention focuses on assessment to design client-centered intervention, rehabilitation, treatment, or controls that use scientific evidence to support best practice. *Work* occasionally publishes thematic issues, but in general, issues cover a wide range of topics such as ergonomic considerations with children, youth, and students, the challenges facing an aging workforce, workplace violence, injury management, performing artists, ergonomic product evaluations, and the awareness of the political, cultural, and environmental determinants of health related to work.
WORLD FEDERATION OF OCCUPATIONAL THERAPY (WFOT) BULLETIN
http://www.wfot.org/Bulletin.aspx The *WFOT Bulletin* is the official publication of the WFOT. Its aim is to promote awareness and understanding of the WFOT and its activities and services, the development of the occupational therapy profession worldwide, and the international exchange of professional knowledge and experience.

6.4 RECORDING INFORMATION FROM RESEARCH ARTICLES

The beginning researcher should develop a system for recording, organizing, and storing information related to a content area in a computer file. It is important to develop this system early in the process by recording bibliographic information from all sources at the time it is obtained, even if the use of the material is questionable. The reconstruction of bibliographic sources later can be time consuming and difficult. Some investigators photocopy studies from periodicals or newspapers that relate to a specific area. Using information obtained from each of these articles, researchers can compile an up-to-date annotated bibliography.

An example of a citation file is shown in Figure 6-5. The file should contain the following information from each study:

- A bibliographical notation that includes all information used in a citation. (See Chapter 10 for examples of citations.)
- Library call number or ERIC number can be helpful also, as this allows the researcher to find the publication quickly.
- Abstract of study including number of subjects, data collection methodology, test instruments, results, and conclusions.
- Important quotations (including page numbers) that can be cited in the literature review.
- Any reactions to the article, such as evaluation of the validity of results or generalizations offered.

By recording this information accurately, the researcher saves time and effort from having to return to the source of the information, whether it be in the library or returning to an information site on the internet. Researchers should obtain information from many different types of publications. While original sources should be used for citation, valuable information can be gleaned from secondary and tertiary sources.

6.5 EVALUATING VALIDITY OF RESEARCH FINDINGS

The finding and citing of research are not the final processes in reviewing literature. A critical analysis is a vital task of the investigator. One of the more difficult tasks in

Braverman, S. E., Spector, J., Warden, D. L., Wilson, B. C., Ellis, T. E., & Bandad, M. J. (1999). Multidisciplinary TBI inpatient rehabilitation programme for active duty service members as part of a randomized, clinical trial. *Brain Injury, 13*(6), 405-415.

Objective: To evaluate the effectiveness of a multidisciplinary rehabilitation program for military service members with moderate brain injury.

Design: Randomized control trial

Setting: Inpatient rehabilitation program in a U. S. military tertiary care hospital

Patients: 67 active-duty individuals with moderate to severe TBI

Intervention: "Eight week rehabilitation program combining group and individual therapies with an inpatient milieu-oriented neuropsychological focus. Group therapies included fitness, planning and organization, cognitive skills, medication and milieu groups, and community re-entry outings. Individual therapy included neuropsychology, work therapy, occupational therapy, and speech and language pathology." (p. 405)

Desired Outcome: Successful return to work and return to duty

Results: At 1-year follow-up, 64 individuals returned to work (96%) and 44/67 (66%) returned to duty.

Conclusion: The multidisciplinary rehabilitation program demonstrated an effective approach to rehabilitate military service members with TBI.

Reaction: May not be generalized to nonmilitary personnel
Doesn't operationally define outcome measures
Can the research design be replicated?

Figure 6-5. An example of a file used in collecting information from articles.

a literature review is the ability to review the articles in an integrated fashion. One cannot evaluate and critique each article separately; rather, the integration of the information must be done by synthesizing the information (Findley, 1989). One outcome of this type of evaluation is that the reader begins to build a conceptual framework, thereby allowing for a more mature evaluation of other literature in the field.

The quality of the research and the validity of the conclusions need to be evaluated before the research can be integrated with other results. When contradictory results arising from different studies occur, the investigator should seek to offer an explanation based on the research methodologies. Occasionally, investigators reviewing literature cite

the results and conclusions of previous research without determining the sample size, data collection procedures, and measuring instruments used. It should be clear to the reader that results of studies involving small samples and using tests that have low reliability are not as valid as large-scale studies in which rigorous methodology and reliable measuring instruments are used. In reporting previous literature, the investigator should consider the following factors in evaluating the validity of the research findings:

- The size of the sample, sampling procedure, and representativeness
- Control of extraneous variables that can potentially affect results
- Evidence of research bias in conclusions that are not consistent with results
- Selection of reliable and valid measuring instruments
- Data collection procedures
- Statistical techniques employed

In addition to these factors, the reader should ask several questions about the article. These questions are summarized in Table 6-5.

6.6 Outlining the Literature Review Section

Whether the researcher is reporting results in a journal article or preparing a thesis, he or she must decide how much of the background literature should be cited. The *Publication Manual of the American Psychological Association* (2011) recommends that a writer of a journal article should:

Discuss the relevant related literature, but do not feel compelled to include an exhaustive historical review. Assume that the reader is knowledgeable about the basic problem and does [not] require a complete accounting of its history. A scholarly description of earlier work in the introduction provides a summary of the most recent directly related work and recognizes the priority of the work of others. Citation of and specific credit to relevant earlier works is part of the author's scientific and scholarly responsibility. … Cite and reference only works pertinent to the specific issue and not those that are of only tangential or general significance. When summarizing earlier works, avoid nonessential details; instead, emphasize pertinent findings, relevant methodological issues, and major conclusions. Refer the reader to general surveys or reviews of the topic if they are available. (p. 28)

In contrast to the journal article, the writer of a master's thesis or doctoral dissertation should include extensive background literature, which demonstrates to the reader that the researcher is cognizant of the important findings with which the present study rests. The continuity of findings should be documented by the researcher. The literature review in a master's thesis or doctoral dissertation serves as a vehicle for presenting chronologically the progression of knowledge in a specific area. Thus, the literature review should reflect the development of a problem by first presenting general background findings and then gradually narrowing to the significant variables identified in the title of the study.

A search of the literature will result in identifying literature that is directly related to the topic at hand, literature less directly related but that should be read, and literature that is unrelated. Although it will be important to peruse all of these, only the articles directly related to the topic will be used in a literature review. Locke, Spirduso, and Silverman (1987) suggested that the literature review "is made to serve the reader's query by supporting, explicating, and illuminating the logic now implicit in the proposed investigation" (p. 59). A well-written literature review allows the reader to (a) understand the significance of the research question, (b) validate the connection between previously conducted research directly related to the present research question, and (c) grasp the reasons for the proposed methodology.

The plan for presenting previous literature should include a logical development that incorporates both a chronological sequence and a topical order. By using an outline, the researcher begins to organize the data found in reviewing the literature. The outline is a working tool; it should change to accommodate new ideas and evidence.

One way to develop an outline is by organizing groups by topic, which makes the writing easier for several reasons. First, by examining and reviewing the literature, important themes and topics may emerge. Second, because the files have been organized by subject, the writer does not waste time looking through the articles and other references for related material. Third, by placing the cards into groups, they can be further organized into a logical outline or sequence.

Although writing the literature review can be challenging, the completed product gives the researcher a sense of accomplishment. The literature review section of a study should represent an extensive process that is the basis for implementing the research design. The worksheet in Box 6-2 describes this process.

TABLE 6-5

CRITICALLY REVIEWING A RESEARCH ARTICLE

INTRODUCTION

- Does the introduction state the hypothesis directly or implied?
- Does the literature review support the hypothesis?
- Are the choices of outcome measures relevant to the study?
- Is the study feasible and furthering knowledge in the field?

METHODOLOGY

- Based on the information presented in the study, can the study be replicated?
- How were the participants chosen for the study?
- Are the demographics of the participants adequately described?
- Were unusual circumstances or extraneous variables (e.g., use of medication, time of testing) described?
- What were the reliability and validity of the outcome measures?
- Were appropriate tests used for the population studied?
- Were the measures free from external bias?
- Were appropriate statistics used?

RESULTS AND DISCUSSION

- Were the results reported in an understandable and clear manner?
- Are the figures and tables clear and consistent with the text?
- Was the discussion related to the findings?
- Was there discussion regarding the acceptance or rejection of the null hypothesis?
- Did the investigator discuss limitations of the study and the need for future research?

Adapted from Maher, B. A. (1978). A reader's, writer's, and reviewer's guide to assessing research reports in clinical psychology. *Journal of Clinical and Consulting Psychology, 46,* 835-838.

Box 6-2. Worksheet for Literature Review

1. State the research problem in question form.

2. Identify variables in the study:

   Independent variables   1.

                                      2.

                                      3.

   Dependent variables   1.

                                      2.

                                      3.

   Target populations   1.

                                      2.

                                      3.

   Specific setting for study (e.g., hospital, clinic)   1.

                                      2.

                                      3.

3. Checklist for locating references (list titles):

   Information retrieval systems   1.

                                      2.

   Directories of references   1.

                                      2.

   Bibliographical indexes   1.

                                      2.

   Annual reviews   1.

                                      2.

   Abstracting periodicals   1.

                                      2.

   Textbooks   1.

                                      2.

   Personal communication from experts   1.

                                      2.

(continued)

Box 6-2. Worksheet for Literature Review (continued)

4. Primary sources utilized (list):

Journals	1.
	2.
Statistical compendium	1.
	2.
Conference proceedings	1.
	2.
Theses and dissertations	1.
	2.

6.7 Summary

In this chapter, the authors discuss the importance of and necessity for a thorough and up-to-date review of the literature as an integral part of a research project. In this process, the researcher needs to locate and retrieve the most important studies relevant to the research project and to evaluate the validity of the methods used in collecting data. While online databases, such as PubMed, are particularly suited for identifying articles from published medical and health related periodicals (both peer-reviewed and non–peer-reviewed), several other resources are identified for retrieving health statistics that are helpful in justifying the need for the study. An up-to-date list of the primary occupational therapy journals that are published internationally is provided in this chapter. The authors also discuss the different types of published literature ,such as research studies, review articles, and theoretical papers. A discussion of how to critically analyze a published research study is described. Finally, a summary worksheet for the literature review is included that can help the reader to organize a systematic search.

7

Research Design and Methodology

The quality of research depends not only upon the adequacy of the research design but also upon the fruitfulness of the data-collection techniques which are employed. The purpose of the various data-collection techniques is simply to produce precise and reliable evidence which is relevant to the research questions being asked. Fulfillment of this purpose, however is rarely simple.

—Johoda, Deutsch, & Cook (1951, p. 92)

OPERATIONAL LEARNING OBJECTIVES

By the end of this chapter the learner will be able to:

- State a research hypothesis or guiding question.
- Operationally define a research variable.
- Identify any assumptions underlying a proposed research study.
- Diagram a research study.
- Identify the possible methodological limitations in a research study.
- State the theoretical rationale underlying a proposed research study.
- Design a procedure for selecting participants for a study.
- Design screening criteria for participant inclusion.
- Define and contrast the terms *random sampling, random assignment, convenience sampling, representative sampling,* and *target population.*
- Define *test reliability* and *test validity.*
- Evaluate the feasibility, reliability, and validity of a published test or measuring instrument.
- Compare and contrast the four scales of measurement.
- Understand the concept of internal validity.
- Design a data collection procedure for a proposed research study.
- Understand ethical principles underlying human research.
- Outline a research proposal including an informed consent protocol.
- Understand the concept of external validity.
- Describe the major research designs and methodological limitations of a study.

Rice, M. S., Stein, F., & Tomlin, G.
Clinical Research in Occupational Therapy, Sixth Edition (pp. 181-208).
© 2019 Taylor & Francis Group.

		TABLE 7-1	
THE RELATIONSHIP BETWEEN A RESEARCH QUESTION, A GUIDING QUESTION, AND A HYPOTHESIS			
	DEFINITION	PURPOSE	EXAMPLE
RESEARCH QUESTION	A broad inquiry into a general area of investigation	Leads researcher into an extensive literature review	What is the relationship between repetitive motion and hand injuries?
GUIDING QUESTION	A statement of inquiry that leads to data collection	Identifies factors that relate to a specific research question	What factors in repetitive motion injury are related to carpal tunnel syndrome?
HYPOTHESIS	A detailed statement that can be tested through inferential statistics	Evaluates effectiveness or significant relationship between variables	There is no statistically significant difference in the use of biofeedback vs. splinting in remediating the symptoms of carpal tunnel syndrome.

7.1 PROPOSING A FEASIBLE RESEARCH QUESTION

The initial step in research is asking the right questions. Science progresses along the continuum of knowledge by researchers seeking solutions to key problems. Historically, researchers gain advanced knowledge by posing feasible questions, such as the following:

- What are the basic anatomical structures and physiological functions of human beings?
- How are diseases transmitted?
- What chemical substances destroy specific microorganisms that cause diseases?
- How can we detect the presence of trace chemicals in food and blood?
- What are the causes of specific diseases?
- What effect does a child with disabilities have on the family?
- What is the effect of including a child with disabilities in a general education classroom?
- What are the most effective methods for rehabilitating individuals with traumatic brain injury?

Scientists have raised numerous questions that have guided research and led to solutions. In the research design section, the investigator raises specific testable or feasible questions that guide the data collection.

In proposing research, the investigator reviews the following six areas:

1. Statements of hypotheses or guiding questions
2. Operational definitions of variables
3. Underlying assumptions of the study
4. Diagrammatical relationship between variables
5. Methodological limitations of the study
6. Overall theoretical rationale guiding the study

7.2 STATEMENT OF HYPOTHESIS

In an experimental design, a *hypothesis* predicts results and can be testable. Hypotheses test the influence of an independent variable upon a dependent variable and can be stated in the directional or non-directional form. For example, a directional hypothesis may be, "Aerobic exercise lowers blood pressure in middle-aged, sedentary men," whereas a non-directional hypothesis may be "Aerobic exercise influences blood pressure in middle-aged, sedentary men." In a correlational design, a hypothesis is a statement predicting the relationship between variables. In logic, it is stated as an *if-then contingency*. For example, consider the hypothesis: "There is a positive, statistically significant relationship between obesity and heart disease in sedentary workers.: In this hypothesis, there is a predicted relationship between obesity and heart disease among sedentary workers expressed as "if obesity (in sedentary workers), then heart disease." The hypothesis contains the question and predicts a directional relationship (a direction can be either positive or inverse).

How does the investigator arrive at a hypothesis or guiding question? The review of literature as discussed in Chapter 6 serves as the generating force in guiding the proposed hypothesis or guiding question. The relationship between a research question, a guiding question, and a hypothesis is described in Table 7-1. The hypothesis is a specific statement that can be derived from a research question or guiding question. Table 7-2 shows the relationship

TABLE 7-2		
THE RELATIONSHIP BETWEEN THE RESEARCH MODEL AND THE HYPOTHESIS		
RESEARCH MODEL	**STATEMENTS**	**EXAMPLES OF RESEARCH QUESTIONS**
Quantitative		
Experimental (prospective research design)	Hypothesis: directional or null	How effective is exercise in reducing symptoms of depression?
Methodological	Guiding question	What factors must be considered in designing a specific instrument or test for measuring pain?
Evaluation	Guiding question	How effective is the occupational therapy department in preventing rehospitalizations?
Heuristic (retrospective research design)	Guiding question	What risk factors are related to the etiology of multiple sclerosis?
Correlational	Hypothesis: directional or null	Is there a statistically significant positive relationship between perceptual motor abilities and reading?
Survey	Guiding question	What are the personality characteristics of the leaders in the field of occupational therapy?
Qualitative		
Individual case study	Guiding question	What are the dynamic factors and processes underlying the cause of schizophrenia in a specific individual?
Operations research	Guiding question	What is the impact of the prospective payment system on the quality of home health care?
Child development studies	Guiding question	What are the sequential steps in a child's development of the palmer grasp?
Longitudinal (prospective research design)	Guiding question	What are the long-term effects on children exposed to cocaine in utero?
Field observation (ethnography)	Guiding question	How do parents' attitudes toward a child with Down syndrome affect the child's development?
Historical research	Guiding question	What are the historical roots of the concept of humanism in occupational therapy?

between a research model and a statement of hypothesis or guiding question.

In quantitative research, the investigator needs to state a guiding question or hypothesis that leads to data collection. In qualitative research, the guiding question or hypothesis can arise during data collection. For example, a researcher who is initially interested in the problems associated with obtaining employment for individuals with schizophrenia may change his or her focus to an examination of the relationship between stress and employment. The qualitative researcher has more flexibility in stating guiding questions or hypotheses than the quantitative researcher who must state the question prior to collecting data. Once the guiding question or hypothesis is stated, the researcher needs to operationally define the variables.

7.3 Operationally Defining a Variable

Variables are operationally defined by stating or describing (a) the treatment procedure (presumed independent variable), (b) the outcome measure (dependent variable), and (c) screening criteria for participant selection. Operational definitions make it possible for researchers to replicate a research study. Many differences arising from the inconsistent results of several investigators often can be traced to different operational definitions of the same stated conceptual variables. For example, the following variables could become ambiguous unless one describes in detail how they are measured or procedurally defined:

- Cognitive rehabilitation (treatment procedure)
- Intelligence (screening criterion for participant inclusion)
- Language disorder (dependent variable or screening criterion for participant inclusion)
- Muscle strength (dependent variable or screening criterion for participant inclusion)
- Spasticity (dependent variable or screening criterion for participant inclusion)
- Sensory-integration therapy (treatment procedure)
- Visual motor ability (dependent variable or screening criterion for participant inclusion)
- Work hardening (treatment intervention)
- Individuals with low back pain (screening criterion for participant inclusion)

Research became rigorous when researchers described experimental procedures in detail so that other investigators could replicate the exact experiment or study as closely as possible. The rigor in operationally defining a variable is associated with internal validity. Results cannot be accepted unless it is known how the investigator defined the variables. Conflicts over the effectiveness of treatment techniques, descriptions of target populations, and measurements of outcome are often caused by comparing seemingly similar variables, which are, in fact, different because of the way they are measured. How many definitions are there for self-perception, cognitive disability, language therapy, manual dexterity, work capacity, and low back pain? The conceptualization of variables described by investigators may be entirely different if they are not operationally defined. Less valuable research is typified by the omission of operational definitions. The problem is compounded when investigators synthesize findings in an area by "lumping" studies. For example, if visual perception is defined operationally through group tests, individual tests, clinical observations, and functional performance, then conflicts will arise when examining the relationship between visual perception and a variable such as activities of daily living performance. A researcher's often fallacious interpretation of the literature and subsequent conclusions of questionable validity are a result of equating variables even though the operational definitions are different.

In operationally defining a variable, the investigator should consider the following questions:

- What is the theoretical rationale underlying the definition?
- What is the accepted definition of a variable as stated in a dictionary or occupational therapy textbook?
- How can the variable be measured?
- Does the investigator need to establish the screening criteria in defining a target population?
- Is the variable defined by a standardized procedure (e.g., employing a treatment technique)?
- Can a mathematical formula be employed in the definition (e.g., in ergonomics when defining work output)?

7.4 Stating Assumptions

A researcher undertaking an investigation may make certain assumptions that are usually unstated. These assumptions can be on a general level, such as:

- All diseases have a cause.
- Intelligence is the result of the interaction between genetic structure and environmental opportunities.
- Language development is maturational.
- Disengagement from social activity is a learned behavior rather than a biological determinant.
- Learning is a complex variable that is not entirely based on external reinforcement.

Other assumptions can be more subtle, such as:

- Rehabilitation of individuals with severe disabilities should have a high priority in a society.
- People with alcohol dependency should be treated as persons with medical problems rather than as criminals.
- Individuals with intellectual disability should be integrated into community schools rather than isolated in large institutions.
- Home health care is more cost-effective than hospitalization.

In designing a research study, the investigator should be aware of all the assumptions underlying the study. Whether the assumptions are made explicit in reporting the results is at the discretion of the researcher. Nonetheless, in preparing a research proposal, the researcher must state all assumptions.

When distinguishing an assumption from established evidence, it should be clear from the previous examples that assumptions are controversial or inconclusive and that they can also reflect the investigator's values or biases. Many assumptions are tacitly implied by an investigator

Figure 7-1. Diagrammatic relationship between variables in experimental research.

who assumes that all people accept certain beliefs or hold certain opinions. A researcher should try to identify all assumptions being made in the study as an indication of his or her own subjective biases and beliefs. Whenever possible, a reference should be used when stating assumptions. The reference could be either theoretical or supported by empirical research.

7.5 DIAGRAMMATICAL RELATIONSHIPS BETWEEN VARIABLES

In clarifying the research design, it is helpful for the investigator to diagram the study, especially in a proposal, showing the relationship among variables, populations sampled, and operational definitions.

7.5.1 Experimental Model

For example, a researcher is interested in testing two therapeutic interventions for students with moderate intellectual disabilities who have difficulty in self-care activities. The experimental model is used in this study. The diagrammatical relationship between variables is depicted in Figure 7-1.

In this hypothetical example, the guiding question is, "Is the cognitive approach more effective than the behavioral approach in increasing self-care abilities among individuals with moderate intellectual disability?"

An operational definition of moderate intellectual disability is required (IQ score obtained on an individual test between 40 and 55, or sub-average adaptive behavior skills in two or more areas [e.g., leisure, communication, social skills] and occurrence in the developmental years). Age, gender, ethnicity, and socioeconomic status should be considered.

7.5.2 Correlational Model

A correlational model could be diagramed in a hypothetical study involving coma. The variables are now considered to have an associational or statistical relationship, not a cause-effect relationship. The hypothetical relationship between variables is diagramed in Figure 7-2. In this model, the independent variable is not experimentally induced; therefore, it is considered to be presumed.

In this model, the guiding question for the hypothetical example is, "Is there a statistically significant relationship between the number of days in a coma and the severity of cognitive deficits?"

Figure 7-2. Diagrammatic relationship between variables in correlational research. (MVA = motor vehicle accident)

An operational definition of the population and the severity of cognition deficits are required. In the hypothetical example, the population is defined as those individuals who (a) have sustained a traumatic brain injury from a motor vehicle accident, (b) are participating in a rehabilitation program, and (c) have gained consciousness after being in a coma for at least 1 hour. Age, gender, socioeconomic status, and handedness must also be considered. Measurement tools include the Glasgow Coma Scale and the Halsted–Reitan Neuropsychological Battery.

7.5.3 Methodological Model

Using methodological research, such as in developing a test, the researcher outlines the study by using the diagram found in Figure 7-3. In this model, there is no hypothesis; rather, the researcher proposes a guiding question.

In the hypothetical question, the researcher wants to design a reliable and valid instrument for assessing the ability to cope with stress. The construct of stress needs to be defined based on theoretical concepts from a literature review. Individuals who deal well with stress and individuals with mental illness who have difficulty dealing with stress participate in the acquisition of normed values for the instrument. Stratification of age, gender, and socioeconomic status could be employed to increase accuracy by examining the differences that may occur because of these variables.

7.5.4 Evaluation Model

In evaluation research, the investigator determines the effectiveness of a health system in meeting the defined objects. This model is diagramed in Figure 7-4. As in methodological research, a guiding question is used by the researcher to propose the research. The researcher must determine the a priori objectives of the system. In the hypothetical example, the investigator would determine the mission statement and the objectives of the Iowa health care system, and then would use these criteria to determine the effectiveness of the system. General criteria for comparison purposes also would be used. In the example, statistical information would be used to compare Iowa's health care system with those of other states.

7.5.5 Heuristic Model

A researcher using a heuristic model seeks to understand and discover the relationship between heuristic factors. In a hypothetical study, such as discovering risk factors for a disease, the researcher seeks to identify the factors that are significantly related to the disability. The hypothetical example, using heart disease, is depicted in Figure 7-5. In this example, the risk factors for heart disease are identified through literature review. The population studied includes individuals with post-coronary heart disease. Control factors include age, gender, socioeconomic status, ethnicity, and severity of disease.

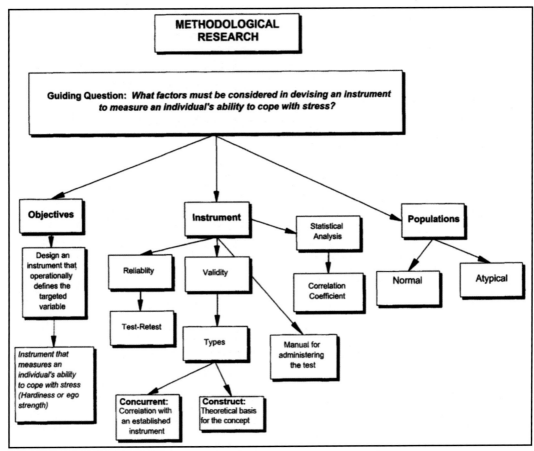

Figure 7-3. Diagrammatic relationship between variables in methodological research.

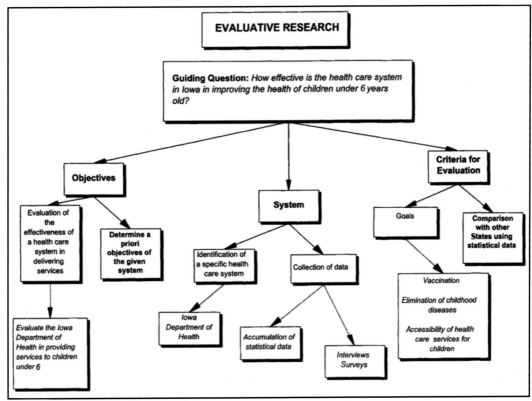

Figure 7-4. Diagrammatic relationship between variables in evaluative research.

Figure 7-5. Diagrammatic relationship between variables in heuristic research.

7.5.6 Survey Model

In this model, the researcher is interested in identifying characteristics of a defined, somewhat homogeneous population. For example, in a hypothetical study, the researcher is interested in examining the level of job satisfaction among occupational therapists in the United States (Figure 7-6). After the survey is completed, the results can be compared with a similar study focusing on another professional group, such as nursing.

The population is identified, but only a sample of the population receives the survey. Of those receiving the survey, it is expected that 50% will respond. Thus, in a population of 60,000 occupational therapists in the United States, only 6000 will receive the survey, and only 3000 are expected to respond.

The survey is sent to a stratified sample of the population giving a representative sample of the distribution of occupational therapists in the United States. Although the stratification is based only on geographical location, the statistical analysis from the results of the survey separates job description (e.g., pediatrics, physical dysfunction, psychosocial) and demographics (e.g., age, gender, socioeconomic status, ethnicity).

In the methodology, the researcher must design a valid and reliable questionnaire. Statistical analysis may consist of descriptive statistics, including a frequency distribution table, a statistical pie chart, histograms, cross-tabulations of variable values, correlational statistics, and even inferential statistics used to examine subgroup differences.

7.5.7 Qualitative Models

Qualitative research (see Chapter 4) models include, but are not limited to:

- Individual case study
- Operations research
- Child development studies
- Longitudinal research (prospective designs)
- Field observation (ethnography)
- Historical research

Figure 7-7 depicts a hypothetical study of a family in which a child has a bipolar disorder. In selecting a family, the researcher would consider the child's diagnosis, severity of illness, family constellation, and cooperativeness of the family to participate in a study. An additional consideration includes the research methods used for data collection and for analyzing the results.

7.6 Theoretical Rationale

Theory generates research, and research generates theory. Research should be a planned activity based on a theoretical rationale. Why are variables correlated? Why do we think this treatment will work? Why do we project these results? What factors justify the conclusions proposed? The researcher is not only interested in the questions "Does it work?" or "Is it curative?" but also "Why is the intervention effective?" "Why is there a relationship between causative factors and the onset of illness?" Theories in science are in a continual state of change. As knowledge progresses in

Figure 7-6. Diagrammatic relationship between variables in survey research.

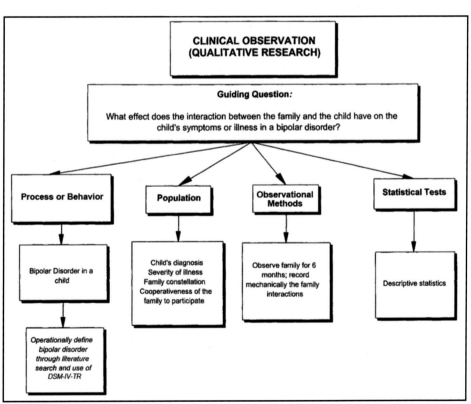

Figure 7-7. Diagrammatic relationship between variables in qualitative research, using an individual case study.

an area, theory evolves to accommodate newly discovered information. Researchers do not assume that theories and knowledge are static. What currently is accepted as accurate may be revised later when new research data are obtained.

The investigator needs to state the underlying theory generating the research design, even if it is meager and incomplete. Research is not justified if we collect meaningless bits of information for analysis. For example, if a researcher working on techniques to improve motor skills in children with severe intellectual disability finds a statistically significant difference between behavior modification and a comparable method in motivating the children to use motor skills but does not explain why behavior modification is effective, the research is incomplete. If, in this example, the group that received behavior modification realized significantly improved motor skills (more than what the control group exhibited), the reader is left to speculate on the causes for the difference. Was the Hawthorne effect controlled? Are there other explanations? The absence of a theoretical explanation leaves a gap in the research and leaves it open to the reader to speculate why motor development was enhanced. Speculations are raised, such as:

- Interpersonal relationships influenced motor learning
- Intervention stimulated motor development
- Reinforcement used in behavior modification was more effective than that used in the comparable methods
- Tests selected were unreliable and inappropriate

The reader can make many speculations in the absence of a theoretical rationale. Research should be guided by theory and explanation rather than merely presenting data that describe the relationships among variables.

7.7 Internal Validity

Internal validity is a theoretical concept that refers to the rigor in an experiment or research design. The degree of internal validity depends on the extent to which the investigator has controlled all variables that can potentially affect the results. If an experiment or research design is judged to have good internal validity, then the experimenter has been able to control for factors that could potentially distort the results. High internal validity is demonstrated by the following:

- A double-blind study in which the investigator eliminates researcher bias and subject influence
- Control of the placebo effect whereby the participant's suggestibility and personal influence are eliminated
- Inclusion of a control group to eliminate the Hawthorne effect
- Matching comparative groups to ensure that all groups compared are not different in variables such as age, gender, degree of disability, intelligence, and socioeconomic status
- Baseline measures of pre-test to ensure that comparative groups are essentially equivalent
- Post-test measures that are compared with pre-test measures
- High reliability and validity of outcome measures or tests to ensure that variables are accurately measured
- Regard for maturational factors that could distort results
- Standardization of administering test and research procedures

- Control for practice effect in test taking to ensure that gain in scores is not attributable to the participant's familiarity with test.

Some ways to increase internal validity are listed in Table 7-3.

7.8 Methods Section

The methodology section of a study includes method of selecting participants, location of study, description of tests and apparatuses used in measuring variables, procedure for collecting data, statistical techniques used for analyzing data, projection of time for completing the study, and procedure of obtaining informed consent from human subjects. Pragmatic and rational considerations guide the investigator in finding the answers to the following questions:

- How many participants should be included in the study?
- Should participants be randomly selected or should they be volunteers or a convenience sample?
- Where should the study take place?
- What tests, diagnostic procedures, questionnaires, or rating scales should be used in the study?
- What are the procedures and time sequence for data collection?
- What are the costs of the study?

The process for the research methodology is shown in Figure 7-8.

7.9 Selection of Participants

One primary purpose of research is to discover relationships among variables in sample groups and to generalize these relationships to a larger population. The ability to generalize results establishes the external validity of a study. Because research usually involves sample groups from populations rather than the total population, the selection of a representative sample is crucial when correctly generalizing results.

In selecting a sample, the first step is to identify a target population. For example, individuals with spinal cord injury, individuals who are juvenile offenders, occupational therapists, graduate students, or administrators of rehabilitation programs are identifiable populations. The target population is narrowed considerably by establishing a screening criteria. Screening criteria contain both inclusional and exclusional factors. For example, a researcher interested in cardiac rehabilitation may want to select a specific population within the area of cardiovascular disease (e.g., individuals who have had heart transplants). The screening criteria will enable the investigator to identify a specific population and to control variables that could

TABLE 7-3

INCREASING INTERNAL VALIDITY

PROBLEM	SOLUTION
Hawthorne effect	• Ensure that control and experimental groups receive equal treatment time
Honeymoon effect	• Do a follow-up study
Placebo effect	• Use motivational techniques to help clients self-improve
Bias of researcher	• Have objective test administrator collect pre-post data
Unreliability of test	• Design new instrument with the goal of high reliability and validity • Use triangulation (e.g., clinical observation, client report, physiological measure)
Insensitivity of test to detecting changes in behavior	• Use criterion-referenced testing • Use triangulation
Unsubstantiated validity	• Do a pilot study to test validity with an established test instrument
Sample is not representative of target population	• Use striated samples • Examine characteristics of sample group for similarities with target population (e.g., age, gender, severity of illness)
Maturational factors affect results	• Use covariance in statistical analysis (ANCOVA) to control for differences in pre- and post-measures
Differences in cognitive abilities of individuals	• Use covariance (ANCOVA) to control for cognitive levels
Comparative groups are not equal	• Set up selection criteria for selection inclusion (e.g., age, gender, socioeconomic status, intelligence, ethnicity)
Treatment method is not stated clearly	• Operationalize treatment method so that it can be replicated

ANCOVA = analysis of covariance

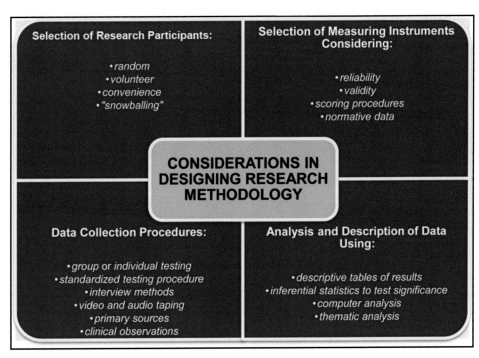

Figure 7-8. Sequential process of research methodology. Notice that there are four basic steps and, within those steps, questions that must be answered.

TABLE 7-4
INCLUSION CRITERIA FOR FOLAN, BARCLAY, COOPER, AND ROBINSON (2015)
• Aged 18 years and above • A diagnosis of tetraplegia with significant upper limb impairment • Beyond acute states of recovery • Either an in-patient at Victorian Spinal Cord Service (VSCS) or had been discharged from the VSCS within the last 18 months and living in the community • Had exposure to assistive technologies for computer access offered by VSCS

potentially affect the results. In setting up a screening criterion for patients with cardiac disease, variables such as age, gender, socioeconomic status, occupation, body type (endomorph, ectomorph, and mesomorph), onset of illness, and range of cardiorespiratory function as indicated by pulse rate and blood pressure should be considered.

Refinement of these variables should narrow the population. Examples of a target population obtained from a priori criteria include the following (inclusionary variable): (a) individuals with coronary disease, (b) male, (c) middle class socioeconomic status, (d) living in urban areas, (e) between the ages of 55 and 65 years, (f) primarily sedentary, and (g) with resting pulse rates below 80 beats per minute. In considering exclusional factors, the researcher specifies variables with values that are used to screen participants out of the study. These variables could include the absence of secondary illnesses (as determined by clinical examination), intellectual disability, or psychosocial dysfunction.

The example from a double case study by Folan, Barclay, Cooper, and Robinson (2015) shows the criteria employed in selecting 7 participants with tetraplegia (Table 7-4). Screening criteria are identified prior to participants selection. The investigator operationally defines the variables identified in the criteria. The rigor in specifying the population to be studied within a narrow domain enables other investigators to replicate the research design by isolating specific variables. By specifying the population and operationally defining the variables in the screening criteria, the investigator has identified a target population.

The next step in selecting participants for the study is to locate all the units in the target population. Studies of the personality characteristics of health science professionals, for example, would entail obtaining annual directories of members from professional associations, noting that not all practicing therapists are members of their professional associations.

Location of populations with disabilities, such as individuals with paraplegia living in the community, may be

obtained through consumer organizations that represent geographic areas. By geographically limiting the representativeness of the study, the investigator controls for social and environmental factors that could potentially affect the results. On the other hand, the investigator may want to guide the scope of the study by identifying *stratified samples*; that is, more homogeneous subgroups of a population based on variables such as geography, educational level, and treatment setting (e.g., community vs. hospital or disability group). Stratified samples are usually determined by previous evidence indicating that the variable identified has a significant effect on a dependent variable. For example, in examining the guiding question, "Does exercise prevent the recurrence of heart disease?" the investigator would control for the variable of smoking because previous evidence has related smoking to heart disease. In using stratified samples, the investigator would separate out populations of smokers who exercise from nonsmokers who do not exercise.

7.9.1 External Validity

External validity refers to the researcher's ability to generalize the results of a research study from a sample to a total population. In general, researchers seek to generalize the results from a study to the sampled population at large. For example, if a researcher found in a clinical study that aerobic exercise is effective in reducing depression in a particular sample, he or she would want to test whether the results could be generalized to all individuals with clinical depression. The extent to which an investigator can with confidence generalize the results of a study depends on the number of participants in the study and whether the study has been replicated, confirming previous results. It is not unusual for government agencies to sponsor extensive clinical trials using large numbers of participants to test the effectiveness of a new vaccine. These types of studies have a high degree of external validity. The example of the development of the polio vaccine during the 1950s demonstrates the ability to obtain external validity from one extensive clinical trial. However, external validity is also dependent on internal validity. In other words, the results of a study cannot be generalized to a population if internal validity is weak.

7.9.2 Random Sampling

Random sampling and random assignment are seen by researchers as methodological virtues. If a study includes a random selection of subjects, it is assumed that the investigator has controlled for researcher bias and selected a representative sample of the population. The concept of random sampling implies that in a population that includes all the components (e.g., all occupational therapists, all individuals with diagnoses of schizophrenia, all nursing homes), units of participants or institutions are representative of the total population. Random sampling is a method to select a representative group from the population. Random sampling does not guarantee a representative group; it serves to eliminate researcher bias in selecting a sample and yield one that is highly probably representative. One method used in random sampling is to assign a number to each population unit and select a representative sample by choosing units from a list of random numbers. For example, an investigator wants to randomly select 40 graduate programs in occupational therapy that are representative of all the accredited programs, totaling more than 150 in the United States. One method the investigator could use is to assign a number from 1 to 150 to each school and then from a list of random numbers select 40 schools. Because the schools are dispersed throughout the country, a representative sample of 40 should reflect the geographical distribution. If a check of the 40 schools reveals that the sample is biased in the direction of a single region, then repeated random selections would be obtained until a fair degree of geographical representativeness occurs. At this point, the reader may ask, why bother with obtaining a sample from random numbers? Why not just merely select a school from each geographical region? The reason this is not valid is because the researcher may overtly or inadvertently select schools that are typical of an educational philosophy or teaching model. Random sampling is simply a method to ensure researcher objectivity. In clinical research on human subjects, this method is sometimes difficult because subjects have the option to participate in the study. Another difficulty is in applying random sampling techniques to potentially large populations of individuals with disabilities situated in a wide geographic area. Is it possible to randomly sample all children with spina bifida, all patients with coronary disease, all prison inmates, all adolescents with attention-deficit/hyperactivity disorder, or all individuals with spinal cord injury in the United States? The complexities and problems in locating every individual in the population do not outweigh the errors that will occur by the very nature of the process. If random sampling of large populations is not practical, are there other objective selection methods that a clinical researcher can use? The answer to this question is yes—if the researcher maintains objectivity by devising systematic methods to obtain subjects and by narrowing the study. By delimiting the population, the investigator can apply random sampling techniques. For example, instead of defining the population as all patients with arthritis in the United States, the researcher delimits the population to all patients with arthritis treated in a specific hospital. The title of the study should describe the population sampled. For example, consider these hypothetical titles:

- Survey of Hand Function in the Patient with Arthritis
- Survey of the Hand Function of Individuals with Arthritis in a General Hospital in the Northeastern United States

In the first example, the investigator implies that the survey represents all patients with arthritis. In the second

example, the investigator has delimited the population to those patients with arthritis receiving treatment in a specific hospital. For most investigators, it is almost impossible to realistically sample a nationwide population of patients with arthritis. The difficulty in locating every member of the population, the cost of the survey, and the extensive time involved in collecting data are practical considerations that would hinder such a study.

7.9.3 Convenience Sample and Volunteers

It is valid to randomly sample from a convenience population (i.e., a population readily available to a researcher) as long as the researcher does not generalize the results to that portion of the total population that was not sampled. In selecting a random sampling of patients with arthritis from an identified population, the researcher would consider the following factors:

- Diagnosis of arthritis operationalized by physician evaluation or by anatomical or physiological evidence
- Age groupings separated into designated units
- Differentiation of gender
- Occupational groupings, such as professional, skilled, unskilled
- Socioeconomic status
- Level of education
- Age of onset
- Presence of stress
- Other relevant variables that could potentially affect the onset and course of arthritis, such as exercise, diet, physical condition, obesity, and weather

These variables can be used to establish screening criteria for subject inclusion in the study or in setting up stratified samples that can be statistically analyzed later for differences.

Another method to counteract researcher bias in selecting subjects is random assignment. For instance, if an investigator is interested in simultaneously comparing two treatment methods for patients with stroke, random assignment would be applied after a population of patients with stroke in a specific rehabilitation center is identified through screening criteria. The investigator would establish two samples by randomly assigning participants to each group from a list of random numbers. In this hypothetical example, the selection of the specific rehabilitation center where the patients with stroke were treated actually provides a convenience sample.

Another frequently used method of obtaining participants in clinical research is to issue a call for volunteers. The limitation of seeking participants in this way is that the volunteers are a self-selected group who may not be representative of non-volunteers, and thus of the larger combined population. The use of screening criteria with

Figure 7-9. Difference between target population, representative sample, and statistic.

volunteers is one method to increasing confidence as to whether the volunteers are representative of the larger, target population. In many studies, volunteers are used to assess normal physiological function, and it is important that the investigator establish criteria for normality by excluding individuals with, for example, vital capacities far above or below average. The relationship between the target population and the representative sample and statistic are presented in Figure 7-9.

Participants can be lost in a study through attrition, such as death, change of residence, or voluntarily dropping out of the study. Any characteristics of a population, such as physiological capacities, personality factors, and demographic information (i.e., social and personal data), are parameters. These values are usually estimated or unknown because most populations are too large to measure in their entirety.

7.10 Size of Sample

Researchers are constantly plagued by the question, "How many participants should I include in the study?" The often repeated response is "As many as possible," because the greater the sample, the more accurately the sample represents the population. A greater sample size also increases statistical power, which is the likelihood of finding via a statistic a real difference or association if one exists. The accuracy of the sample depends only on the variability in the sample and the size of the sample. Statistical power takes into account the confidence level desired (95% or 99%; higher means less power), the variability in the sample (greater means less power), the strength of the association or the magnitude of the difference (greater means more power), and the sample size (greater means more power). In the statistical tables for the *t*-test, analysis of variance, and correlation coefficient, it is clear that the number of participants affects statistical significance because the degrees of freedom, which determine the critical value of the statistic to be exceeded, are derived from the number of participants in a study. For example, in applying the Pearson correlation coefficient to a study using a two-tailed design, a small *r*

of .20 can be statistically significant at alpha level of .05 level with samples sizes over 100. On the other hand, the researcher needs an *r* of .58 with a sample of 10 subjects to obtain statistical significance at the .05 level.

Another consideration in determining sample size is the length of the study and the financial resources available to collect data from participants. For example, if the researcher has only 3 months to collect data, the number of participants is limited to the time it takes within this period. If the researcher assumes that he or she needs as many participants as possible, then the costs and the time for collecting data for each participant should be calculated as part of the research proposal. Many times, these pragmatic considerations are the sole criteria for determining sample size, especially when one is awarded a grant for the research.

It is possible to have too small of a sample, which could possibly lead to a Type II error. A power analysis is a method by which an educated estimation can be made of mustering an adequate sample size. While there are different power analysis strategies based upon the research design, one of the most common types is to calculate for a simple experimental design where there are two conditions. This type of power analysis will calculate the number of required persons within each condition to obtain a certain level of probability of establishing a relationship if one exists. Care must be taken to consider the total number of required participants based upon the number of conditions within the study. It is important to keep in mind when determining the sample size includes the following concepts. Type I error is the probability of concluding that there was a difference in the dependent variable(s) across conditions when in truth there was not; Type II error is the probability of concluding that there was no difference in the dependent variable(s) across conditions when in truth there was. Statistical power is the probability of concluding there is a difference in the dependent variable(s) when in truth there is a difference. Type I error is associated with the Greek letter alpha (α); Type II error is associated with the Greek letter beta (β) and power is 1-β. Traditionally α is set at .05, and β is set at .2, with the power thus being .8. (See Chapter 8 for more information.)

7.11 Selection of Measuring Instrument

7.11.1 Selecting a Specific Test for a Research Study

Whether to select a published test or to construct a new test is a frequent dilemma for the researcher. Figure 7-10 describes this process. Further discussion on this topic is in Chapter 10.

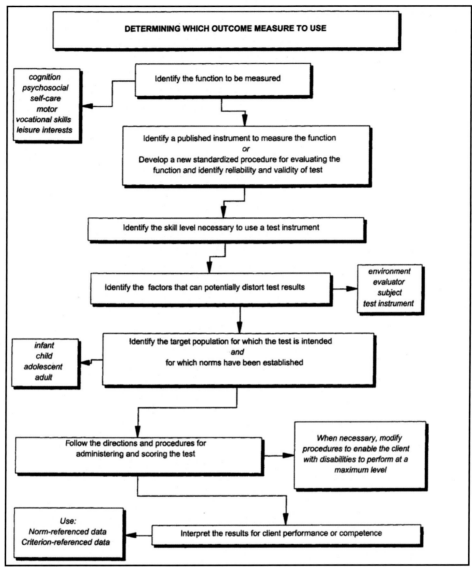

DETERMINING WHICH OUTCOME MEASURE TO USE

cognition
psychosocial
self-care
motor
vocational skills
leisure interests

Identify the function to be measured

Identify a published instrument to measure the function
or
Develop a new standardized procedure for evaluating the
function and identify reliability and validity of test

Identify the skill level necessary to use a test instrument

Identify the factors that can potentially distort test results

environment
evaluator
subject
test instrument

infant
child
adolescent
adult

Identify the target population for which the test is intended
and
for which norms have been established

Follow the directions and procedures for
administering and scoring the test

When necessary, modify
procedures to enable the client
with disabilities to perform at a
maximum level

Use:
Norm-referenced data
Criterion-referenced data

Interpret the results for client performance or competence

Figure 7-10. Steps in choosing a test instrument and the process of deciding what to use as the outcome measure. The researcher must decide whether to construct a new test or use a previously published test based on several factors.

The conceptual definition of a variable should lead the investigator to a specific test that is the most appropriate one once the variable is operationally defined. In clinical research, it is critical for the investigator to select a measuring instrument that has high reliability and is a valid measure of outcome. Measuring improvement or change in areas such as cognition, psychosocial, self-care, motor, vocational skills, and leisure interests depends directly on the adequacy and sensitivity of the instrument. A crude measuring instrument that does not have the capacity to detect subtle changes in an individual's functioning or behavior is of less value to the researcher if the purpose of the study is to establish the effectiveness of an intervention in bringing about a detectable change in performance.

7.11.2 Concept of Measurement and Numbers: Data

Data in statistics are derived from empirical observations. These observations are the result of a standardized measurement procedure, such as simple counting, interviews, observations, standardized test results, or machine monitoring of physiological functions. *Measurement* is the assignment of numbers to objects, persons, or events according to rules. Measurement transforms certain attributes of the world into numbers, which can then be summarized, organized, and analyzed by statistical procedures.

The properties or characteristics of objects, persons, or events are called *variables* (e.g., height, weight, intelligence). A variable must be able to assume two or more different values, reflecting the fact that objects, persons, or events vary in the level they show of certain characteristics. This concept of *individual differences* is central to most scientific disciplines. One of the purposes of statistics is to reflect and summarize such individual differences in the values of variables.

7.11.3 Measurement Scales

Measurement scales are a system for the numerical representation of the values of a variable. Four basic types of measurement scales are distinguished in statistics.

7.11.3.1 Nominal Scale Data

Nominal scale measurement is the most discrete and simplest level of data. With nominal scale data, observations are arranged into various classes or categories. Observations falling into the same class or category are considered qualitatively equivalent, whereas observations in different classes are considered qualitatively different. For example, eye color, as classified into blue, brown, hazel, or gray, is an example of nominal scale data.

Numbers are assigned usually to each class or category, but these numbers merely reflect a label for the classes. The numbers do not reflect arithmetical magnitude or order; they only distinguish one class or category from another.

With nominal scale measurement, categories and classes are determined, and a count is made of the number of observations in each category. Because nominal data constitute the most elementary level of measurement, the only arithmetic operation that can be performed on the data is counting the number of observations in a category and then analyzing proportional differences between categories. Examples of nominal scale data in health research include diagnostic categories, sub-specialization areas, geographic locations, leisure interests, and health care environments (e.g., hospitals, nursing homes, rehabilitation clinics).

7.11.3.2 Ordinal Scale Data

Ordinal scale data is the next level of measurement where objects or individuals are not only distinguished from one another, but also are arranged in order or rank. The numerical values of a variable are arranged in a meaningful order to indicate a hierarchy of the levels of the variable or to show relative position. Examples of ordinal scale data are birth order among siblings, the order of finish in a race, or the relative academic standing of university students in a class. The numbers assigned in these examples not only distinguish between individuals, but also indicate the order or rank of the individuals relative to one another.

The major limitation of ordinal scales is the inability to make inferences about the degree of difference between values on the scale. Numbers assigned in ordinal scale measurement have the properties of both distinctness and order, but the difference between the numbers may not be equal. For example, the difference between 1st and 3rd place in a race may not be equivalent to the difference between 25th and 27th place in the race. There may be wide or narrow differences between each rank. With ordinal scale data, it is only possible to state that one individual or object ranks above or below another. Examples in health care include the degree of improvement, muscle strength categories (e.g., good, fair, poor), a self-care index, the severity of illness or injury, and the degree of pain.

7.11.3.3 Interval Scale Data

Interval scale measurement extends ordinal scales by adding the principle that equal differences between scale values have equal meaning. Thus, the difference between each variable score (e.g., 1, 2, 3, 4 ...) is equivalent. With interval measurement, numbers serve two purposes: (a) to convey the order of the observations and (b) to indicate the distance or degree of differences between observations. Numbers are assigned so that equal differences in the numbers correspond to equal differences in the property or attribute measured. However, the zero point of the interval scale can be placed arbitrarily and does not indicate absence of the property measured.

Examples of interval scale data are calendar years and the temperature scales of Celsius and Fahrenheit. In a temperature scale, the difference between 10°C and 15°C is the same quantitative difference as between 20°C and 25°C, but 20°C is not twice as warm as 10°C because 0°C is not a true zero point, representing the absence of all heat.

Interval scales are important in scientific research. Many human characteristics and attributes, such as intelligence scores, range of motion (ROM), dexterity, coordination, and standard scores, are scales with approximately equal intervals. In addition, more sophisticated inferential statistical procedures may be performed with interval scale data compared with the lower level nominal and ordinal data.

7.11.3.4 Ratio Scale Data

Ratio scale data is the highest level of measurement and includes the maximum amount of information. The ratio scale is named as such because the ratio of numbers on the scale is meaningful. Because there is a genuine zero point, equal ratios between scale values have equal meaning (i.e., the ratio 40:20 is equivalent to 100:50 or 120:60, that is, twice as much of the attribute). The zero point on a ratio scale indicates total absence of the property measured. With ratio scale data, all arithmetic operations (addition, subtraction, multiplication, and division) are meaningful. Measurement of variables such as height, weight, heart rate, and respiratory rate are all ratio scaled. Figure 7-11 illustrates the differences between the four basic types of measurement scales, and Table 7-5 illustrates their characteristics and properties.

Progress in scientific research gained momentum with the design of tests and instruments that measured and recorded human performance accurately. The measuring instrument is the sine qua non of quantitative research. Without an adequate measuring instrument, a problem

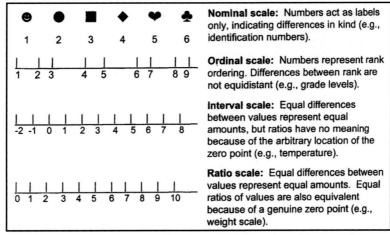

Figure 7-11. Steps in choosing a test instrument and the process of deciding what to use as the outcome measure. The researcher must decide whether to construct a new test or use a previously published test based on several factors.

remains unquantifiable. The adequacy of a measuring instrument is determined by its reliability (i.e., consistency in measurement) and validity (i.e., soundness in measurement).

Various examples of measurable variables in health and education research are described in Table 7-6. "In its broadest sense, measurement is the assignment of numerals to objects or parts according to rule" (Stevens, 1951, p. 1).

In the foregoing example (see Table 7-6) of measurable variables, numbers can be assigned to indicate the degree of improvement, strength, perceptual ability, and quality of life. Rating scales can also be devised using a continuum of measurement, equal intervals, or item ranking. Likert-type scales using descriptor adjectives are another alternative. In this scale, it is not assumed that there are equal intervals between numbers (e.g., 1 to 2 is not assumed to be the same distance as 2 to 3) or that there is an absolute zero. Nonetheless, measurement at this level is an improvement over a clinician subjectively stating, on the basis of treatment, that the patient has either improved or not improved. Measurement enables the clinical researcher to operationally define and objectively evaluate an outcome variable. Without objective measurement, clinicians have no criteria or standards to compare the effects of various treatment modalities.

For example, an investigator is interested in comparing two methods of increasing self-care skills in patients who have experienced a stroke. After establishing two groups based on screening criteria and random assignment, the researcher operationally defines self-care skills, such as independence in dressing. The operational definition includes the test and procedure in measuring the dependent variable, self-care. In another example involving retrospective research, an investigator is interested in determining the correlation between disengagement in social decision making and choice of housing for individuals who are older (e.g., nursing home care, independent community living).

The presumed variable, housing arrangements, is hypothesized to affect social decision making. Screening criteria are established in operationally defining the two housing arrangements. The researcher would then select the settings, and participants would be selected randomly from each institution. The crux of the research is in operationally defining the concept of social decision making by selecting an objective standardized test.

In selecting a measuring instrument, the researcher is faced with two basic questions:

1. Does the instrument measure a variable consistently?

2. Is the instrument an accurate measure of the variable?

The first question seeks a reliability index, and the second question raises issues of validity.

7.11.4 Reliability

If one assumes that a specific characteristic of an individual remains stable over time, then a reliable measuring instrument should reflect the stable characteristic through repeated trials. For example, an electron microscope, sensitive enough to enlarge chromosomes so that a researcher can perceive them, maintains a consistency in measurement. In the physical sciences, where comparison constitutes the foundation of measurement, the reliability of instruments has progressively evolved. Nonetheless, the individual using a sensitive measuring instrument can affect what is being measured. This is conceptually similar to the Heisenberg Uncertainty Principle. For example, astronomers observed that the individual's reaction time in viewing the movement of stars affects the calculations done to determine the distances between the stars. In response to this human factor, astronomers developed photographic means of recording the movement of stars over time. The control of personal agency in measurement is an important factor to consider in every research study where there is an

		TABLE 7-5		
		CLASSIFICATION OF SCALES OF MEASUREMENT		
MEASUREMENT SCALE	**TYPE OF VARIABLE**	**RESEARCHER APPLICATION**	**PURPOSES**	**EXAMPLES**
Nominal	Discrete	Sorting of items	Establishing mutually exclusive groups	Occupations, diagnostic groups
Ordinal	Discrete	Rank ordering of items	Determination of greater or lesser	Patient improvement, clinical performance of students
Interval	Continuous	Equal ordering of items	Establishing equal intervals on a continuum	Intelligence, perceptual-motor abilities, work capacities
Ratio	Continuous	Equal ordering of items with an absolute zero point	Establishing continuous measurement with zero point	ROM, muscle strength, weight, height, auditory and visual acuity

	TABLE 7-6
	MEASURABLE VARIABLES
VARIABLE TO BE TESTED	**EXAMPLES OF MEASURING INSTRUMENTS**
Hand strength	Dynamometer
ROM	Goniometer
Attitudes toward individuals with disabilities	Attitudes Toward Disabled Persons Scale
Clinical performance of students	American Occupational Therapy Association's Fieldwork Performance Evaluation for the Occupational Therapy Student
Psychological improvement	Tennessee Test of Self Concept
Social values and life goals	Life Satisfaction Index
Stress management	Stress Management Questionnaire
Sensory integration	Sensory Integration and Praxis Tests
Cognitive functioning	Allen's Cognitive Level
Self-care	Functional Independence Measure
Developmental levels	Miller Assessment Profile
Eye-hand coordination	Developmental Test of Visual-Motor Integration
Perceptual ability	Test of Visual Perceptual Scales (non-motor)
Instrumental activities of daily living	Executive Function Performance Test
Hand function	Jebsen-Taylor Hand-Function Test

interaction between the person or object observed and the investigator.

Researchers strive to reduce the error in measurement by increasing the reliability of an objective test or instrument and reducing the variability of extraneous factors in the individual. Instruments, such as the electrocardiograph, electroencephalograph, radiograph, electromyograph, positron emission tomography scan, magnetic resonance imaging, and single-photon emission computed tomography are usually reliable indicators of bodily functions. On the other hand, questionnaires, surveys, rating scales, attitude inventories, interest tests, and objective psychological tests may be less reliable. The nature of the test affects the reliability index. Automatic instruments that record bodily functions need to be mechanically sound or calibrated to be reliable. In devising a reliable instrument, the investigator is concerned with eliminating items that are ambiguous or that can be answered in more than one way. Reliability is not a simple concept that merely reflects the consistency of the instrument. In any test administered to subjects, individual differences e.g., level of reading ability, need to conform, desire to please the examiner, motivation, test anxiety) are important factors that could potentially increase the error variance and decrease the consistency of response. Because human beings are constantly reacting to internal and external factors, reliability must be interpreted in a relative degree when considering psychological tests, questionnaires, and attitude scales. Most researchers with human subjects accept a reliability coefficient of approximately $r = .80$ or above to be an acceptable level of a test's consistency in measuring a variable.

7.11.4.1 Techniques for Measuring Test Reliability

Test reliability is usually measured by correlating two sets of scores and arriving at a correlation coefficient. For example, an investigator is interested in devising a test of perceptual-motor ability with school-age children from 8 to 11 years old. In the process of devising the test, the investigator constructs 50 items that measure perceptual-motor ability. The items are screened for clarity in a pilot study with 24 children as subjects. The investigator seeks to determine split half reliability and test-retest reliability. In split half reliability, the test is broken into two equal parts (in this example, 25 items each) and correlated with each other. In test-retest reliability, a test is given twice within a short period of time (usually within 2 weeks) and the scores on the two tests are correlated.

In the hypothetical example shown in Table 7-7, there is a perfect positive correlation (+1.00) between the scores on the first and second tests. The scores also reflect a practice effect, which is typical of test-retest reliability. A practice effect exists when scores increase consistently as a function of the participant's familiarity with the content of the test and his or her reduced anxiety. In many published tests, the practice effect is controlled when developing normative data.

7.11.5 Item Analysis

When devising a test or assessing students, a researcher may be interested in the effectiveness of individual test items that differentiate between high and low achievers. The researcher may also be interested in eliminating those items that are ambiguous and have a low discriminative level. Item analysis is a method of gauging the difficulty value and ambiguity of each item. In item analysis, the percentage of passes and failures are calculated for each item. For example, if items 1, 2, and 3 are passed by 80%, 60%, and 40% of the subjects, respectively, we can infer

TABLE 7-7
HYPOTHETICAL DATA FOR TESTING RELIABILITY

TEST-RETEST RELIABILITY

Subject	Test 1	Test 2
01	69	72
02	34	37
03	71	74
04	20	23
05	95	98
06	10	13
07	99	102
08	81	84
09	92	95
10	49	52
11	97	100
12	63	66
13	86	89
14	9	12
15	96	99
16	81	84
17	20	23
18	69	72
19	81	84
20	24	27
21	97	100
22	55	58
23	54	57
24	97	100
25	68	71

that item 3 is either more difficult or more ambiguous than item 1 or 2. Another method is analyzing items to determine which items were passed by high overall scorers and failed by low overall scorers. This analysis will enable the researcher to separate out those items that have discriminative value. Items that are passed by all examinees have little discriminative value but may indicate the level at which all members of the group are functioning. This may be particularly important in criterion-referenced tests where the test administrator is most concerned with issues related to competency.

7.11.6 Validity

Validity reflects the authenticity and accuracy of a test. Does the test measure what it purports to measure? A test may measure a concept consistently but it may not, in fact, measure what the researcher identifies as the intent of the test. Psychological tests purporting to measure general intelligence, self-image, body defensiveness, and attitude toward individuals with disabilities may be measuring other concepts. The degree to which a test is valid is the degree of empirical evidence that corroborates the results of a test. Tests or instruments that collect primary data, such as an electromyograph, radiograph, goniometer, ergometer, and magnetic resonance imaging, are more easily verified and corroborated. By contrast, tests that collect secondary data derived from multiple factors in the individual, such as visual perception, are more difficult to validate. Personality, attitude, values, perception, and interests are complex variables derived from many facets of the individual's life that are related to genetic predisposition, social learning, cultural identification, and physiological factors. The researcher seeking to validate a visual-perceptual test is limited by the ability to corroborate the findings. Traditionally, validity is established on the following bases:

- *Content validity*: The degree to which the test appears to measure a concept to experts in the field.
- *Concurrent validity*: The degree of correlation with another standardized instrument. A new test may be derived because it is less time-consuming and less expensive than another established validated instrument. What is the correlation between the established test and the new test?
- *Face validity*: The degree to which the test appears to measure a concept by a logical analysis of the items. Does each item appear to relate to the content being tested?
- *Predictive validity*: The degree to which a test can predict accurately over a period of time (longitudinally). For example, a test devised to predict success in a graduate program for occupational therapists or success in a rehabilitation program for patients with stroke are examples of predictive validity. In the examples, follow-up data from longitudinal studies would determine the correlation between the initial test predictor score and subsequent success in a program.
- *Construct validity*: Considered to be the highest form of empirical evidence that is most sought after by scientific researchers. Construct validity assumes a theoretical rationale underlying the test instrument. In testing an instrument for construct validity, the researcher seeks the statistical analysis of empirical data to substantiate the position that the test is in fact measuring the defined variable. For example, an investigator devising a test to measure self-image would first construct a theory that underlies the concept. The theory would include developmental factors, relationships with other variables, and behavioral observations supporting the evidence for construct validity. In another example, the electroencephalogram, which records brain waves and is used indirectly for diagnosing brain damage, can be checked for construct validity through dissection of an animal brain or through postmortem examination.

7.12 Ethical Principles Guiding Human Research

Boxes 7-1 through 7-3 give examples of documents related to ethical issues guiding clinical research.

7.12.1 Human Subjects Review Protocol

Any institution actively involved with research involving human subjects needs to establish an institutional review board (IRB) as outlined in the US Federal Policy 45 CFR 46. Research involving human participants falls into one of three categories: convened, expedited, or exempt. The determination is based upon the risk to human subjects. A basic rule of thumb is that research protocols that have more than minimal risk are required to be assigned to the convened application process. Minimal risk is defined as "... the probability and magnitude of harm or discomfort anticipated in the research are not greater in and of themselves than those ordinarily encountered in daily life or during the performance of routine physical or psychological examinations or tests" (U.S. Department of Health and Human Services, 2005, §46.102 Definitions, para. i.). If there is risk associated with the research protocol, but the risk is no more than minimal, then the protocol will be assigned to an expedited review. In protocols where there is no risk involved, then the IRB review designation will be exempt. Exempt status is generally applied to studies involving de-identified preexisting data or observations being made in public.

Box 7-1. Indiana Wesleyan University Research Application

IRB PROPOSAL FORM

(March 2017)

Proposals must be submitted as a Microsoft Word document to irb@indwes.edu. The IRB cannot adequately review proposals or supporting documents submitted as PDFs, JPGs, Google Docs, HTML, etc. The only exception is that pages which require a signature (the title page, the IRB Proposal Checklist and the Principal Investigator Assurances) may be submitted in a PDF format. Please see the document Guidelines for the Preparation of a Proposal for additional guidance in completing this form. Please delete all prompts/instructions in red text before submitting the final proposal.

Title: _____

Check One:

_____   Faculty-Staff Research

_____   Student Research

Division/Department:

Principal Investigator(s):

Street address and city, state and zip code are not required for IWU community members (students, faculty, staff)

_____

Street Address

_____

City, State, Zip Code

_____

E-mail Address

_____

Phone Number

_____

Investigator Signature: _____

Research Advisor: _____

Research Advisor E-mail: _____

Research Advisor Signature: _____

(continued)

Box 7-1. Indiana Wesleyan University Research Application (continued)

Purpose of the Research

(This statement should be easily understood by reviewers with no prior knowledge of the area of study. The statement should be brief but long enough for reviewers to understand the purpose of the project. What are you trying to learn from the study? Avoid all jargon. Please delete all prompts/instructions in red text before submitting the final proposal.)

Methodology

Please describe the steps that will be taken to complete the project. Provide enough detail so that reviewers will understand how the study participants will be involved. Include information about the study population that will be sampled. Explain how the privacy and confidentiality of each participant will be protected. Explain how the data will be stored, e.g. in a locked filing cabinet in a locked office or on a secure server. State that electronic copies of all signed consent forms will be sent to the IRB in one electronic file at the completion of the study. State that all other study documents (hard copy or electronic) will be retained for a minimum of three years after close of the study by the principal investigator. Remember to attach survey instruments, if applicable, and permission to use copyrighted survey instruments, when applicable.

Participant Recruitment Strategy

Discuss in detail how subjects will be approached to participate in the research. What recruitment methods will be used to select subjects?

Potential Risks Involved And Methods of Minimizing Risks, Inconveniences, or Discomforts

What risks may participants face? Remember that just because a study is anonymous does not mean that the participants will not face risks. What will be done to alleviate discomforts? Is there someone the participants can speak with if they so desire about discomforts they may experience while being part of the study? What are the costs to participants to be in the study, e.g. loss of time, travel expenses, etc.?

Anticipated Benefits and Importance of Gained Knowledge

Are there any benefits that participants will receive for being in the study? Note: Payments to research subjects for participation in the study are not considered benefits. What does the study add to scholarship and knowledge?

Known Conflicts of Interest

Does the Principal Investigator, Research Advisor, or anyone else involved in the research have an equity interest in a company that is a sponsor of the research or owner of products being evaluated in the research. Does anyone involved in the research have a financial interest in a particular outcome of the research? Is there any other circumstance that might cause the investigator(s) to be unduly biased toward a particular outcome of the research? If a conflict of interest is recognized, does the research design adequately protect human subjects and study integrity from bias? If there are no known conflicts of interest, state so in this section.

References

Please cite the literature that you have used to develop your proposal.

All required forms

Reproduced from Indiana Wesleyan University and available at Indiana Wesleyan University's Office of Research Integrity, 4201 South Washington Street, Marion, Indiana 46953-4974.

BOX 7-2. INDIANA WESLEYAN UNIVERSITY INFORMED CONSENT FORM

Research Participant Consent Form

Title of Project:

Principal Investigator's Name:

Research Advisor's Name:

Academic Division/Department:

This form is to be used to obtain consent from the participant. Please remove all text in red prior to submission of the proposal package to the IRB.

Purpose of Research

This statement should be easily understood by individuals with no prior knowledge of the area of study—avoid all jargon. It is best that the first person be used consistently throughout each section of the informed consent document rather than just cutting and pasting from other sections of the proposal. For example, begin sentences with "I understand that …" or "I acknowledge that …." The goal is to make sure the potential human subject completely understands the study and the nature of her or his involvement. Consistently using the first person in the consent form will help comprehension.

Specific Procedures to be Used

This should include each step of the procedure the participants would either observe or experience.

Duration of Participation

This should inform the potential participants of the amount of time (number of days/hours) they will need to commit to the project (including travel time).

Risks to the Individual

Each study has some amount of risk. If the risk is minimal or similar to that of everyday life, state that fact. If the respondent is asked to answer personal questions, e.g. about self-concept, emotions, or health conditions, note that this can cause discomfort. The fact that a study is anonymous does not preclude risk. When applicable, note that if there is a chance you may become privy to information that must be reported, such as child abuse, child neglect, elder abuse or intent to harm self or others, this must be disclosed as a risk to participants.

Benefits to the Individual or Others

Benefits refer to direct benefits to the participants. They need to be clearly stated. Not all studies will have direct benefits to the participants and if this is the case, it needs to be stated as so. Compensation is not a benefit.

Compensation

If there is compensation, it needs to be listed here; it is not to be considered a benefit. Put N/A in this section if not applicable.

Extra Costs to Participate

This may include, but is not limited to, transportation costs for travel to the site of research, costs of medicine, etc. If there is no cost to the participant, state that fact.

(continued)

Box 7-2. Indiana Wesleyan University Informed Consent Form (continued)

Injury or Illness

This should explain what the plan is for any medical situation that may occur during the research process. Explain who will be contacted and what the participant's rights are in terms of medical compensation. A plan for medical care should also be included.

Confidentiality

Explain how the privacy and confidentiality of each participant will be protected. Include where, how, and for how long documents related to this study will be kept and how they will be eventually disposed of. Explain how the data will be stored, e.g. in a locked filing cabinet in a locked office or on a secure server. State that electronic copies of all signed consent forms will be sent to the IRB in one electronic file at the completion of the study. State that all other study documents (hard copy or electronic) will be retained for a minimum of three years after close of the study by the principal investigator. Include the process of keeping audio/video media confidential (if applicable). It also needs to be stated if confidentiality is limited. For example, if you are meeting in focus groups, information shared may not be kept confidential by other group members. Also, there may be some information that is brought to light that you are required, by law, to report. If subjects will be paid, the statement, "I understand that my name, social security number and address may be provided to the business office of Indiana Wesleyan University for the purpose of facilitating payment to me for participating in this study," should be included in this section as well.

Voluntary Nature of Participation

I do not have to participate in this research project. If I agree to participate I can withdraw my participation at any time without penalty.

Explain how a participant would withdraw from participating without any penalty. If there is any circumstance that would make withdrawing difficult, that must be explained. If a participant is an employee who is part of a study related to the participant's work, include a statement to the effect that willingness to participate or not participate in the study and decision to withdraw from the study will have no effect on the person's employment. Similarly, if the participant is a student who is part of a study related to his or her education site, include a statement to the effect that willingness to participate or not participate in the study and my decision to withdraw from the study will have no effect on my standing at the institution of higher education where I am enrolled.

Release

I participate of my own accord in this research project and release any claim to the collected data, research results, publication in any form including thesis/dissertation, journal article, conference presentation or commercial use of such information or products resulting from the collected information.

All consent forms must contain the above statement.

Contact Information:

If I have any questions about this research project, I can contact:

Insert Investigator's name and phone number (students are encouraged to use departmental phone numbers rather than private numbers) plus any additional research personnel that participants may find appropriate to contact along with said persons' contact information. Also, for student research, include the research advisor's name and contact information.

If I have concerns about the treatment of research participants, I can contact the Institutional Review Board (IRB) at Indiana Wesleyan University, 4201 South Washington Street, Marion, IN 46953. (765) 677-2090.

I have had the opportunity to read this consent document, ask questions about the research project and am prepared to participate in this project.

(continued)

Box 7-2. Indiana Wesleyan University Informed Consent Form (continued)

Participant's Signature:

Participant's Name (Type or Print):

Date:

Investigator's Signature:

Date:

* Please note that all consent forms that are longer than one page must provide a place for the participant to initial and date all non-final pages. A format such as the following may be added to the bottom of each non-final page:

I have read this page _____ (initials here)

Continue to next page.

For principal investigators who are using electronic consent:

Some studies allow for electronic consent, e.g. when potential participants are solicited through an email or social media. In that case, the preamble/cover letter/email should include all of the information contained in the above informed consent document template.

Additionally, the following clause or similar wording as befits the proposal shall be included in electronic informed consent documents if participants will take an electronic survey: "The survey is designed not to collect e-mail addresses or Internet protocol (IP) addresses. To further maintain confidentiality of the survey, please do not include your name or any other information by which you can be identified in any of the comment boxes in the survey."

Under no circumstances shall electronic informed consent be used for studies that include children under the age of 18 years.

Reproduced from Indiana Wesleyan University and available at Indiana Wesleyan University's Office of Research Integrity, 4201 South Washington Street, Marion, Indiana 46953-4974.

Box 7-3. Indiana Wesleyan University Checklist for Complying With Institutional Review Board Standards

INDIANA
WESLEYAN
UNIVERSITY

IRB Proposal Checklist

Check all items that have been completed and sign. Research Advisor must sign as well.

_____ 1. Completed Proposal Title Page

_____ 2. Purpose of the research

_____ 3. Methodology

　_____ a. Subjects (how many, how selected or excluded)

　_____ b. Description of instruments

　_____ c. Procedures (including steps for retention of records and consent forms)

(continued)

Box 7-3. Indiana Wesleyan University Checklist for Complying With Institutional Review Board Standards (continued)

____ 4. Participant recruitment strategy

____ 5. Potential risks involved and methods of minimizing risks, inconveniences, or discomforts

____ 6. Describe anticipated benefits and importance of the knowledge that may reasonably be expected to result.

____ 7. Known conflicts of interest

____ 8. All required forms

____ a. Consent forms

____ b. Letters of permission

____ c. Copies of all instruments to be used

____ 9. Signed copy of Principal Investigators Assurance form

____ 10. Copy of Certificate of Completion of the CITI Program's Human Subjects Research course for all persons (investigators and research advisors) whose names appear on Page 1 of the proposal form

____ 11. IRB proposal checklist

By signing below, I confirm that I have read and followed the IWU IRB's Guidelines for the Preparation of a Proposal (March 2017 edition).

Investigator Signature: _____

Research Advisor Signature: _____

CITI = Collaborative Institutional Training Initiative

Reproduced from Indiana Wesleyan University and available at Indiana Wesleyan University's Office of Research Integrity, 4201 South Washington Street, Marion, Indiana 46953-4974.

Convened reviews require more effort by the entire IRB and are thus more carefully scrutinized than the other two types of review. Whereas the expedited review generally involves less scrutiny, it still requires a thorough review by one or more IRB members for approval. The exempt review usually involves fewer IRB members than the other two types of review but still requires a thorough IRB review. The IRB application process usually includes an application (see Box 7-1), an informed consent form and procedure (see Box 7-2), the research protocol, and a financial disclosure and conflict of interest form, as well as any supporting data collection tools, instruments, advertisement flyers/brochures, and letters of support. A full IRB application is a thoughtful process and requires that all individuals associated with the research protocol have documented training in the following:

- Health Insurance Portability and Accountability Act
- Federal assurance for the protection of human subjects
- Protecting human research participants online course
- Collaborative institutional training initiative program

Box 7-1 is an example of an application for an IRB review used by Indiana Wesleyan University; Box 7-3 is an example of a checklist from Indiana Wesleyan University that can be used by the research to conform with IRB guidelines. However, it is important for researchers to follow the guidelines established by the IRB at the institution with which they are affiliated.

7.13 Data Collection Procedures

The time schedule for collecting data, the costs of the study, the setting for administering group or individual tests, a cover letter to prospective subjects explaining the nature of the study, an individual data collection sheet recording descriptive information and test scores, an informed consent agreement between the researcher and the participant, and the statistical techniques used to analyze the data are all factors for the investigator to consider in the prospectus for the study.

The checklist in Table 7-8 should guide the investigator in preparing a data collection procedure. The reader should review this frequently to ensure that all parts of the data collection have been considered.

7.13.1 Informed Consent and Forms

The informed consent is a legal document that informs participants about the procedures that are to occur, the place in which the data collection will occur, the amount of time required for participation, and the potential risks or hazards of the study. Informed consent must be documented (U.S. Department of Health and Human Services, 2009). A copy of the signed informed consent form must be obtained for the principal investigator's files from each participant, or in the case of a minor, the parent, guardian or surrogate parent. A copy should be given to each participant. The participant's copy should include the name, address, telephone number, and e-mail address of the person to whom requests for information or results may be addressed. It must also include the name, address, telephone number, and e-mail address of the person to whom complaints may be addressed. The informed consent form should be written in language that is easily understood by all participants.

The following is described in detail in the informed consent form:

- The procedure for obtaining informed consent.
- A brief statement regarding the objectives of the study
- The amount of time each participant will be asked to devote to the study
- The compensation, remuneration, or other rewards, if any, to be received by the participants
- A description of any expected benefits that may be obtained by the participant
- A description of the procedures and methods to be used in the study
- The identification of potential risks or hazards that might occur during the study
- The identification of any costs to the participant
- The procedures that will minimize any identified risks or hazards
- The procedures that will ensure confidentiality of the participants

When children are used in research, additional procedures must be used. According to the *Code of Federal Regulations* (U.S. Department of Health and Human Services, 2009), permission must be obtained from the parents, guardians, or surrogate parents to enlist the child and assent must be obtained from the child:

TABLE 7-8

CHECKLIST FOR GUIDING DATA COLLECTION

TIME SCHEDULE

- Have you determined the length of time needed for administering individual or group testing?
- Have you considered travel time and time for interviewing?
- Have you determined the length of time for scoring tests?

INFORMED CONSENT

- Have you prepared a form describing to the subject the procedure, tests, information, and length of time involved?
- Have you informed the participant that he or she may decline from the study without any implied penalty?
- Does the participant have a signed form in his or her possession?

DATA COLLECTION SHEET

- Have you prepared a data collection sheet for each subject, coding the name to guarantee anonymity and providing room for every datum item collected?

COMPUTER ANALYSIS

- Have you considered using computer time in analyzing the data?

STATISTICAL TECHNIQUES

- Does the study meet the assumptions of a parametric statistic?
  - If not, what specific nonparametric statistics will be used to analyze the data?
- Have you done a statistical analysis of the hypothetical data?

COST ANALYSIS

- Have you considered the costs of purchasing tests or instruments?
- Have you considered the costs of postage, address labels, and mailings?
- Have you considered the costs of analyzing data?
- Have you considered the costs of travel?
- Have you considered the costs of telephone calls?
- Have you considered payment for participants?

[W]hen in the judgment of the IRB the children are capable of providing assent. In determining whether children are capable of assenting, the IRB shall take into account the ages, maturity, and psychological state of the children involved. This judgment may be made for all children to be involved in research under a particular protocol, or for each child, as the IRB deems appropriate. If the IRB determines that the capability of some or all of the children is so limited that they cannot reasonably be consulted or that the intervention or procedure involved in the research holds out a prospect of direct benefit that is important to the health or well-being of the children and is available only in the context of the research, the assent of the children is not a necessary condition for proceeding with the research. Even where the IRB determines that the subjects are capable of assenting, the IRB may still waive the assent requirement under circumstances in which consent may be waived in accord with Sec. 46.116 of Subpart A. (§46.408, para a)

Although not required, the investigator may want to develop a written assent for children rather than just asking the child to verbalize assent. Care should be taken to ensure that the reading level is appropriate for the age and ability level.

Box 7-2 depicts a model for an informed consent form that was developed by the Indiana Wesleyan University Office of Research Integrity.

7.14 Methodological Limitations of a Study

Researchers can assume that most studies have limitations in selecting a sample, using a measuring instrument, collecting data, or analyzing results. A section devoted to the limitations of a study is an objective means for discussing flaws in research methods. This section is not meant to be an excuse or rationalization for not obtaining acceptable results or confirming predicted hypotheses, but rather is meant to be an unbiased analysis of shortcomings in the research. These flaws in methodology do not necessarily mean that the research is worthless or inadequate; on the contrary, it serves to guide future researchers in avoiding the same mistakes when the research is replicated or when another research design is proposed. Research often involves trial-and-error methods with factors of risk and uncertainty. Results are important if the researcher has been objective and unbiased. The honesty and integrity of the researcher are enhanced when both the merits and deficiencies of a study are objectively reported. Likewise, the limitations of a study can serve as the basis for recommending further research.

7.15 Summary

After the researcher selects a meaningful problem, the next step is to narrow the focus of the research into a feasible study. This chapter on research and methodology describes the step-by-step procedures in implementing a study from stating a testable hypothesis, operationally defining the independent and dependent variables, diagramming the study by showing the relationship between variables in the research models, and discussing the theoretical rationale underlying the study. All these steps should be well-thought through before the researcher actually begins collecting data. Those steps are the foundation for the study and the preparatory work must be done before the study is implemented. The next part of planning a research study is the methods section, which comprises selecting the participants, determining the location of where data will be collected, determining the assessment tools that will be used in the study, and creating the strategy for increasing the internal validity of the study, such as controlling for extraneous variables that can affect outcomes. The ethics of performing research is discussed in detail and an example of an informed consent procedure is included. This chapter is a pragmatic approach that delineates the essential factors in planning a research study.

8

Data Analysis and Statistics

Statistical interpretation depends not only on statistical ideas, but also on "ordinary" thinking.
Clear thinking is not only indispensable in interpreting statistics, but is often
sufficient even in the absence of specific statistical knowledge.

—Wallis & Roberts (1962, p. 29)

OPERATIONAL LEARNING OBJECTIVES

By the end of this chapter the learner will be able to:
- Define *statistics*.
- Describe the importance of statistics in contemporary society.
- Understand the difference between descriptive and inferential statistics.
- Understand the concept of measurement and data.
- Understand the difference between discrete and continuous data.
- Identify seven statistical models for analyzing clinical research data.
- Distinguish between parametric and nonparametric statistical tests.
- Understand when to apply specific statistical tests to clinical research designs.

Rice, M. S., Stein, F., & Tomlin, G.
Clinical Research in Occupational Therapy, Sixth Edition (pp. 209-270).
© 2019 Taylor & Francis Group.

8.1 Definition and Meaning of Statistics

Statistics, as a practical discipline, is defined as the application of statistical tests and procedures for organizing, analyzing, and interpreting results or data according to mathematical formulas. Statistics is taught, at some level, in almost every university and college around the globe. Although statistics is derived from mathematics, it is taught in many academic departments with application to economics; agriculture; medicine; natural, physical, and social science; nursing; health science professions; and education. The rapid evolution of mainframe and personal computers has expanded the role of statistics to almost every aspect of our lives, including banking, retailing, education, manufacturing, farming, politics, communication, transportation, and health care. Through the availability of the internet and email, statistical programs and databases are easily accessible to researchers. Computer programs using sophisticated statistical models have enabled pollsters to predict election results based on representative sampling procedures and insurance companies to set up actuarial tables based on the presence or absence of risk factors for morbidity and mortality.

Statistics is also an essential component of clinical research, enabling the investigator to objectively describe and infer logical conclusions from the results. In general, statistical analysis of the data strengthens the impact of the results and allows the investigator to compare current findings with previous research. The researcher in occupational therapy should have a basic understanding of descriptive statistics and the most frequently used inferential statistical tests and procedures. Common inferential statistics include *t*-test and analysis of variance (ANOVA) for comparing sample means, Pearson correlation coefficient and Spearman rank order correlation for testing relationships between variables, and Chi-square for testing the differences between observed and expected frequencies. The researcher should be able to calculate the incidence (initial occurrences) and prevalence (prevailing rates) of diseases and be able to read and interpret vital statistics related to morbidity and mortality. Quantifiable or measurable data are counted as statistics. For example, the total number of individuals with a spinal cord injury, the number of workers with disabilities, or the number of occupational therapists working in public schools are all identifiable statistics.

Historically, the earliest statistics amassed by local authorities were census counts. Statistical occurrences also replaced subjective descriptions of populations, such as "abundant," "flourishing," and "enormous," to describe epidemics and population density. The first use of statistics recorded factual information, such as the annual rate of births, deaths and marriages. During periods of epidemics, such as the Black Death (bubonic plague) in Europe during the 16th and 17th centuries, statistics were used to tabulate the number of deaths and their presumed causes. Also, tax collectors used statistics in Europe before the Middle Ages to assess wealth and agricultural holdings. In the latter half of the 18th century, census taking became a systematic governmental function. The U.S. Constitution of 1790 includes provision for a regular population census every 10 years. The application of probability theory to the prediction of death rates (actuarial tables among populations) and the use of sampling procedures advanced the science of statistics. In the mid-19th century, statistical societies were founded (e.g., the American Statistical Association was organized in Boston in 1839). Vital statistics became more accurate, and methods were developed to analyze health data and to correlate injuries and diseases with occupation and social class. The emergence of modern statistics based on probability theory led to the application of statistical methods in laboratory and clinical research. R. A. Fisher, a geneticist, extended statistics from small samples where inferences were made to large populations. The work of Fisher and his colleagues in the early part of the 1900s led the way to quantifiable analysis of research data in the biological, physical, and social sciences. Currently, hundreds of textbooks are published on the application and theory of statistics in a wide range of professional disciplines. Despite this, the field of statistics is as much of an art as an empirical science. There are many points of disagreement on the correctness of applying specific statistical tests to research data. The student learning and applying statistics must decide which statistical tests are most appropriate for analyzing the results. How the variable is measured (e.g., continuous or discrete), the probability level required, and the direction of the hypothesis stated will help the researcher to select a specific statistical test. The material presented in this chapter is organized to aid the student in reading and understanding statistics presented in research articles and to follow a step-by-step procedure in calculating statistical results. Each step in the process of deciding on the statistical test to be employed, the analysis of the raw data, and the interpretation of the statistical results should be carried through in a problem-solving, reflective manner.

8.2 Relationship of Statistics to Clinical Practice

Statistics as a methodology enables the researcher to organize, analyze, and interpret data. In the context of a research design, statistical application does not change the quality of the data or influence the validity of the results. In conducting research, the investigator should have an overall concept of the meaning of the projected results and how a statistical test will be used to accept or reject a hypothesis. For example, an investigator wishes to compare attitudes of health professionals and nonhealth professionals toward individuals with disabilities utilizing a survey

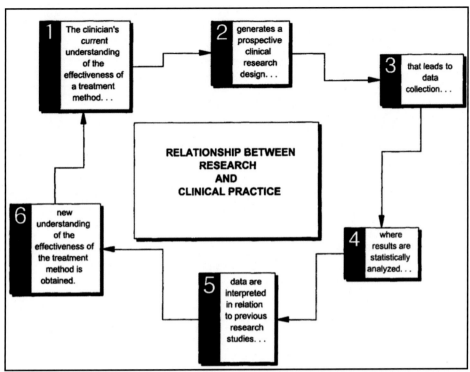

Figure 8-1. Relationship between research and clinical practice. Notice that the relationship is continuous; the completion of Step 6 leads back to Step 1. A clinician should be continually involved in practices that lead to research that can be applied to clinical practice.

questionnaire. He or she has hypothesized that health professionals will have more positive, realistic attitudes toward individuals with disabilities than will nonhealth professionals. Then the researcher would apply a statistical test, such as an ANOVA, to accept or reject the hypothesis.

The process of statistical analysis and its relationship to clinical practice is illustrated in Figure 8-1. In this example, a clinician proposes to test the effectiveness of a specific treatment method. Six stages may be distinguished in this process:

1. A hypothesis is conceived.
2. A research plan is devised to study the effects of a treatment method or procedure traditionally used by clinicians.
3. Quantifiable data are collected from a patient group.
4. The data are statistically processed and analyzed.
5. The results are interpreted.
6. Conclusions are drawn, and the information is disseminated back to the scientific community and clinical practitioners.

The cycle continues with new treatment methods introduced and ineffective methods discarded. Hopefully, the process leads to the evolution of clinical efficacy. This example demonstrates the importance of statistics to clinical research. What are the most common statistical procedures employed in clinical research?

Statistical procedures employed in clinical research are based on descriptive and inferential statistics. Figure 8-2 outlines the specific descriptive and inferential statistical tests.

- *Descriptive statistics* are procedures for reducing, summarizing, and describing results or data. For example, in descriptive statistics a large set of data are reduced to summary values, graphs, frequency polygons and scatter diagrams, measures of central tendency (i.e., mode, median, mean), measures of variability (i.e., range, standard deviation, variance), and incidence and prevalence rates.

- *Inferential statistics* are methods for generalizing data collected from a representative sample to a larger target population that includes all subjects or observations. The essence of inferential statistics is to sample a representative portion of a population to infer information representative of the whole population. Inferential statistics are applied for two main purposes: (a) to estimate the characteristics of a population (parameters) and (b) to test hypotheses about populations. In inferential statistics, a sample is drawn from the target population, the characteristics of this sample are measured, and inferences or estimates about the corresponding characteristics are made to the population at large.

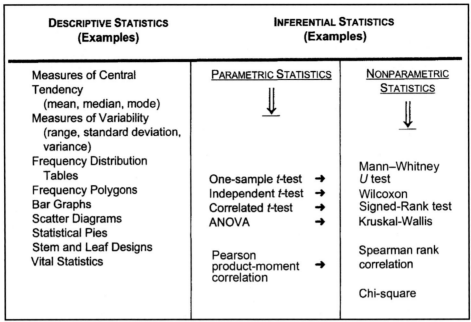

DESCRIPTIVE STATISTICS (Examples)	INFERENTIAL STATISTICS (Examples)	
	PARAMETRIC STATISTICS	NONPARAMETRIC STATISTICS
Measures of Central Tendency (mean, median, mode) Measures of Variability (range, standard deviation, variance) Frequency Distribution Tables Frequency Polygons Bar Graphs Scatter Diagrams Statistical Pies Stem and Leaf Designs Vital Statistics	One-sample *t*-test ➔ Independent *t*-test ➔ Correlated *t*-test ➔ ANOVA ➔ Pearson product-moment correlation ➔	Mann–Whitney *U* test Wilcoxon Signed-Rank test Kruskal-Wallis Spearman rank correlation Chi-square

Figure 8-2. Statistical procedures and tests used in the analysis of data.

- A *parameter* is a descriptive value attributed to the sample population. Parameters are usually unknown. For example, in the population of individuals with spinal cord injury in North America, the parameter value of age would be inferred or estimated because it would be almost impossible to survey all individuals in North America who have spinal cord injury. The parameter value is usually estimated through descriptive studies of representative samples in more than one geographical area. The data from a representative sample are extrapolated to the target population. The reliability of the estimate increases with the number of descriptive studies that show concurrence.

- A *statistic* is a quantitative measure of a sample. For example, the average heart rate of a sample of college students is 72 beats/minute. This is a statistic with a summary value representing the average heart rate in the sample. When a total population is available and every individual is measured, a parameter value may be computed directly. Population data usually are not available, so researchers use a representative sample drawn from a population to compute a statistic and employ inferential statistics to estimate or extrapolate parameter values. Vital statistics are used to estimate the incidence or prevalence rates of a specific disability in a population. For example, if an investigator is interested in determining the number of individuals with a diagnosis of muscular dystrophy in the United States, he or she can carry out epidemiological studies with representative samples in specified geographic areas, such the Midwest. Frequently, epidemiological studies are replicated in other geographical areas to test the

validity of previous results and to monitor trends in the incidence and prevalence rates of specific diseases.

8.2.1 The Process of Statistical Analysis

The important steps for researchers are to develop a hypothesis, select the appropriate statistical test, calculate the results, and interpret the data. The decision process in applying statistics and interpreting the results is shown diagrammatically in Figure 8-3.

8.3 KEY DEFINITIONS OF STATISTICAL CONCEPTS

The first step in understanding statistics is to understand the definitions of statistical terms. With a conceptual understanding of statistics, one can critically understand published studies that use statistical designs. The bases on which hypotheses are substantiated or rejected and on which conclusions are generated are derived from a statistical analysis of the results. The following definitions are essential to understand statistics. They are listed alphabetically and are intended to be used as a reference aid.

- *Continuous variables* are examples of interval or ratio scale measurement. Weight, height, age, muscle strength, blood pressure, and hearing acuity are all examples of continuous variables. It is assumed that, in measuring continuous variables, there are an infinite number of values between each pair of scores.

Figure 8-3. The process of statistical analysis.

- *Data* are the numerical results of a study. In a descriptive study of a population, data are enumerated totals, such as the number of emergency patients in a hospital clinic or the number of health care workers in a rural area. Descriptive statistics of populations, such as the mean and median, are data. In small sample research in which inferential (probability) statistics are used, data represent comparative results derived from the research. These results are the bases of discussion and interpretation. The singular of data is datum or statistic.

- *Degrees of freedom* (*df*) is a mathematically derived value used in reading statistical tables. It is often calculated by subtracting 1 from the total number (N) of subjects in a group. It is defined as the number of observations in the calculation of a statistic that are free to vary.

- *Dichotomous variables* contain only two subsets, such as male and female subjects, improvement or no improvement, experimental and control group, or any other two variable sets created by the investigator or found naturally.

- *Discrete variables* identify separate categories, such as diagnostic groups, allied health professions, occupations, vitamins, pharmaceutical drugs, and treatment methods. Discrete variables belong to a set of objects sharing some trait or characteristic. They are examples of nominal scale measurements.

- A *directional hypothesis* predicts one of the following:
  - There will be a statistically significant difference in a specified direction between two groups after applying a treatment in experimental research
  - There will be a statistically significant relationship (positive or inverse) between two variables

- *Frequency* is the number of times that a result occurs. A frequency distribution table of results describes the number of times a variable falls into a discrete category.

- *Measures of central tendency* are descriptive statistics (e.g., mean, median, mode) that measure the center or location of a data distribution.

- *Measures of dispersion* or *variability* are descriptive statistics that indicate the spread of scores in a data distribution. The range, variance, and standard deviation scores are measures of dispersion. Factors such as the difference between the highest and lowest scores and the number of scores that deviate from the mean influence measures of dispersion.

- *Nonparametric statistics* are sometimes referred to as *distribution-free statistical tests* because they are applied to data for which no assumptions are made regarding the normal distribution of the population and interval scale measurement. The advantages of nonparametric statistics are that they can be applied to small sample data without having to meet the stringent assumptions of parametric statistics. Examples of nonparametric tests include, but are not limited to, Chi-square, Spearman rho, Mann–Whitney *U* test, Wilcoxon test for correlated samples, and Kruskal-Wallis test.

- The *normal (Gaussian) distribution* or *bell-shaped curve* represents a theoretical distribution that approximates the range and frequency of many normal human functions and anatomical descriptions, such as blood pressure, lung capacity, height, and weight. The major assumption underlying the concept of a normal curve is that variables are distributed along a continuum with the greatest frequency in the middle and the least frequency at the outer edges of the distribution. Figure 8-4 indicates the percentage of cases found within each

z-scores	- 3 SD		-2 SD		-1 SD		0 SD		+1 SD		+2 SD		+3 SD
Percentile	0.1	0.4	1	2	5	9	16	25	37	50	63	75	84	91	95	98	99	99.6	99.9
IQs		55		70		85		100		115		130		145
Standard Scores (Based on Wechsler's Scales)	1	2	3	4	5	6	7	8	9	10	11	12	13	14	15	16	17	18	19

Figure 8-4. The bell-shaped curve, which illustrates the percentage of population at each level. Included in this figure are the relationships between the standard deviations (*z*-scores), percentiles, IQ scores, and standard scores (based on Wechsler's scaled scores).

area of the normal curve. For example, 68% of cases are distributed toward the center of the curve in a symmetrical pattern. The basis of inferential parametric statistics rests on the assumption that the sample data are derived from a population that is normally distributed.

- A *null hypothesis* predicts that there will be no statistically significant difference or correlation between two or more specified groups, that is, after experimentally manipulating a variable or when testing the relationships between variables.
- *Parametric statistics* are applied to data in which certain underlying assumptions have been made. Examples of parametric statistics are *t*-test, ANOVA, and Pearson product-moment correlation coefficient.
- *Probability theory* is a branch of mathematics upon which inferential statistics is based. It is a theory that speaks to the likelihood of something being true.
- A *research hypothesis* is a prediction of results.
- *Standard deviation* is a statistical measure of the dispersion of scores from the mean.
- *Standard error of measurement* is a statistical value that indicates the band of error surrounding a test score. For example, a raw score of 90 with a standard error of measurement of 4 represents a score ranging from 86 to 94.
- *Statistical assumptions* are preconditions that are required before a specific statistical test can be applied. Nearly all inferential statistics have their own set of assumptions, some of which are unique to that statistic

and some of which are shared among several statistics. Examples of common assumptions include:
  - ◦ The variables measured approximate a normal distribution in the target population sampled.
  - ◦ The sample is a random selection or is representative of the target population.
  - ◦ Each data point occurrence is independent from other data point occurrences.
  - ◦ The variance, such as the standard deviation, within the compared groups are approximately the same.
- *Statistical tables* contain critical levels and values of probability for accepting or rejecting a hypothesis. By using a statistical table, the investigator determines whether the statistical value obtained is significant compared with the critical value. Using statistical tables, the investigator decides the level of significance, such as .05 or .01.
- *Statistically significant results* means that there are differences between two or more groups that are not due to chance. In every statistically significant result, there is a comparison between the effects on two or more groups. In clinical research, statistically significant results are traditionally accepted at the .05 or .01 level, which means that the results are not due to chance in 95/100 cases or 99/100 cases. In using the concept of statistical significance, the investigator performing experimental clinical research assumes an explanation that is sometimes confusing to students who think that statistics is an exact science that can be used to determine cause-effect relationships. Conclusive cause-effect relationships are only meaningful when an investigator can control every variable that may affect the results. The closest that medical research comes to the control of extraneous variables is in experimental animal research where environmental and sometimes genetic factors can be rigorously controlled. In clinical research with human subjects, it is almost impossible to obtain results that are 100% conclusive because of the interactional effects between the therapist, patient, treatment method, and environment. Inferential statistics, which are based on probability theory, are applied to data derived from samples of populations so that everyone in a population is not tested or measured. Samples per se indicate inconclusive data and an uncertainty even if a representative sample has been selected. In summary, a statistically significant result in experimental clinical research implies the following:
  - ◦ Probability theory is assumed in interpreting the data.
  - ◦ A sample of population is used rather than the entire population.
  - ◦ There is an allowance for error based on a researcher's inability to control all variables that may possibly influence the results.

- Conclusiveness of results is not assumed, and the investigator can only suggest that a cause-effect relationship exists.
- *Test of statistical significance* is based on the characteristics of the normal curve and probability theory.
    - *Two-tailed tests of statistical significance* are used in analyzing data if the researcher has stated the hypothesis in a null form.
    - *One-tailed tests of statistical significance* imply that the researcher has predicted a directional hypothesis, and there is prior evidence, either through a literature review or clinical observation, that there will be a statistically significant difference between the groups or a statistically positive correlation between variables.
- *Variables* are factors that can be operationally defined, categorized, and measured. Variables can be homogeneous groups, such as undergraduate university students, patients with hemiplegia, or hospital administrators. Variables are also conditions or behaviors, such as group therapy, cardiovascular disease, or activities of daily living (ADL) training. In experimental research, the *independent variable*, which is manipulated by the investigator, is the direct cause of the *dependent variable*, which is the resultant effect. Variables can be discrete, dichotomous, rank order, or continuous. (Refer to Chapter 7 for further discussion about variables.)
- *Variance* is a measure of the average of each score's deviation from the mean. Variance is an intermediate value used in calculating the standard deviation.

8.3.1 Universal Symbols Used in Statistics

α   alpha, associated with hypothesis testing, the probability of a Type I error

β   beta, associated with hypothesis testing and the chance of a Type II error

χ^2 Chi-square statistical test

df   degrees of freedom

f   frequency of cases in a distribution

F   statistic associated with ANOVA

μ   mu, the population or parameter mean; oftentimes, this value is unknown and estimated by the mean

H_0 null hypothesis or the concept that there is no statistically significant relationship between two or more variables (e.g., $\mu_1 = \mu_2$)

H_1 alternative hypothesis, opposite of null hypothesis (e.g., $\mu_1 \neq \mu_2$)

n   number of subjects within a designated sample

N   total of number of subjects in a group or population

P   probability of a chance occurrence

P-value   obtained or observed significance value (e.g., if $P < \alpha$, H_0 is rejected)

r   the Pearson product-moment correlation coefficient indicating the degree of relationship between two variables or two sets of data

r_s the Spearman rank order correlation for ordinal data (formerly rho [ρ])

s   the standard deviation of a sample (SD)

σ   lowercase sigma, the standard deviation of a population, usually estimated by s

Σ   uppercase sigma, sum of an arithmetic calculation

t   *t*-test statistic

t_{obs} *t* observed, *t* value derived from the *t*-test

t_{crit} *t* critical, the value derived from a statistical table of values found through α levels

z   standard score measured in standard deviation units

≠   not equal to

≥   greater than or equal to

≤   less than or equal to the mean value of a sample

8.4 Seven Statistical Models for Clinical Research

Seven statistical models for analyzing data are outlined in Table 8-1. These models represent the most frequently used statistical tests for clinical researchers. The format in presenting each model is to define the model and the statistical tests that the models represent, analyze an example of the statistical test from the literature, outline sequential steps in calculating the statistical results, and follow through with a hypothetical stepwise example. Many statistical tests are not covered in these models. References to textbooks on statistics are provided throughout the chapter as a guide for those researchers inspired to further explore the world of statistics. As one becomes adept in using statistical software programs for personal computers, the options for selecting statistical tests broaden. However, it is first important for the clinical researcher to understand the concepts underlying the statistical applications. Doing statistical tests with a calculator and doing exploratory data analysis aids the researcher to better understand statistical processes that are done later through computer software programs.

8.4.1 Model I: Descriptive Statistics

In this model, the researcher calculates descriptive statistics based on data collected from a representative sample or the total population. The statistical procedures include the following:

- Frequency distribution tables
- Frequency polygons
- Histograms and bar graphs
- Scatter diagrams

		TABLE 8-1	
		SEVEN STATISTICAL MODELS	
	STATISTICAL MODEL	**PURPOSE**	**EXAMPLES OF STATISTICAL TESTS OR PROCEDURES**
I.	Descriptive statistics	Describe the statistical characteristics in samples or populations	Measures of central tendency (mean, mode, median), measures of variability (range, standard deviation, variance), frequency distribution table, frequency graph, scatter diagram, statistical pie, stem and leaf, vital statistics
Inferential Statistics			
II.	One-sample problems	Test the difference between a sample mean and a parameter mean	One-sample *t*-test
III.	Two independent samples	Test the differences between sample means from two independent groups	Independent *t*-test (parametric statistic) Mann–Whitney *U* test (nonparametric statistic)
IV.	Paired-data sample	Test the differences between two conditions (means) in the same sample	Correlated *t*-test (parametric statistic), Wilcoxon signed rank test (nonparametric statistic)
V.	*k*-independent samples	Test the differences between means from two or more independent groups	ANOVA (parametric statistic), Kruskal-Wallis (nonparametric statistic)
VI.	Correlational sample	Test the relationship between two variables	Spearman rank order (nonparametric statistic), Pearson correlation coefficient (parametric statistic), regression line, correlation matrix
VII.	Observed minus frequencies expected	Test the differences between observed minus expected frequencies	Chi-square (nonparametric statistic)

Adapted from Larson, R. J. (1975). *Statistics for the allied health sciences.* Columbus, OH: Merrill Publishing.

- Statistical pies
- Stem-and-leaf displays
- Measures of central tendency
- Measures of variability
- Vital statistics

8.4.2 Model II: One-Sample Problems

The purpose of this statistical model is to compare data collected from a representative sample of a population and then to compare the obtained value with a parameter value that is known or estimated or to a standard value. Examples include comparing air samples from a metropolitan area to a standard accepted for clean air. The research question that this model answers is whether the mean of the representative sample and the established parameter mean value are statistically significantly different. The statistical procedure for this model is the one-sample *t*-test.

8.4.3 Model III: Two Independent Samples

The purpose of this statistical model is to test whether the means for two representative samples are statistically significantly different. An example in clinical research is determining whether one treatment method (e.g., sensory integration therapy) is more effective in reducing hyperactivity than a comparable treatment method (e.g., relaxation therapy) in two independent groups. The statistical test (independent *t*-test) is applied to determine whether there is a statistically significant difference between the two treatment methods. The Mann–Whitney *U* nonparametric statistical test is another example used to evaluate data using this model.

8.4.4 Model IV: Paired-Data Sample

The primary purpose of this statistical model is to examine the difference between mean values in one sample group with two data points, such as pre- and post-test. This statistical model employs the correlated *t*-test to test whether there will be a statistically significant difference between the means in two conditions. This statistical model is frequently used in clinical research to determine if a treatment method is effective when compared to a baseline measure of a dependent variable. The Wilcoxon nonparametric statistical test is an alternative to the parametric one-sample correlated *t*-test.

8.4.5 Model V: k-Independent Samples

If the researcher is comparing the means of more than two independent samples, then he or she applies an ANOVA. The ANOVA is similar to the independent test when two independent samples are compared. If the results of the ANOVA are statistically significant, then the researcher employs post-hoc tests to determine which groups are statistically different from each other. Examples of these post hoc tests (similar to *t*-tests) include the Scheffé, Duncan multiple analysis, or Tukey tests. The nonparametric alternative to ANOVA is the Kruskal-Wallis statistical test.

8.4.6 Model VI: Correlational Sample

In this statistical model, the researcher measures the degree of relationship between two variables, such as in a study examining the relationship between perceptual motor skills and functional abilities in self-care. The relationship can range from 0, indicating that the two variables are completely independent and do not affect each other, to ±1.00, indicating a perfect relationship between two variables. An example of a perfect correlation is the effect of temperature on the expansion of the chemical element mercury. As the temperature goes up, mercury expands; as the temperature goes down, mercury contracts. A perfect correlation can be positive (+1.00) when both variables change in the same direction, or it can be negative or inverse (-1.00) when the variables change in inverse directions (i.e., as one variable goes up, the other variable goes down). An example of an inverse relationship is the presence of serotonin, a neurotransmitter, and symptoms of depression. As serotonin is depleted in the blood, the symptoms of depression increase.

The relationship between two variables can be described in a scatter diagram. The Pearson correlation coefficient for interval scale data and the Spearman rank order correlation for ordinal scale data are applied to evaluate the degree of relationship (*r*) between two variables. A regression line can be calculated when there is a high correlation between two variables. The regression line is calculated by using the results of the Pearson correlation coefficient and plugging the values into a formula for the regression line. In this formula, variable values are estimated from known X variable values. This is illustrated in Figure 8-5.

8.4.7 Model VII: Observed Minus Expected Frequencies

In this model, the investigator compares groups or conditions based on frequency or nominal data. Chi-square is the statistical test used when comparing the differences between observed frequencies and expected frequencies based on probability. For example, Chi-square is used frequently in drug research to compare the differences in the number of patients who have improved with an experimental drug as compared with the number of patients taking a placebo who have improved.

8.5 MODEL I: DESCRIPTIVE STATISTICS: ORGANIZATION AND TABULATION OF DESCRIPTIVE DATA

8.5.1 Table of Percentage

Statistical analysis begins with organizing data into summary tables and diagrams. In descriptive studies, as in survey research, tabular summaries of data provide the results. For example, Table 8-2 summarizes data from three different mental health diagnostic groups who were earning at least minimum wage. The table reports the percentage of people employed at least minimum wage who either had a single or who had multiple hospital admissions. The data are also stratified by age group. Three striking trends can be observed from this table. First, there is an inverse relationship between age and employment. Second, males have a higher employment rate than females, and third, higher employment rates are associated with single admissions compared to multiple admissions.

However, another method of displaying data is to compare results between periods of time, distances, or events. For example, Table 8-3 lists cancer sites and the frequency of distribution in percentage across categories of cancer stages. When examining the data, the reader can note that some types of cancer are evenly distributed across the various stages (e.g., digestive system and liver, intrahepatic bile duct, and lung and bronchus), whereas other frequencies are clustered within one or two stages (e.g., melanoma of the skin, brain and other nervous system, and myeloma).

Figure 8-5. Example of a scattergram showing the relationship between two variables. When the value of X is known, then the value of Y can be predicted by the use of the regression line.

These examples demonstrate the importance of descriptive statistics in summarizing results from a research study. Several methods can be used to describe data. Some of the most frequently used methods for organizing descriptive data are discussed in the following section.

8.5.2 Frequency Distribution Table

A *frequency distribution table* is organized into columns of data that include the number or frequency of cases (and the equivalent percentages) that fall into a designated category. In the research study in Table 8-4, a frequency distribution table describes the age and gender of the population sampled in the study

The first column of a frequency distribution table includes the class intervals (in this example, age group by years). It could also represent data such as range of motion (ROM) in degrees, scores on perceptual tests, or diastolic blood pressure. The class intervals are separated into equal 10-year intervals in the previous example (e.g., 15 to 24 and 25 to 34). The second column of a frequency distribution includes the number of classes tallied within the class intervals as with 36 males between the ages of 5 and 14. The third column includes the percentage of cases within a class interval. For example, there are 52 females in the class interval of 25 to 34, which represents 52 over a total of 228 females in the study for 22.8%, which is rounded to 23%. We can also determine the *cumulative frequency* of each class interval and the *cumulative relative frequency* with the

data provided in the study. The following data are reorganized into a frequency distribution table to include relative frequency and cumulative relative frequency for males only:

Frequency Distribution Table for Males

CI	f	Relative f (%)	Cumulative f (Cf)	Cumulative Relative f (%)
5 to 14	36	6	36	6
15 to 24	147	24	183	30
25 to 34	200	33	383	63
35 to 44	105	17	488	80
45 to 54	60	10	548	90
55 to 64	41	7	589	97
>65	21	3	610	100
Unknown	4	.006	614	100
Total	*614*	*100%*	*614*	*100%*

In summary:

- *Class interval* is the category of score values in a distribution. The number of class intervals is determined by the number of subjects in the study and the range of values or scores.

- *Frequency of cases* includes the total number of cases within an assigned class interval.

- *Relative frequency* or *percentage* is the percentage of cases falling within the class interval and is calculated by dividing the number of cases within the class interval by the total number of cases in the distribution.

- *Cumulative frequency* represents the total number of scores within a class interval that is added cumulatively from the lowest to the highest class interval. The grand total of the cumulative frequency equals the total number of scores or cases in the distribution.

- *Cumulative relative frequency* or *cumulative percentage* is the percentage of cases added from the lowest class interval through the highest class interval. The percentage should total 100%.

Table 8-2

Percent Earning Minimum Wage or Above in the Three Diagnostic Groups and in the General Population in December 2010

AGE GROUP		RHEUMATOID ARTHRITIS		SPINA BIFIDA		NEUROFIBROMATOSIS		GENERAL POPULATION
		Single Admission (% Employed)	*Multiple Admissions (% Employed)*	*Single Admission (% Employed)*	*Multiple Admissions (% Employed)*	*Single Admission (% Employed)*	*Multiple Admissions (% Employed)*	
Total category, N		3876	16,083	4704	6670	988	3352	3,835,406
21 to 30	Males	18.6	8.7	31.2	18.6	34.7	26.3	48.3
	Females	13.1	4.5	23	10.2	34.3	18.1	37.2
31 to 40	Males	19.8	9	37.8	31.2	52.8	40.9	64.7
	Females	11.3	7.4	30.5	13	44.5	30.2	47.8
41 to 50	Males	14	5.7	31.5	22	37.3	34.2	64.4
	Females	6.5	3.7	21.4	10.2	34.3	24.3	49.2
51 to 60	Males	6.8	2.3	20.7	15.1	26.9	16.6	47.7
	Females	5.4	2	13.1	4.5	14.7	13.5	35.7

Adapted from Davidson, M., Kapara, O., Goldberg, S., Yoffe, R., Noy, S., & Weiser, M. (2015). A nation-wide study on the percentage of schizophrenia and bipolar disorder patients who earn minimum wage or above. *Schizophrenia Bulletin, 42,* 443-447.

TABLE 8-3
STATE DISTRIBUTION BY CANCER SITE, ALL AGES, ALL RACES, BOTH SEXES, 2000 TO 2007

CANCER SITE	LOCALIZED	REGIONAL	DISTANT	UNSTAGED
Digestive system	31.9	32.7	25.6	9.8
Liver and intrahepatic bile duct	37.7	25.0	18.0	19.4
Lung and bronchus	16.4	21.9	52.9	8.8
Melanoma of the skin	83.8	8.3	3.7	4.2
Brain and other nervous system	72.9	15.8	2.2	9.0
Myeloma	4.7	0.0	94.2	1.0

Note. Cancer sites include invasive cases only unless otherwise noted. *Localized* means the cancer is only located at the organ where it began with no spreading. *Regional* means the cancer has spread beyond the primary site to nearby lymph nodes or organs and tissues. *Distant* means the cancer has spread from the primary side to distant organs or distant lymph nodes and *unstaged* means cancer for which there is not enough information to indicate a stage.

Reprinted with permission from Young, J. L., Roffers, S. D., Ries, L. A. G., Hurlbut, A. A. (Eds.) (2001). *SEER summary staging manual—2000: Codes and coding instructions.* National Cancer Institute. NIH Pub. No. 01-4969, Bethesda, MD.

8.5.2.1 Constructing a Frequency Distribution Table

The table below displays hypothetical ungrouped raw scores on resting heart rate for 50 healthy young adults.

Step 1. Record raw scores from ungrouped data.

Subject	Score	Subject	Score	Subject	Score	Subject	Score
01	54	14	67	27	54	40	79
02	72	15	74	28	73	41	85
03	80	16	76	29	72	42	52
04	53	17	79	30	78	43	56
05	75	18	77	31	78	44	67
06	53	19	48	32	56	45	55
07	78	20	76	33	80	46	79
08	47	21	47	34	84	47	81
09	72	22	50	35	72	48	72
10	54	23	65	36	68	49	67
11	66	24	83	37	57	50	71
12	68	25	55	38	57		
13	68	26	76	39	63		

Step 2. Identify the highest and lowest values in the distribution. Subjects 08 and 21 have heart rate scores of 47 (lowest score). Subject 41 has a heart rate score of 85 (highest score).

Step 3. Calculate the range (highest score to lowest score). In our example, the range is 85 - 47 = 38.

Step 4. Determine the number of class intervals. Determining the number of class intervals depends on the number of scores in the frequency distribution and the range of scores. Too many or too few class intervals may not give adequate information to describe the distribution. Determining the number of class intervals is a trial-and-error process. For example, compare the three frequency distributions using the same scores but with class intervals of too many, too few, and approximately correct. These data are shown in Table 8-5. As a general rule, most researchers constructing frequency distributions establish 6 to 15 class intervals.

Step 5. Determine the size of a class interval. The size of the class interval is determined through estimation by dividing the range of scores by the number of class intervals. Using the same example, the range of 38 is divided by 13 (the number of class intervals) to yield a class interval size of 3. It is recommended that an odd number be selected for the class interval so that the midpoint of the class interval is a whole number. For example, the midpoint of the class interval of 83 - 85 is 84. Later, in calculating group means from a frequency distribution table, the reader will find that it is easier to work with whole numbers than with fractions in calculating values.

On the other hand, if we determine that the size of a class interval in the previous example is 5, how many class intervals would be established? In this case the range of scores (38) is divided by the size of the class intervals (5) to arrive at 8 class intervals.

TABLE 8-4

PERCENTAGE OF RESPONDENTS REQUIRED TO PERFORM MANUAL TRANSFERS AND PERCENTAGE OF THOSE WHO SUSTAINED AN INJURY WHILE TRANSFERRING A PATIENT IN THEIR FACILITY

FACILITY	NUMBER OF RESPONDENTS (N)	RESPONDENTS REQUIRED TO PERFORM MANUAL TRANSFERS (%)	RESPONDENTS WHO SUSTAINED INJURY DUE TO MANUALLY TRANSFERRING OF PATIENT WITHIN THE PAST YEAR (%)
Acute care	19	100.0	10.0
Home health	14	100.0	0.0
LTC/SNF	87	92.0	4.6
Hospital inpatient rehab.	34	91.2	11.8
Private practice	8	87.5	0.0
Community center	8	87.5	25.0
Outpatient rehab.	29	82.8	3.3
School system	48	60.4	4.2
Psych-based	5	60.0	0.0
Work hardening/ industrial rehab.	7	57.1	0.0
Academia	10	30.0	0.0

LTC = long-term care; SNF = skilled nursing facility

Reprinted with permission from Rice, M. S., Dusseau, J. M., & Miller, B. K. (2011). A questionnaire of musculoskeletal injuries associated with manual patient lifting in occupational therapy practitioners in the state of Ohio. *Occupational Therapy in Health Care, 25,* 95-107.

CI	Midpoint
81 to 85	83
76 to 80	78
71 to 75	73
66 to 70	68
61 to 65	63
56 to 60	58
51 to 55	53
46 to 50	48

Step 6. Tally the number of scores within each class interval. Check to determine if the number of tallies total up to the number of scores in the frequency distribution.

CI	Real Limits[a]	Midpoint	Tally	f	Cf
83 to 85	82.5 to 85.5	84	|||	3	50
80 to 82	79.5 to 82.5	81	|||	3	47
77 to 79	76.5 to 79.5	78	|||||||	7	44
74 to 76	73.5 to 76.5	75	|||||	5	37
71 to 73	70.5 to 73.5	72	|||||||	7	32
68 to 70	67.5 to 70.5	69	||	2	25
65 to 67	64.5 to 67.5	66	||||||	6	23
62 to 64	61.5 to 64.5	63			1	17
59 to 61	58.5 to 61.5	6	0	0	16
56 to 58	55.5 to 58.5	57	||||	4	16
53 to 55	52.5 to 55.5	54	|||||||	7	12
50 to 52	49.5 to 52.5	51	||	2	5
47 to 49	46.5 to 49.5	48	|||	3	3
Total				50	50

[a]How to define upper and lower real limits of the class interval follows.

TABLE 8-5		
INTERVALS FOR CLASS DATA		
NUMBER OF CLASS INTERVALS		
Too Many (20 Class Intervals)	*Too Few (4 Class Intervals)*	*Approximate Correct (13 Class Intervals)*
84 to 85	75 to 85	83 to 85
82 to 83	65 to 74	80 to 82
80 to 81	55 to 64	77 to 79
78 to 79	45 to 54	74 to 76
76 to 77		71 to 73
74 to 75		68 to 70
72 to 73		65 to 67
70 to 71		62 to 64
68 to 69		59 to 61
66 to 67		56 to 58
64 to 65		53 to 55
62 to 63		50 to 52
60 to 61		47 to 49
58 to 59		
56 to 57		
54 to 55		
52 to 53		
50 to 51		
48 to 49		
46 to 47		

The upper real limit of a class interval is the highest value contained in the interval. Conversely, the lower real limit of a class interval is the lowest value contained in the interval. In dealing with numbers having at least two decimals, round the number up to include it in the nearest class interval. For example, 82.50 or greater would be tallied in the class interval 83 - 85. On the other hand, 82.44 would be tallied into the class interval 80 - 82 as shown in the example.

Step 7. Determine the relative frequency or percentage. Calculate the relative frequency of the scores in each class interval by dividing the number of cases or scores in the class interval by the number of cases in the frequency distribution. This is illustrated in Table 8-6.

Percentage = frequency of cases in the class interval/total cases in the frequency distribution

Step 8. Determine cumulative frequency. Calculate the cumulative frequency by adding the total frequency in each class interval consecutively from the highest class interval to the lowest. In the previous example, the number of cases in the class interval 83 - 85 is 3. This number is added to the number of cases in the class interval 80 - 82, which is also 3, giving a cumulative frequency of 6. The completed frequency distribution table is shown in Table 8-7.

Summary of Construction of Frequency Distribution Table

1. Organize raw scores from ungrouped data by arranging values from the lowest to the highest scores.
2. Identify the lowest and highest scores in the distribution.
3. Calculate the range, which is the difference or distance from the lowest to the highest scores in the distribution.
4. Determine the number of class intervals, using the rule of thumb of selecting within a range of 6 to 15 categories of intervals.
5. Determine the size of each class interval. First, estimate the size of class intervals by dividing the range by the number of class intervals. Try to select an odd number so that the midpoint of the class interval will be a whole number.
6. Count or tally the number of scores within each class interval.
7. Calculate the relative frequency or percentage of scores in each class interval.
8. Calculate the cumulative frequency by adding in succession the frequencies in each class interval. Check that the number of cases counted in succession is equal to the total number of cases or scores in the distribution.
9. Determine the cumulative relative frequency, which is the percentage of cumulative frequency sitting in each class interval. It is customary to start from the lowest class interval when calculating cumulative values.

8.5.3 Graphs and Other Pictorial Representations

In addition to presenting data in tables, many researchers use pictorial presentations to display results and describe data. These presentations can be in the form of frequency polygons, histographs, bar graphs, pie graphs, and stem-and-leaf display.

8.5.4 Frequency Polygon

A frequency polygon is a line graph displaying the frequency of data by categories. The categories compared are on the horizontal axis (abscissa), and the frequencies of occurrences are on the vertical axis (ordinate).

The frequency polygons in Figure 8-6 show the percentile of respective hypothetical body mass index (BMI) for males and females from 2004 through 2016. The BMIs are listed on the x-axis, the abscissa, and the year groupings are on the y-axis, the ordinate. Observations from this figure illustrate that BMIs included in the 50th percentile or smaller remained relatively similar through the years; however, the BMIs within percentiles greater than 50 tended to increase, particularly from 2010 through 2016.

8.5.5 Histograms and Bar Graphs

Histograms and bar graphs are often used by investigators to display frequency of data within categories, similar to frequency polygons. In histograms, the bars are attached to each other and represent number ranges, whereas in bar graphs, each bar is detached from one another and represent categories. The distinction sometimes is based on aesthetic reasons. The bar graph shown in Figure 8-7 illustrates the number of reported injuries by occupational therapy practitioners to various body parts due to manually transferring patients.

8.5.5.1 Constructing a Frequency Polygon, Histogram, or Bar Graph

A frequency polygon, histogram, or bar graph graphically depicts the data provided in a frequency distribution table. The data provided in Table 8-7 will be used in the following examples.

Step 1. Identify the x-axis (abscissa) and the y-axis (ordinate). This is illustrated in Figure 8-8.

Step 2. Label the abscissa descriptively. In the example in Table 8-7, the heart rate values range from the lowest score of 47 to the highest of 85. The midpoints of each class interval are located on the abscissa (Figure 8-9). The class intervals are extended on both ends to include zero frequency intervals. The lowest class interval with zero frequency is 44 to 46, with a midpoint of 45. The highest class interval with zero frequency is 86 to 88, with a midpoint of 87. There are now 15 class intervals including the zero frequency intervals.

Step 3. Organize the ordinate into frequency of occurrence. In the previous example, frequencies of occurrence range from 0 to 7. As a rule of thumb, the number of class intervals for frequency should be between 8 and 15. In this case, there will be 8 class intervals including 0.

The frequency polygon is depicted in Figure 8-9 with the data from Table 8-7. The histogram is depicted in Figure 8-10 with the same data used in constructing the frequency polygon. Bar graphs are similar to histograms, differing only in that the bars are detached (McCall & Kagan, 1986).

TABLE 8-6

CALCULATION OF CUMULATIVE FREQUENCY

CLASS INTERVAL	FREQUENCY	PERCENTAGE	CUMULATIVE PERCENTAGE
84	3	3/50 = 6%	100 %
81	3	3/50 = 6%	94%
78	1	7/50 = 14%	88%
75	5	5/50 = 10%	74%
72	7	7/50 = 14%	64%
69	2	2/50 = 4%	50%
66	6	6/50 = 12%	46%
63	1	1/50 = 2%	34%
60	0	0/50 = 0%	32%
57	4	4/50 = 8%	32%
54	7	7/50 = 14%	24%
51	2	2/50 = 4%	10%
48	3	3/50 = 6%	6%
Total	**50**	**50/50 = 100%**	**100%**

TABLE 8-7

FREQUENCY DISTRIBUTION OF HEART RATE SCORES FOR A HYPOTHETICAL POPULATION

CLASS INTERVAL	MIDPOINT	FREQUENCY	CUMULATIVE FREQUENCY	RELATIVE FREQUENCY (%)	CUMULATIVE RELATIVE FREQUENCY (%)
83 to 85	84	3	50	6	100
80 to 82	81	3	47	6	94
77 to 79	78	7	47	14	88
74 to 76	75	5	37	10	74
71 to 73	72	7	32	14	64
68 to 70	69	2	25	4	50
65 to 67	66	6	23	12	46
62 to 64	63	1	17	2	34
59 to 61	60	0	16	0	32
56 to 58	57	4	16	8	32
53 to 55	54	7	12	14	24
50 to 52	51	2	5	4	10
47 to 49	48	3	3	6	6

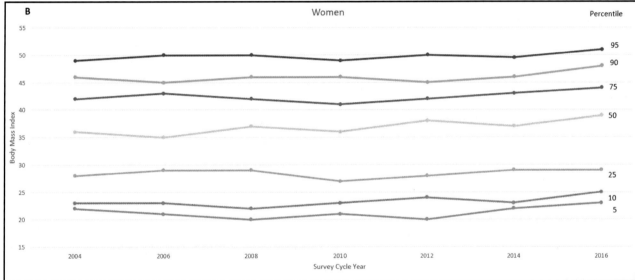

Figure 8-6. Selected weighted percentiles of BMI by survey cycle: NHANES 2005 to 2014. (Source: Flegal, Kruszon-Moran, Carroll, Fryar, & Ogden, 2016.)

There are several software programs that create any number of graph styles. For instance, spreadsheet programs often have a graphing module and a statistical module that can conveniently facilitate the creation of graphs.

8.5.6 Cumulative Frequency Distributive Polygon

A cumulative frequency distribution polygon is a line graph that shows the total number of observations or cases up to the upper real limit of a given class interval. For example, in Section 8.5.2, Step 8, determining cumulative frequency, the data for the heart rates for 50 subjects are displayed. In Figure 8-11, the cumulative frequency distribution polygon is constructed from the previous table of hypothetical heart rate values (see Table 8-7).

Cumulative frequency curves are useful in specifying the individual subject's relative position or standing in a total distribution of scores. For example, someone with a heart rate of 80 in the previous distribution is in the 94th percentile, or upper 6% of the distribution. Cumulative frequency curves often are useful in plotting group test data, such as grip strength, ROM, blood pressure, and achievement test scores. Individual test data plotted on a cumulative frequency curve can be used to evaluate an individual's function and diagnosis.

In designing a cumulative frequency curve, the ordinate axis is used to display cumulative frequencies, cumulative percentages, or cumulative proportions. The abscissa shows the score values as midpoints or individual scores.

The shape of the cumulative frequency curve reflects the form or shape of the original frequency distribution. As a

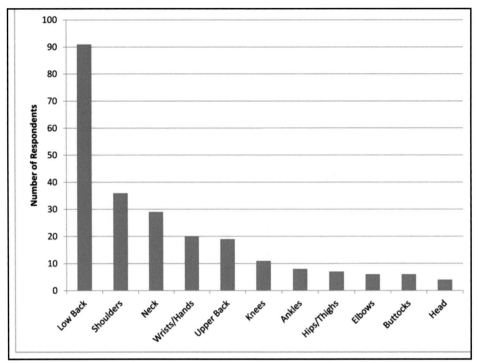

Figure 8-7. Example of a histogram depicting the maximum number of injuries related to various body parts associated with manually transferring patients. (Reprinted with permission from Rice, M. S., Dusseau, J. M., & Miller, B. K. [2011]. A questionnaire of musculoskeletal injuries associated with manual patient lifting in occupational therapy practitioners in the state of Ohio. *Occupational Therapy in Health Care, 25*[2-3], 95-107.)

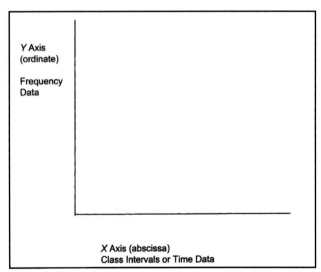

Figure 8-8. Parts of a frequency polygon, histogram, or bar graph. The frequency data are plotted along the vertical axis or ordinate (y-axis), while the class intervals or time data are plotted along the horizontal axis or abscissa (x-axis).

Figure 8-9. Frequency distribution polygon illustrating the frequencies of heart rate scores for a hypothetical population. The data used to plot this polygon are from Table 8-7.

general rule, the cumulative frequency curve will have the greatest slope or most rapid rate of rise at the point where there is the greatest accumulation of the scores in the original frequency distribution. The cumulative frequency curve levels off and shows the lowest slope for the class intervals when there are fewer scores. Cumulative curves do not describe variations in the data as well as histograms and should not be used to draw conclusions about the form

or shape of the data. The original frequency distribution is best used for this purpose.

8.5.7 Statistical Pie

A statistical pie is a pictorial representation of the relative percentage of discrete variables or nominal categories, such as health professions, distributions of disease, occupational role functions, types of work injuries, or treatment

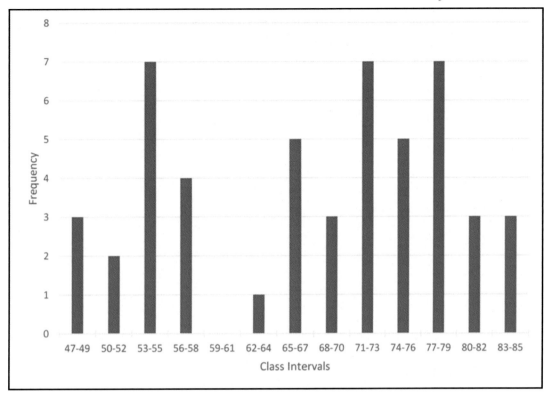

Figure 8-10. Histogram of heart scores in a hypothetical population. The data from Table 8-7, depicted in Figure 8-9 in a frequency polygon, are depicted in a histogram here.

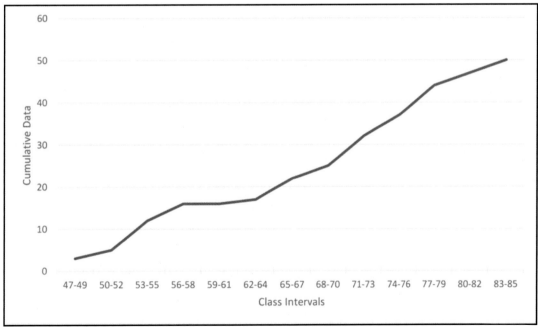

Figure 8-11. Cumulative frequency distribution polygon using data from Table 8-7.

techniques applied. It is particularly useful to quickly assess the relative percentage of each category. In Figure 8-12, the percentage of placement of students with special needs in each type of educational placement is graphically displayed in a statistical pie.

8.5.7.1 Constructing a Statistical Pie

Step 1. Make sure the statistical pie is relevant for describing data. The statistical pie is appropriate when there are between 3 and 10 discrete categories. If there are more than 10 categories, the data will be better presented in a frequency distribution table. The data collected should

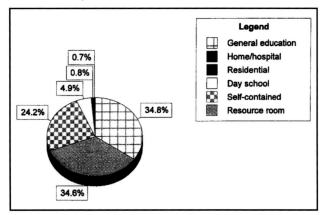

Figure 8-12. An example of a statistical pie graph that illustrates the hypothetical percentages of specialty practice areas of female physicians.

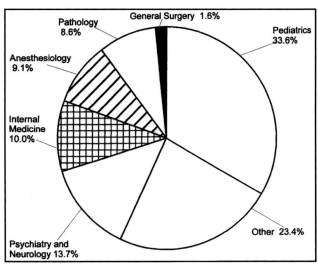

Figure 8-13. Statistical pie graph illustrating data from the hypothetical data of female physicians.

be categorical and inclusive. For example, data collected regarding the cause of death should include all major causes for a designated population and should add up to 100%. Unknown causes should be included in the statistical pie.

Step 2. First organize data into a frequency distribution table deriving relative percentages for each category. In the hypothetical example that follows, specialty areas for female physicians are described. A sample of 250 female physicians was surveyed.

Medical Specialty	f	Relative Percent
Pediatrics	84	33.6
Psychiatry and neurology	34	13.7
Internal medicine	25	10.0
Anesthesiology	23	9.1
Pathology	22	8.6
General surgery	4	1.6
Other	58	23.4
Totals	*250*	*100*

Step 3. Transform relative percent into the degrees of a circle, which is the proportion of 360 degrees. The relative percent is multiplied by 360 degrees.

Step 4. Use software with graphing capabilities to construct the pie chart. Divide the statistical pie with a protractor into seven segments running clockwise starting with the largest category at 12 o'clock, which in this example, is pediatrics (33.6% or 121 degrees), other (23.4% or 84 degrees), and psychiatry and neurology (13.7% or 49 degrees). Continue with the other specialty areas in completing the 360 degrees circle.

Step 5. Label each segment category with the relative percent rather than the degrees of arc. The completed statistical pie is shown in Figure 8-13.

8.5.8 Scatter Diagrams

A scatter diagram is a graphic representation of the relationship between two variables. In this example, the scatter plot depicts the relationship between age (presumed independent variable) and life expectancy (presumed dependent variable) in males and females between the age of 0 and 100 years (Figure 8-14). The size of the class interval for age (x-axis) is 20 years, and the size of the class interval for life expectancy (y-axis) is 10 years. The highest life expectancy is approximately 80 for females and is a few years less for males. This is associated with the youngest age on the y-axis (0). Visual examination of scatter diagrams often reveals a trend. In Figure 8-14, the trend is that as age increases, the life expectancy (meaning the number of years one is expected to continue to live at a given age) decreases. The points located on the scatter diagrams are coordinates in which the two variables intersect. For example, in this graph, the expected life expectancy at age 100 is approximately 2 years.

8.5.8.1 Constructing a Scatter Diagram

In a hypothetical example, a researcher collects the following data, examining the relationship between grip strength as measured by a Jamar dynamometer and Functional ADL scores as measured by the Klein-Bell Test for patients with muscular dystrophy.

Step 1. Record raw data for hypothetical example of grip strength and ADL scores in patients with muscular dystrophy.

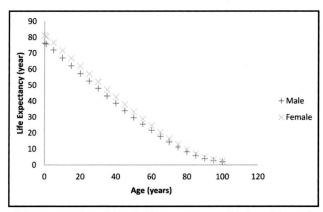

Figure 8-14. Male and female life expectancy in the United States for all races in 2013.

Subject	Grip Strength (abscissa)	ADL Score (ordinate)
01	15	20
02	40	95
03	30	50
04	30	80
05	10	20
06	25	15
07	10	15
08	20	42
09	20	15
10	15	75
11	40	70
12	30	60
13	20	45
14	10	30
15	40	85

Step 2. Determine the range along the abscissa (grip strength) and ordinate (ADL scores). The range for grip strength is 30 (highest value [40] minus lowest value [10]). The range for ADL scores is 80 (highest value [95] minus lowest value [15]).

Step 3. Determine the number of the class intervals for each variable. Using the convention of 6 to 15 class intervals, we would establish 8 class intervals for grip strength, with the size of the interval being 5. The actual score values are 5, 10, 15, 20, 25, 30, 35, and 40 (along the abscissa). For ADL scores, the class interval is 20, with a range from 15 to 95. The actual score values plotted along the ordinate are 0, 20, 40, 60, 80, and 100.

Step 4. Design the scatter diagram (Figure 8-15) with the score value on the abscissa (grip strength) and ordinate (ADL scores). For example, Subject 01 had a grip strength score of

Figure 8-15. Example of a scattergram. Hypothetical example showing the relationship between grip strength and ADL scores in patients with muscular dystrophy.

15 and an ADL score of 20. The investigator plots the coordinates for all 15 subjects.

In this example, a positive relationship is noted because as scores on one variable increase, scores on the other variable increase correspondingly. A negative, or inverse, relationship is obtained when scores on one variable increase while the corresponding scores on the other variable decrease. The degree of relationship between the two variables of the correlation coefficient will be discussed later in this chapter (Section 8.11).

8.5.9 Measures of Central Tendency

The first step in organizing data is usually to design a frequency distribution table or graph. The table or graph provides information concerning the form of the data. The properties of a set of data can be further described by calculating a summary statistic, such as a measure of central tendency. Measures of central tendency describe typical or average values in a distribution of data. An index of central tendency provides one value that best captures the distribution as a whole. There are generally three ways to do this:

1. *Mode*: The most frequent score in a distribution
2. *Median*: The point halfway between the top and bottom halves of a distribution (50th percentile)
3. *Mean* (M): The arithmetic average of all the scores

8.5.9.1 Mode

The mode is the easiest measure of central tendency to compute and the simplest to interpret. It may be used to describe any distribution, whether the data is nominal, ordinal, interval, or ratio.

8.59.1.1 Definition

The mode is the most frequent score (raw or ungrouped data) or the midpoint of the interval containing the most scores (grouped data). In a frequency distribution graph,

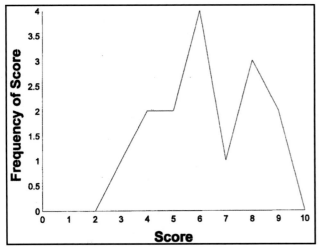

Figure 8-16. Illustration of a mode. The highest point is the mode.

Figure 8-17. Example of data where there is no mode. Note that the frequency of each score is the same.

the mode is the highest peak in the graph. Figure 8-16 illustrates the mode using the following data on a distribution of scores in which there is only one mode:

Score (X)	f	
3	1	
4	2	
5	2	
6	4	Mode=6
7	2	
8	3	
9	2	

There is no mode in a distribution of scores if all the scores occur with the same frequency (Figure 8-17). For example:

Score (X)	f
1	2
2	2
3	2
4	2

When two adjacent scores have the same frequency and this frequency is higher than any other scores in the distribution, the mode is the average of the two adjacent scores (Figure 8-18). For example:

Score (X)	f	
1	1	
2	2	
3	4	
		Mode=3.5
4	4	
5	2	
6	1	

For grouped data, it is necessary to first calculate the midpoint of each class interval before computing the mode. The mode is then the midpoint of the interval containing the most scores (Figure 8-19).

Score (X)	Midpoint	f	
10 to 12	11	2	
13 to 15	14	2	
16 to 18	17	3	
19 to 21	20	5	Mode=20
22 to 24	23	4	
25 to 27	26	2	
28 to 30	29	1	

The mode is the simplest measure of central tendency, but it has two primary limitations:

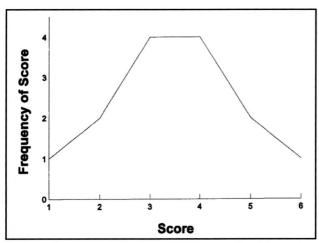

Figure 8-18. Example illustrating the mode when the data has two adjacent numbers with the same frequencies. In this case, the mode is equal to the average of the two adjacent numbers

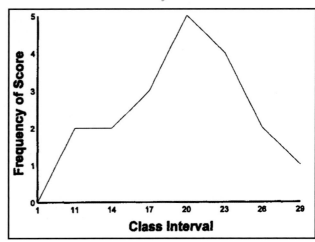

Figure 8-19. Example of a mode when grouped data are used.

1. Frequency distributions may have more than one mode, such as a bimodal or even trimodal distribution. In this case, there may be ambiguity about which mode to report, especially if the two (or more) peaks in the distribution are nearly equal. Often, one mode is reported as the *primary* or *major mode* (slightly higher peak), and the other peak reported as the *secondary* or *minor mode* (Figure 8-20).

2. When data are grouped, the mode is sensitive to the size and number of class intervals. By changing the class intervals for a distribution, the mode will change—sometimes drastically.

8.5.9.2 Median

A second and more sophisticated measure of central tendency is the median. The median is appropriate as a measure of central tendency for ordinal, interval, or ratio data but not for nominal or categorical data from which the mode is the only measure of central tendency that can be calculated.

8.5.9.2.1 Definition

The median is the 50th percentile in an ordered group of scores, that is, the point in an array of scores that has 50% of the cases below it and 50% of the cases above it. The median divides the ranked scores into halves, with one half of the scores below the median and one half of the scores above the median.

The calculation of the median is a simple procedure for raw or ungrouped data:

Step 1. When the number of cases (N) is odd, the median is the score of case (N + 1)/2 after scores are ranked (either

in ascending or descending order). For example, consider the following array of nine scores:

6, 2, 17, 5, 11, 8, 3, 13, 10

To calculate the median, the nine scores are ranked in order as follows:

Rank of Score	Score (X)	f	
1	2	1	4 scores below median
2	3	1	
3	5	1	
4	6	1	
5	8	1	Median = 8
6	10	1	4 scores above median
7	11	1	
8	13	1	
9	17	1	

Median = (score for rank N + 1)/2
= (score for rank 9 + 1) / 2
= score for rank 5.

Therefore, the median is equal to the score for rank #5, which is equal to the score of 8.

Step 2. When N is even, the median is the score midway between the scores after all scores are ranked. For example, consider the following scores (N = 8):

2, 1, 10, 7, 0, 15, 8, 5

The first step in calculating the median is again to rank order the scores.

Rank of Score	Score (X)	f	
1	0	1	3 scores below median
2	1	1	
3	2	1	
4	5	1	Median = 6 (midpoint of 5 and 7)
5	7	1	
6	8	1	3 scores above median
7	10	1	
8	15	1	

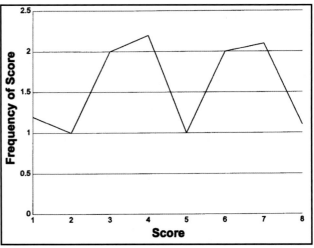

Figure 8-20. Example of scores with an ambiguous mode. The slightly higher peak is considered the primary or major mode, while the next highest peak is considered the secondary or minor mode.

For grouped data, the median is the point in a distribution at or below which exactly 50% of the cases fall. The median is calculated by constructing a cumulative frequency distribution. The median is then calculated from the cumulative frequency distribution with the following formula:

$$\text{Median} = \text{LL} + \left(w_i \left[\frac{(N/2)-cf}{f_i}\right]\right)$$

Where:
LL = lower real limit of the median interval
w_i = width of class interval
N = number of cases
cf = cumulative frequency up to the median interval
f_i = frequency within the median interval

The first stage in calculating the median is to construct a cumulative frequency distribution beginning with the lowest class interval and proceeding in ascending order to the highest class interval. The next step is to locate the interval that contains the 50th percentile or the median by examining the cumulative frequency column. For example:

CI	Real Limits	F	Cf	Cumulative Percentile	
12 to 14	11.5 to 14.5	2	2	10	
15 to 17	14.5 to 17.5	4	6	20	
18 to 20	17.5 to 20.5	3	9	45	
21 to 23	20.5 to 23.5	5	14	70	The median is in the CI in which the 50th percentile rests.
24 to 26	23.5 to 26.5	3	17	85	
27 to 29	26.5 to 29.5	2	19	95	
30 to 32	30.5 to 32.5	1	20	100	

Inspection of this cumulative frequency distribution shows that the median, or 50th percentile, must fall in the class interval of 21 to 23 because the previous interval of 18 to 20 has cumulated only 9 of the 20 total cases, that is, 45% or 45th percentile.

LL = lower real limit of median interval = 20.5

w_i = width of class interval = 3

N = total number of cases in the frequency distribution = 20

cf = cumulative frequency *up to* median interval = 9 (starting from the lowest to the highest score)

f_i = frequency within median interval = 5

Therefore:

$$\text{Median} = \text{LL} + \left(w_i \left[\frac{(N/2) - cf}{f_i} \right] \right)$$

$$= 20.5 + \left((3) \frac{[(20/2) - 9]}{5} \right)$$

$$= 20.5 + [3 (1/5)]$$

$$= 20.5 + 3 (.20)$$

$$= 20.5 + .6$$

$$= 21.1$$

This formula can be used to calculate the median for any grouped frequency distribution, as well as for ungrouped distributions (with or without tied scores).

8.5.9.2.2 Calculation of the Raw Score from the Percentile Rank

A modification of the formula allows a generalized method for calculating raw scores corresponding to a given percentile rank (PR).

$$\text{LL} + \left[(w_i) \left(\frac{\{[(PR)(N)/100] - cf\}}{f_i} \right) \right]$$

Where:

LL = lower real limit of the interval containing the given raw score, that is, (PR)(N)/100

w_i = width of the class interval

PR = percentile rank

N = number of cases in the distribution

cf = cumulative frequency up to the given class interval containing the raw score

f_i = number of cases within the class interval containing the raw score.

In the next example, what is the raw score corresponding to the 90th PR?

$$\text{Raw score } (rs) \text{ at 90th PR} = 26.5 + \left[(3) \left(\frac{\{[(90)(N)/100] - cf\}}{f_i} \right) \right]$$

Where:

LL = 26.5	Cf = 17
w_i = 3	f_i = 2
N = 20	PR = 90

$$rs = 5 + \left[(3) \left(\frac{\{[(90)(20)/100] - 17\}}{2} \right) \right]$$

$$rs = 26.5 + [(3) * \{[(1800 / 100) - 17] / 2\}]$$

$$rs = 26.5 + \{(3) * [(18 - 17) / 2]\}$$

$$rs = 26.5 + 3 (1 / 2)$$

$$rs = 26.5 + 1.5$$

Therefore, a PR of 90 corresponds to a raw score of 28.

8.5.9.2.3 Calculation of the Percentile Rank From the Raw Score

A researcher may also want to calculate the PR from the raw score. For example, given a raw score of 19 in a group distribution, what is the PR?

$$PR = \frac{[(f_i)(rs - \text{LL})] + [(w_i)(cf)]}{(N)(w_i)}$$

Where:

f_i = 3	r_s = 19
LL = 17.5	w_i = 3
cf = 6	N = 20

$$PR = \frac{[(3)(19 - 17.5)] + [(3)(6)]}{[(20)(3)]}$$

$$= \{[(3) (1.5) - 17.5)] + (18)]\}/ 60$$

$$= (4.5 + 18) / 60$$

$$= 22.5 / 60$$

$$= 37.5 \text{ PR}$$

Therefore, a raw score of 19 equals a PR of 37.5.

8.5.9.3 Mean

The mean is the most widely used and familiar index of central tendency. The mean is the arithmetic average of all the scores in a distribution and is calculated by summing all scores and dividing by the total number of scores.

The general formula for the mean ($\overline{X}$) is

$$\overline{X} = X_1 + X_2 + X_3 \ldots X_n/N$$

$$\overline{X} = \Sigma X/N$$

Where:

$\overline{X}_1$ = first raw score

$\overline{X}_2$ = second raw score

$\overline{X}_3$ = third raw score

$\overline{X}_n$ = nth raw score

Σ = summation or sum of scores

N = number of subjects in the distribution

The mean may be conceptualized as a center of gravity or balance point in which the scores, or weights, on one side exactly balance the scores or weights on the other side. Each weight represents a score from a distribution of scores. The arithmetic mean of all the scores or weights is the center of gravity or balance point. The deviation of scores in one direction exactly equals the deviation of scores in the other direction.

8.5.9.3.1 Calculating the Mean for Raw or Ungrouped Data

The mean is readily calculated for a distribution of raw scores in which each score occurs only once. The mean is simply the sum of the raw scores divided by the number of scores. For example, consider the following distribution of eight scores:

3, 6, 7, 8, 11, 15, 16, 22

$\Sigma X = 88$

$N = S$

$\overline{X} = \Sigma X / N$

$= (3 + 6 + 7 + 8 + 11 + 15 + 16 + 22)/8$

$= 88 / 8$

$= 11.0$

The mean or average value is calculated as 11.0.

For ungrouped data with a small sample of scores, the previous procedure may be used to calculate the mean. Alternatively, for grouped data, a frequency distribution should be set up. Then the mean is calculated from the frequency distribution table by multiplying each score by the frequency of occurrence and summing the total across all scores before dividing by the total number of scores.

In the following example, several scores occur more than once:

2, 3, 3, 4, 5, 5, 6, 6, 6, 7, 8, 8, 9, 9, 9

Step 1. The first stage in computing the mean is to form a frequency distribution table.

X	f	fX
2	1	2
3	2	6
4	1	4
5	2	10
6	3	18
7	1	7
8	2	16
9	3	27
		$\Sigma (fX = 90)$

The number in the third column is obtained by multiplying each raw score by the frequency of occurrence. The symbol fX represents the product of the scores multiplied by the frequency of scores. This column is then summed and divided by the total number of scores—in this example, 15 scores.

$\overline{X} = \Sigma fX/N$

So:

$\Sigma fX = 0$

$N = 15$

$= 90/15$

$= 6.0$

8.5.9.3.2 Calculating the Mean for Grouped Data

When working with grouped data, first find the midpoint of each score interval before calculating the mean.

The general formula to determine the mean for grouped data is

$\overline{X} = \Sigma fX/N$

As an example, consider the following scores grouped into six class intervals:

CI	Midpoint (X)	f	fX
3 to 5	4	2	8
6 to 8	7	1	7
9 to 11	10	4	40
12 to 14	13	6	78
15 to 17	16	3	48
18 to 20	19	4	76
		$\Sigma f = 20$	$\Sigma fX = 257$

Therefore,

$\overline{X} = 257/20$

$\overline{X} = 12.85$

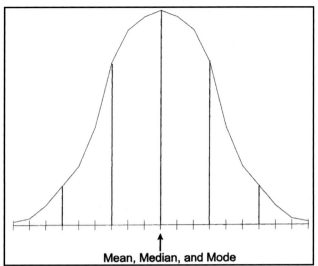

Figure 8-21. The normal unimodal curve depicting the mean, median, and mode. All three fall at the same place on a bell-shaped curve.

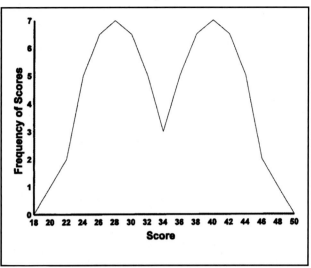

Figure 8-22. Comparison of mean, median, and mode in a bimodal distribution. The two modes have the value of 28 and 38. The median and the mean have the same value, 34.

In this example, the midpoint of each class interval (X) was multiplied by the frequency in each interval. This product was summed over all the class intervals to give a value equal to 257. This value (ΣfX) is then divided by the total number of scores or the sum of the frequencies (i.e., $\Sigma f = 20$) to yield the final calculated mean of 12.85.

The mean calculated from a grouped frequency distribution will differ slightly from the mean calculated from raw scores. When scores are grouped, information is lost and a certain amount of inaccuracy introduced. As a general rule, the coarser the grouping of scores, the more the grouped mean will differ from the raw score mean. Nonetheless, for most situations in which 10 to 20 class intervals are typically used, the agreement is close enough between the two calculated means.

8.5.9.3.3 Comparing the Mode, Median, and Mean

As a measure of central tendency, the mean takes into account all the scores of distribution and is affected by each single value. One extreme score, or outlier, can influence the mean to a large degree, especially with small samples. For example, in the following distribution of 10 scores, both the mean and median have a value of 6.0; when an extreme score of 50 is added as the 11th score, the mean dramatically increases to 10.0, while the median changes only to 7.0:

Scores: 2, 3, 4, 4, 5, 7, 8, 8, 9, 10

Mean = 6.0   Median = 6.0

The mean is changed when an extreme score of 50 is added:

Scores: 2, 3, 4, 4, 5, 7, 8, 8, 9, 10, 50

Mean = 10.0   Median = 7.0

Therefore, when extreme scores or outliers are present in a frequency distribution of scores, the median may be a more appropriate measure of central tendency than the mean.

In distributions that are symmetrical in shape, the mean equals the median, and both are equal to the mode if the distribution is unimodal. This is illustrated in Figure 8-21.

In distributions that are symmetrical but not unimodal, it is important to report the mode, mean, and median to provide a clearer picture of the shape and central tendency of the distribution. In Figure 8-22, which depicts a bimodal distribution, there are two modes (at 28 and 40) that should be noted. The mean equals the median and both equal 34.

In distributions that are skewed to the left or right, the mode, median, and mean will have different values. Note that the mean is pulled either to the right or to the left by the outliers or extreme scores on one end of the skewed distribution. The median is the preferred measure of central tendency for skewed distributions, especially when the degree of skewness increases. Figures 8-23 and 8-24 illustrate the locations of the three measures of central tendency for right- and left-skewed distributions.

8.5.10 Measures of Variability

Measures of variability are descriptive statistics that indicate how scores in a distribution differ from each other and from the mean. For example, in a distribution with the scores 7, 7, 7, 7, the measure of variability is 0 because the scores do not differ from each other and from the mean of 7. The measure of variability increases from zero as the scores vary from each other and from the mean. The *measures of variability* are the range, variance, and standard deviation.

8.5.10.1 Range

The range is the value derived from subtracting the largest score in the distribution from the smallest scores. In the distribution 21, 23, 24, 26, 28, 30, the range is 9. The range is

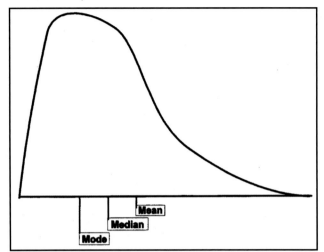

Figure 8-23. A positively skewed distribution. Notice that the figure is pulled to the left, indicating that the scores with the largest frequencies are at the lower end of the distribution.

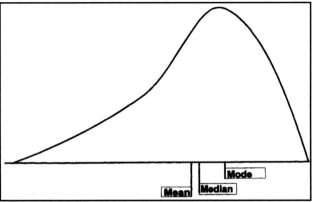

Figure 8-24. A negatively skewed distribution. The figure is pulled to the right, indicating that the scores with the largest frequencies are at the upper end of the distribution.

a crude measure of variability because only the highest and the lowest scores of a distribution are used.

8.5.10.2 Variance

The variance is a measure of the variability of scores in a distribution that takes into account all the scores in that distribution. The computational formula for the variance is:

$$s^2 = [N \Sigma X^2 - (\Sigma X)^2]/N (N-1)$$

Where:

N = total number of subjects or scores in the distribution

ΣX^2 = raw scores are squared and then the values are totaled

$(\Sigma X)^2$ = the value which equals the square of the summation of the scores.

8.5.10.2.1 Example of Calculating the Variance

Subject	Score (X)	X²
01	2	4
02	4	16
03	7	49
04	9	81
05	10	100
06	12	144
07	14	196
N = 7	$\Sigma X = 58$	$\Sigma X^2 = 590$

8.5.10.2.2 Computational Formula for the Variance

$$s^2 = [N \Sigma X^2 - (\Sigma X)^2] / [N (N-1)]$$

$$s^2 = [(7)(590) - (58)^2] / [7(7-1)]$$

$$s^2 = [4130 - 3364] / 42$$

$$s^2 = 766 / 42$$

$$s^2 = 18.238$$

8.5.10.3 Standard Deviation

The *standard deviation* is the square root of the variance. In the previous example, the variance equals 18.23. Therefore, the standard deviation equals 4.27. The standard deviation is an important value that is analogous to the mean. It is used in inferential statistics, such as the *t*-test.

8.5.11 Stem-and-Leaf Display

Stem and leaf is a method of displaying data developed by Tukey (1977) and is an alternative to the frequency distribution. It derives its name from its display: Any given number is divided into two parts, a stem and a leaf. The first part, the stem, represents a large class into which the number falls, while the second number, the leaf, designates the actual placement in the larger class. For example, the number 15 can be divided into 1 (the stem) and 5 (the leaf), while the number 216 can be divided into 2 or 21 (the stem) and 16 or 6 (the leaf). When the stem and leaves are displayed in a column, the researcher can easily visualize the organization of the data. The researcher is able to identify the specific scores obtained, as well as the frequency of the class of scores. Once the data have been organized into a stem and leaf display, a graph is drawn, allowing the researcher to visualize the structure of the data.

An example of unpublished data helps to explain the concept. Pre- and post-test data were collected to determine the change in understanding of collaboration techniques. The pre- and post-test scores, as well as the ranks for each of the scores, are reproduced in Table 8-8.

The stem-and-leaf display is as follows:

Pre-Test Scores	Pre-Test Leaf	Stem	Post-Test Leaf	Post-Test Scores
59	9	5*		
63, 62	32	6	53	65, 63
71	1	7	16	71, 76
82	2	8	724	87, 82, 84
99, 96, 92, 95	9625	9	46	94, 96
106, 108, 118, 136, 133, 140, 100	06, 08, 18, 36, 33, 40, 00	1**	02, 02, 01, 14, 48, 40	102, 102, 101, 114, 148, 140
152, 151, 192	52, 51, 92	1	59, 75, 86, 98	159, 175, 186, 198
		2	22	222

The asterisks (**) that follow the number in the stem indicate the number of digits that are included in each leaf. For example, 5* means one digit is added to the stem and 1** means two digits are added to the stem. Although commas are not necessary between the leaves, we have chosen to use them. Notice that the number of digits in the leaf can change within a single display. The use of asterisks indicates a change in digits. In this display, the pre-test leaves are displayed on the left, and the post-test leaves are displayed on the right. The stem is placed in the center with the leaves on either side. This allows the researcher to compare sets of data easily. For the reader's convenience, the pre- and post-test scores have been listed.

This system has advantages. First, the leaves do not have to be placed sequentially beside the stems. However, when the numbers are ranked later (necessary for the graph), the researcher will want to put them in sequential order. Second, not only is the researcher able to tell the shape of the data, but he or she can obtain the specific scores. This is not possible in a frequency distribution graph.

When building a stem-and-leaf display, the number of stems is only limited by the data. The researcher does not want to use so many stems that the data are too spread out or too few lines so that the data are too crowded. Trial and error may be necessary to determine the appropriate number of stems. In general, the last digit of a given number becomes the leaf, whereas the first digit(s) will be used as the stem. Sometimes, when there are too many leaves on one stem, the stem may be split into parts. By splitting the stem, the leaves may be divided. An example of a split stem can be seen by the repetition of the digit 1.

Once a stem and leaf display has been produced, the researcher needs to make a graph. The graph is called a *box-and-whisker plot* because of the way in which it is drawn. The graph consists of a box that has lines (the whiskers) connected to either side. A box-and-whisker plot uses the ranks of median or middle score, the ranks of the extremes, and the ranks of the hinges. An examination of Table 8-8 shows the median for the pre-test to be 100 (rank of 10) and the median of the post-test to be 101.5 (rank of 10.5). The extremes are the ranks of the highest and lowest scores. The pre-test extremes are 59 and 192, ranked at 1 and 19. The post-test extremes are 63 and 222, ranked at 1 and 20. The hinges or quartile ranks lie halfway between the median and the extremes. They are obtained by the following formula:

Lower hinge = ½ (lower extreme + median)
Upper hinge = ½ (upper extreme + median)

When the rank of a median is not a whole number, drop the decimal (e.g., 10.5 becomes 10). The upper and lower hinges become the upper and lower limits of the box. The whisker is a line that connects the hinges to the extremes. An example of this is seen in Figure 8-25. An examination of the two box plots in this figure reveals that there is little difference between the two scores. Although the upper extreme and the upper hinge is higher on the post-test, the medians, lower extreme, and lower hinge are similar. There is more variability on the post-test.

TABLE 8-8

HYPOTHETICAL PRE-TEST AND POST-TEST SCORES

	PRE-TEST		POST-TEST	
Subject	Score	Rank	Score	Rank
1	28	18	37	18
2	16	2	35	16
3	18	4	28	8
4	20	9	19	2
5	24	13	25	5
6	23	11	28	9
7	25	15	22	3
8	19	6	31	12
9	23	12	33	13
10	29	20	38	20
11	15	1	34	14
12	19	7	29	10
13	19	8	18	1
14	25	16	26	6
15	22	10	27	7
16	26	17	23	4
17	18	5	30	11
18	24	14	34	15
19	28	19	37	19
20	16	3	35	17

Figure 8-25. An example of a box-and-whisker plot using the data from Table 8-8.

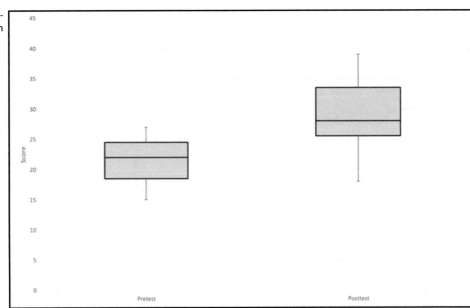

8.5.11.1 Construction of a Stem-and-Leaf Display and Box Plot

Step 1. Make a stem-and-leaf display. The following scores have been collected from post-tests. Because the scores are between 72 and 97, both the stem and leaf will consist of a single digit. Because of the number of scores that fall between 80 and 89, the stem will be divided into two.

Scores: 88, 82, 75, 93, 96, 81, 83, 82, 97, 96, 87, 88, 72, 75, 95, 82, 80, 87, 89, 88

Stem	Leaf	Cumulative Rank	Scores Repeated	# of Leaves
7*	525	3	75, 72, 75	3
8	213220	9	82, 81, 83, 82, 82, 80	6
8	878798	15	88, 87, 88, 87, 89, 88	6
9	36765	20	93, 96, 97, 96, 95	5

*The asterisk is placed after the 7 to denote that only one digit is used in the leaf.

Step 2. Find the median score. Because there are 20 scores, the median rank will be 10.5. The score that falls at this rank is 87.

Step 3. Find the extremes. The extremes are the ranks of the highest and lowest scores or, in this case, those scores with a rank of 1 and 20. The scores for rank 1 and rank 20 are 72 and 97, respectively.

Step 4. Calculate the hinges. The hinges or quartile ranks lie halfway between the median and the extremes. They are obtained by adding the rank of the extremes to the rank of the median and dividing by 2. When the median rank has a decimal, drop the decimal.

Lower hinge = (1 + 10)/2 = 11/2 = 5.5. The rank for the lower hinge is at 5.5. The score that would fall at this rank is 81.5, obtained by finding the halfway point between the scores that rank at 5 and 6, respectively (e.g., 81, 82).

Upper hinge = (20 + 10)/2 = 15. The score at this rank is 89.

Step 5. Draw a box using the lower and upper hinges as the outer limits of the box and connect the extremes to the box with a solid line. Notice that the box can be drawn horizontally or vertically.

An examination of this box plot suggests that the scores are negatively skewed; that is, more scores are at the upper end of the distribution than the lower end.

8.5.12 z-Scores and the Normal Curve

The *z*-scores are summary values that indicate the distance between a raw score and the mean, using standard deviation units. For example, a *z*-score of 0 is equal to the mean. The *z*-scores are important to describe the relative standing of a raw score. For example, a raw score of 40 is equal to a *z*-score of +1 in a normal distribution with a mean equal to 30 and one standard deviation equal to 10. Figure 8-26 illustrates the *z*-score for a raw score of 40.

In this example, a raw score of 40 is equal to a PR of 84, which means that an individual with a *z*-score of +1 did better than, or is above, 84% of the individuals in that distribution.

The formula for calculating *z*-scores is:

z = (raw score - mean)/standard deviation or $z = (r_s - \overline{X})/s$

In the previous example:

$z = [40 - 30]/10$

$z = 10/10$

$z = +1$

The *z*-scores can be positive or negative depending on whether the raw score is above or below the mean. These scores are widely used in psychometric testing and are helpful in interpreting raw scores.

8.5.12.1 Normality and the Normal (Gaussian) Curve

For the occupational therapist, one of the most difficult decisions is to decide whether a physiological or psychological function is within normal limits. What is normal blood pressure, heart rate, muscle strength, height, visual-perceptual function, or intelligence? Is normality a function of personality or behavior or is it a statistical value?

When an individual goes to a physician for a physical examination, the physiological and neurological functions are tested to determine whether they are within normal limits. Predetermined values are used by the physician to compare with the patient's results. Individual differences within a range of normality are accepted by the physician to determine whether a function is abnormal. The same judgments are made by the occupational therapist in testing ROM in a specific joint or evaluating muscle strength.

On the other hand, the statistician's definition of normality and abnormality will depend on the frequency of occurrences within designated class intervals. Abnormality is interpreted by the statistician as a variance from the mean value, such as 1 or 2 standard deviation units from the mean of a normally distributed variable. In research, scores or values that are abnormal are outliers, or scores that vary widely from expected values. Often, those outliers or abnormal scores are considered at variance with the test of values in a distribution. Consider the scatter diagram in Figure 8-27. Four of the five scores are consistent with a positive relationship with the X and Y variables. However, one coordinate (50, 5) seems to be an outlier and does not

Figure 8-26. Normal curve depicting raw score of 40, mean of 30, and standard deviation of 10. Notice that a raw score of 40 lies one standard deviation above the mean (e.g., *z*-score of + 1) and at a percentile of 84.

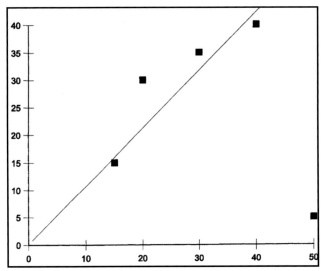

Figure 8-27. Scattergram showing an outlier at the coordinates of 50, 5. The outlier is the score that appears to be significantly different from the other scores.

fit into the pattern. The outlier or abnormal score should be discussed separately by the researcher.

The normal curve (see Figure 8-26) is the statistician's guide for examining the relationship between normal values and outliers. In the normal curve, it is expected that 68% of the cases will lie within -1 to +1 standard deviation units and 96% of the cases will lie within -2 to +2 standard deviations units. If we know that a characteristic is normally distributed, then we will be able to determine how many of the cases will be within -2 to +2 standard deviation units from the mean by calculating the mean and standard deviation of a population. For example, if we know that the resting heart rate is normally distributed and that the mean value for adults is 72 beats/minute with a standard deviation of 5, then we can determine the PR from the raw scores. For example, what is the PR of an individual with a resting heart rate score of 78?

The normal curve in Figure 8-28 shows the relationship between the raw score of 78 and the normal values for resting heart rate. We estimate that, based on the diagram, the PR for a raw score of 78 will be slightly above the 84th PR.

8.5.12.1.1 Calculation of Percentile Rank

First calculate *z*-scores from raw scores:

$z = (r_s - \overline{X})/s_z$
$= (78 - 72)/5_z$
$= 6/5 = 1.2$
$z = 1.2$

Look up the PR from the statistical table (see Table C-2) for the *z*-score of 1.2. Note that in Table C-2 in Appendix C, a *z*-score of 1.2 is equal to the PR of .8849.

8.5.13 Vital Statistics

The quality of a health care system in a country is usually described by vital statistics, such as the infant mortality rate, rates of illnesses and diseases, life expectancy, and mortality rates from specific diseases. In justifying the need for a research study in a clinical area, the researcher first reports the incidence and prevalence rates of a disability or illness to establish the significance of the study. What are some of the most common vital statistics?

8.5.13.1 Crude Mortality (Death) or Morbidity (Disease) Rates

The crude mortality or morbidity rate is calculated by dividing the frequency of deaths or illnesses by the total number of individuals in the population. This number is then multiplied by 1000, 10,000, or 100,000 so it can be used as a comparative figure. For example, if a certain population has a mortality rate of 9.3/1000 population per year, how does this compare with another population where there are 180,000 deaths in a population of 24,000,000?

8.5.13.1.1 Calculation of Crude Mortality Rate

Crude death rate = (180,000/24,000,000) (1000)
            = .0075 × 1000
            = 7.5 per 1000 population

In this hypothetical case, the investigator would conclude that there is a lesser mortality rate in the sample of 180,000 deaths/24,000,000 population than in the 9.3/1000 population.

8.5.13.2 Prevalence and Incidence Rates of Disability or Disease

The terms *prevalence rate* and *incidence rate* are often confused with each other. Prevalence rate refers to the number or proportion of a population who have a given condition. Incidence rate is the number of new cases of a condition within a given time period.

In 2012, the estimated population in the United States was about 313,000,000. In that same year, there were an estimated 1,218,400 people in the United States living with HIV infection (Centers for Disease Control and Prevention, 2014). In the same year, the estimated incidence for new cases of HIV infection was approximately 48,000 (Center for Disease Control and Prevention, 2014).

8.5.13.2.1 Calculation of Prevalence and Incidence Rates

Incidence rate = (48,000/313,000,000) (100,000)

       = .000153 (100,000)

       = 15.3 per 100,000 population

Prevalence rate = (1,218,400/313,000,000) (100,000)

       = .0038 (100,000)

       = 380 per 100,000 population

8.5.13.3 Adjusted Rate

Researchers are also interested in obtaining statistics for specific populations. In these examples, the calculation of rates are adjusted. For example, an investigator is interested in comparing infant mortality rates adjusted for gender. In a hypothetical population, there are 40,000 births of males and 35,000 births of females. In this population, 150 males and 180 females die at birth. What are the adjusted infant mortality rates for females compared with the total crude rates per 1000 population?

8.5.13.3.1 Calculation of Crude Rate

Crude rate = [(150 + 180)/(40,000 + 35,000)] [1000]

       = (330/75,000) (1000)

       = (.0044) (1000)

       = 4.4 per 1000 (for both males and females)

8.5.13.3.2 Adjusted Rate for Females

Adjusted rate = (180/35,000) (1000)

       = (.0051) (1000)

       = 5.14 per 1000

For this hypothetical example, it appears that the infant mortality rate is higher in females compared with the total population.

8.6 INFERENTIAL STATISTICS AND TESTING A HYPOTHESIS

8.6.1 Probability and Clinical Research

When an investigator predicts a statistically significant relationship between two variables, it is assumed that the relationship will not exist by chance alone. In other words, the researcher is predicting that X factor is related to Y

Figure 8-28. Normal curve depicting the relationship between the heart beat rate of 78 when the mean is 72 and the standard deviation is 5. What is the z-score of this heartbeat? Is it above or below normal?

factor, or that the independent variable, whether manipulated or not, is related to the dependent variable. In clinical research, however, it is difficult to control for all possible factors that could affect the dependent variable. For example, if a researcher discovers through a thorough search of the literature that arthritis is a psychophysiological disorder, then a set of research investigations would be generated based on this assumption. In a retrospective correlational study, the researcher could select a group of patients with arthritis and investigate personality relationships and the incidence of arthritis. If a statistically significant relationship is found between the incidence of arthritis and personality relationships, it will be beyond a certain probability level but will not necessarily be a one-to-one relationship. This means that not all individuals with a certain described characteristic are arthritic. This leads us to the question, why do we accept a partial relationship rather than a 100% probability in clinical research? Several factors in clinical research impinge on statistically significant results that prevent the perfect 100% probability relationships. They are:

- Complex interrelationships among variables in which more than one factor contributes to a disability that can affect results in clinical research. For example, in arthritis a multifactorial etiology is assumed. In clinical research, however, we may be able to identify only some portion of the variance associated with the onset of arthritis.

- Diseases in which genetics, age, diet, and numerous other factors influence the course of a disorder can affect research results. There may be individual factors occurring in the individual that are difficult to identify in clinical research during a study.

- The problem of accurately formulating a diagnosis in chronic disabilities such as arthritis, diabetes mellitus, multiple sclerosis, cardiovascular disease, schizophrenia, or ulcerative colitis may affect the results in clinical research. Moreover, the sample may not be a homogeneous group, which could contaminate results.
- The error variance existing in all clinical research, such as measurement of variables, control of experimental conditions, uniformity of subjects, and data collection procedures, that could affect results.

In short, all statistical analyses using hypothesis testing are based on probability. When inferential statistics are applied in a clinical research study, the investigator bases results and conclusions on the probability that any differences between the experimental and control groups are either attributable to chance or are statistically significantly different.

8.6.2 Procedure for Statistically Testing a Hypothesis

Step 1. State the hypothesis. A null hypothesis is stated unless the researcher is replicating a previous study or has research evidence to support a directional hypothesis.

1. Null hypothesis is $\mu1 = \mu2$ or $r = 0$. *Stated in clinical research study*: There is no statistically significant difference between means or no significantly statistical relationship between variables.
2. Non-directional hypothesis is $\mu1 \neq \mu2$ or $r \neq 0$.
3. Directional hypothesis is $\mu1 > \mu2$, or r is statistically significantly > 0, or statistically significantly < 0.

Step 2. Select a level of significance. The researcher usually selects the .05 level of significance in the social sciences. This means that the researcher accepts an error level of 5%. The researcher can also state that at $\alpha = .05$, there is a 95% confidence level that results are not due to chance.

Step 3. Apply inferential statistics and select a procedure or a parametric or nonparametric statistical test based on the assumptions underlying the test, such as randomness, normal distribution of data, and homogeneity of variance.

Step 4. Obtain the critical value from the appropriate table for statistical tests based on whether it is a one- or two-tailed test, the level of statistical significance, and the *df.*

Step 5. Calculate the value of test statistics, such as f-observed, *F*-observed, chi-square or correlation coefficient through a mathematical formula.

Step 6. Accept or reject the research hypothesis (null or directional).

8.6.3 Potential Sources of Research Errors Affecting Statistical Significance

One important aspect of clinical research is to reduce the possible errors in an experiment that could impact on the results. These errors include:

- *Hawthorne effect*: Attention given to subjects may increase positive outcomes and camouflage the true effects of the independent variable or treatment method. When a Hawthorne effect is present, the subjects' improvement is caused by the attention received from the researcher rather than the direct result of the treatment intervention.
- *Placebo effect*: The suggestion that subjects receiving a treatment, such as medication or a procedure, may produce positive expectations that the treatment will be effective. The subjects may will themselves to improvement. The placebo produces in the subject a desire for improvement. There is some evidence that a psychophysiological effect occurs from the placebo effect.
- *Honeymoon effect*: A short-term effect of a new treatment procedure that subjects hope will impact on a disease. The initial enthusiasm disguises the true effects of the treatment procedure.
- *Researcher bias*: The researcher carrying out a clinical treatment program affects the results through his or her enthusiasm and desire for the treatment to be effective. The researcher's knowledge of the study may affect its outcome.
- *Test administrator bias*: The individual testing the outcome of treatment method is aware of which subjects are in the experimental group and which are in the control group.
- *Sampling errors*: If the researcher's results are based on a sample from a population that is not representative, the results will be skewed or biased to the research sample selected.
- *Systematic variance*: The researcher fails to control for extraneous variables that could possibly affect the results, such as age, gender, intelligence, education, socioeconomic status, or degree of disability.
- *Error variance*: The researcher overlooks or minimizes the effects of anxiety, lack of motivation, inattention, distractive environments, and other unexpected problems in the test environment.

8.6.3.1 Type I and Type II Errors

All of the previously discussed factors and other sources of error in an experiment can potentially affect the results of research. The errors in testing a hypothesis are identified as either a *Type I* or *Type II* error, and result from the researcher accepting or rejecting a hypothesis based on the statistical results. The probability of a Type I error in hypothesis testing is typically accepted at the .05 or .01 level. The researcher has confidence that the results are not attributable to chance 95% or 99% of the time. Nonetheless, it is possible that the results are false in 5/100 tries or 1/100 tries purely based on chance errors. Table 8-9 summarizes the relationship between decision errors and hypothesis testing.

TABLE 8-9

TESTING THE NULL HYPOTHESIS, DECISION ERRORS, AND CLINICAL ANALOGY IN MEDICINE

Null hypothesis H_0 predicts that there is no statistically significant difference between means (1 = 2) or no statistically significant relationship between variables ($r = 0$).

DECISION BY RESEARCHER	TRUE SITUATION	ANALOGY IN MEDICINE
1. Reject Null Hypothesis: • $\mu_1 \neq \mu_2 \neq \mu_3 \neq \mu_4 \ldots$ • $r \neq 0$	**Type I Error (a):** Researcher rejects the null hypothesis when it should be accepted. There is no significant difference between means or significant relationship between variables. • $\mu_1 = \mu_2$ • $r = 0$ Researcher should accept the null hypothesis	**False Positive:** Clinician falsely detects the presence of disease or condition when in reality no disease exists. For example, falsely diagnosing breast cancer through mammography screening when breast cancer is not present.
2. Reject Null Hypothesis: • $\mu_1 \neq \mu_2 \neq \mu_3 \neq \mu_4 \ldots$ • $r \neq 0$	**No Error:** Researcher rejects null hypothesis and concludes that there is a statistically significant difference between the means or that $r > 0$.	**Correct Diagnosis:** Clinician correctly detects presence of disease and concludes a correct positive diagnosis of a pathological condition.
3. Accept Null Hypothesis: • $\mu_1 = \mu_2 = \mu_3 = \mu_4 \ldots$ • $r = 0$	**Type II Error (β):** Researcher accepts null hypothesis when it should be rejected. There is a significant difference between means or a significant relationship between variables. • $\mu_1 \neq \mu_2$ • $r \neq 0$ Researcher should reject null hypothesis.	**False Negative:** Clinician falsely concludes that based on test results, no disease is present when a disease exists.
4. Accept Null Hypothesis: • $\mu_1 = \mu_2 = \mu_3 = \mu_4 \ldots$ • $r = 0$	**No Error:** Researcher accepts null hypothesis.	**Correct Diagnosis:** Clinician correctly concludes that no disease is present.

The concept in medicine of a false positive or false negative is analogous to describing a Type I or Type II error. A false positive in medicine occurs when a disease is falsely detected, whereas a false negative exists when a disease is overlooked or not detected. Errors in clinical medicine can occur because of human error due to mistaken judgments in interpreting results, the unreliability of the test equipment or procedure, or unexplained or temporary variables in the patient's condition that can lead to a false diagnosis. Often, clinicians will use more than one test, as well as repeat tests, to confirm or validate a diagnosis. Researchers, on the other hand, try to reduce Type I and Type II errors by replicating experiments with representative samples from different geographical areas.

In summary:

- A Type I error is when a hypothesis is accepted when it should be rejected.

- A Type II error is when a hypothesis is rejected when it should be accepted.

8.6.4 Exploratory Data Analysis

Tukey (1977) stated, "It is important to understand what you CAN do before you learn to measure how WELL you seem to have done it" (p. v). In clinical research, the question that is usually raised is, how effective is a treatment procedure? For example, are sensory integration techniques more effective than neurodevelopment treatment? The researcher must determine at what level of significance the hypothesis would be accepted. If the researcher is using a standardized test, such as the Sensory Integration and Praxis Tests (Ayres, 1989), then a definition of significance should be decided in advance. Guidelines for the degree of differences between the mean at post-test after intervention should be established. For example, one standard deviation above the mean will show significance. If Group 1 had a mean of 100 and Group 2 had a mean of 85, on a test in which one standard deviation equaled 15, significance has been demonstrated before a *t*-test or ANOVA was been applied to the data. This exploratory data analysis is a method of eyeballing the data before applying a statistical test to the results. Exploratory data analysis involves the following:

- Calculating group means and standard deviations to determine if the results are clinically significant
- Screening results by collapsing data in nominal categories and performing a chi-square test
- Describing results in scatter diagrams showing the relationship between variables
- Using stem-and leaf-displays and box plots to tally the frequency count within designated categories

For a more detailed account of exploratory data analysis, see Hoaglin, Mosteller, and Tukey (1991) and Tukey (1977).

8.6.5 The Concept of Statistical Power and Effect Size

Statistical power is the ability of a statistical test to accurately reject the null hypothesis and to detect a difference between groups when one exists. Statistical power is related to the occurrence of a Type II error when the researcher finds that there is no statistically significant difference between the groups when, in reality, there is a significant difference. It is affected by the size of the sample, the probability level of significance, such as .05 or .01, and the magnitude of the relationship between the variables measured. When large samples are used in a clinical study, any statistical analysis will be powerful. For example, a sample of 100 subjects in a clinical study will be more powerful than a sample of 25 subjects. The researcher will have more confidence in rejecting the null hypothesis with a larger number of subjects than with small-size samples. However, statistical significance at a .05 level with large numbers of subjects may or may not demonstrate clinical significance. The power of a test, indicating the ability to reject the null hypothesis, also increases when the researcher is willing to accept a higher probability of error (e.g., .05 level has more power than the .01 level). What this means is that the researcher is willing to accept more error in interpreting the statistical results. Some researchers recommend a power level of .80 (Ottenbacher & Barrett, 1990). Nonetheless, a major question for a clinical researcher still remains: Is this treatment method effective? Statistical power should not be manipulated to camouflage clinical

results. Clinical research study results should be analyzed to determine if the treatment method is promising, if it is effective with specific patients, and if it can be refined to improve its effectiveness. Statistical confidence should not be compromised to justify the use of treatment methods when they have not demonstrated effectiveness.

Additional concepts associated with determining sample size include the respective means of the dependent variable in each condition as well as their respective variance. There is a formula that takes all of these concepts into account that is called *Lehr's Equation* (Lehr, 1992). For example:

$$ n = \frac{16}{(\frac{\mu_0 - \mu_1}{\sigma})^2} $$

Where

n = number of participants in each condition
μ_0 = the mean of the first condition
μ_1 = the mean of the second condition
σ = the homogenous variance of the means.

The number 16 is a constant and is part of Lehr's Equation. This equation assumes α is set at .05 and β is set at .2.

To use this equation, it is necessary to have access to some data. This can occur through pilot testing where a researcher can obtain some preliminary data, or it could come from other studies that have investigated similar dependent and in dependent variables. As an example, consider a similar study investigating the efficacy of two types of splints (a hard splint and a soft splint) upon the ability to grasp clothes pins. Say the mean of the hard splint groups was 11 and the mean of the soft splint group was 17. The homogenized variance between the two means is 8. Lehr's equation would give the following:

$$ n = \frac{16}{\left(\frac{11 - 17}{8}\right)^2} $$

Therefore

n = 28.44

According to this formula, the research would need to recruit 29 participants for each condition (i.e., 58 for the entire study).

8.6.5.1 Effect Size

In clinical research, the effect size is presented by researchers to demonstrate the difference between treatment methods and their impact on improvement. For example, if a researcher is comparing the effectiveness of two types of hand exercise programs to increase grip strength, the researcher should apply an independent *t*-test to evaluate statistical significance. The researcher also may be interested in looking at the clinical impact of the two treatment techniques. Effect size is an important concept that reflects both the variance between the groups and the variance within the groups.

The formula for effect size is

Effect Size $= (\mu_0 - \mu_{01})/s$

where s is the pooled standard deviation of both groups.

The effect size is zero when the null hypothesis is true (Cohen, 1988). The effect size also serves as an index of the degree of departure from the null hypothesis. For example, a relatively large effect size can be interpreted to mean that the study has high statistical power in accurately rejecting the null hypothesis. Most researchers have defined small, medium, and large effect sizes. Small effect sizes are about .2, medium effect sizes are about .5, and large effect sizes are about .8 (Cohen, 1988).

8.7 MODEL II: ONE-SAMPLE PROBLEMS (ONE-SAMPLE *T*-TEST)

One-sample *t*-tests are applied to research studies in which the investigator is testing whether a sample mean is equal to, less than, or greater than a given value. An example from environmental science is the sampling of air or water to determine if the air or water is polluted. Scientists concerned with the quality of air and water use one-sample *t*-tests to compare samples with parameter values. These parameter values are health standards that have been predetermined by scientific evidence to be at acceptable health levels. At which point is the air considered to be polluted? What are the accepted levels of bacteria for water consumption? These are problems for one-sample *t*-tests. We can also use one-sample *t*-tests for screening populations. For example, is a group sample above or below normal values in height, weight, cholesterol level, blood pressure, heart rate, and hearing acuity? The procedure for applying a one-sample *t*-test is to compare the sample mean with a hypothetical parameter value.

8.7.1 Hypothetical Example for Testing for Statistically Significant Differences Between Sample Mean and Parameter Mean Values

Step 1. State the research hypothesis.

1. *Null Hypothesis*: There is no statistically significant difference between the height (μ) of adult Japanese American men and the standard height (μ_0) of all adult American men.

$\mu = \mu_0$ (mu, parameter mean value)

$N = 10,000$

2. *Alternative Hypothesis*: There is a statistically significant difference between the height (μ) of adult Japanese-American men and the height (μ_0) of all adult American men.

$\mu \neq \mu_0$ (mu, parameter mean value)

Step 2. Select the level of statistical significance: $\alpha = .05$

Step 3. Select test statistics. Use *t*-test.

The formula for a *t*-test is

(Note: *s* divided by square root of N)

Step 4. Identify the t_{crit} from the *t* distribution table.

  a. significance level: $\alpha = .05$

  b. two-tailed test of significance

  c. $df = N - 1 = 10,000 - 1 = 9999$

    $t_{crit} = .196$

(For t_{crit}: Because $df = 9999$, which is larger than 120, t_{ctit} may be obtained from Appendix C, Table C-2 Normal Curve)

Step 5. Calculate the test statistic value. From a random sample of 10,000 adult Japanese-American men living in the United States, the following data were collected. An $\overline{X}$ is used rather than a μ because only a sample of the total number is used. In this case, the $\overline{X}$ is a value obtained from a representative sample of the population (μ).

$\overline{X} = 64$ in.

standard deviation (s) $= 1.8$ in.

Step 6. Identify parameter values. The parameter values (i.e., hypothetical values set to explain concepts) for the average adult American men are:

$\mu_0 = 69$ in.

$s = 1.9$ in.

In this case, μ is used because the total population is being considered.

Step 7. Graph normal curve for parameter value. Because the parameter values are a constant, we can use the normal curve to describe the distribution of parameter values. This is shown in Figure 8-29. For a normal distribution with a mean of 69 and a standard deviation of 1.9, we will expect 68% of adult American men to have heights between 67.1 and 70.9 inches.

Step 8. Graph normal curve for sample. This is shown in Figure 8-30. For the sample distribution with a mean of 64 and a standard deviation of 1.8, we will expect 68% of the adult Japanese-American men to have heights between 62.2 and 65.8 inches.

Step 9. Calculate the t_{obs} using the formula for *t*-test (see Step 3).

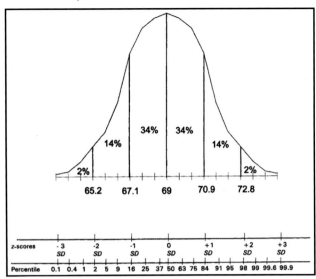

Figure 8-29. Hypothetical data for typical adult American men depicting a normal distribution in which the mean height is 69 inches and the standard deviation is 1.9. Sixty-eight percent of the adult population should fall between +1 and -1 standard deviation, or heights of 67.1 and 70.9 inches.

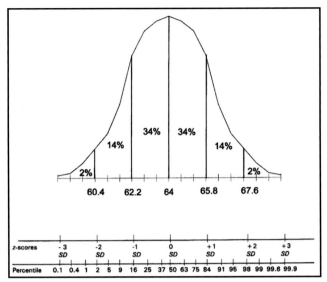

Figure 8-30. Hypothetical data for a sample of 10,000 adult Japanese-American men depicting a normal distribution in which the mean height is 64 inches and the standard deviation is 1.8. Sixty-eight percent of the adult population should fall between +1 and -1 standard deviations, or heights of 62.2 and 65.8 inches.

$$t = \frac{\overline{X} - \mu_o}{s / \sqrt{N}}$$

Where
$\overline{X}$ = sample mean = 64
s = sample standard deviation = 1.8
μ_0 = parameter mean = 69
N = sample number of subjects = 10,000

$$t = (64 - 69) / 1.8\sqrt{10,000}$$

$$= (-5)/(1.8/100)$$
$$t_{obs} = -5/.018$$
$$t_{obs} = -277.77$$

Step 10. Compare t_{obs} with t_{crit}

$t_{obs} = -277.77$

$t_{crit} = 1.960$

$t_{obs} > t_{crit}$

Thus, the researcher rejects the null hypothesis and concludes that there is a statistically significant difference between the height of adult Japanese-American men compared with the average heights of all adult American men.

8.8 MODEL III: TWO INDEPENDENT GROUPS

8.8.1 Independent t-Test

The purpose of this statistical model is to test whether there is a statistically significant difference between the means of two independent samples. This frequently is used to test the differences between two clinical techniques applied to an experimental group and a control or comparative group. For example, if a researcher is examining the comparative effectiveness of two treatment techniques in two independent groups, such as progressive relaxation exercise vs. transcutaneous electrical nerve stimulation in reducing pain, then an independent *t*-test will be applied to the outcome measure for pain (dependent variable). The *t*-test is also applied when the researcher examines whether there is a statistically significant difference in the characteristic abilities of two groups. In the example that follows from Sin and Lee (2013), the authors compared performances of a group of stroke survivors who were randomly assigned to an experimental or a control group. The experimental group was enrolled in a virtual reality Xbox Kinect

TABLE 8-10				
COMPARISON OF PERFORMANCE ON PERCEPTUAL SPATIAL ORIENTATION TASKS				
SKILL	MAXIMUM SCORE	SDAT GROUP *(n = 15)* M (SD)	CONTROL GROUP *(n = 15)* M (SD)	P^*
Figure-ground perception (total)	48	26.33 (6.61)	36.47 (4.63)	≤.0001
Figure-ground perception (Part 1)	24	16.00 (3.59)	20.53 (1.19)	<.0002
Figure-ground perception (Part 2)	24	10.33 (4.15)	15.93 (3.90)	≤.001
Shape (visual)	10	9.67 (0.82)	10.00 (0.00)	ns
Shape (tactual)	10	6.13(2.26)	8.93 (1.34)	≤.0005
Size (visual)	6	6.00 (0.00)	6.00 (0.00)	ns
Size (tactual)	15	14.33 (1.23)	14.87 (0.35)	ns
Position in space (total)	16	11.93 (4.01)	15.33 (0.82)	≤.004
Position in space (Part 1)	8	7.20(1.42)	7.93 (0.26)	≤.06
Position in space (Part 2)	8	4.73 (2.92)	7.4 (0.74)	≤.002
Spatial relations	15	1 1.47 (2.67)	14.73 (0.59)	≤.0002
Left-right discrimination	10	9.67 (0.72)	10.00 (0.00)	ns

ns = not significant; SDAT = senile dementia of the Alzheimer type.

*Two-tailed *t*-test for independent samples.

Reprinted with permission from Liu, L., Gauthier, L., & Gauthier, S. (1991). Spatial disorientation in persons with early senile dementia of the Alzheimer type. *American Journal of Occupational Therapy, 45*(1), 67-74.

(Microsoft) training regime whereas the control group was enrolled in a traditional occupational therapy regime. The outcome variables (i.e., dependent variables) included upper extremity ROM, the Fugl-Meyer Assessment, and the Box and Block Test. The independent *t*-test analysis compared the amount of change observed in each group for each of the outcome variables. Table 8-10 contains the outcome means for these variables.

Of the 12 variables tested, only 4 did not reach statistical significance at the $P < .05$ level. The researchers used a two-tailed test for determining the critical level of significance with a total of 30 subjects (15 in each group), at a *df* of n - 2. In a two-tailed test with 28 *df*, the critical value of *t* is 2.0484 (see Table C-3 in Appendix C). The observed *t* was above 2.0484 in 8/12 variables tested. The *t* values reflected the differences between the group means and the comparative homogeneity of the two independent sample standard deviations. In general, a *t* value is statistically significant when there is a relatively large difference between the group mean and a small difference within the groups. On the other hand, if the differences within the groups are larger than the differences between the groups, then there will likely not be a statistically significant difference between the groups as reflected in the observed *t* value. For example, in examining the first variable, figure-ground perception (total), the SDAT group mean was 26.33 and the control group mean was 36.47. The mean difference between the groups was 10.14. The standard deviations of 6.61 and 4.63 were comparatively homogeneous. Thus, there was a statistically significant difference between the two independent groups. In examining the variable shape (visual), note that the differences between the group means is .33 (10.00 - 9.67), while the standard deviation for the SDAT group is .82, thus indicating no statistically significant difference between the two independent group means.

8.8.1.1 Operational Procedure for Testing for Statistically Significant Differences Between Two Independent Samples

Step 1. State the research hypothesis.

a. *Null Hypothesis:* There is no statistically significant difference between the mean of Group 1 vs. the mean of Group 2:

H_0: $\mu_1 = \mu_2$

b. *Directional Hypothesis:* Mean one is significantly statistically different from mean two in a stated direction:

$\mu_1 > \mu_2$

c. *Alternative Hypothesis:* Mean one does not equal mean two, and there is a statistically significant difference between the two means (nondirectional):

H_1: $\mu_1 \neq \mu_2$

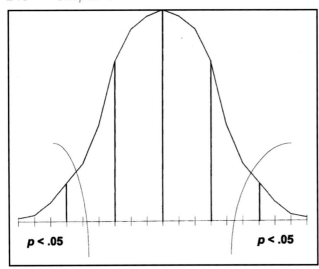

Figure 8-31. Model for a two-tailed test. A one-tailed test would use only one of the two marked areas.

Figure 8-32. Graph to visualize values of scores to estimate possible statistical significance between the group means.

$$t_{obs} = \frac{\overline{X_1} - \overline{X_2}}{\sqrt{\{[(n_1 - 1)(s_1^2) + (n_2 - 1)(s_2^2)] / (n_1 + n_2 - 2)\}[(1/n_1) + (1/n_2)]}}$$

Step 2. Select the level of statistical significance. In social sciences research, the .05 level of significance is traditionally selected.

Step 3. Select the statistical test. Use independent *t*-test.

Step 4. Decide whether to use a one- or two-tailed test for statistical significance. A two-tailed test is used with a null hypothesis to determine if there are statistically significant differences in either direction of the tail. The model for a two-tailed test are the tails in a normal curve (Figure 8-31). A one-tailed test is used with a directional hypothesis when the researcher predicts that the experimental group mean will be either statistically greater or lesser than a comparison mean.

Step 5. Look up the critical value (t_{crit}) from the published statistical table. The critical value is determined by:
a. The *df*
b. The level of significance ($\alpha < .05$ or $< .01$)
c. The direction of the test (one-tailed or two-tailed)
d. The value of t_{crit} as indicated in the statistical table (see Table C-3 in Appendix C).

Step 6. Calculate the group means and standard deviations.

Step 7. Do an exploratory data analysis to determine if the differences between the two means are clinically significant and that the standard deviations in both groups are approximately equal.

Step 8. Plot a graph. Use the graph mean and raw scores of Groups 1 and 2 to visualize whether there seems to be a statistically significant difference between the group means (Figure 8-32). If there appears to be a difference between the two group means, then go to Step 8 and calculate the values.

Step 9. Calculate the t_{obs} using the formula.

The formula for t_{obs} is:

Where
$\overline{X}_1$ = mean value of Group 1
$\overline{X}_2$ = mean value of Group 2
n_1 = total number of cases in Group 1
n_2 = total number of cases in Group 2
s_1^2 = variance (the standard deviation squared) for Group 1
s_2^2 = variance for Group 2

Step 10. Compare the two values: t_{obs} and t_{crit}.
a. Accept the null hypothesis if t_{obs} is less than t_{crit}
b. Reject the null hypothesis if t_{obs} is equal to or greater than t_{crit}
c. Accept the directional hypothesis if t_{obs} is greater than or equal to t_{crit} in the direction that is hypothesized
d. Reject the directional hypothesis if t_{obs} is less than t_{crit} or if the mean value that is predicted to be greater is less than the mean value of the control or comparative group. For example, a researcher predicts that cognitive training is more effective than behavioral therapy in increasing attention span. The results show a statistically significant difference between the two means, but behavioral therapy demonstrates to be more effective. Because the researcher predicted that cognitive therapy is more effective than behavioral therapy, the directional hypothesis is rejected.

8.8.1.2 Two Independent Groups Example

Is there a statistically significant difference between stress management and group psychotherapy in reducing anxiety scores in patients with clinical depression?

Hypothetical Post-Test Scores on the State-Trait Anxiety Inventory

Stress Management Group			Psychotherapy Group		
Subject	Score (X_1)	$X_1{}^2$	Subject	Score (X_2)	$X_2{}^2$
01	35	1225	01	51	2601
02	41	1681	02	48	2304
03	38	1444	03	52	2704
04	42	1764	04	43	1849
05	43	1849	05	49	2401
06	36	1296	06	54	2916
07	32	1024	07	61	3721
08	40	1600	08	56	3136
09	41	1681	09	54	2916
10	43	1849	10	60	3600
11	42	1764	11	48	2304
12	34	1156	12	46	2116

$\Sigma X_1 = 467$

$\Sigma X_1{}^2 = 18333$

$(\overline{X}_1) = 38.9$

$\Sigma X_2 = 622$

$\Sigma X_2{}^2 = 32568$

$(\overline{X}_2) = 51.8$

Grand Mean $= (\Sigma X_1 + \Sigma X_2) / 24 = (467 + 622)/24 = 45.37$

Smaller score indicates less anxiety

Step 1. State the research hypothesis. There is no statistically significant difference between a stress management group and a psychotherapy group in reducing anxiety in a sample of depressed patients. The hypothesis is stated in null form ($\mu_1 = \mu_2$).

Step 2. Select the level of statistical significance. The $\alpha = .05$ level of statistical significance will be accepted.

Step 3. This is a nondirectional two-tailed test for statistical significance because a null hypothesis was stated. Decide the test statistic. Independent *t*-test will be used.

Step 4. Determine the critical value for *t* from published statistical tables (see Table C-3 in Appendix C).
- a. $df = n_1 + n_2 - 2 = 22$
- b. level of significance $\alpha = .05$
- c. $t_{crit} = 2.0739$

Step 5. Calculate the mean and standard deviations.

Stress Management Group	Psychotherapy Group
$(\overline{X}_1) = \Sigma X_1/n = 467/12 = 38.9$	$(\overline{X}_2) = \Sigma X_2/n = 622/12 = 51.8$
$(\overline{X}_1) = 38.9$	$(\overline{X}_2) = 51.8$
$s_1 = 3.80$	$s_2 = 5.45$

8.8.1.3 Computational Formula for Standard Deviation

$$s = \sqrt{[n\Sigma X^2 - (\Sigma X)^2] / [n(n - 1)]}$$

$$s_1 = \sqrt{[(12)(18333) - (467)^2] / [12(12 - 1)]}$$

$$s_1 = \sqrt{(219996 - 218089) / [12(12 - 1)]}$$

$$s_1 = \sqrt{1907 / 132}$$

$$s_1 = \sqrt{14.44}$$

$$s_1 = 3.80$$

$$s_2 = \sqrt{[(12)(32568) - (622)^2] / [12(12 - 1)]}$$

$$s_1 = \sqrt{(390816 - 386884) / [12(12 - 1)]}$$

$$s_1 = \sqrt{3932 / 132}$$

$$s_1 = \sqrt{29.78}$$

$$s_1 = 5.45$$

Step 6. Exploratory data analysis.
$(\overline{X}_1) - (\overline{X}_2) = 38.9 - 51.8 = 12.9$
$s1 = 3.80$
$s2 = 5.45$
The mean difference is greater than the standard deviation for Groups 1 or 2. Standard deviation difference between the two groups is 1.65. There is a relative homogeneity of variance for the two groups.

Step 7. Exploratory graph analysis. Figure 8-33 shows the graph obtained from the analysis. There appears to be a significant difference between the two groups.

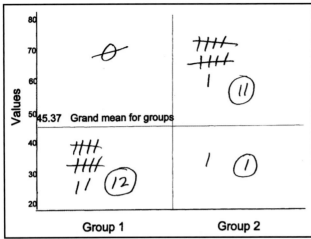

Figure 8-33. Exploratory graph analysis for hypothetical post-test scores on the State-Trait Anxiety Inventory. The graph shows the difference in scores between two independent groups of patients with clinical depression receiving either stress management training or group psychotherapy. The test being performed is an independent *t*-test.

Step 8. Calculate t_{obs}

$$t_{obs} = \frac{\overline{X_1} - \overline{X_2}}{\sqrt{\{[(n_1 - 1)(s_1^2) + (n_2 - 1)(s_2^2)] / (n_1 + n_2 - 2)\}[(1/n_1) + (1/n_2)]}}$$

Where

Group 1	Group 2
$\overline{X_1} = 38.9$	$\overline{X_2} = 51.8$
$n_1 = 12$	$n_2 = 12$
$s_1^2 = (3.80)^2 = 14.44$	$s_2^2 = (5.45)^2 = 29.70$

$$t_{obs} = \frac{38.9 - 51.8}{\sqrt{\{[(12 - 1)(14.44) + (12 - 1)(29.78)] / (12 + 12 - 2)\}[(1/12) + (1/12)]}}$$

$$t_{obs} = \frac{-12.9}{\sqrt{[(158.84 + 327.58) / 22][1.667]}}$$

$$t_{obs} = \frac{-12.9}{\sqrt{[(486.12)/22][1.667]}}$$

$$t_{obs} = -12.9/\sqrt{3.685}$$

$$t_{obs} = -12.9/1.9196$$

$$t_{obs} = -6.72$$

Step 9. Compare t_{obs} and t_{crit}

$t_{obs} = -6.72$

$t_{crit} = 2.0739$

The examination shows $|t_{obs}| > t_{crit}$. (Note: $|t_{obs}|$ is an absolute value that disregards the sign. The parallel lines indicate absolute value.) Reject the null hypothesis. There seems to be a statistically significant difference between the two means, indicating that the stress management group was significantly more effective that the psychotherapy group in the reduction of anxiety in patients with clinical depression.

8.8.2 Mann–Whitney U Test

8.8.2.1 Rationale

The Mann–Whitney *U*, a nonparametric alternative to the independent *t*-test, is used to test whether two independent groups have been drawn from the same population. In practice, the Mann–Whitney *U* is used with ordinal scale data.

1. The null hypothesis states that the two independent groups have the same population distribution.
2. An alternative, directional hypothesis is that there is a significant difference between the group means (when the distributions are approximately the same).

8.8.2.2 Assumptions

1. Random selection of each group
2. Two mutually independent groups are compared
3. The measurement scale is at least ordinal
4. n for each group is < 20

8.8.2.3 Computation

1. Rank order every raw score combining the two groups, (e.g., lowest score in both groups is assigned the rank of 1).
2. When two or more raw scores are the same, average the ranks.
3. Add the ranks for one group, obtaining T_A value.

8.8.2.4 Formula for Mann–Whitney U Test

$U_{obs} = (n_A n_B) + [(n_A)(n_A + 1)/2] - [T_A]$

Where

n_A = number of subjects in Group 1

n_B = number of subjects in Group 2

8.8.2.5 Example

Language intelligibility scores were compared between an experimental and control group after a 6-month treatment period. There was no significant difference between the groups on the pre-test (two-tailed test α = .05).

The following data were collected:

Experimental Group A			Control Group P		
Subject	*Score*	*Rank*	*Subject*	*Score*	*Rank*
101	33	12	201	35	13
102	30	10	202	32	1 1
103	25	8	203	27	9
104	24	6.5	204	24	6.5
105	22	5	205	21	4
106	19	3	206	18	2
			207	16	1
	$T_a = 44.5$			$T_b = 46.5$	
	$n_A = 6$			$n_B = 7$	

$U_{obs} = [(6)(7)] + [6(6+1)/2] - [44.5]$

$U_{obs} = 42 + 21 - 44.5$

$U_{obs} = 63 - 44.5$

$U_{obs} = 18.5$

Obtain U_{crit}: from table for Mann–Whitney U test (see Table C-7 in Appendix C).

$n_A/n_B = 6/7$

$U_{crit} = 6/36$

If U_{obs} is between 6 and 36, do not reject null hypothesis.

8.8.2.6 Conclusion

Null hypothesis is not rejected because $U_{obs} = 18.5$, which is between 6 and 36. Thus, the researcher concludes that there is no statistically significant difference in the experimental and control groups in language intelligibility post-test scores.

8.9 MODEL IV: PAIRED DATA SAMPLE

8.9.1 Correlated t-Test

The correlated *t*-test, often called a *paired t-test*, is applied to data when a researcher compares a group's performance or characteristic on two measures. For example, a researcher compares the difference between pre-test and post-test scores of an observed variable. Another example is to compare the difference of two variables in one group, such as intelligence and perceptual motor test scores. The difference between the correlated *t*-test and the independent *t*-test is that the correlated *t*-test is applied with one independent group and two variables, whereas the independent *t*-test is applied to scores for two independent groups.

An example of a correlated *t*-test was found in a study by Van Heest, Mogush, and Mathiowetz (2017). The authors compared the difference in the score on the same test between a pre- and post-test performance on several measures, including energy conservation, fatigue, self-efficacy, and quality of life. The table that follows describes the means, standard deviations, and the *P*-values for the pre-post and the pre-follow-up comparisons, respectively.

Correlated t-Tests Between Pre-Test and Post-Test Scores

Subtests	Pre-Test	Post-Test	Follow Up	Pre-Post
	Mean (s)	Mean (s)	Mean (s)	Pre-Follow up
				P-Value
FACIT FS	22.7 (8.2)	29.5(10.4)	29.4 (11.0)	<.001; .315
FACT-G[a]	69.0 (16.8)	77.7 (16.6)	77.8 (17.6)	<.001; .085
Physical Well-Being	17.1 (4.8)	20.2 (4.9)	20.2 (5.4)	<.001; .237
Social Well-Being	19.4 (6.1)	20.1 (6.3)	20.0 (6.6)	.186; .361
Emotional Well-Being	16.2 (4.0)	18.3 (3.8)	18.5 (4.0)	<.001; .164
Functional Well-Being	16.5 (5.2)	19.1 (4.9)	19.2 (5.1)	<.001; .108
SEPECSA	7.2 (1.7)	8.3 (1.1)	8.4 (1.1)	<.001; .439

For pre-test vs. post-test, n = 49; for post-test vs. follow-up, n = 36.

FACIT FS = Functional Assessment of Chronic Illness Therapy–Fatigue Scale; FACT–G = Functional Assessment of Cancer Therapy–General; SEPECSA = Self-Efficacy for Performing Energy Conservation Strategies Assessment.

[a]Subscales of the FACT–G.

There was a statistically significant difference between pre-test and post-test means on all the variables except for Social Well-Being, and there were no significant differences between the post-test and follow up for any of the variables. These finding suggest that in persons with chronic conditions and fatigue, the fatigue management course was successful in improving various aspects of well-being and that these improvements were maintained through the follow up period.

8.9.1.1 Operational Procedure for Testing for Statistical Significance in a Paired Data Sample

Step 1. State the research hypothesis.
  a. *Null Hypothesis*: H_0: $\mu_1 = \mu_2$
  b. *Alternative Hypothesis*: $\mu_1 \neq \mu_2$
  c. *Directional Hypothesis*: H_1: $\mu_1 > \mu_2$

Step 2. Select the level of statistical significance.
  $\alpha = .05$ or $.01$ level of significance

Step 3. Decide the test statistic and whether to apply a one- or two-tailed test for statistical significance.

Step 4. Look up the critical value for t_{crit} from statistical table.

    a. Determine the degrees of freedom: $df = N - 1$

    b. Level of significance $\alpha = .05$ or $.01$

    c. One-tailed or two-tailed test

    d. t_{crit} derived from table of values (see Table C-3 in Appendix C).

Step 5. Calculate the group means and standard deviations for each variable.

Step 6. Do an exploratory data analysis by determining if mean differences are greater than standard deviations for each variable.

Step 7. Plot a graph (see Independent *t*-test).

Step 8. Calculate t_{obs} using the formula:

$$t_{obs} = \frac{\Sigma D_1}{\sqrt{[N\Sigma D_1^2 - (\Sigma D_1)^2]/N - 1}}$$

Where

$\Sigma D_1 =$ sum of differences between each subject's score on measured variable

$\Sigma D_1^2 =$ sum of the squared differences on each score

$N =$ total number of subjects

Step 9. Accept the null hypothesis if $t_{obs} < t_{crit}$

Step 10. Reject the null hypothesis if $t_{obs} \geq t_{crit}$

8.9.1.2 Paired Data Sample

Hypothetical example of correlated *t*-test. Is there a statistically significant difference between performance IQ scores in adults with traumatic brain injury (TBI) after undergoing an intensive cognitive retraining program?

Performance IQ Scores

Subject	Baseline (Pre-Test)	X_1^2	After Treatment (Post-Test)	X_2^2
01	97	9409	113	12769
02	106	11236	113	12769
03	106	11236	101	10201
04	95	9025	119	14161
05	102	10404	111	12321
06	111	12321	121	14641
07	115	13225	121	14641
08	104	10816	106	11236
09	90	8100	110	12100
10	96	9216	126	15876
	$\Sigma X_1 = 1022$	$\Sigma X_1^2 = 104988$	$\Sigma X_2 = 1141$	$\Sigma X_2^2 = 130715$

Step 1. State the research hypothesis. There is no statistically significant difference between pre- and post-test IQ performance scores in adults with TBI who have undergone an extensive cognitive retraining program. This is a null hypothesis (H_0: $\mu_1 = \mu_2$).

Step 2. Group 1: The level of statistical significance is $\alpha = .05$.

Step 3. Decide whether to use a one- or two-tailed test. This problem requires a two-tailed test because the hypothesis is stated in null form and the researcher is examining statistical significance without direction.

Step 4. Look up t_{crit} (see Table C-3 in Appendix C).

    a. $df = N - 1 = 9$

    b. $\alpha = .05$

    c. two-tailed test

    d. $t_{crit} = 2.2622$

Step 5. Calculate the group means and standard deviations for the baseline and retest conditions.

Group 1	Group 2
$\overline{X}_1 = \Sigma/N = 1022/10 = 102.2$	$\overline{X}_2 = \Sigma/N = 1141/10 = 114.1$
$s_1 = 7.74$	$s_2 = 7.65$

Standard deviation computation formula

$$s = \sqrt{[N\Sigma X^2 - (\Sigma X)^2]/[N(N-1)]}$$

$$s_1 = \sqrt{[(10)(104988) - (1022)^2]/[(10)(10-1)]}$$

$$s_1 = \sqrt{[1049880 - 1044484]/90}$$

$$s_1 = \sqrt{5396/90}$$

$$s_1 = 7.74$$

$$s_2 = \sqrt{[(10)(130715) - (1141)^2]/[10(10-1)]}$$

$$s_2 = \sqrt{[(1307150 - 1301881]/90}$$

$$s_2 = \sqrt{5269/90}$$

$$s_2 = \sqrt{58.54}$$

$$s_2 = 7.65$$

Step 6. Exploratory data analysis

$\overline{X}_1 - \overline{X}_2 = 102.2 - 114.1 = 11.9$

    $s_1 = 7.74$

    $s_2 = 7.65$

The mean difference between pre- and post-test scores is greater than the standard deviations for pre- and post-test scores. The difference between the standard deviations is relatively small, indicating a homogeneity of variance for the two groups of scores.

Step 7. Exploratory graph. This is displayed in Figure 8-34.

From the exploratory data analysis, there appears to be a significant difference between the pre- and post-test scores.

Step 8. Calculate t_{obs}

$$t_{obs} = \frac{\Sigma D_1}{\sqrt{[N\Sigma D_1^2 - (\Sigma D_1)^2]/N - 1}}$$

Subject	Baseline Test	Retest	D_1	D^2
01	97	113	-16	256
02	106	113	-07	49
03	106	101	+05	25
04	95	119	-24	576
05	102	111	-09	81
06	111	122	-11	121
07	115	121	-06	36
08	104	106	-02	4
09	90	110	-20	400
10	96	126	-30	900
	1022	142	$\Sigma D_1 = -120$	$\Sigma D^2 = 2448$
				$(\Sigma D_1)^2 = 14400$

$$t_{obs} = \frac{-120}{\sqrt{[(10)(2448) - (14400)]/10 - 1}}$$

$$t_{obs} = \frac{-120}{\sqrt{(24480 - 14400/9)}}$$

$$t_{obs} = \frac{-120}{\sqrt{10080/9}}$$

$$t_{obs} = (-120)/\sqrt{1120}$$

$$t_{obs} = (-120)/33.460$$

$$t_{obs} = -3.586$$

Step 9. $t_{obs} = $ -3.586. Using Table C-3 in Appendix C, we find that $t_{crit} = 2.2622$. The researcher rejects the null hypothesis and concludes that there appears to be a significant difference between the pre- and post-test scores and that cognitive rehabilitation appeared to be effective in raising Performance IQ scores in this sample of individuals with TBI. (Note that the negative sign in -3.5 does not affect the value. Both positive and negative values are interpreted equally when compared with the t_{crit} value for the table.)

Figure 8-34. Exploratory graph analysis using hypothetical data. The graph shows differences between pre- and post-test performance IQ scores for a group of adults with traumatic brain damage after cognitive retraining. The statistical test being performed is a correlated *t*-test.

8.9.2 Wilcoxon Test for Paired Data Samples

The Wilcoxon signed rank test is a nonparametric alternative to the *t*-test for correlated samples.

8.9.2.1 Assumptions in Applying Wilcoxon Test

1. Random selection or random assignment of subjects
2. Measurement scale is at least ordinal.

8.9.2.2 Example of Applying Wilcoxon Test

An investigator is interested in comparing the pre- and post-test scores for a group of nine subjects. The null hypothesis is stated with $\alpha = .05$. The data for this example are as follows:

Subject	Pre-Test Raw Score	Post-Test Raw Score	Difference	Rank Difference
01	10	12	-2	(-) 4
02	12	15	-3	(-) 7
03	8	6	2	4
04	6	10	-4	(-) 8
05	14	12	2	4
06	7	6	1	1
07	10	12	-2	(-) 4
08	14	16	-2	(-) 4
09	12	18	-6	(-) 9

8.9.2.3 Stepwise Procedure for Wilcoxon Signed-Rank Test (Example)

Step 1. Calculate the difference between the pre- and post-test raw scores, subtracting the post-test raw scores from the pre-test raw scores.

Step 2. Rank order the differences between raw scores from smallest to largest, ignoring the negative or positive signs. Notice that in tied ranks, such as with 2 as a difference, the midpoint of the rank is 4 (2, 3, 4, 5, 6).

Step 3. Sum the positive rank differences.

4
4
+1
9

Step 4. Sum the negative rank differences.

-4
-7
-8
-4
-4
(+) -9
-36

Step 5. Determine T value. T is the absolute value of the smaller sum of the rank differences.

$T = 9$

Step 6. Compare the T_{obs} with T_{crit} from the table for critical values to T (see Table C-8 in Appendix C).

$N = 9$

$\alpha = .05$

two-tailed test

$T_{crit} = 5$

Step 7. If the T_{obs} is equal to or less than T_{crit}, then reject the null hypothesis and conclude that there is a statistically significant difference between the pre- and post-test scores. Because $T_{obs} = 9$ is greater than $T_{crit} = 5$, we accept the null hypothesis and conclude that there are no statistically significant differences between the pre- and post-test scores.

8.10 Model V: *K*-Independent Samples

8.10.1 Analysis of Variance

ANOVA is a widely used statistical test equivalent to the independent t-test when testing for significant differences between two means. ANOVA is applied to statistical data when two or more independent group means are being compared. The statistic for the ANOVA is F. (k refers to the number of independent groups or conditions in the study.)

F = variance between groups/variance within groups

The concept of the ANOVA is that if there are large differences between the group means compared with relatively small differences within the variances or scores within the group, then a statistically significant result is evident. ANOVA answers the question: Is there a statistically significant difference between the independent groups being tested? For example, does $\mu_1 = \mu_2 = \mu_3 = \mu_k$? ANOVA is always tested by a null hypothesis. When there is a statistically significant result, the researcher then carries out a post hoc analysis, such as the Scheffé, Duncan Multiple Range, Neuman-Keuls, and Tukey's procedures. These post hoc tests are similar to t-tests for independent measures, applied to the data after attaining a significant F.

8.10.1.1 One-Way Analysis of Variance

A one-way ANOVA simply analyzes the group means for statistically significant differences. The hypothetical table of results that follows is a typical example of a one-way ANOVA for comparing the effectiveness of 3 handwriting programs among 19 children with handwriting problems.

ANOVA Summary Table for Comparing Two Treatment Groups

Source of Variance	df	SS	MS	F
Between treatment groups	2	16	8	4.0*
Within treatment groups	16	32	2	
Total	18			

*$P = < .05$, $F_{crit} = 3.63$

Where

SS = sums of squares

MS = mean squares

k = number of treatment groups

N = total number of subjects in all groups

F is a derivative value equivalent to F_{obs} that is compared with the F_{crit} derived from a statistical table of values. For example, the F_{crit} for 2 df (treatment groups - 1) and 16 df [number of subjects (19) - number of groups (3)] with 2/16, $\alpha = .05$ is 3.63. The df is derived from between treatment groups (k - 1) and within treatment groups (N - k).

The result in this hypothetical example shows that there is a statistically significant difference between the three treatment methods for handwriting disorders. F_{obs} 4.00 > F_{crit} 3.63. Thus, the researcher will reject the null hypothesis.

8.10.1.2 Example of Two-Factor ANOVA From the Literature

A one-way ANOVA analyzes the group means for statistically significant differences. The two-factor ANOVA looks at the variables from a two-dimensional perspective. It analyzes interactive effects, such as treatment method and therapist personality or treatment method and patient diagnosis. Lin et al. (2015) investigated upper extremity motor control under challenging vs. easier cognitive tasks. The design involved a 2 X 2 (Condition X Group) design, with the Condition factor being either the single task or the dual task and the Group factor being either participants with schizophrenia or the healthy controls. Results are shown in the following table.

Summary Table of ANOVA on Condition and Group

Source of Variance	df	F	P-Value
Condition (Single, Dual Task)	1	33.49	<.001*
Group (Schizophrenia, Control)	1	47.59	<.001
Condition X Group	1	6.15	.02

*P<.05 significant

The results show that there was a significant difference in upper extremity motor performance between the single and dual tasks conditions and between the two population groups and that there was a significant interaction between the Condition and Group factors, meaning that the differences between the single and dual task performances were significantly different depending on the population.

8.10.1.3 Stepwise Procedures for One-Way ANOVA (Hypothetical Example)

Step 1. State the research hypothesis. The hypothesis is always stated in the null form when using ANOVA. For example, there is no statistically significant difference between electrical stimulation (ES), acupuncture (A), and proprioceptive neuromuscular facilitation (PNF) in improving upper extremity function in patients with chronic hemiplegia.

$H_0 = \mu_1 = \mu_2 = \mu_3$

Step 2. Select the level of statistical significance.

$\alpha = .05$

Step 3. Identify F_{crit} from table (see Table C-4 in Appendix C).

  a. *df* for the numerator = 2 (3 treatment groups - 1)
    df for the denominator = 15 (number of subjects - the number of groups 18 - 3 = 15)
    df = 2/15

  b. $\alpha = .05$

  c. $F_{crit} = 3.68$

Step 4. Calculate means and standard deviations. (The Fugl-Meyer Poststroke Motor Recovery Test scores were used for the example. Range is from 0 to 60.)

ES Group

Subject	Score (X)	X_1^2
01	23	529
02	31	961
03	16	256
04	27	729
05	32	1024
06	18	324
07	38	1444
$\Sigma X_1 = 185$	$\Sigma X_1^2 = 5267$	
$(\overline{x1}) = 26.4$		

A Group

Subject	Score (X)	X_2^2
01	13	169
02	19	361
03	19	361
04	25	625
05	18	324
$\Sigma X_2 = 94$	$\Sigma X_2^2 = 1840$	
$(\overline{x2}) = 18.8$		

PNF Group

Subject	Score (X)	X_3^2
01	33	1089
02	42	1764
03	30	900
04	38	1444
05	44	1936
06	41	1681
$\Sigma X_3 = 228$	$\Sigma X_3^2 = 8814$	
$(\overline{x3}) = 38.0$		

$$s = \sqrt{N\Sigma X^2 - (\Sigma X)^2 / N\,(N-1)}$$

$$s_1 = \sqrt{7(5267) - (185)^2 / 7(7-1)}$$

$$s_1 = \sqrt{2644\,/\,42}$$

$$s_1 = \sqrt{62.95}$$

$$s_1 = 7.93$$

$$s_2 = \sqrt{5(1840) - (94185)^2 / 5(4)}$$

$$s_2 = \sqrt{364/20}$$

$$s_2 = \sqrt{18.2}$$

$$s_2 = 4.26$$

$$s_3 = \sqrt{6(8814) - (228)^2 / 6(5)}$$

$$s_3 = \sqrt{(900/30)}$$

$$s_3 = \sqrt{30.00}$$

$$s_3 = 5.48$$

Step 5. Exploratory data analysis.

$\overline{X}_1 = 26$	$s_1 = 7.93$
$\overline{X}_2 = 18.8$	$s_2 = 4.26$
$\overline{X}_3 = 38.0$	$s_3 = 5.48$
$\overline{X}_1 - \overline{X}_2 = 7.6$	$s_1 - s_2 = 3.67$
$\overline{X}_1 - \overline{X}_3 = -11.6$	$s_1 - s_3 = 2.45$
$\overline{X}_2 - \overline{X}_3 = -19.2$	$s_2 - s_3 = -1.22$

There appears to be a statistically significant difference between the means and a relatively homogenous variance.

Step 6. Exploratory graph analysis. This graph is shown in Figure 8-35.

$$\text{Group mean} = (\Sigma(\overline{X}_1) + \Sigma(\overline{X}_1) + \Sigma(\overline{X}_1))/(N_1 + N_2 + N_3)$$
$$= (185 + 94 + 288)/(7 + 5 + 6)$$
$$= 507/18$$
$$= 28.17$$

There appears to be a statistically significant difference between Group 2 and Group 3.

Step 7. Calculate *F*.

Summary Table for One-Way ANOVA

Source of Variance	df	SS	MS	F
Between groups	2	1039.98	519.99	12.99
Within groups	15	600.52	40.03	
Total	17			

8.10.1.4 Formulas for ANOVA

a. $F = MS$ between groups/MS within groups
b. *df* between groups (df_{bg}) = Number of groups - 1 = (3 - 1) = 2
c. *df* within groups (df_{wg}) = Total number of subjects in all groups minus the number of groups = 18 - 3 = 15
Mean Square between groups = SS_{bg}/df_{bg}
Mean Square within groups = SS_{wg}/df_{wg}
d. Sum of Squares between groups:

$$SS_{bg} = \Sigma\left[(\Sigma X_1)^2 / n_1\right] + \left[(\Sigma X_2)^2 / n_2\right] + \left[(\Sigma X_3)^2 / n_3\right] - \left[(\Sigma X_1 + \Sigma X_2 + \Sigma X_3)^2 / \Sigma N\right]$$

Group 1
$(\Sigma X_1)^2 = (185)^2 = 34225$
$n_1 = 7$
$(\Sigma X_1)^2/n_1 = 4889.29$

Group 2
$(\Sigma X2)2 = (94)^2 = 8836$
$n_2 = 5$
$(\Sigma X_2)^2/n_2 = 1767.2$

Group 3
$(\Sigma X_3)^2 = (228)^2 = 51984$
$n_3 = 6$
$(\Sigma X_3)^2/n_3 = 8664.0$

$Total = (4889.29 + 1767.2 + 8664.0) = 15320.49$
$(\Sigma X_1 + \Sigma X_2 + \Sigma X_3)/\Sigma N) = 257049/18 = 14280.5$
$SS_{bg} = [(4889.29 + 1767.2 + 8664.0)] - [(257049)/18]$
$SS_{bg} = 15320.49 - 14280.5$

Figure 8-35. Exploratory graph for ANOVA using hypothetical data. The graph shows differences in scores between three different groups.

$SS_{bg} = 1039.99$
e. Sums of Squares within groups.
$SS_{wg} = \Sigma (\Sigma X_2^2 + \Sigma X_2^2 + \Sigma X_3^2) - 15320.49$
$SS_{wg} = \Sigma (5267 + 1840 + 8814) - 15320.49$
$SS_{wg} = 15921 - 15320.49$
$SS_{wg} = 600.51$
f. Mean Square between groups.
$SS_{bg}/df_{bg} = 1039.99/2 = 519.99$
g. Mean Square within groups
$SS_{bg}/df_{wg} = 600.51/15 = 40.03$
$F = MS_{bg}/MS_{wg} = 519.99/40.03 = 12.99$
Step 8. Compare F_{obs} with F_{crit}
$F_{obs} = 12.99$ $F_{crit} = 3.68$

Thus, we reject the null hypothesis and conclude that there is a statistically significant difference between the three groups. This confirms our exploratory data analysis.

Step 9. Conduct a post hoc test. If there is a significant *F* (i.e., the mean values are statistically significant) then the researcher carries out a post hoc analysis. This analysis is parallel to doing independent *t*-tests and determine which pairs of means have statistically significant differences.

There are several post hoc tests that are available to the researcher, such as:

- Tukey's Honestly Significant Differences (HSD)
- Neuman-Keuls
- Duncan Multiple Range
- Scheffé

8.10.1.5 Example of a Post Hoc Analysis

In the previous example, it was found that F_{obs} is statistically significant when

$$\overline{X}_1 = 26.4$$
$$\overline{X}_2 = 18.8$$
$$\overline{X}_3 = 38.0.$$

H_0: Null hypothesis is rejected and we conclude that all the means are not the same. We can now compare each pair of means, such as:

$$\overline{X}_1 \text{ compared to } \overline{X}_2$$
$$\overline{X}_1 \text{ compared to } \overline{X}_3$$
$$\overline{X}_2 \text{ compared to } \overline{X}_3$$

A significant F means that at least one pair of means are significantly different (e.g., the highest and lowest mean). Therefore, $\overline{X}_2$ compared to $\overline{X}_3$ has a statistically significant difference. We do not know whether there is a statistically significant difference between $\overline{X}_1$ and $\overline{X}_2$ and/or $\overline{X}_1$ and $\overline{X}_3$. A post hoc analysis tests for a statistically significant difference in these two situations.

In this example the Tukey HSD, a widely used post hoc analysis, was selected. The formula for the Tukey is (Gravetter & Wallnau, 2009):

$$HSD = q\sqrt{MS_{wg}/n}$$

Where

q = a derived table value (see Table C-9 in Appendix C). In this case, q = 3.67

MS_{wg} = the value calculated for mean squares within groups and is taken from the ANOVA table. In this example, this value is 40.03.

n = the average of the number of cases in each group. In this example, $n_1 = 7$, $n_2 = 5$, and $n_3 = 6$. The average is 6.

k = number of groups (k) = 3

df for $MS_{wg} = 15$

α = .05

$$HSD = q\sqrt{MS_{wg}/n}$$

$$HSD = 3.67\sqrt{40.03/6}$$

$$HSD = 9.479$$

Therefore, the mean difference between any two group scores must be at least 9.48 to be statistically significant.

a. $(\overline{X}_1) - (\overline{X}_2) = 26.4 - 18.8 = 7.6$. Therefore, the null hypothesis is accepted and $(\overline{X}_1) = (\overline{X}_2)$
b. $(\overline{X}_1) - (\overline{X}_3) = 26.4 - 38.0 = 11.6$. Therefore, the null hypothesis is rejected and $(\overline{X}_1) \neq (\overline{X}_3)$
c. $(\overline{X}_2) - (\overline{X}_3) = 18.8 - 38.0 = 19.2$. Therefore, the null hypothesis is rejected and $(\overline{X}_2) \neq (\overline{X}_3)$

In conclusion, a post hoc analysis test determines the pairs of means that have statistically significant differences.

8.10.2 Kruskal-Wallis Test for k Sample

The Kruskal-Wallis test is a nonparametric alternative to the one-way ANOVA when comparing three or more independent groups.

8.10.2.1 Assumptions

a. Random selection or random assignment of subjects to each independent group
b. Ordinal scale measurement
c. Each group should have at least five subjects

8.10.2.2 Example of Applying Kruskal-Wallis

Step 1. The investigator hypothesizes that there is no statistically significant difference between the three groups.

Group 1		Group 2		Group 3	
Subject	Raw Score	Subject	Raw Score	Subject	Raw Score
101	10	201	14	301	12
102	8	202	12	302	14
103	6	203	10	303	7
104	10	204	8	304	6
105	12	205	9	305	10
106	14				

Step 2. Rank order every raw score, combining all groups (in this example, three groups), with the lowest score assigned a rank of 1. In this example, the raw score of 4 made by Subject 303 is assigned the rank of 1.

Subject	Raw Score	Rank	
101	10	8.5	
102	8	4.5	
103	6	2.5	
104	10	8.5	
105	12	12	
106	14	15	$\Sigma_{ranks} = 51$
201	14	15	
202	12	12	
203	10	8.5	
201	8	4.5	
205	9	6	$\Sigma_{ranks} = 46$
301	12	12	
302	14	15	
303	4	1	
304	6	2.5	
305	10	8.5	$\Sigma_{ranks} = 39$

n = 16

Step 3. Sum the ranks for each group.

Group 1		Group 2		Group 3	
8.5	15	12	14	301	12
4.5	12	15	12	302	14
2.5	8.5	1	10	303	7
8.5	4.5	2.5	8	304	6
12	6	8.5	9	305	10
15					
$\Sigma_1 = 51$		$\Sigma_2 = 46.0$		$\Sigma_3 = 39.0$	
$n_1 = 6$		$n_2 = 5$		$n_3 = 5$	

Step 4. Calculate the formula for Kruskal-Wallis (Hobs)

$$H_{obs} = 12 / [N(N+1)] [(T_1^2 / n_1) + (T_2^2 / n_2) + (T_3^2 / n_3)] - [3(N+1)]$$

Where

$N = n_1 + n_2 + n_3 = 16$
$T_1^2 = (\Sigma_{1\text{-ranks}})^2 = 51^2 = 2601$
$T_2^2 = (\Sigma_{2\text{-ranks}})^2 = 46^2 = 2116$
$T_3^2 = (\Sigma_{3\text{-ranks}})^2 = 39^2 = 1521$
$H_{obs} = 12/[16(17)] [(2601/6) + (2116/5) + (1521/5)] - [3(17)]$
$\quad = [12/272] [433.5 + 423.2 + 304.2] - [51]$
$\quad = [.044] [1160.9] - [51]$
$\quad = 51.08 - 51$
$\quad = .08$

Step 5. Calculate H_{crit} for $\alpha = .05$, $df =$ number of groups (k) - 1 = 2.

$H_{crit} = 5.99$. (Use Chi-Square, Table C-10 in Appendix C, to test for statistical significance.)

Step 6. Compare H_{obs} (.08) with H_{crit} (5.991). If H_{obs} is equal to or more than H_{crit}, reject the null hypothesis. In this example, the null hypothesis is accepted, and we conclude that there is no statistically significant difference between the three groups tested.

8.11 MODEL VI: CORRELATION (PEARSON AND SPEARMAN CORRELATION COEFFICIENTS)

What is correlation? What is the difference between an associational relationship and causality? How do we graph the relationship between variables? What is a correlational matrix? What is a regression line? What is the difference between the Pearson correlation coefficient and the Spearman rank order correlation coefficient? All these questions relate to the correlational model in statistics.

8.11.1 Definition of Correlation

Correlation is the reciprocal relationship between two variables. It is a general concept that assumes that variables can be measured and correlated. The index of the degree of relationship between two variables is the correlation coefficient. This index can range from 0, which indicates no relationship, to +1.00 or -1.00, which indicates a perfect correlation between two variables. For example, a correlation coefficient of .30 indicates a low correlation, whereas .90 is a high correlation. The symbol for correlation is *r*. A correlational relationship indicates an association between variables; it does not indicate a causal relationship.

8.11.2 Example of a Correlation in the Literature

Table 8-11 displays the relationship between occupational disruption and autism service characteristics. Participants in this study were mothers of children with autism who returned surveys (n = 139) about their experience and ability to receive services for families of children with autism.

In this example from Hodgetts, McConnell, Zwaigenbaum, and Nicholas (2014), 64 correlation coefficients (*r*) were completed to construct the correlational matrix table. The researchers used the $\alpha = .05$ for level of statistical significance. It is important to note that with correlations, statistical significance is not as important as establishing a clinical level of correlation. For example, in establishing an acceptable reliability for a test, many researchers will accept Pearson correlation coefficients of

TABLE 8-11

CORRELATION MATRIX: OCCUPATIONAL DISRUPTION AND AUTISM SERVICE CHARACTERISTICS

	1	2	3	4	5	6	7	8
1. DISRUPTED EMPLOYMENT								
2. DISRUPTED LEISURE	0.124							
3. MULTIPLICITY	0.106	0.095						
4. FREQUENCY	0.118	0.009	0.553**					
5. CONTINUITY	−0.207*	−0.301**	0.197*	0.233*				
6. RESPONSIVENESS	−0.014	−0.152	0.177	0.161	0.495			
7. RECEIVES HOME-BASED SERVICES	0.141	0.161	0.505**	0.436**	0.115	0.091		
8. RECEIVES OCCUPATIONAL THERAPY/SPEECH PATHOLOGY	0.045	−0.103	0.627**	0.652**	0.303**	0.192*	0.412**	
9. RECEIVES BEHAVIOR SUPPORT	0.059	−0.096	0.632**	0.339**	0.252**	0.073	0.461**	0.518**

Note: * <.05; ** <.01

Reprinted with permission from Hodgetts, S., McConnell, D., Zwaigenbaum, L., & Nicholas, D. (2014). The impact of autism services on mothers' occupational balance and participation. *OTJR: Occupation, Participation and Health, 34*(2), 81-93.

$r = .80$ or above as acceptable. In the example in Table 8-11, $r = .60$ is considered by some researchers to be low to moderate in clinical significance. In understanding the correlational results, the square of r is the proportion of variance in one variable that is associated with another variable. If $r = .60$, then the proportion of variance accounted for is only .36, which means that .64 is that portion of the variance that is not accounted for. Correlation is a measure of predicting the value of one unknown variable (Y) if another variable (X) is known. If there is a high correlation between the two variables (e.g., $r = .90$), then the researcher has a high degree of confidence in predicting "if X, then Y." The degree of confidence in the relationship is more important in clinical research than is the statistical r value.

In the example illustrated in Table 8-11, there are comparatively low correlations between the disruption factors (i.e. employment and leisure) with the autism service characteristics. Whereas, there are moderate associations amongst several of the autism service characteristics (i.e., multiplicity with receiving occupational therapy and speech-language pathology, multiplicity with behavior support). In other words, it appears that there is little association between the mothers' occupational disruption and the autism service characteristics. Based on these results, the researchers should conclude that there is not a strong relationship between occupational disruption and autism service characteristics even though there is a statistically significant relationship at the .05 level.

8.11.3 Stepwise Procedure for Correlation

Step 1. State the research hypothesis. For example, there is no statistically significant relationship between variable X and variable Y. (Null hypothesis, $r = .00$ or below predetermined level of correlation.)

Step 2. Determine the degree of relationship that will be acceptable for significance.

a. In establishing test-retest reliability, a correlation coefficient of $r = .80$ or above is considered acceptable (Anastasi, 1988).

b. In clinical research, a correlation coefficient of below $r = .60$ is moderate to low.

Step 3. Collect data and arrange raw scores into a table. For example:

Subjects	Variable X Raw Score	Rank	Variable Y Raw Score	Rank	d (difference in ranks between X and Y)	d² (difference squared)
1	31	7	45	5	2	4
2	22	5	58	8	−3	9
3	19	4	57	7	−3	9
4	16	3	48	6	−3	9
5	78	8.5	61	9	−0.5	0.25
6	3	1	36	4	−3	9
7	93	10	18	3	7	49
8	78	8.5	88	10	−1.5	2.25
9	23	6	9	1	5	25
10	15	2	12	2	0	0
	$\Sigma X = 378$		$\Sigma Y = 432$		$\Sigma d = 0^a$	$\Sigma d^2 = 116.5$

Step 4. Rank order each raw score, with lowest score being assigned rank of 1. Note: for tied ranks, take the midpoint of the rank. For example, a raw score of 78 occupies ranks 8 and 9 and becomes rank of 8.5.

Step 5. Do exploratory data analysis. Note in Figure 8-36 that each point in the scatter diagram is a coordinate value. It appears from the scatter diagram that there is a low-to-moderate correlation between the two variables.

Step 6. Calculate Spearman rank correlation coefficient and estimate degree of relationship between the two variables (X and Y). The formula for Spearman r_s is:

$r_s = 1.00 - [(6)(\Sigma d^2)/(N^3 - N)]$

$= 1.00 - [(6)(116.5)/(1000 - 10)]$

$= 1.00 - [699/990]$

$= 1.00 - .71$

$r_s = .29$

The exploratory data analysis indicates that there is a low correlation between the X and Y variables.

Step 7. Calculate the Pearson *r* correlation coefficient. The Spearman (rank order) is a good screening test for the Pearson (product-moment), which is a more accurate test because the Pearson *r* computes raw scores, whereas the Spearman r_s computes ranks that are transformed scores. The reader shall note that the Pearson *r*, which is a parametric test, should be applied to interval or ratio scale data. The Spearman r_s is a nonparametric statistical test that can be used with ordinal scale data. As the reader will note, interval scale data can be transformed to ranks (ordinal scale data).

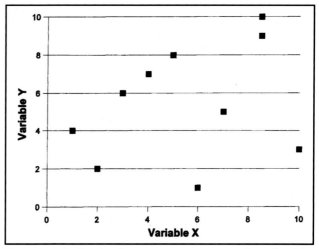

Figure 8-36. Exploratory data on a scattergram using the ranks of the scores. Notice that each point is a coordinate value. There appears to be a low-to-moderate correlation between the two variables.

The formula for the Pearson *r* product-moment correlation is:

$$r = [N\Sigma XY - (\Sigma X)(\Sigma Y)] / \sqrt{N\Sigma X^2 - (\Sigma X)^2][N\Sigma Y_2 - (\Sigma Y)^2]}$$

8.11.3.1 Calculation for Pearson *r* Product-Moment Correlation

Subject	X	X²	Y	Y²	XY
01	31	961	45	2025	1395
02	22	484	58	3364	1276
03	19	361	57	3249	1083
04	16	256	48	2304	768
05	78	6084	61	3721	4758
06	3	9	36	1296	108
07	93	8649	18	324	1674
08	78	6084	88	7744	6864
09	23	529	9	81	207
10	15	225	12	144	180
	378	23642	432	24252	18313
	$\Sigma X = 378$	$\Sigma X2 = 23,642$	$\Sigma Y = 432$	$\Sigma Y2 = 24,252$	$\Sigma XY = 18,313$

$N = 10$ $\Sigma X^2 = 23,642$

$\Sigma XY = 18,313$ $\Sigma Y^2 = 24,252$

$\Sigma X = 378$ $\Sigma X^2 = 142,884$

            t

$\Sigma Y = 432$ $(\Sigma Y)^2 = 186,624$

$r = [(10)(18313) - (378)(432)] / \sqrt{(10)(23642) - (142884)][(10)(24252) - (186624)]}$

$= [183130 - 163296] / \sqrt{(236420 - 142884)(242520 - 186624)}$

$= 19834 / \sqrt{(93536)(55896)}$

$= 19834 / 72317$

$r = .274$

The Pearson r of .274 is similar to the Spearman r_s of .29. In both computations, the correlation is low and will not be clinically significant because only a small portion of the variance is accounted for.

Step 8. Calculation of regression line. A regression line describes the relationship between variable X and variable Y. The formula for the regression line is

$\overline{Y} = a + bX$

Where

Y is a predicted variable from the known X value

b is the slope of the line

a is the Y intercept.

The regression line that is calculated assumes that if a perfect correlation 1.00 exists between two variables, then one could predict the Y value if the X value is known. For example, suppose we derive the formula for a specific regression line to be:

$Y = 1.50 + .30X$

and $X = .500$

$Y = 1.50 + .30 (.500)$

$= 1.5 + .15$

$Y = 1.65$

Therefore, if $X = 5.00$, then $Y = 3.00$ in this example. The calculation of a regression line is useful when there is a high correlation between two variables. On the other hand, a low correlation of $r = .29$ would not warrant constructing a regression line.

The computational formula for the slope is:

$b = [N (\Sigma XY) - (\Sigma X)(\Sigma Y)] / [N (\Sigma X^2) - (\Sigma X^2)]$

The formula for the Y intercept is

$a = Y - bX$

Step 9. Identify the critical values for the Spearman Rank Order Correlation Coefficient.

    a. Determine number of subjects (N)

    b. Significance level, such as $\alpha = .05$, .01

    c. Directional or nondirectional hypothesis

For example, with $N = 10$, $\alpha = .05$, nondirectional test, $r_{s(crit)} = .648$ (see Table C-6 in Appendix C). In the previous example, $r_{s(obs)} = .29$. In this result, the researcher will accept the null hypothesis and conclude that there is no statistically significant relationship between the two variables.

Step 10. Identify the critical values for the Pearson product-moment correlation.

    a. $df = N - 2$

    b. Significance level

    c. Directional or nondirectional hypothesis

In the example as shown, $df = 8$, $\alpha = .05$, nondirectional test, $r_{crit} = .6319$ (see Table C-5 in Appendix C). Because $r_{obs} = .27$, the null hypothesis is accepted and the researcher concludes that there is no statistically significant relationship between the two variables.

The reader should note that as the N increases, the r_{crit} decreases. For example, for 100 df, $\alpha = .05$ level of significance, $r_{crit} = .1966$, whereas for 20 df, $r_{crit} = .4227$.

8.12 MODEL VII: OBSERVED FREQUENCIES (CHI-SQUARE)

When researchers work with nominal data, they frequently are concerned with differences in the number of cases falling into discrete categories, such as improved vs. not improved or active versus disengaged. The major purpose of this statistical model is to test whether there are statistically significant differences between the observed and the expected frequencies of two independent groups. For example, this model could be applied if a researcher is interested in determining whether there is a gender difference in the distribution of individuals with multiple sclerosis in a population where there are 51% female subjects and 49% male subjects. Is there a statistically significant difference between the number of men as compared with women who have a diagnosis of multiple sclerosis? In this hypothetical example, the researcher will compare the observed differences between the number of men and women diagnosed with multiple sclerosis with the expected prevalence (i.e., 51% for women and 49% for men).

8.12.1 Example of Chi-Square

In an example from the literature, the investigators examined the factors influencing the successful outcome of tracking individuals with severe psychiatric illnesses in the community compared with those in hospitals (Dean & Gadd, 1990). In Table 8-12, the investigators compared the patients treated at home with patients admitted to a hospital in relation to where they were assessed during a psychotic episode.

8.12.1.1 Formula for Chi-Square (χ^2)

$\chi^2_{obs} = \Sigma [(O - E)^2] / E$

$\chi^2_{obs} = [(51 - 42)^2/42] + [(3 - 11)^2/11] + [(11 - 10)^2/10] + [(0 - 2)^2/2] + [(13 - 22)^2/22] + [(13 - 6)^2/6] + [(5 - 5)^2/5] + [(3 - 1)^2/1]$

$\chi^2_{obs} = 1.92 + 5.81 + .09 + 2 + 3.68 + 8.16 + 0 + 4$

$\chi^2_{obs} = 25.66$

$\chi^2_{crit} = 7.82$ (3 df, $\alpha = .05$)

LOCATION OF ASSESSMENT DURING A PSYCHIATRIC EPISODE					
	PATIENTS TREATED AT HOME		PATIENTS ADMITTED TO HOSPITAL		
LOCATION OF ASSESSMENT	*Observed*	*Expected*	*Observed*	*Expected*	*Total Patients*
Home	51	42	13	22	65
Hospitals	3	11	13	6	16
Outpatient Clinic	11	10	5	5	16
Police Station	0	2	3	1	3
	65	65	34	34	99

TABLE 8-12

Reprinted with permission from Dean, C., & Gadd, E. M. (1990). Home treatment for acute psychiatric illness. *British Medical Journal, 201,* 1023.

8.12.1.2 Conclusion

Dean and Gadd (1990) rejected the null hypothesis and concluded that there is a statistically significant difference where patients are assessed if they are treated at home or admitted to a hospital. From the results, the researchers concluded that if patients are assessed at home, they will have significant less probability of hospitalization for a psychiatric illness. The results of the study reinforced their hypothesis that home treatment is a feasible alternative to hospital treatment for many individuals with psychiatric illness. The application of chi-square is an appropriate statistical test when comparing nominal categories of data. It is a simple but powerful statistic that can be applied to outcome studies of clinical populations.

8.12.2 Operational Procedure of Observed Versus Expected Frequencies (Chi-Square)

Step 1. State the research hypothesis. The null hypothesis is: There is no statistically significant difference between the observed vs. expected frequencies in normal groups ($\chi^2_{obs} < \chi^2_{crit}$). The alternative hypothesis is: There is a statistically significant difference between the observed versus expected frequencies in nominal groups ($\chi^2_{obs} - \chi^2_{crit}$)

Step 2. Select the level of statistical significance. This is usually $\alpha = .05$.

Step 3. Determine the *df* for the contingency table.

$df = (r - 1)(c - 1)$

r = number of rows in the table

c = number of columns in the table

For example, in a 2 X 2 contingency table, $df = 1$. In a 3 X 6 contingency table, $df = 10$.

Step 4. Identify χ^2_{crit} (chi-square critical) from the statistical table of values. The critical value is determined by:

  a. Level of significance

  b. *df*

For example, $\chi^2_{crit} = 18.307$ for $\alpha = .05$, nondirectional test, with $df = 10$ (see Table C-10 in Appendix C).

Step 5. Identify the discrete nominal categories being compared. For example, diagnostic groups, gender, and health care settings.

Step 6. Determine the number of columns and rows in the chi-square contingency table. Chi-square contingency tables are based on the number of columns and rows being compared. Contingency tables range from 2 rows and columns (2 x 2 contingency table) to larger number of rows and columns, such as 2 x 3, 3 x 5, or 6 x 8.

Step 7. Tabulate the observed number of frequencies within each discrete category or group.

	Nonsmokers		Smokers		
	O	E	O	E	Total
Lung Cancer	500	1000	1500	1000	2000
No Lung Cancer	4500	4000	3500	4000	8000
Total	5000	5000	10,000	5000	10,000

The researcher counts the number of individuals with lung cancer who were smokers or nonsmokers in a population.

Step 8. Calculate the expected frequencies based on the probability of chance. The expected frequencies in a cell are computed by multiplying the total frequencies of a row that contains the cell by the total frequencies of the column that contains the cell and dividing this product by the total number of cases in the population. In this example, the expected frequencies for nonsmokers with lung cancer is equal to:

(2000) (5000)/10,000 = 1000

Step 9. Calculate chi-square (χ^2_{obs}). The formula for chi-square is:

$\chi^2_{obs} = \Sigma \ [(O - E)^2/E]$
Where
Σ = grand sum of all the cells
O = observed frequency in each cell
E = expected frequency in each cell

Step 10. Compare the two values: χ^2_{obs} and χ^2_{crit} (see Table C-10 in Appendix C for critical score).

Accept the null hypothesis if χ^2_{obs} is less than χ^2_{crit}

Reject the null hypothesis if χ^2_{obs} is equal to or more than χ^2_{crit}

8.12.2.1 Observed Frequencies, Chi-Square Example

Research Problem. Is cognitive-behavioral treatment as effective as antidepressant medication in treating individuals with clinical depression?

Step 1. Research hypothesis. Null hypothesis: There is no statistically significant difference between the number of individuals with depression who improve with medication (Med) compared to those who receive cognitive-behavioral treatment.

Step 2. Level of significance: $\alpha = .05$.

Step 3. Determine the *df* from the contingency table.
$df = (r - 1) \ (c - 1)$
$df = (2 - 1) \ (3 - 1) = 2$

Step 4. Identify χ^2_{crit} from the statistical table of values.
a. $\alpha = .05$
b. $df = 2$
c. $\chi^2_{crit} = 5.99$ (See Table C-10 in Appendix C.)

Step 5. Identify the nominal categories. In this example, the nominal categories are the following:
a. Those individuals treated with cognitive-behavioral treatment who regressed.
b. Those individuals treated with cognitive-behavioral treatment who showed no improvement.
c. Those individuals treated with cognitive-behavioral treatment who improved.
d. Those treated with medication who showed no improvement.
e. Those treated with medication who improved.

Step 6. There are two rows and three columns: (2 x 3 contingency table).

Step 7. Enumerate the observed number of frequencies within each nominal category and place in a 2 x 3 contingency table.

	Regressed		No Improvement		Improvement		
Treatment	O	E	O	E	O	E	Total
Cognitive-Behavioral	20	24.70	40	57.64	150	127.64	210
Medication	40	35.29	100	82.35	160	182.35	300
Total	60		140		310		510

In this example, 210 individuals received cognitive-behavioral treatment and 300 individuals received medication. A total of 510 individuals with depression were included in the study. Of the 310 individuals who improved, 160 received medication and 150 received cognitive-behavioral treatment. The rest of the group (200 individuals) showed either no improvement (remained the same) or regressed.

Step 8. Calculate the expected frequencies for each nominal category or cell based on the formula.

To complete the expected frequency of any cell, multiply the marginal total for the row that contains the cell by the marginal total for the column that contains the cell and divide this product by the total number of cases in the table (McCall & Kagan, 1986).

Cognitive-behavioral treatment (Regressed) = (210)(60)/510 = 24.70

Cognitive-behavioral treatment (No Improvement) = (210) (140)/510 = 57.64

Cognitive-behavioral treatment (Improved) = (210)(310)/510 = 127.64

Medication (Regressed) = (300) (60)/510 = 35.29

Medication (No Improvement) = (300) (140)/510 = 82.35

Medication (Improved) = (300) (60)/510 = 182.35

Step 9. Calculate chi-square (χ^2_{obs}).

$\chi^2_{obs} = \Sigma \ [(O - E)^2/E$

$\chi^2_{obs} = [(20 - 24.70)^2/24.70] + [(40 - 57.64)^2/57.64] + [(150 - 127.64)^2/127.64] + [(40 - 35.29)^2/35.29] + [(100 - 82.35)^2/82.35] + [(160 - 182.35)^2/182.35]$

$\chi^2_{obs} = .89 + 5.39 + 3.91 + .62 + 3.78 + 2.73$

$\chi^2_{obs} = 17.32$

Step 10. Compare χ^2_{obs} with χ^2_{crit}

$\chi^2_{obs} = 17.32$

$\chi^2_{crit} = 5.991$

Reject the null hypothesis. There is a statistically significant difference between cognitive-behavioral treatment and medications in the treatment of depression. It appears that cognitive-behavioral treatment is more effective than medication in the improvement of depression in this hypothetical example. For this example, 150 (71%) of the 210 individuals in the cognitive-behavioral treatment group improved, whereas 160 (53%) of the 300 individuals of the medication group improved.

8.12.3 Kappa

8.12.3.1 Purpose

The purpose of kappa is to determine the degree of agreement between two or more judges independently ranking a variable. It can be used to measure inter-rater reliability. Kappa can range from +1.00 to -1.00

8.12.3.2 Assumptions

a. The units are independent (i.e., completed by independent observations).
b. The categories are nominal scale measurements, fully mutually exclusive, and exhaustive.
c. The judges operate independently.
d. There is no criteria for correctness, choices, clinical judgment, or client attitudes.
e. Judges have equal competence, education, or ability to make ratings.
f. There are no restrictions placed on ranking or rating the variable.

8.12.3.3 Formula for Kappa

Kappa $= P_0 - P_c / 1 - P_c$

Where

P_0 = the observed proportion of agreement

P_c = the proportion of agreement expected by chance alone

8.12.3.4 Example

In a hypothetical observation, two independent observers rate the level of depression indicated by a behavioral scale. One individual is observed by two independent raters during 10 sessions to evaluate the level of depression (i.e., low depression [LD], medium depression [MD], and severe depression [SD]). Each category of depression is operationally defined, and each rater has been trained

previously using a standardized rating scale. They independently observe a patient on a ward applying a behavior rating scale. Is there a high inter-rater relationship between the two observers using a standardized rating scale? The data from the observations follow:

Sessions	Observer 1	Observer 2	Agreement
1	LD	MD	no
2	MD	MD	yes
3	LD	LD	yes
4	MD	MD	yes
5	LD	LD	yes
6	LD	LD	yes
7	MD	MD	yes
8	LD	MD	no
9	MD	MD	yes
10	LD	LD	yes
Totals	6 LD, 4 MD, 0 SD	4 LD, 6 MD, 0 SD	Agreements: 8/10 = 80%

8.12.3.5 Stepwise Procedure for Kappa

Step 1. Place data into a 3 x 3 contingency table to display agreements. Use three categories of depression: MD, LD, and SD.

	LD	MD	SD	Marginal Totals
LD	4	2	0	6
MD	0	4	0	4
SD	0	0	0	0
Marginal Totals	4	6	0	(10)

Notice that there were four instances of both observers agreeing on low depression and four instances of both observers agreeing on moderate depression. There were no observations of severe depression. The agreements will always be the numbers in the diagonal cells when there are 2 observers and 1 subject. Also note that, when adding frequencies in cells, Observer 1 usually is on the y-axis and Observer 2 is on the x-axis of the table. In this example, the discrepancy between the two raters occurred in the cell containing 2. This is where Observer 1 rated subject twice as low depression and Observer 2 rates the same subject for sessions 1 and 8 as moderate depression.

Step 2. Calculate for kappa applying the formula.

Kappa $= P_0 - P_c / 1 - P_c$

P_0 is obtained by adding all the frequencies in the cells that both observers agree.

	Observer 2		
	11	12	13
Observer 1	21	22	23
	31	32	33

Each cell is numbered to represent the rating of each observer. For example, cells 11, 22, and 33 represent agreements of Observers 1 and 2. On the other hand, cell 21 represents discrepancy between Observers 1 and 2.

$P_0 =$ the frequency of agreement over the total number of observations (N).

The formula is

$P_0 = (n_{11} + n_{22} + n_{33} + n_{ii})$/Sum of Marginal Cells

Where

$n_{ii} =$ and other cells

The marginal total is the sum of each row or column.

$n_{11} = 4$

$n_{22} = 4$

$n_{33} = 0$

$P_0 = 8/10 = .80$

$P_c =$ marginal totals of Observer 1 times marginal totals of Observer 2, divided by the total number of observation periods of sessions squared.

$P_c = \{[(6)\ (4)] + [(4)\ (6)] + [(0)\ (0)]\}/10^2$

$P^c = [(24) + (24) + (0)]/100$

$P_c = 48/100$

$P_c = .48$

$Kappa = P_0 - P_c/1 - P_c$

$Kappa = (.80 - .48)/(1 - .48)$

$Kappa = 32/52$

$Kappa = .61$

A kappa of .70 is considered to indicate an acceptable level of agreement (Sattler, 1988). The results indicate a slightly lower inter-rater agreement than what statisticians consider acceptable inter-rater reliability. Note that the percentage of agreement (i.e., 80%) is uncorrected for chance. From a pragmatic perspective, kappa should always be interpreted in terms of its value to the clinician. In this example, the clinical researcher would interpret a kappa of .61 as acceptable.

8.12.4 Rasch Analysis

Rasch analysis is a statistical method that calculates the likelihood of something being true based upon the probabilities of how strong effects are while considering the probabilities of the effectiveness of control variables. Rasch analysis is particularly suited for evaluating psychometric concepts such as attitudes, abilities, and personality traits. This statistical method has been used frequently for testing the validity and reliability of psychometric scales and assessments (Velozo, Kielhofner, & Lai, 1999).

A good example in occupational therapy that uses the Rasch method is the Assessment of Motor and Process Skills (AMPS Project International, 2010; Fischer, 1994). In this instance, the Rasch model predicts the probability of how well an individual performs a task based on many different factors, including but not limited to the person's ability to perform the task, the skill required to complete the task, how simple the task is, and the leniency associated with the examiner. The Rasch model is able to take into account all of these factors, and more, and predict the probability of how well a person performs a certain task.

Another example using Rasch analysis is from a study by Lehman, Sindhu, Shechtman, Romero, and Velozo (2010) comparing the effectiveness of two separate upper extremity assessments to measure change. Based upon the results from the Rasch analysis, these researchers determined that there was no clear advantage of using the Disabilities of Arm, Shoulder, and Hand (DASH) over the Upper Extremity Functional Index to measure clinical change.

8.13 STATISTICAL SOFTWARE PACKAGES

Although the authors have used hand calculations to solve the examples presented in this book many statistical problems can be solved through one of several statistical packages available for computers. Three widely used computer programs designed for the health and social sciences are detailed in the following sections.

8.13.1 Statistical Product and Service Solutions

IBM SPSS produces a data analysis package for research scientists. It has been widely used within the social science fields as well as other disciplines. Statistical Product and Service Solutions (IBM SPSS) includes the capabilities to perform basic analyses (e.g., frequencies, correlations) and more advanced analyses (e.g., regression, ANOVA, general linear models, contingency tables, factor and discriminant analysis, nonparametric statistics, and time series).

8.13.1.1 Statistical Product and Service Solutions Example

Statistical software packages such as IBM SPSS make it possible to obtain statistical results with relative ease. The following is an example of an IBM SPSS printout of an ANOVA, first discussed in an earlier section: 8.10 Model V: k-Independent Samples. The data comes from the hypothetical Fugl-Meyer Poststroke Motor Recovery Test Scores listed in Section 8.10.1. IBM SPSS version 17.0.1 was used (http://www-01.ibm.com). In this experiment, a comparison was being made between the performance of subjects on the Fugl-Meyer test based upon their random assignment to the electrical stimulation (ES), acupuncture (A), or the proprioceptive neuromuscular facilitation (PNF) groups.

To have the software calculate various statistical procedures, data need to be arranged in a specific manner depending on the type of statistical procedure. Generally, for IBM SPSS, data can be arranged by columns or by rows depending on the data collected. In this example, the data representing the dependent variable are listed in a column format labeled as "SCORE," whereas the independent variable is organized by rows. For example, the factor labeled "GROUP" represents the independent variable and is listed as being either ES, A, or PNF, depending on the row. If this example had contained two dependent variables, there would be two columns representing the dependent variables.

A typical manner in which to enter these types of data into an IBM SPSS spreadsheet (i.e., IBM SPSS Statistics Data Editor) would look like the following:

Subject	Group	Score
1	ES	23
2	ES	31
3	ES	38
4	ES	27
5	ES	32
6	ES	28
7	A	17
8	A	13
9	A	19
10	A	19
11	A	25
12	A	18
13	PNF	33
14	PNF	42
15	PNF	30
16	PNF	38
17	PNF	44
18	PNF	41

Note that all the subjects are labeled from 1 to 18. Once the data are entered, it is important to make sure the column labeled "SCORE" is categorized as "NUMERICAL." This can be done using the "VARIABLE VIEW" within the IBM SPSS Statistics Data Editor. Next, it is good practice to make sure the data have a bell-shaped distribution, also referred to as being normally distributed. If data are not normally distributed, then they may be skewed. If the skewness measure is greater than 1 or less than -1, the data are skewed; however, if the skewness measure is between --1 and +1 then the data are not skewed. If the data are skewed, apply a nonparametric statistic, such as Kruskal–Wallis (see Section 8.10.2).

Calculating the Skewness: This can be done in the IBM SPSS Statistics Data Editor.

1. Under the "ANALYZE" pull-down menu, select "DESCRIPTIVE STATISTICS."
2. Choose "EXPLORE."

3. Once the "EXPLORE" window opens, identify the "DEPENDENT LIST" (i.e., score) and the "FACTOR LIST" (i.e., Group).

4. Click "OK." This action will open the IBM SPSS Statistics Viewer and, among other things, a "DESCRIPTIVES" table that lists various descriptive statistics. See the following descriptive table for this set of data:

Group				Statistic	Standard Error
Score	A	Mean		18.5000	1.58640
		95% confidence interval for Mean	Lower Bound	14.4220	
			Upper Bound	22.5780	
		5% Trimmed Mean		18.4444	
		Median		18.5000	
		Variance		15.100	
		Standard Deviation		3.88587	
		Minimum		13.00	
		Maximum		25.00	
		Range		12.00	
		Interquartile Range		4.50	
		Skewness		.537	.845
		Kurtosis		2.056	1.741
	ES	Mean		29.8333	2.08833
		95% confidence interval for Mean	Lower Bound	24.4651	
			Upper Bound	35.2015	
		5% Trimmed Mean		29.7593	
		Median		29.5000	
		Variance		26.167	
		Standard Deviation		5.11534	
		Minimum		23.00	
		Maximum		38.00	
		Range		15.00	
		Interquartile Range		7.50	
		Skewness		.467	.845
		Kurtosis		.629	1.741

Group			Statistic	Standard Error
PNF	Mean		38.0000	2.23607
	95% confidence interval for Mean	Lower Bound	32.2520	
		Upper Bound	43.7480	
	5% Trimmed Mean		38.1111	
	Median		39.5000	
	Variance		30.000	
	Standard Deviation		5.47723	
	Minimum		30.00	
	Maximum		44.00	
	Range		14.00	
	Interquartile Range		10.25	
	Skewness		-.602	.845
	Kurtosis		-1.308	1.741

5. Examine the skewness. The skewness is .537 for Group A; .467 for Group ES; and -.602 for PNF. Because all skewness values are ≥ 1 and < 1, it is safe to assume that these data are appropriate for an ANOVA regarding skewness.

Calculating the ANOVA:

1. Go back to the IBM SPSS Statistics Data Editor, select the "ANALYZE" menu pull-down and select "GENERAL LINEAR MODEL."

2. Select "UNIVARIATE."

3. Move the "SCORE" variable to the "DEPENDENT VARIABLE" box and the "GROUP" variable to the "FIXED FACTOR" box using the little arrow buttons.

4. Click "OK." The IBM SPSS Statistics Viewer will reopen and display several tables including one labeled, "Tests of Between-Subjects Effects."

Source	Type III Sum of Squares	df	Mean Square	F	Sig
Corrected Model	1150.78[a]	2	575.39	24.22	.000
Intercept	14906.89	1	14906.89	627.51	.000
Group	1150.78	2	575.39	24.22	.000
Error	356.33	15	23.76		
Total	16414.00	18			
Corrected Total	1507.11	17			

[a]R Squared = .764 (Adjusted R Squared = .732)

8.13.1.1.1 Discussion of Specific Results from SPSS Analysis

Notice that some of the same information in this table is identical to that shown in the Summary Table for one-way ANOVA in Section 8.10.1. As a part of interpreting the results, it is important to consider whether the observed F value is larger than the critical F value. IBM SPSS does not automatically provide a table of critical F values, but more conveniently produces the associated P-value, which is labeled in the table as "SIG," meaning significance. In this comparison, the important items to consider are the F and P-values associated with the variable labeled "GROUP," which in our case is labeled as 24.22 and < .001, respectively.

Because the P-value is < .05, it can be assumed that there is a statistically significant difference among the three groups. However, this test does not say which groups are significantly different from each other. To determine which groups are significant from each other, a post hoc comparison is necessary.

If the original research hypothesis was not to just determine whether there would be a significant difference among the three groups, but rather to determine which individual groups are significantly different from the other individual groups, then this should be stated in the original statistical plan. Proper protocol stresses that it is only appropriate to execute a post hoc comparison if statistical significance exists among the three groups. In our hypothetical example, this is indeed the case because of having a P-value < .05.

8.13.1.1.2 Post Hoc Tests of ANOVA

1. To run a post hoc comparison, go back to the IBM SPSS Statistics Viewer or the IBM SPSS Statistics Data Editor and select the "ANALYZE" pull-down menu, then select the "GENERAL LINEAR MODEL," then select "UNIVARIATE." If this is done after completing the previous steps, the "DEPENDENT VARIABLE" and "FIXED FACTOR(s)" won't need to be redefined again.

2. In the UNIVARIATE window, select the "POST HOC" button.

3. At the top of the "UNIVARIATE: POST HOC MULTIPLE COMPARISONS FOR OBSERVED MEANS" window select the "GROUP" factor and move it to the "POST HOC TESTS FOR:" window using the little arrow button.

4. Once this occurs, you will notice that all the post hoc options are no longer grayed out. You will notice that there are approximately 20 different options from which to choose. Each option is unique and should be chosen depending upon specific statistical assumptions and strategies. Common options include the Bonferroni, Tukey, Scheffé, and Dunnett comparisons.

5. For this example, the Bonferroni option was chosen before clicking the "CONTINUE" button. This will bring you back to the "UNIVARIATE" window where the arrangement of the dependent variable and the fixed factors should be the same as you recently left them.

6. Click the "OK" button to run the new analysis. The IBM SPSS Statistics Viewer will generate an ANOVA table identical to the one without the post hoc analysis. The bottom of the ANOVA table should be a section labeled as "POST HOC TESTS." You should see a "MULTIPLE COMPARISONS" table that also identifies "BONFERRONI" at the top. The "MULTIPLE COMPARISON" table for this set of data is shown here.

(I) Group	(J) Group	Mean Difference (I-J)	Standard Error	Sig.	Lower Bound (95% CI)	Upper Bound (95% CI)
A	ES	-11.3333*	2.81399	.003	-18.9135	-3.7532
	PNF	-19.5000*	2.81399	.000	-27.0801	-11.9199
ES	A	11.3333*	2.81399	.003	3.7532	18.9135
	PNF	-8.1667*	2.81399	.033	-15.7468	-.5865
PNF	A	19.5000*	2.81399	.000	11.9199	27.0801
	ES	8.1667*	2.81399	.033	.5865	15.7468

Based on observed means.

The error term is Mean Square (Error) = 23.756.

*The mean difference is significant at the 0.05 level.

This table individually compares each intervention group with the other intervention groups. There is some redundancy within the table. The left columns are labeled (I) Group and (J) Group. The (I) group is compared with the other groups (J). In the first row, the A group is being compared to the ES and the PNF groups. The third column is the mean difference between the "I" and "J" groups and the fourth column is the associated standard error. The fifth column is labeled as "Sig" (significance), which is how IBM SPSS labels the P-value.

The IBM SPSS multiple comparison table for this example shows that there are statistically significant differences between all possible comparisons of these three treatment approaches. In this table, the P-values have 3 decimal places. In this case, it would not be accurate to report the P-value as being = .000. The P-value, while being very small, is actually > 0; it's just that it would require more than 3 decimal points to give the exact value. Therefore, the proper way to report this would be "< .001." The 95% confidence intervals (both the lower and upper bounds) for the comparisons are listed in the two most right columns.

When examining the remainder of the Multiple Comparisons table, we learn that there are statistically significant differences between the A and the PNF groups, the ES and the PNF groups, and the A and the ES groups. This knowledge, considered along with the means of the respective groups, allows one to interpret with confidence (within the bounds of at least 95% certainty) that the PNF group significantly outperformed the ES group, which in turn outperformed, at a statistically significant level, the A group on the Fugl-Meyer Poststroke Motor Recovery Test.

8.13.2 SAS System

This statistical package is an integrated system of data access, management, analysis, and presentation, which is not limited to a particular computer system. The software is available for mainframes and personal computers. Basic and advanced statistics are available, and the analysis can be integrated into a presentation for any type of reporting needs. Training and support are available.

8.13.3 SYSTAT

This statistical package is available through the website at https://systatsoftware.com. A menu-driven data analysis tool enables data to be analyzed in basic statistics (e.g., descriptive, t-test, correlation) and more advanced statistics (e.g., ANOVA, multiple regression, and factor analysis). As with most packages, graphics are available.

8.13.4 UNISTAT

This statistical program for Microsoft Windows was first made available in 1984. It is described by the company as a "fully fledged spreadsheet for data handling, a wide range of statistics and powerful 2D and 3D presentation quality graphics." It can be used alone or combined with Excel.

8.14 SUMMARY

In this chapter, the authors have presented the basic statistical concepts and tests that are applied in clinical research. Statistics is both an art and a science. The art of statistics is the decision-making involving the selection of the appropriate statistical test for a research study. There are several possibilities in this decision, based on the level of measurement, the probability level for statistical significance, and the number of subjects in the study. The science of statistics is based on mathematical reasoning and use of statistical tables. Mastery of statistics means approaching the subject with an objective attitude and open mind. Statistics should not be applied mechanically such as throwing data in a computer. The researcher should use statistics in a reflective manner while interpreting and analyzing the results. In this way, statistical analysis is integrated into the research study.

9

Single-Case Experimental Design

Every clinical therapist providing service, however, has the responsibility to document, in a systematic manner, the effectiveness or non-effectiveness of the service provided to any given client …
The primary tool advocated for achieving this goal is the small-N or "intensive" design.

—Ottenbacher (1986a, pp. 5-6)

OPERATIONAL LEARNING OBJECTIVES

By the end of this chapter the learner will understand:

- The unique contribution of single-case experimental design (SCED) studies to evidence-for-practice in occupational therapy.
- The most common terms used in SCED.
- SCED as a type of controlled experimental design.
- The process of operationally defining the intervention (independent variable), and the measurement of the outcome (dependent variables) in an SCED.
- The types of demonstrable changes in performance in an SCED (level, slope, variability) through figures.
- Approaches to an analysis of the results through visual and statistical methods and through interpretation of the findings.
- The strengths and limitations of SCED pertaining to measurement, statistical, and generalizability issues.
- The historical contributions of SCED in the occupational therapy literature and its application to professional practice.

Rice, M. S., Stein, F., & Tomlin, G.
Clinical Research in Occupational Therapy, Sixth Edition (pp. 271-289).
© 2019 Taylor & Francis Group.

9.1 A Hypothetical Example

Imagine an occupational therapist providing services to a client with an inability to dress independently after a stroke. First, the therapist will evaluate the client to determine current functioning. The therapist notices an inability to close buttons due to a lack of fine motor coordination in the affected hand. The therapist decides on the intervention of providing a buttonhook. During the intervention, the therapist keeps track of the client's performance with the buttonhook each day to monitor progress. After two sessions, the client can dress independently, including using fasteners in a blouse or shirt.

The evaluation was equivalent to collecting baseline data (called *Phase A*), and the intervention was like the treatment phase (called *Phase B*). Though the client improved, was it because of the therapy? Consider the two extremes of possible situations: in one scenario, the therapist just treated the patient without evaluating the client (performed Phase B only). Suppose the client does better after a couple of sessions. The therapist claims it was the treatment that caused the improvement. But, wouldn't you be skeptical? In the second scenario, the therapist evaluates the client and establishes the client's stable functional performance level (Phase A). Then, the intervention is applied and the client's performance improves (Phase B). Next, the therapeutic effect is removed (the buttonhook is taken away), and the performance declines to what it was before (return to Phase A). The intervention is reapplied and the performance improves again (second Phase B). Removal, decline, reapplication, improvement (A, B, A, B)—after a few cycles anyone would be persuaded that the intervention does indeed cause the improved performance. Furthermore, the client is convinced and refuses to have the therapeutic intervention removed again.

This scenario was meant to illustrate the essence of an SCED and to show how much it resembles the occupational therapy process itself.

A clear distinction needs to be made among terms that are similar sounding and often confused. An SCED is not the same as a *case report*, a *case study*, or a *case series*, which are considered to be basic descriptive research, according to the research pyramid model of evidence (Tomlin & Borgetto, 2011). SCED studies represent a type of controlled experimental design, specifically level E4 in the pyramid model (Tomlin & Borgetto, 2011) or level IV in the American Occupational Therapy Association (AOTA, 2014) levels of evidence hierarchy.

9.2 Typology: Single-Case Experimental Design as a Type of Experimental Research

SCED study designs have many similarities to traditional group experimental designs:

- They are inspired by an important research question that can be applied to a single client or a small group of clients, such as "Do alternative seating devices lead to greater classroom attention in elementary school-aged children with autism spectrum disorder (ASD)?"
- They seek to justify the claim of a likely causal relationship between an intervention and an improved outcome in the client, such as "Does constraint-induced movement therapy bring about greater functional use of the affected upper extremity in an individual who has had a stroke?"
- They identify demographic characteristics of the research participant(s), such as age, sex, diagnosis, performance challenges, and the occupational profile.
- Their design involves the manipulation of conditions to isolate a causative factor (i.e., what is the effect of the independent variable, or intervention, on the dependent variable, or outcome?).
- They contain an operationalization of the independent and dependent variables, the procedure used for collecting data, and the conditions under which data are collected.
- They are concerned with procedural reliability (i.e., fidelity) in the application of the designated intervention.
- They are concerned with procedural reliability of measurements of the dependent variable in the baseline and intervention phases, as well as intra- and inter-rater reliability.
- They often triangulate data collection by measuring multiple types of dependent variables, such as a physiological measure, a standardized test of skills/performance/behavior, and a self-evaluation.
- Experimental control can be applied in SCED by participants acting as their own control (baseline phase or phases).
- Control of confounding variables (e.g., history effects) or their documentation is incorporated into the design to enhance the accuracy of the interpretation of results.
- Blinding of evaluators or test administrators is sometimes possible, even if blinding of participants and therapists may not be possible.

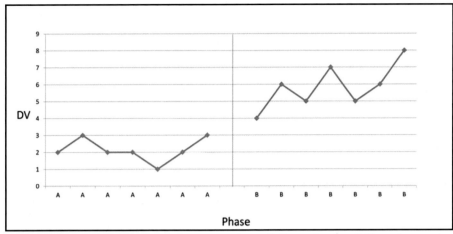

Figure 9-1. Typical data plot of a single case experiment (A Phase = baseline; B Phase = intervention; DV = dependent variable)

- Outcomes are often appropriate for statistical analysis.
- Analysis, interpretation, and generalization of the results and their limitations are stated and clinical implications are projected.
- Conclusions can suggest a possible cause-effect relationship between the independent and the dependent variables. In most cases, the study should be replicated to strengthen the dependability of the conclusions and their generalizability.

SCEDs can be used as pilot projects to explore the relationship between variables and to test intervention protocols for later revision. In addition, whenever it is too costly, too time-consuming, or simply infeasible to conduct a study using group experimental design because a sufficient number of individuals with like challenges is not available in a setting, much can be gained through an SCED (Ottenbacher, 1986a). Their minimum recommended structure (Lane, Ledford, & Gast, 2017; Tate et al., 2016) now is a baseline phase followed by an intervention followed by a return to baseline followed by another phase of intervention (ABAB, see below). In this structure, they closely mimic the sequence of the occupational therapy process itself (ABAB: evaluation, intervention, reevaluation, adjusted intervention) (AOTA, 2014). SCED can present a feasible means for therapists to scientifically evaluate the effects of their work with individual clients.

9.3 STRUCTURE OF SINGLE-CASE EXPERIMENTAL DESIGNS: DESIGN CONSIDERATIONS TO STRENGTHEN CAUSAL CLAIMS

9.3.1 AB Structure

The simplest SCED has the structure AB. That is, a baseline (A) phase of a certain length of time is followed by an intervention (B) phase, also of a certain length of time. Each phase involves multiple measurement occasions to provide confidence that the researcher has an accurate estimate of the client's actual performance level during this phase. Typically, data are measured three to eight times per phase, each time on a different day (Figure 9-1). Statistically speaking, a minimum of six is recommended so that any one data point does not overly influence the findings. For example, Mulcahey, Smith, Betz, and Weiss (1995) studied the hand dexterity before and after tendon transplant surgery of an 11-year-old boy with tetraplegia due to a spinal cord injury. The surgery, postoperative care, and 4 weeks of hand therapy coincided with an immediate and steady improvement in hand function and activities of daily living performance (Mulcahey et al., 1995). Sufficient data were assembled in this study to provide persuasive evidence that the surgery and therapy caused the improvement in function.

Whenever a marked difference in performance is apparent after the intervention is started (the transition to Phase B), then the researcher could formulate the claim that the intervention caused the improved performance. However, it is possible that something else may have happened just at the phase change that was the actual cause of the improvement. This actual cause might be another intervention being started by a different practitioner, a developmental milestone being naturally reached by the client, or an event in the living situation of the client (e.g., changing residence, absence or return of a family member, or recovery from an illness).

9.3.2 ABA Structure

Thus, a stronger causal claim could be made if data were further collected during a return-to-baseline phase, where the client's performance sharply returns to that in the original baseline phase when the intervention is removed. This design would be called an *ABA* (Figure 9-2). For interventions providing a non-permanent effect, one expects the dependent variable to decline when the intervention is stopped, such as in the provision of assistive technology.

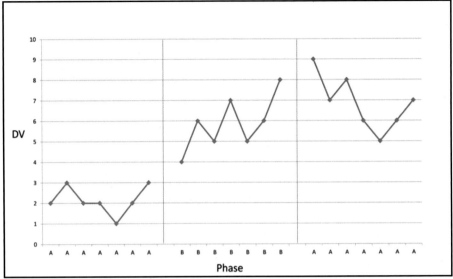

Figure 9-2. ABA design. Each A is a data collection occasion in baseline, each B an occasion during intervention. The phases are separated slightly for clarity.

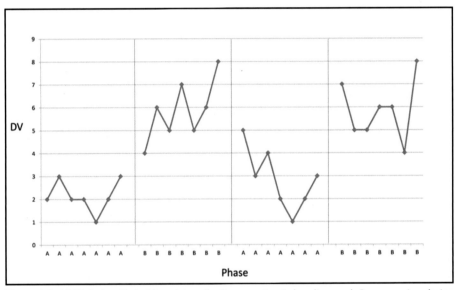

Figure 9-3. ABAB design. Each A is a data collection occasion in baseline, each B an occasion during intervention. The phases are separated slightly for clarity.

Alternatively, if the intervention seeks to make a permanent change in the client, then one would expect the better performance to be maintained in the return to baseline (the second Phase A). For example, Dickerson and Brown (2007) studied the effects of constraint-induced movement therapy on upper extremity use and the quality of functional movement in a 24-month-old child with hemiparesis. Upon application of a constraint on the unaffected arm of the child (Phase B), performance improved in 6/7 outcome variables. After the constraint was removed, performance was better than baseline in 7/8 recorded variables (Dickerson & Brown, 2007).

9.3.3 ABAB Structure

Stronger yet would be if data were also measured during a second Phase B (ABAB; Figure 9-3). If performance improvement was observed both times there was an A-to-B transition, then the researcher could be much more confident that the change was caused by the intervention. Hence, the SCRIBE (Single-Case Reporting Guideline In Behavioural Interventions) recommendation for contemporary SCED to have a design at least as thorough as ABAB (Tate et al., 2016). For example, Watling and Deitz (2007) studied the classroom behaviors of four 3- to 4-year-old boys with ASD before and after providing two separate

Figure 9-4. Alternating treatment design. Each A is a data collection occasion. The blue line is standard intervention, and the red line is new intervention.

phases of Ayres Sensory Integration intervention. Although no immediate clearly beneficial changes were observed in undesired behavior or task engagement, parents noted more positive behaviors at home and therapists documented new, positive behaviors for each boy during therapy (Watling & Deitz, 2007).

9.3.4 ABC/ABAC Structure

Phase pairs AB could be repeated further, but more common is the introduction of a second, different intervention, called C. The simplest design with a Phase C would be ABC. Here, the baseline phase is followed by a period of intervention B followed by a period of intervention C. Performance during B might not show an improvement over that in A, but perhaps with the onset of C does show improvement. For example, Gustafson, Patterson, Marshall, Bennett, and Bower (2016) examined whether compression bandaging (Phase B) and compression gloves (Phase C) could reduce edema in the stroke-affected upper limb of four individuals. They found the bandaging was accompanied by reduced edema at all five measured anatomical sites for each of the four participants; however, edema in Phase C rebounded in most sites for most participants, calling into question the effectiveness of a glove that was not custom fitted (Gustafsson et al., 2016).

It would be better if Phase C had been preceded by a return to baseline, or ABAC. Stronger still would be the design ABACA, where a final return to baseline tests whether the intervention of C was actually effective. That is, what happens when it is removed? Does the client's performance drop back to that of the original baseline? It is also possible to design a study where interventions are applied separately and then together (ABACA, then B+C simultaneously). Each additional comparison made

between phases offers the opportunity to make a stronger causal case because coincidences are even more unlikely to have caused the changes in performance.

9.3.5 Alternating Treatment Design Structure

A different approach is used in the SCED, called *alternating treatment design* (ATD). In this design, two interventions are compared on several occasions (usually at least six). On each occurrence of measurement, one intervention is applied first and then the other is applied; the resulting performance level of the client is then measured. If one intervention is clearly superior to the other, the plotted lines will diverge and remain separate. Tanta, Deitz, White, and Billingsley (2005) used an ATD design (with a preparatory Phase A) to determine whether five children with developmental play delays showed more initiation and more response during play when paired with a higher functioning child or a lower functioning child (Figure 9-4). The three boys and two girls (aged 3 to 6 years old) had play ages of 2.5 to 4.4 years. Generally, the initiation and response of all five participants was greater when they played with a higher-level playmate, contrasting the findings of some earlier research (Tanta et al., 2005).

9.4. MULTIPLE BASELINES

To enhance the portrayal of a client's performance and to strengthen the internal validity of the study, another addition is undertaken in some SCED: multiple baselines. This term refers to the presence of more than one dependent variable on which the research participant is tracked.

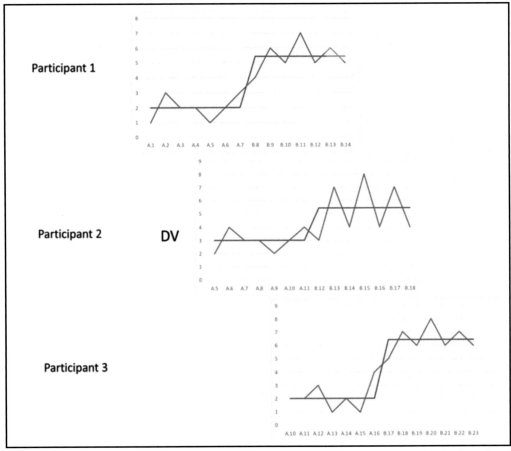

Figure 9-5. Multiple baseline design (multiple participants). Numbers after A or B represent calendar dates. A and B are phases of baseline and intervention, respectively. Blue lines represent data, and horizontal red lines are mean levels in each phase. Diagonal red lines represent jump in level. The jumps occur not on the same calendar day, but as intervention is begun, on different days for each participant.

The differential effect of the independent variable on the various dependent variables can be carefully weighed in the interpretation of findings. For example, Watling and Deitz (2007) tracked both undesirable behavior and task engagement as separate dependent variables in four children with ASD receiving Ayres Sensory Integration therapy. They also staggered the transition from the baseline phase to intervention phase to control for history effects. A single dependent variable might also be measured in multiple settings (e.g., home, school, neighborhood park), and thus under different contextual conditions. Multiple baselines (settings) can show how widely applicable the performance improvement is, strengthening the external validity (generalizability) of the findings to more aspects of the participant's life.

Another example of multiple baselines is the inclusion of more than one participant in an SCED. Recently, a higher proportion of published SCED in the *American Journal of Occupational Therapy* (AJOT) contained data from more than one participant. (The average number of cases per SCED in AJOT has increased from 2.5 in the 1990s, to 3.0 in the 2000s, and to 5.0 in the 2010s.) If each participant

is started into their Phase A on a different calendar day and then transitioned to Phase B on a different day, possible history effects are strongly mitigated (Figure 9-5). A multiple-case SCED can sometimes suggest patterns that help explain why the intervention worked for some but not for others (McGruder, Cors, Tiernan, & Tomlin, 2003). The essence of such a comparison is shown in Figure 9-6. Comparing data from multiple participants can allow for the discovery of the effects of various demographic characteristics or hidden differences on the outcome variables.

9.5 OPERATIONALIZATION OF VARIABLES

Just as a precise description of the protocols in group experimental studies is crucial for future replication, so it is for SCED. This precise definition of the applied intervention (e.g., amount, frequency, by whom, conditions) and of how the outcomes are measured is called *operationalization of variables*.

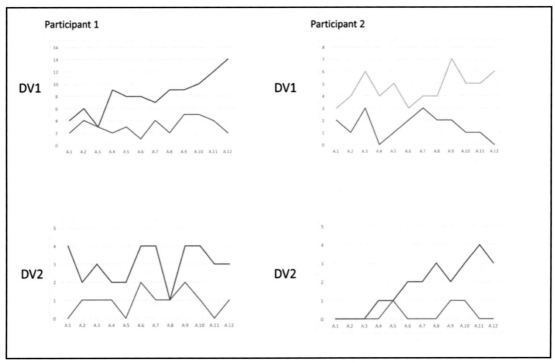

Figure 9-6. ATD, multiple baseline design (two interventions tested across two participants and two dependent variables).

9.5.1 Operationalization of the Independent Variable

To replicate or generalize an SCED, readers must be informed about the exact nature of the intervention that was delivered to the participant. First, to ensure that the intervention was delivered as intended to the participant, procedural reliability is monitored. Typically, this monitoring is done via a checklist of every pertinent detail of the setup and delivery of the therapy, as well as of the surroundings. Is furniture exactly in its intended place? Are supplies laid out the same each time a data measurement occasion occurs? Are seating, lighting, temperature, and background noise standardized from session to session? Is the intervention provided in exactly the intended manner (also called *treatment fidelity*)? The demands of fidelity can run the gamut from a precisely specified protocol (e.g., ABA therapy for a child with ASD) to a globally outlined procedure, such as "intervention was applied according to the professional judgment of the treating therapist." If the intervention is provided under requirements more similar to the latter description, then the representativeness of the occupational therapy practitioner providing the intervention becomes of greater importance. Would the average therapist implement such an intervention in approximately the same way? To the extent the answer to this question is "no," the generalizability of the findings to other settings is correspondingly weakened.

Of course, if the SCED protocol includes the provision of more than one type of intervention (either separately or combined), then each intervention must be operationalized.

9.5.2 Operationalization of the Dependent (Outcome) Variables

See Chapter 8 for information on operationalizing outcome variables in a group experimental study.

Just as crucial as operationalization of the independent variable is the precise definition of how the outcome variable (dependent variable) was collected. When were measurements taken (what time of day, day of the week, intervals, any interruptions; what were conditions before, during, and after)? By whom were the measurements made (occupational therapist, parent or caregiver, teacher, paid graduate student, the researcher)? Did the research protocol include provisions for controlling observer drift (i.e., maintenance throughout the study of intra-rater reliability)? If more than one data gatherer or rater were involved, did the researcher take steps to establish, measure, and maintain inter-rater reliability? These reliabilities are more important in SCED due to the repeated measurement of the same individuals in the generation of the data. If observer drift occurs, then an apparent change in the performance displayed by the data might not have been caused by the intervention, but rather could be attributable to the drift (systematic measurement error) instead.

9.6 SPECIFIC CONSIDERATIONS FOR COLLECTING DATA IN SINGLE-CASE EXPERIMENTAL DESIGN

Often in SCED, the dependent variable is a repeatedly occurring behavior or performance of a task. Whether such a behavior or performance can be reliably observed and measured is influenced by the following considerations.

9.6.1 Counting

If the outcome is a behavior to be counted, what is and is not an occurrence? a separate occurrence? a double occurrence? For example, suppose an SCED is testing whether a specific sensory approach in the classroom is effective for reducing the biting behavior of a child with a developmental disorder. What, exactly, counts as a bite? Bear in mind, this definition of *bite* must be such that a bite can be observed and counted in a reliable way. Part of the operationalization of a bite must be to describe when a bite occurs as opposed to a non-bite or a near-bite. What counts as two bites vs. a double-bite? The operationalization is not as simple as it might at first appear.

One possible operationalization would be to define a bite as happening when the teeth visibly touch the skin of the child (easy to observe), regardless of how much pressure may be applied (which would be difficult to judge reliably by observation alone). The bite ends when the teeth cease to have contact with the skin. If contact is made with the skin immediately thereafter, then that counts as two (separate) bites. If, however, after contact the jaws seem to clamp down on the skin twice, with the teeth never breaking contact with the skin, then that counts as only one bite. A motion toward the skin with the mouth open but where the teeth never touch the skin does not count as a bite.

In this way, the counting of bites can be made more reliable among raters or within a single rater over many data collection occasions. This reliability is crucial for the internal validity of an SCED due to the multiple times of measurement. The researcher and the reader must both be confident that plotted changes in the dependent variable are due to actual changes and not to spurious variability introduced by unreliable measurement.

9.6.2 Timing

The researcher has several alternatives when employing timing of behaviors in an SCED. Is the total amount of time the participant is engaged in a behavior to be measured? Or is the longest single occurrence of the behavior what is most important in the study? Perhaps it is the average length of engagement in a behavior over a given span of time that is of greatest functional importance. It might also be that the frequency of the behavior is most important: how many times did it occur in a 5-minute period? a 45-minute classroom session? during recess? (in which case, see Section 9.6.1, Counting). How is the timing exactly to be done? When does the timing of the behavior start? When does it stop? The more precisely these moments can be defined in advance, including all the complicating contingencies that might occur, the more thoroughly operationalized the dependent variable is, the more accurate the data will be, and the greater the internal validity of the study.

In some SCEDs, the behavior of interest occurs too rapidly for a timing of it or an accurate frequency count. In this case, a time sampling of behavior may be indicated. For example, exactly every 5 minutes the data gatherer looks to see whether the participant is engaged in the behavior. The outcome is recorded as a 0 (no) or a 1 (yes). If observations take place each day for 1 hour, then 12 5-minute intervals will be sampled, yielding a possible total score of 0 to 12. An occupational therapy practitioner might have a set performance as the client's long-term goal (e.g., 10 times of every 12 opportunities the behavior is manifested). The SCED researcher is interested in documenting whether the independent variable brings about any reliable improvement in the dependent variable over the duration of the study.

Time sampling is often used when the participant is engaged in a group activity. Can the observer reliably pick the participant out of the group? Can the observer reliably observe the participant's behavior or do others block the view? These questions are best answered empirically through a pilot data collection session (often with similar individuals not in the study itself to avoid contamination). Based on the findings from the pilot test, the operationalization of the dependent variable collection of the SCED can be adjusted.

9.6.3 Graphing the Data

The report of results from an SCED almost always includes one or more graphs of the data. The multiple times of measuring the dependent variable per participant, separated into phases where the phase transition is of great importance, lend themselves to a pictorial display. In a simple AB study, the appearance of the plotted data points and of how they differ from Phase A to Phase B provide a direct avenue for a visual interpretation of the results. (See Ottenbacher [1986b] and the following for how visual analysis alone under certain circumstances can be misleading.)

9.6.3.1 Setting up the Axes of the Graph

By convention, moving along the x-axis (horizontal axis) from left to right represents the passage of time. Each time an outcome behavior or performance is collected, it is noted on the graph as a single point. The amount of the variable that was measured at this time x is plotted along the y-axis (vertical axis). This axis represents the dependent variable (see Figure 9-1). The y-axis almost always indicates a linear (equal interval) scale. Most commonly, the x-axis also shows a scale of equal intervals where each measurement occasion is an interval. However, these equal intervals may not represent equal intervals of time. That is, if measurements are made on a Monday/Wednesday/Friday schedule for 3 weeks, then there are nine data points appearing on the graph. They are plotted at equal distances horizontally from one another; however, the points representing a Friday and the subsequent Monday have two non-data days between them (Saturday, Sunday), whereas those collected during the week are separated by only one day (Tuesday, Thursday). This simplification in the graph may have implications for the findings as explained below. In addition, by convention adjacent data points are connected by a solid line. Connecting the points through time indicates an assumption of an underlying potential to produce this behavior or achieve this performance that is continuous or ongoing. The actual data points represent the results when this potential is sampled at discrete points in time. If an intended data collection point is missing (e.g., due to illness in the participant), then some researchers advocate breaking the data line, or indicating it by a dotted line between the data points on either side of the missing point.

With an ATD, both conditions (with or without adaptive equipment, as in McGruder et al. [2003] or playing with child A or child B, as in Tanta et al. [2005]) are typically plotted on the same graph so that a visual comparison can easily be made. In standard SCEDs (e.g., ABA, ABAB), there is usually only one dependent variable per graph plotted, although more are possible, as in Dickerson and Brown (2007). However, a single figure of the published article may contain two or more graphs aligned for easier visual comparison by the reader (Figure 9-6). These graphs may show an alignment of all dependent variables from one participant, the results on one dependent variable from more than one participant, or the dependent variable data from one participant measured in different settings.

The researcher should unambiguously state for each graph whether up (more of y) represents better. For example, when functional behaviors or positive performance is plotted, up is better and a rising graph is what the researcher hopes for. In contrast, in the case of dysfunctional behaviors, the hope is that what is plotted will decline. Likewise, if "time taken to perform a task" or "number of errors committed" or "amount of assistance needed" is how the dependent variable was operationalized, then a decline in scores is desirable. Care must be taken when a study measures multiple dependent variables and for some of them "up" is better and for others "down" is better.

9.6.3.2 Indicating the Phases

Even the simplest design in an SCED has a phase change between Phase A (baseline) and Phase B (intervention). This change is usually displayed as a vertical line at the point of phase change (halfway between the last baseline data point and the first intervention phase data point). In an ABA design, there would be two vertical dashed lines separating A from B and B from the return to Phase A. In an ABAB design, there will be three phase transitions (see Figure 9-3).

Ordinarily, each phase would be an equal length of time. For any statistical analysis, having an equal or near-equal number of data points in the phases to be compared is advantageous. However, there is one circumstance where equal length of phases is not sought. If the participant's behavior or performance in the baseline phase is extremely variable, some researchers continue Phase A until the behavior stabilizes. The measurement logic of this elongation of phase is based on sampling theory. A sample will be a more accurate representation of the actual capabilities of the participant if it is larger and less variable. For example, if you only observed a child on the playground twice and one time the child played with classmates appropriately and the other time the child withdrew from them and hid, you could not feel confident stating that the regular experience of the child at recess was to hide 50% of the time. If, however, you had observed the child 20 times during recess and the child hid twice, you could be more confident in saying that the worrisome behavior occurred approximately 10% of the time.

Thus, the goals of the study are to enable the researcher to make some inferences about the relationship between the independent and the dependent variables and to draw some conclusions about the effectiveness of the interventions. Because the data analysis rides on the picture that the data points form, the reliability in their determination is crucial. Accuracy in plotting the points is also of vital importance. In the section following, the three types of changes between phases that can be identified will be discussed, along with the various techniques (statistical and non-statistical) of quantifying these changes in a dependable way.

9.7 VISUAL AND STATISTICAL ANALYSIS

A valuable aspect of SCED is that three types of changes between phases can be detected: change in level, change in slope, and change in variability. These changes could occur one at a time, two at a time, or all three at once. Note that in traditional group experimental design, the main attention is placed upon changes in level (i.e., a difference in the means of the two groups being compared). Much less often is attention placed in a group design on differences in slope (differences in the change in the dependent variable over time) between the groups or on differences in variability between the two groups. There is nothing that prevents a researcher from building these analyses into a group design. However, an SCED more readily lends itself to examining both level and slope, and sometimes in addition variability, given the way data are collected and displayed.

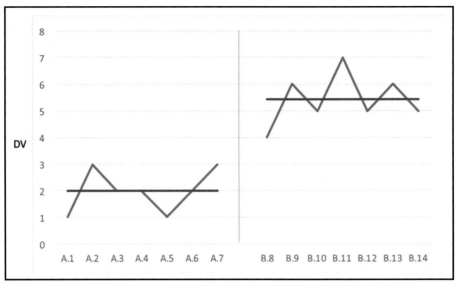

Figure 9-7. Change in level, baseline to intervention phases. Each A is a data collection occasion in baseline, each B an occasion during intervention. The phases are separated slightly for clarity.

9.7.1 Change in Level

A change in level of the dependent variable from one phase to the next would be indicated by a bump in the graphed line upward or downward (Figure 9-7). Assuming that up is better in this case, the researcher would want to know two things about this bump. First, could it have happened purely by chance (through random variation in the behavior or performance of the participant) and not be due to the independent variable? Second, if the level change upward seems to be the new norm for the participant, is the performance now at a level that is functional, akin to normal, or meeting a criterion for task completion, habit consistency, or maintenance of a routine? In other words, as with group experiments, the researcher must appraise both the statistical validity and the clinical or occupational validity of the change. Statistical procedures adapted for SCED can help answer the first question. Only knowledge of human occupation and of the goals of the participant and family can help answer the second. Tools for the analysis of level will be discussed in the following section.

9.7.2 Change in Slope

During the baseline phase, there could be any of three types of slope in the data points. They could show essentially no change in level over time (i.e., a zero slope); they could slope upward (assuming still that up is better); or they could be sloping downward. Now assume the intervention has begun and data are being collected during Phase B. For each of the slopes of Phase A (-, 0, +), there could arise a negative, zero, or positive slope in the subsequent Phase B. Consider what the importance of each of these combinations might be. If the baseline slope is zero and the intervention slope is also zero (so there would be no change

in level), we would tend to conclude that the intervention had no effect. If the baseline slope is zero and the intervention was accompanied by an upward slope, then we might conclude that the intervention probably had a positive effect on the participant's outcome. If the baseline slope was already upward, it would take a sharp ramping up of that slope to persuade us that the intervention had a beneficial effect (Figure 9-8). After all, in this case the participant was already performing better over time in the baseline phase. If the baseline slope were downward, we might consider it a victory for the intervention to have changed that slope to zero (that is, help a person whose behavior was in decline to level off). Of course, the researcher would be most happy if a negative baseline slope were changed by the intervention into a positive, upward slope (Figure 9-9). Tools to help the researcher determine whether these changes in slope could have merely happened by chance are discussed later in this chapter.

9.7.3 Change in Variability

Variability itself is not often a concern in therapy situations; however, it may be the key consideration. Suppose a young man or a young woman had a flat affect due to an emotional trauma. Little to no variation in facial expression could lead to notable disadvantages in social communication and participation. The goal for therapy, and thus the focus of analysis in a corresponding SCED, would be to increase the variability of facial expression. A different situation would be where a person is experiencing marked role dysfunction due to alternating periods of mania and depression. Here, the therapist, and likewise the SCED researcher, would seek to dampen the variability of mood experienced by the person (Figure 9-10). Thus, it may be beneficial for the variability of behavior to be increased in

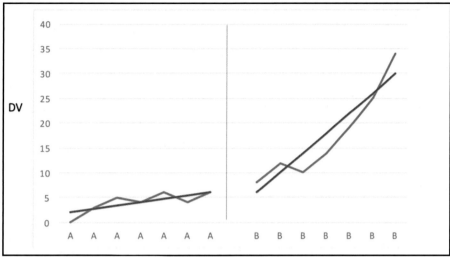

Figure 9-8. Change in slope upward, baseline to intervention phases. Each A is a data collection occasion in baseline, each B an occasion during intervention. The phases are separated slightly for clarity. Red lines are slope for that phase.

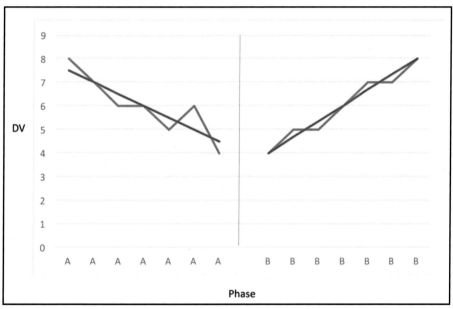

Figure 9-9. Change in slope from downward to upward, baseline to intervention phases. Each A is a data collection occasion in baseline, each B an occasion during intervention. The phases are separated slightly for clarity. Red lines are slope for that phase.

some studies and decreased in others, depending on the condition and the situation. In either case, an SCED, with its repeated measurements, could be the means for persuasively demonstrating that the intervention probably had the desired effect.

9.7.4 Change in Level With a Positive or Negative Baseline Slope

Assume the slope in the data during baseline phase is upward and the intervention was accompanied by a positive bump to the natural healing, learning, or developmental process, without the slope changing. That would probably

indicate an intervention that was successful. If the baseline slope was downward (as in a chronic, progressive disease) and the intervention gave a decline stalling bump to the process, it could also be considered a positive effect, even if the long-term downward trend continues.

Occasionally, an intervention will temporarily have a negative effect on a client's performance but will result in greater benefits in the long run. Ayres (1972) claimed that traditional Ayres Sensory Integration therapy for children with learning disabilities would sometimes cause an immediate disorganization in the child's movement. However, after some weeks of therapy, the child would have improved at such a pace (despite the momentary bump downward) that the current performance was superior to where it

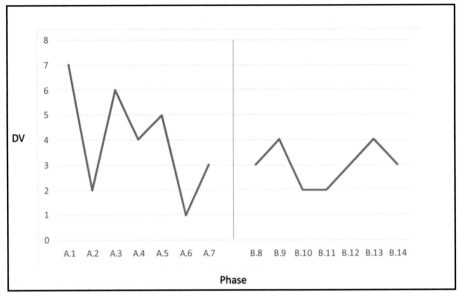

Figure 9-10. Change variability downward, baseline to intervention phases. Each A is a data collection occasion in baseline, each B an occasion during intervention. The phases are separated slightly for clarity.

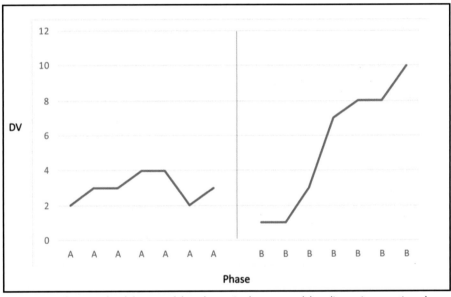

Figure 9-11. Change in level downward, but change in slope upward, baseline to intervention phases. Each A is a data collection occasion in baseline, each B an occasion during intervention. The phases are separated slightly for clarity.

would have been without therapy. In an SCED graph, this scenario might look like Figure 9-11.

Changes in level, slope, and variability must be interpreted considering the salient factors pertaining to the particular situations studied in the SCED. Furthermore, when multiple graphs are available, either because of multiple participants or because of multiple baselines, there are more opportunities to examine and interpret similarities and differences or to point out where the data fulfilled the expectations of the researcher and where they did not. Such detailed "narratives" interpreting client changes in functional performance with respect to level, slope, and variability—within a participant

as well as across participants—virtually never occur in a group experimental design study, with its focus on the comparison of group mean scores.

9.7.5 Statistical Analysis

Despite some early objections to using statistical approaches for the analysis of SCED data, doing so is now widely accepted. Some mathematical assumptions of the statistical procedures are not met; thus, it is prudent to interpret any statistical analysis cautiously, with a recognition of where limitations may exist.

Figure 9-12. Two-standard deviation band method of statistical analysis. Each A is a data collection occasion in baseline, each B an occasion during intervention. The phases are separated slightly for clarity. Two consecutive circled points mean performance improved in Phase B ($P < .05$).

There are three basic statistical approaches to the analysis of data in SCEDs: (1) the two-standard deviation (2-SD) band method (when there is a zero slope in the baseline phase); (2) the split-middle/binomial test (when the baseline data do show a slope up or down); and (3) the C-statistic (showing whether there is a trend in the baseline phase and, if not, whether the intervention data in the subsequent Phase B differ from the baseline data; Portney & Watkins, 2009). There are additional, less common statistical methods that are not covered in this chapter, such as the non-overlap techniques described by Parker, Vannest, and Davis (2011).

9.7.5.1 Two-Standard Deviation Band Method

If the data in the baseline phase are stable (have a zero slope) and are about six or more in number, then the 2-SD band method may be used. The analysis is based on the logic of the null hypothesis, which would declare that any difference in level seen between the baseline phase and the intervention phase data is due solely to chance (random variation). If the data of Phase B show enough difference that it is improbable it would have happened by chance, then we can reject the null hypothesis and claim that the difference seen is probably real.

To use the 2-SD band method, the mean value for the points in the baseline phase is found (add the value of the points together and divide by the number of points). A solid line is drawn across Phase A at this level on the graph, then the SD of the Phase A points is calculated. Only include the Phase A data points (not A and B) when calculating the SD. The size of the SD is then doubled, and this amount is added to and subtracted from the mean value found earlier. Dashed or dotted lines are drawn at these two levels across

Phase A, forming a band. This band is 2 SDs above the mean and 2 SDs below the mean (or actually 4 SDs wide). The dashed lines of the 2-SD band are now drawn across Phase B. If two consecutive data points from Phase B fall outside the band, then one can reject the null hypothesis of there being no real difference between Phases A and B. Having two consecutive points outside the band is held to be too unlikely for the null to be retained. If the points outside the band are outside in the desired direction, then one may claim that the Phase B performance level is better than the Phase A level (Figure 9-12).

9.7.5.2 Split-Middle/Binomial Test Method

If there appears to be a slope in Phase A then using the 2-SD band method is not valid because the slope, left alone as it continues across Phase B, would result in higher data points. Even if the conditions in the 2-SD band method for rejecting the null hypothesis were triggered, it would not enable a valid claim that the Phase B performance was higher due to the intervention. The Phase A slope indicated that the participant was already improving before the intervention began. Under this condition, a difference in the level between Phases A and B would not be evidence of an effective intervention.

In this case, the split-middle/binomial test method can be used. Here, the null hypothesis is used once again, but this time with respect to the existing slope in the data across Phase A. If the intervention had no effect, then this slope would be expected to continue unchanged across Phase B, except for random variation. However, if the Phase B points show enough of a deviation from this expectation, then we can reject the null and claim that a change did take place when the intervention was instituted.

Figure 9-13. Split-middle method of analysis with binomial test. Each A is a data collection occasion in baseline, each B an occasion during intervention. Red line is slope of data in Phase A projected across Phase B. With 8 points above the red line and 1 point beneath, one could conclude that Phase B performance is improved (*P* < .05).

To find the line representing the overall slope of Phase A, count the number of data points in the baseline, divide the total number of data points in half, and draw a dashed vertical line between the two adjacent points between the first half of points and the second half of points. (If baseline had an odd number of points, then draw the vertical line through the middle point, leaving an equal number of points to the left and right of it.) Within each of these half-phases, find the median value of the points in that half-phase. Plot this median value at the position on the x-axis representing the mid-point of time in this half-phase. Then do this for the second half of Phase A. Draw a solid line connecting these two points. If necessary, adjust this line upward or downward (but keeping it parallel to its original alignment) so that there are an equal number of Phase A points above and below the line. (This adjustment is often not necessary.)

Now extend this solid line into and across Phase B. Phase B points will lie on either side of this line (Figure 9-13). If the null hypothesis is true, 50% of the points would appear above and below the line (the intervention made no difference). However, it would also not be unlikely if the points divided 60%/40% or even 70%/30% in cases where there are not many data points in Phase B. Indeed, with only 4 to 8 data points in Phase B, they would all need to be above the solid line drawn from the baseline phase to reject the null. If there are 9 points in Phase B, then one of them could be below the solid line and we could reject the null at an alpha of .05. For 12 points in Phase B, two of them could be below the solid line and we could still reject the null hypothesis at α = .05. These decisions are based on the probability values in a binomial test statistical table (see Table C-11).

If the evidence is present to reject the null, then the claim can be made that we are 95% confident that performance in Phase B is better (or worse, if the points went that direction) than in Phase A—and not from pure chance. The strength of any argument that the intervention itself caused this difference would need to be built up with supporting evidence. For example, if a return to baseline conditions was accompanied by a decline in performance and then a reapplication of the intervention caused an increase, the researcher could be more confident that the intervention is causing the increases. Nonetheless, this evidence does not constitute proof that the intervention was the cause. It just makes it more plausible that the intervention caused the change.

9.7.5.3 C-Statistic

A less-often used alternative analytic method for SCED data is the C-statistic. The C-statistic estimates trends in a time series. It needs a minimum of 8 data points in Phase A (Tryon, 1982). First, it determines whether there is no trend in the baseline. Then, if there is not, it determines whether there is a difference between the baseline (A) and the treatment (B) phases. For more detail on the C-statistic, see Ottenbacher (1986a), Portney and Watkins (2015), and Tryon (1982).

All three of the approaches described can be equally used to test for changes from Phase B to a return to baseline or from the second Phase A to the second Phase B, and so on. Most authors explicitly warn that these analyses should only be used to compare adjacent phases in the data stream. The most important reason for this warning is that the logic of the null hypothesis only applies between a given phase and the immediately preceding phase of data.

9.7.5.4 The Phenomenon of Serial Dependency (or Autocorrelation)

In many group statistical comparisons, one assumption of the statistical test is that the data points are independent of one another (e.g., in an independent *t*-test or an analysis of variance). An example of non-independence of data would be if children were given a motor test where those waiting their turn could see the children being tested before them. The performance of one child could influence the performance of another, contaminating the independence of the data. In SCED, since the entire data stream is derived from the same individual, it is likely that the assumption of independence of data is violated. If it is, there could exist the situation of serial dependency or autocorrelation. Ottenbacher (1986a) and others recommend testing for autocorrelation in any data set in SCED. Its presence would not affect the C-statistic but could affect the accuracy of the 2-SD band method or the split-middle/binomial test method.

Therefore, although it is advisable to use statistical analyses to avoid some of the pitfalls of a pure visual analysis, these analyses have their own limitations. They should always be interpreted in context and with caution.

9.8 INTERPRETATION OF RESULTS IN SINGLE-CASE EXPERIMENTAL DESIGN

9.8.1 Immediate Interpretation

Applying visual and statistical analyses to the data points of an SCED puts the researcher in a position to make justifiable inferences about what the experiment has shown. These inferences should only be made while keeping in mind the following possible limitations.

Did the measuring instrument for the dependent variable (or the operationalization of the dependent variable) have noteworthy limitations? Larger than desirable random measurement error in the dependent variable might manifest itself as larger than expected variability in the plotted data. If the 2-SD band method of analysis was used, then the larger variability in Phase A would result in a wider SD band. This greater width would make it less likely for any improvement to have produced two consecutive Phase B points outside the band. This disadvantage is analogous to greater variability in a group experimental design, lessening statistical power.

According to the scale used for the dependent variable, it might display a floor or ceiling effect. A *floor effect* means that the dependent variable scale cannot measure below a certain performance or behavior level. Suppose the

researcher is seeking to show statistically that the intervention diminished a negative behavior. The plotted data from Phase A give rise to a 2-SD band that is below the lowest possible score on the dependent variable. It would then be impossible for Phase B to produce two consecutive data points outside the SD band. It will appear that the intervention had no noteworthy effect. If the change sought is upward, then a *ceiling effect* would likewise prevent the researcher from using a 2-SD band method to demonstrate the intervention's effectiveness.

Another interpretive limitation occurs when there are missing data points. The participant may be ill one day so no data were collected. Should the x-axis be collapsed across that missing day? Whether the researcher compresses the x-axis could influence the outcome if a split-middle/binomial test is used in the analysis. Similarly, if there are only a few data points in Phase A, then the 2-SD band will be based on such a small number of points that confidence in its accuracy will be weakened. Likewise, the split-middle/binomial test method, when used with only a few data points in Phase A, may become unstable and thus be potentially misleading. When there are few points in Phase B (fewer than 9), it is difficult or impossible to reject the null hypothesis.

Mid-phase changes in level, slope, or variability pose additional challenges for interpretation. First, there arises the question, What could have caused this change? It is convenient to think that only the independent variable could cause a change in the dependent variable, but we know that for matters of human performance, this assumption is far too simple. Such mid-phase changes also create the following dilemma: Should only the data after the change be used to examine subsequent changes between Phases A and B? Or should all the Phase A points still be averaged together to form a representative 2-SD band or sloped line? There is no mathematical answer to these questions. The researcher must make the case logically, with reference to the context of the participant being studied.

9.8.2 Long-Term Interpretation

Once the decision has been made whether the Phase A to Phase B transition is accompanied by improved performance, no change, or a decline in performance, and once parallel decisions have been made for every other phase transition (e.g., B to A, A to B), there remains the need to interpret the meaning of the SCED as a whole. In a multi-participant SCED, this task would also involve considering why the intervention seemed to work for some individuals but not for others (McGruder et al., 2003; see Figure 9-6). Having demographic and diagnostic information about the participants to hypothesize about possible causes of a difference can be helpful here.

9.9 Global/Social/ Ecological Validity

Even clear and persuasive inferences from the experimental data of SCED, with their selected, operationalized outcomes, do not automatically translate to the actual contextualized, occupational life of the individual participant. One way to improve external validity is to collect data in multiple settings and on several participants. A final inference needs to be made, ultimately, about whether the intervention holds promise for similar individuals in their own unique naturalistic settings.

9.10 Strengths

The strengths of SCEDs are multiple. The intervention usually takes place in naturalistic (non-contrived) settings, such as a school, the community, or the home. The intervention is individualized, which accords with client-centered practice. In some SCEDs, the intervention is graded up or down as necessary. They offer the possibility of enlisting multiple cases or collecting data in multiple settings or under multiple conditions to reveal how variables may interact. Indeed, by focusing attention on a single individual case, an SCED can reveal the cumulative and complex interactions among all variables that are measured, giving rise to new insights, hypotheses, or theories.

A strength of SCEDs is their ability to display changes in the level of the dependent variable, in the change in the dependent variable over time (slope), and in the variability of the dependent variable during control (A) and experimental (B) phases. This detail allows for a more sophisticated investigation of the relationship between the independent and dependent variables in the context of existing knowledge about them. Further illustration of this relationship follows.

Historically, SCEDs have been criticized for lacking generalizability. Of course, as an N-of-1 study, an SCED cannot have the type of statistical generalizability that a group experiment can have when its sample has been randomly selected from a population. Such a claim is rarely made by the authors of an SCED. However, these authors themselves often underestimate the strength of generalizability that an SCED can have. That is, one therapist achieving a positive outcome with one client using a specified intervention demonstrates that it is at least a possibility that other therapists can achieve this same result by applying the insights gained. The knowledge that a possibility exists can be particularly valuable for intervention decisions for clients who have a rare condition, multiple diagnoses, unusual impairments or challenges, or for whom standard approaches have not been successful.

Some SCEDs (e.g., ATD) offer a fast, reliable comparison of equipment options, tool options, postural or technique options, or options in environmental conditions or modifications, allowing for a persuasive argument to be made for the superiority of one over another.

Finally, SCED can suggest why an intervention works with one individual and not with another, or which intervention works better for which individuals. This aspect of discovering knowledge for customized therapy is often not pursued in group experimental studies.

9.11 Weaknesses

Nonetheless, there are certain inherent weaknesses in SCEDs. Chief among them is a challenge with external validity. Is the participant in an SCED representative of other clients? The random selection of a sample, sometimes possible in group experimental studies, strengthens the external validity of group studies. As mentioned previously, SCEDs do not have the statistical models of traditional group experimental designs with adequate degrees of freedom and statistical power to support internal validity. Additionally, the influence on the outcome of the therapeutic relationship between the independent variable provider and the client may be difficult to assess. Indeed, practitioner bias should be addressed in SCEDs but is difficult to control in this design. Measurement limitations may also exist. Although not exclusive to SCEDs, these consist of floor and ceiling effects, insensitivity in the dependent variable to small but important changes, an unknown relationship of the outcome performance or behavior to the norms in society, or an unknown amount of the dependent variable that would be the criterion for independent performance in a population.

In the analysis of SCED data, there is often a bending of certain statistical assumptions, especially independence among data points. The data display of SCED is vulnerable to graphing contingencies, such as missing data.

Finally, a dependable argument for the causal relationship between the independent and the dependent variables can be complicated. It is often built upon several component inferences, unlike in a group experiment. In the latter, rejecting the null via a single statistical test can be taken as a sufficient reason to confidently claim that the intervention caused the better outcome in the clients receiving it, compared to the control group. Due to the possible honeymoon, or short-term Hawthorne effect in the client upon receiving a novel treatment, SCEDs need to be replicated to strengthen any causal claim.

For these and other reasons, SCED researchers have recently issued the SCRIBE Guidelines (Tate et al., 2016) to protect against some of the possible flaws in SCED and to provide better detail and transparency so that replication by other researchers is more straightforward.

9.12 WHEN IS A SINGLE-CASE EXPERIMENTAL DESIGN APPLICABLE?

It is feasible to undertake an SCED when:
- Maintaining a baseline period is ethical and can be done long enough to establish a relatively stable picture of the typical range of performance on the dependent variable for this individual before intervention begins.
- The desired outcome performance is measurable.
- Repeated measurements of the individual are feasible and not contraindicated by limited endurance or a measurement tool that is affected by repeated administration.
- Intervention creates an immediate or a near-immediate effect on outcome.
- The case can be followed long enough to establish a persuasive pattern in the data.
- Constructs of interest (whether occupation-based or client-centered factors) are feasible to quantify.

9.13 WHEN IS A SINGLE-CASE EXPERIMENTAL DESIGN NOT APPLICABLE?

An SCED is not applicable for studying a case when:
- The baseline measures show great instability.
- It is not feasible, ethical, valid, or safe to measure the dependent variable repeatedly.
- There is a long or unknown lag time between the intervention and a demonstrable effect.
- An interaction of the intervention studied with other simultaneous interventions is present.
- Uncontrollable outside events or dramatically changing external conditions occur.
- Only a brief period is available for intervention and measuring its effect (except for SCEDs using the ATD).
- The selected occupation-based constructs are difficult to measure through repeated data collection.

See Figure 9-14 for a flowchart showing the design and implementation of a SCED.

9.14 ROLE OF SINGLE-CASE EXPERIMENTAL DESIGN IN THE PROFESSION: CONTRIBUTIONS TO RESEARCH AND PRACTICE

Of 53 SCEDs published in AJOT during 1990–2017, 34 (64.2%) pertained to pediatric clients and 19 (35.8%) to adults. Of the total, 7 (13.2%) were concerned with classroom seating and weighted clothing, 6 (11.3%) with computers, 6 (11.3%) with sensory integration intervention, 5 (9.4%) with pediatric splinting, 3 (5.7%) with oral function in young children, 3 (5.7%) with vision, 3 (5.7%) with edema treatment, 2 (3.8%) with pediatric constraint-induced movement therapy, 2 (3.8%) with intervention for adults with traumatic brain injury, 11 (20.8%) with miscellaneous pediatric topics, 3 (5.7%) with the elderly, and 3 (5.7%) with miscellaneous adult topics.

These SCEDs made notable contributions to knowledge in the field in many ways. As their participant selection was rarely anything other than a convenience sample, one cannot make a statistical projection about the generalizability of their findings to the larger population. However, their findings do offer other evidence about practice that is of value to therapists. First, some SCEDs allow a generalization from one or a few cases to a hypothesis—that is, why a certain intervention was effective for a person or why there was a difference in response among different individuals. For example, in McGruder et al. (2003), wearing a weighted wrist cuff was accompanied by taking less time to self-feed in 4/5 participants with a static acquired brain lesion. In 2/5 participants, the tremors themselves occurred at a statistically reduced rate during feeding. However, the mechanism of reduction for one participant seemed to be greater proprioceptive input but was greater biomechanical inertia for the other. The participant who showed no statistically significant improvement on any outcome variable had had surgery to remove a brain tumor. Other symptoms seemed to mask her tremors (McGruder et al., 2003). From these differences among participants, several hypotheses about the complex effects of using weighted cuffs could be devised. Such insights could then inform practitioners making decisions about the type of intervention to try with future clients.

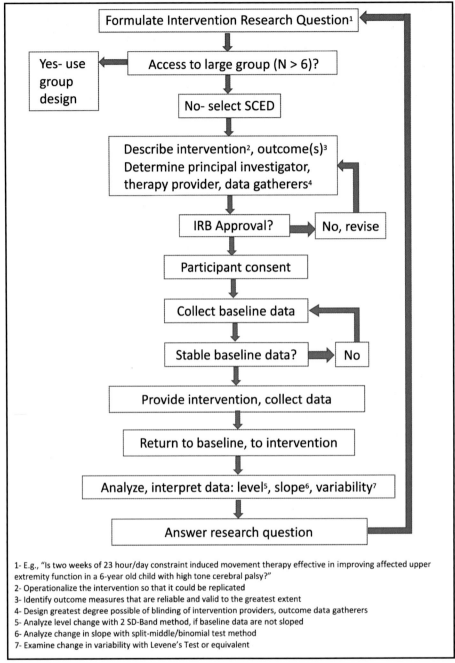

Figure 9-14. SCED process.

Other SCEDs provide the opportunity to generalize from a case to the idea of an innovative possibility. For example, Casby and Holm (1994) discovered that in 2/3 elderly individuals with dementia, playing music via personal earphones was accompanied by a significantly diminished number of disruptive vocalizations. Even if this intervention was effective for only a minority of clients, its ease and low cost would indicate that practitioners should certainly try it.

It is also possible for an SCED to demonstrate how occupationally important variables can be operationalized and reliably measured (Watling & Deitz, 2007). The authors

defined *undesired, interfering behavior,* and *engagement* for four 3- to 4-year-olds who were video-recorded during structured play sessions. Inter-rater reliability for these two constructs was 95% and 91%, respectively. Although the provision of sensory integration treatment did not result in immediate statistically significant effects in the children, their parents and their treating therapists reported greater social interaction and easier transitioning between activities after the treatments (Watling & Deitz, 2007).

Just as group experimental studies, SCEDs can indicate what amount of improvement in client performance might be expected from a given intervention over a certain period of time. DeVries, Deitz, and Anson (1998) demonstrated that in two clients with spinal cord injury, neither a mouthstick nor a head-mounted pointer allowed word processing speeds at a vocationally competitive rate for text entry. Gutman, Raphael-Greenfield, and Rao (2012) demonstrated that the greatest amount of learning of social skills in 15- to 17-year-olds with ASD occurred in the first phase of the program—namely, a 150% increase in the appearance of targeted positive behaviors. Mulcahey et al. (1995) documented how an 11-year-old boy improved from 0 lateral pinch to 3.5 pounds of pinch after 1 year, subsequent to tendon transfer surgery and occupational therapy treatment. In all three cases, the SCED showed what is possible in magnitude of outcome following the intervention.

SCED can be effective in showing how durable improvements may be over time. Gustafsson et al. (2016) presented findings that indicated the reduction in post-stroke edema accompanying the use of finger to axilla compression bandages for 7 days was not maintained after bandage removal. Furthermore, when circular-knit compression gloves were used after bandage removal, success was mixed. Only at the mid-proximal phalanx of the third digit were edema gains sustained; the reductions were reversed at the other four more proximal points of the upper extremity. Such SCED inform practitioners which interventions are likely not to provide client benefit.

Another important purpose of SCED is to serve as a pilot project, where promising results would justify further research. Crocker, MacKay-Lyons, and McDonnell (1997) found that after 3 weeks of splinting the less-involved upper extremity, a 2-year-old girl with cerebral palsy had better quality, quantity, and variety of use in the more involved extremity, persisting at a 6-month follow-up. Dickerson and Brown (2007) discovered that gains in spontaneous reach, pushing a button for sound, and pulling a toy in the more involved upper extremity of a 2-year-old boy with prenatal stroke accompanied 3 weeks of constraint-induced movement therapy. Most of the gains were sustained at a 1-month follow-up. In the ensuing 10 years, at least 5 group experimental studies on pediatric constraint-induced movement therapy have been published in AJOT. The SCED showed the feasibility, operationalization of procedures, and promising outcomes from this approach, enabling the later, larger studies.

Also of value, SCEDs can inform practitioners of the possibility that a certain intervention gives rise to no measurable effect in the type of client studied. Ross (1992) found that early versions of visual scanning computer applications, popular at the time in rehabilitation facilities, were not actually accompanied by increased performance in functional tasks by three adults with a traumatic brain injury. Umeda and Deitz (2011) found no measurable

improvements in classroom behaviors of two kindergarten pupils with ASD when therapy cushions were used for seating. Nonetheless, because they were simple to use and showed no noticeable negative effects, the classroom teacher involved in the study wanted to keep them available. He reported that the cushions sometimes appeared to help the students' attention to task. These SCEDs serve as a reminder that findings might become outdated (given the increase in sophistication of software between 1992 and now), and that an intervention with no known harmful effects can be perceived as useful to have at hand.

Finally, SCED can serve as a model for collaboration between practitioner and academician where the practitioner provides the clinical case and the academician assists in the research methodology, improving the control over confounding variables (Sharpe & Ottenbacher, 1990). In fact, given the thin coverage of the 53 SCEDs published in AJOT over the 27 years covered, one could cogently advocate for far more collaboration between researchers and practitioners in documenting these small-scale but important advances in occupational therapy practice.

9.15 SUMMARY

In this chapter, the authors describe various components of an SCED. SCEDs can be used in occupational therapy clinical research to provide evidence for assessing the effectiveness of an intervention. As a type of experimental design, SCED studies apply a research hypothesis, operationally define an independent variable (intervention), control extraneous variables, and measure outcomes (dependent variable) by using reliable and valid assessments with one or a small number of participants. Their design structures range from the simple (AB) to the complex (ABABAB). Internal validity of the findings of an SCED can be strengthened by multiple phase changes, multiple baseline starting times, multiple outcome measures, and multiple contexts of investigation. One of the advantages of an SCED is that it can be used to portray changes in level, slope, and variability in the data, a more detailed analysis than usually available with other methodologies. Another advantage is that with one or two participants, it can serve as a pilot study to justify further research. The 53 SCEDs reviewed for this chapter, appearing in AJOT from 1990 to 2017, have made several distinctive contributions to the occupational therapy literature. They identified interventions that may be effective, even in individuals with severe or complex conditions. They have suggested why a particular therapy works for some individuals and not for others. Last, they have documented the magnitude of effect that an intervention may have.

10

Selecting a Test Instrument

For all such areas of research—and for many others—the precise measurement of individual differences made possible by well-constructed tests is an essential prerequisite.

—Anastasi (1988, p. 4)

OPERATIONAL LEARNING OBJECTIVES

By the end of this chapter the learner will be able to:

- Define key concepts in testing.
- Discuss the early history in the development of testing.
- Identify the major purposes of testing.
- Know where to look for bibliographies of tests in books, test catalogues, and online.
- Know how to select a test for a specific function and target population.
- Know how to evaluate reliability and validity of tests.
- Know how to incorporate tests into a research study.
- Determine the skills necessary in:
  - Administering tests
  - Scoring tests
  - Interpreting results of tests
- Develop an objective attitude in selecting a test instrument and evaluating its effectiveness.
- Identify the potential sources of error in testing.

Rice, M. S., Stein, F., & Tomlin, G.
Clinical Research in Occupational Therapy, Sixth Edition (pp. 291-338).
© 2019 Taylor & Francis Group.

TABLE 10-1

KEY CONCEPTS IN TESTS AND MEASUREMENTS

- Assessment refers to the entire process of obtaining, interpreting, and documenting an individual's functional status (American Occupational Therapy Association [AOTA], 2014). Assessment involves gathering data from client records, the client, family members, administration of one or more assessment tools or procedures, and integrating the information so that appropriate therapy can be planned (Powell, 2008).
- Evaluation refers to "gathering data on performance, such as activities of daily living (ADLs) or observation, or using a specific tool or tools in one or more areas" (Powell, 2008, p. 390).
- Measurement is "a process of assigning quantitative values to objects or events according to certain rules" (Sattler, 2008, p. 92).
- A measurement scale is a system of assigning scores to a trait or characteristic.
- A test is essentially an objective and standardized measure of a sample of behavior (Anastasi & Urbina, 1997).
- A major purpose of a test is to predict future performance based on a current sample of behaviors.
- An extremely important quality of a test is to accurately detect change in an individual's behavior (e.g., improvement).
- The value of a test depends on its purposes, ability to predict outcome, and the degree of consistency and precision in defining a variable.
- The degree of accuracy of a test is based on its ability to be consistent (reliability) and to test what it claims to measure (validity).
- The sources of error in measurement are derived from factors such as the unreliability of the instrument, bias of the test administrator, behavior from the client, and adverse test environment
- Distributions of data from heterogeneous populations tend to be normally distributed, while data from homogeneous populations tend to be skewed.
- A norm-referenced test (NRT) is a standardized sampling of behavior that uses data from a heterogeneous group of individuals in interpreting results.
- A criterion-referenced test (CRT) is a standardized sampling of behavior that bases performance on accepted standards of competency.

Adapted from Anastasi, A., & Urbina, S. (1997). *Psychological testing* (7th ed.). Englewood Cliffs, NJ: Prentice Hall; Sattler, J. M. (1992). *Assessment of children* (3rd ed., Rev.). San Diego, CA: Author.

10.1 KEY CONCEPTS IN TESTING

To understand testing and evaluation, one should be able to define the key concepts. How is a test defined? How does the evaluator determine what is normal behavior and what is atypical behavior? Why are tests used? What are potential sources of error in testing? What is the difference between norm- and criterion-referenced tests? These key concepts, listed in Table 10-1, are elaborated upon in this chapter.

10.2 EARLY HISTORY OF TEST DEVELOPMENT

Tests have been used for generations for problem solving and decision making. For example, in the 12th century, the Chinese used civil service examinations to make hiring

decisions (Teng, 1943). The ancient Greeks administered physical and intellectual tests as part of the educational process. In Europe, from the time of the Middle Ages, universities gave tests as part of the process of awarding professional degrees and bestowing honors. In the United States, procedures for testing applicants to the U.S. Civil Service were introduced in 1883. Not until the 19th century, however, when an interest in providing humane treatment to individuals with intellectual disabilities and mental illness arose, were tests developed that could identify and distinguish between intellectual disabilities and emotional disturbance (Anastasi & Urbina, 1997; Sattler, 2008; see Table 10-2 for a summary of major events in test development during the 19th and 20th centuries).

Traditionally, test theorists have taken the viewpoint that human characteristics and abilities are normally distributed. Thus, researchers involved in early test development sought to demonstrate what was normal to identify those individuals who differed significantly from the

TABLE 10-2

EARLY HISTORY OF THE TEST MOVEMENT

THEORIST	OCCUPATION	CONTRIBUTION TO TESTING
Jean-Étienne Dominique Esquirol (1838)	Physician	Classified individuals with intellectual disabilities into various levels of intellectual disability; believed that language provided the best measure of intelligence.
Paul Broca (1864)	Surgeon	Proposed a relationship between the volume of the brain and intelligence.
Sir Francis Galton (1883)	Biologist	Theorized that physical traits (i.e., visual and hearing acuity, muscular strength) and reaction speed could serve as a measure of gauging intellectual abilities.
James McKeen Cattell (1890)	Psychologist	Developed norms in sensory, motor, and simple perceptual processes for comparing individuals, helping to create the concept of mental measurement.
Emil Kraepelin (1895)	Psychiatrist	Developed assessment of daily living skills based on perception, memory, attention, and motor functioning. Interested in the clinical examinations of psychiatric patients. Tests of critical functions were designed to measure practice effects in memory and susceptibility to fatigue and to distraction.
Charles E. Spearman (1904)	Psychologist	Proposed that intelligence was comprised of a primary factor (g) and specific factors (s).
Alfred Binet (1905)	Psychologist	Along with Simon, developed a test that identified children who could not benefit from formal education. This instrument consisted of short tests measuring perception, judgment, comprehension, and reasoning.
Lewis M. Terman (1916)	Psychologist	Popularized and revised Binet's scale by including tasks to identify superior adult intelligence and by assigning age equivalents to items.
H. H. Goddard (1919)	Educator	Introduced Binet's scale in the United States, adding categories of intellectual ability and disability.
Robert M. Yerkes (1921)	Psychologist	Instrumental in developing the Army Alpha, a verbal test, and the Army Beta, a visual test, for group testing. He also espoused the idea of point scales rather than age scales.
Louis L. Thurstone (1938)	Psychologist	Proposed that intelligence was comprised of several different factors, which he called *primary mental abilities*, all of which could be considered equally important.
David Wechsler (1939)	Psychologist	Developed the Wechsler-Bellevue, the precursor to the Wechsler Scales. This test had a verbal scale and a performance scale.
Raymond B. Cattell (1979)	Psychologist	Along with John Horn, proposed that intelligence was comprised of fluid (nonverbal, novel, relatively culture-free) and crystallized (acquired skills strongly dependent upon culture) reasoning.

(continued)

TABLE 10-2 (CONTINUED)		
EARLY HISTORY OF THE TEST MOVEMENT		
THEORIST	**OCCUPATION**	**CONTRIBUTION TO TESTING**
Jagannath Das (1963)	Psychologist	Used an information-processing model to describe cognitive functioning. Information is obtained through two distinct methods: simultaneously and sequentially.
J. P. Guilford (1967)	Psychologist	Attempted to link theory to test development by proposing a three-dimensional structure of intellect with 120 factors that led to a test that measured each factor.
Howard Gardner (1983)	Psychologist	Proposed that there are several autonomous intellectual competencies or multiple intelligences, which are manifested differently in different individuals.

typical population. Sir Francis Galton (1883), advocating the importance of individual differences, postulated that differences in physical characteristics such as vision, hearing, reaction time, and physical strength could be used to determine mental capabilities. He tried to validate his beliefs through the use of statistical methods developed by Karl Pearson (1900). Although he was unsuccessful in showing that mental abilities were related to physical characteristics, our use of a normative sample is a direct result of his hypothesis (Swanson & Watson, 1989). James McKeen Cattell (1890), an assistant to Galton, supported Galton's views that "mental tests" measuring sensory and physical abilities differentiated individuals. Although he found no relationship between these abilities and school achievement, he contributed to the understanding of tests and measurement by demonstrating that mental ability could be examined empirically (Sattler, 2008).

Eduardo Séquin (1997) also believed that individuals could be differentiated by sensory and motor-control abilities. Galton had believed that the differences were inherent and unchangeable; however, Séquin believed that training in these areas could improve one's intellectual potential. Currently his materials, such as the form board (a task in which individuals place wooden or plastic shapes into puzzle frames) are used as a part of a test battery for young children (Swanson & Watson, 1989).

One of the first attempts to classify individuals with intellectual disabilities was made by Jean-Étienne Dominique Esquirol (1838). He recognized that individuals with intellectual disabilities had diverse abilities and concluded that language development was the most important characteristic for distinguishing between degrees of intellectual capacity. His appreciation for the importance of language in the development of intellectual capacity influenced the development of intelligence tests (Anastasi & Urbina, 1997).

While researchers in the United States tried to measure intellectual development through performance on sensory and motor tasks, clinicians in Germany turned toward more complex and abstract tasks as a means of measuring

aptitude. Emil Kraepelin (1919), recognizing the importance of measuring skills needed for daily living, developed a battery that measured such skills as perception, memory, motor function, and attention. H. Ebbinghaus (2013), after teachers in Germany requested that he develop an aptitude test, produced a timed completion task consisting of reading passages from which words had been left out. This test was a forerunner of group intelligence tests. He also produced tests that assessed arithmetic and memory skills. Carl Wernicke (1970), noted for his work on aphasia and brain localization, investigated individual differences in verbal conceptual thinking and generalization.

10.2.1 Influence of Binet on IQ Testing

In 1905, Alfred Binet (, a French psychologist, and a colleague, Theodore Simon (1873–1961), were commissioned by the French government to develop a test that would identify those children who could not benefit from formal education (Binet & Simon, 1916). The content of Binet's test came from educational research and through a deductive analysis of the factors that underlie academic achievement. The Binet-Simon test was developed pragmatically, without a theory of intelligence to guide its contents. Nonetheless, the influence of individuals such as Esquirol and Séquin was apparent in that Binet included items measuring sensory perception, motor control, and language. In addition, the Binet-Simon intelligence test:

> had several unique characteristics: (1) questions were arranged in a hierarchy of difficulty, (2) levels were established for different ages (establishment of mental age), (3) a quantitative scoring system was applied, and (4) specific instructions for administration were built into the test. (Swanson & Watson, 1989, p. 9)

The initial test consisted of 30 items related to following simple directions, defining words, constructing sentences, and answering judgmental questions of a psychological nature.

Binet's test was translated into English by H. H. Goddard (1920) in 1910; Lewis Terman (1877–1956) revised the Binet-Simon Intelligence test in 1916 for use in the United States (Sattler, 2008; Swanson & Watson, 1989; Terman & Merrill, 1960). While Binet had perceived his instrument as a way to identify those students who needed to be instructed through alternative methods, Goddard, in the early 19th century, linked intelligence test scores to occupation and social status (Gould, 1996). Terman extended Binet's test by adding additional items suitable for testing adults and by adding the concept of "mental quotient" to that of mental age. Terman's revision became known as the *Stanford-Binet*, so named because he was a professor at Stanford University in California.

10.2.2 Alternative Tests to the Binet

Binet's test and the revisions by Terman were developed on the premise that one's ability to successfully complete a particular task was related to developmental level. Thus, in a heterogenous set of items arranged in a developmental sequence, age scores could be assigned based on the ability of a majority of children at a given age level to do a particular task. Mental ability was determined by obtaining a ratio between the obtained age score and one's chronological age. Tests that use this format to find mental abilities are said to have an age scale.

Discontent with age scores led individuals such as Robert M. Yerkes (1921, 1930) and David Wechsler (1939) to develop tests with a radically different scoring format. Rather than using age score, similar items were put together and points were assigned to each item. Then, the raw score, determined by the number of points received, was converted into standard scores and an overall score. Scales with this type of scoring are known as a point scale. The IQ scores derived in this manner are called *Deviation IQs*. At this time, most tests developed for school-age children, adolescents, and adults use the point scale, whereas developmental scales, developed for infants, toddlers, and preschoolers, use an age scale.

Another concern regarding intelligence testing was the emphasis on verbal reasoning seen on the Stanford-Binet. Tests such as the Leiter International Performance Scale (Leiter, 1948), the Arthur adaptation of the Leiter International Performance Scale (Arthur, 1949), the Kohs Block Design Tests (Kohs, 1923), and the Culture-Fair Intelligence Scale (Cattell, 1950) were developed to counterbalance the highly verbal influence of the Stanford-Binet. The Wechsler-Bellevue, developed in 1939 by Wechsler, consisted of a verbal and a performance scale. This test, based on Wechsler's conception that intelligence was global, included tasks from various sources (e.g., Kohs Block Design Test, Army Alpha, Army Beta). Although the items have changed over time, many of the same types of items are included in the present-day Wechsler scales (Sattler, 2008).

10.2.3 Factor Analytical Theories of Intelligence

With the development of computers and more advanced statistical methods (e.g., factor analysis), the concept of intelligence has changed drastically. Although both Binet and Wechsler believed that intelligence was composed of many different abilities, neither one had proposed a theory that identified the components of intelligence. Binet had used items that he believed would assess skills necessary to succeed in an academic setting. Wechsler, on the other hand, had borrowed from a number of available tests, all of which he believed were factors in the construct of intelligence (Sattler, 2008). It fell to theorists like Charles E. Spearman (1863–1936; Spearman, 1927), Edward L. Thorndike (1874–1949; Thorndike, Bregman, Cobb, & Woodyward, 1926), and Louis L. Thurstone (1938) to suggest the components contained in the construct of intelligence. In general, there were three viewpoints regarding the structure of intelligence:

1. Intelligence was composed of a primary factor called *g* made up of complex mental tasks, such as reasoning and problem solving, and specific factors called *s* that required less complex processes, such as speed of processing, visual-motor, and rote learning (Spearman, 1927).

2. Intelligence was multifactorial and similar abilities clustered to form more complex skills (Thorndike et al., 1926).

3. Intelligence was comprised of primary factors (e.g., verbal, perceptual speed, inductive reasoning, work fluency, space or visualization) rather than a single unitary factor (Thurstone, 1938).

More recently, others (e.g., Gardner, 2011; Guilford, 1967; Sternberg, 1985) have proposed alternative theories to account for the nature of intelligence. In an effort to link theory to intelligence tests, J. P. Guilford proposed in *The Nature of Human Intelligence* (Guilford, 1967) that human intellect could be understood by a three-dimensional model, which he called the *Structure of Intellect*. This structure contained (a) five operations, which defined the way we process information (e.g., divergent or convergent); (b) four contents, which defined the manner in which the material is presented (e.g., visual or verbal), and (c) six products, which defined the outcome of the mental process (e.g., units or classes). By using combinations of one attribute from each dimension, 120 factors of intelligence can be identified (5 operations × 4 contents × 6 products). Theoretically, if one were to assess a student in each of these 120 factors, one would have a better understanding of how the student learned and could provide an appropriate educational program for that student. Unfortunately, Guilford's model has not been widely accepted, nor has it been used in many research studies.

Raymond B. Cattell (1963) and John L. Horn (1968) agreed with Guilford (1967) that intelligence was not a unitary concept but disagreed in the specific components comprising intelligence. They suggested, instead, that intelligence is made up of two constructs: fluid (*Gf*) and crystallized (*Gc*). Tasks considered to be fluid intelligence include unlearned, culture-free, novel experiences in which adaptation or generalization of previously learned tasks is required (e.g., nonverbal analogies, block building, speed of processing, problem solving). Crystallized intelligence, on the other hand, is defined as acquired knowledge, such as what is learned in school or in cultural experiences. Examples of tasks measuring crystallized intelligence include vocabulary tests, verbal analogies, rote learning, and rule learning. Two tests that were developed using the concept of crystallized and fluid intelligence are the *Stanford-Binet Intelligence Scale-Fifth Edition* (SB5; Roid, 2003) and the *Kaufman Adolescent and Adult Intelligence Test* (Kaufman & Kaufman, 1993). The most recent revisions of the Wechsler scales have also incorporated this concept.

In 1993, John Carroll at Cambridge, England proposed that intelligence "could be understood best via three strata that differed in breadth and generality" (Miller, 2009, p. 104).

Each stratum represents a different level of abstraction. Stratum I includes approximately 70 narrow abilities derived from more than 400 data sets; Stratum II represents Carroll's groupings of differentiated broad abilities that are similar to the *Gf-Gc* factors recognized by Horn and others; Stratum III represents the construct of general intellectual ability (*g*). (Schrank, Miller, Wendling, & Woodcock, 2010, p. 2)

The integration of Cattell-Horn and Carroll's work has resulted in the Cattell-Horn-Carroll theory. As a result of continued research by McGrew (2005) and McGrew, Flanagan, Keith, & Vanderwood (1997), the theory has become the framework for the development of the Woodcock-Johnson (Woodcock, McGrew, Mather, & Schrank, 2003) assessment family (e.g., WJ-III Tests of Cognition, WJ-III Tests of Achievement). These assessments are widely used in education to determine eligibility for special education services.

10.2.4 Alternative Theories of Intelligence

Although factor analysis theories of intelligence are still the most widely accepted, two additional approaches to intelligence should be mentioned. One approach, information processing, involves the understanding of the ways in which individuals take in and transform the information so that it can be used. While information processing is frequently linked with memory processes, the concept has been extended by individuals such as Das, Kirby, and Jarman (1975) and Campione and Brown (1978). Das et al. (1975) conceptualized intelligence as having two processes: (1) simultaneous, in which information is processed in a spatial, gestalt manner, and (2) sequential, in which material is sequenced in temporal order. Campione and Brown (1978) theorized that intelligence consisted of structures that enabled learning (e.g., memory, efficiency) and an executive system that controlled and managed the components involved in problem solving (e.g., knowledge, metacognition, use of learning strategies). The latter theory has led special educators to emphasize the use of strategies in the learning process as a means of improving problem solving and learning. Continued research is needed to identify ways to teach learning strategies so that learners can benefit from the process.

A second approach to intelligence other than factor analysis is that proposed by Howard Gardner. In *Frames of Mind: The Theory of Multiple Intelligences*, Gardner (2011) proposed that there are several autonomous competencies, each of which can be thought of as separate intelligences. Although he only identified seven of these separate intelligences (linguistic, musical, logical-mathematical, spatial, bodily-kinesthetic, interpersonal, and intrapersonal), he suggested that there may be others. Gardner (2000) has added naturalist to his list and has considered spiritual, existential, and moral intelligences. Gardner's theory has taken hold in many educational circles, and curriculums have been developed to encourage development of each of these.

Another important influence has been emotional intelligence, defined as the ability or capacity to identify, assess, and control one's emotions (Mayer, Salovey, & Caruso, 2008). Although the idea was first introduced by Thorndike (1920) as social intelligence, the concept has been expanded by Salovey and Mayer (1990) and Goleman (1995). Proponents of emotional intelligence suggest that emotional intelligence may be more important than IQ in predicting success in the corporate field:

IQ washes out when it comes to predicting who, among a talented pool of candidates within an intellectually demanding profession will become the strongest leader. In part this is because of the floor effect: everyone at the top echelons of a given profession, or at the top levels of a large organization, has already been sifted for intellect and expertise. At those lofty levels a high IQ becomes a threshold ability, one needed just to get into and stay in the game. (Goleman, 1995, xiv-xv)

10.2.5 Group Aptitude and Achievement Tests

Although the early IQ tests were administered individually, the advent of World War I resulted in a need for group aptitude (mental ability) testing. In 1917, Yerkes, an American psychologist and professor at Yale, was appointed by the American Psychological Association (APA) to develop group mental tests that could effectively evaluate military recruits. Working with Goddard and Terman, Yerkes developed the Army Alpha, a verbal test, and the Army Beta, a perceptual test, to be administered to recruits who failed the Army Alpha. Although the army made little use of their tests, the major result was the obtaining of normative data on 1.75 million men and the recognition that levels of intelligence could be obtained through group testing. What transpired after that was the massive development and the multiplication of group testing for all groups in society. Students and job applicants were routinely administered tests to determine aptitude and achievement. Two factors led to this phenomenon of mass testing: (a) individuals could be tested simultaneously with less time and personnel needed to administer the tests and (b) simplified instructions enabled individuals without professional training in testing to administer the tests. Thus, many professionals working with groups (e.g., teachers, therapists, counselors, personnel directors) are able to administer group tests (Anastasi & Urbina, 1997; Gould, 1996).

Although group testing developed because of the need to determine intellectual ability, issues regarding academic achievement soon became a concern of the nation. Group written examinations were first introduced in the Boston schools in 1845 as a substitute for individual oral examinations. The Stanford Achievement Test, developed in 1923, was the first achievement test to be standardized by using statistical principles of measurement (Sattler, 2008). The practice of mass educational testing continues today at the national level, where students enrolled in public schools are administered a group achievement test during the spring semester (*No Child Left Behind*, 2002). Entrance into post-secondary schools is partially based on the results of the American College Test (ACT) and the Scholastic Aptitude Test (SAT) tests. Entrance into a profession is routinely accompanied by a test (e.g., Graduate Record Exam [GRE], Graduate Management Admissions Test [GMAT], Law School Admissions Test [LSAT]) developed specifically to evaluate proficiency and knowledge of the profession.

10.3 OUTLINE OF OVERALL EVALUATIVE PROCESS OF TESTING

The steps in the overall evaluative process of testing are listed in Table 10-3 and are elaborated upon in the following section.

The first step in the process of testing is to determine what will be measured and to operationally define the variable. The researcher must be precise and state clearly what

TABLE 10-3

STEPS IN THE EVALUATION PROCESS

1. Identify the function to be measured.
2. Identify a published instrument to measure a condition or develop a new standardized procedure for evaluation of function.
3. Identify the skill level necessary to use a test instrument.
4. Identify the possible factors in the environment, tester, subject, or test instrument that can potentially distort the test results.
5. Identify the target population for which the test is intended and for which norms have been established.
6. Strictly follow the directions and procedures for administering and scoring the test or for modifying the test procedure to enable the client with disabilities to perform at a maximum level.
7. Interpret the results based on one of the following:
   a. Norm-referenced data based on the general population
   b. Criterion-referenced data for client performance or competence

is to be discovered. For example, a clinical researcher is interested in evaluating visual perception. Visual perception consists of several different skills, such as discrimination, spatial orientation, form-constancy, memory, figure ground, closure, and visual-motor integration. Although it is possible to evaluate visual perception, effective treatment necessitates an understanding of the individual's ability in each of the various components.

Once the researcher has identified the function to be measured, he or she selects an instrument to measure that function. Often a published instrument is available. Sometimes published instruments may be better because of the known psychometric properties; however, it may be that there is no instrument, and the researcher has to develop one. This is frequently true when designing an interview or survey questionnaire (see methodological research in Chapter 3).

If the clinical researcher chooses to use a published instrument, then it will be necessary to determine what qualifications are needed to administer the test. Qualification levels are set by the APA Standards for Educational and Psychological Testing (American Educational Research Association [AERA], APA, & National Council on Measurement in Education [NCME], 1999), and most test publishers adhere to this policy (Pearson Assessments, 2010, para. 4-6).

- Level A: There are no special qualifications to purchase these products.
- Level B: Tests can be purchased by individuals with (a) certification by or full active membership in a professional organization (ASHA [American Speech-Language-Hearing Association], AOTA, APA, AERA, ACA [American Counseling Association], AMA [American Medical Association], NASP [National Association of School Psychologists], NAN [National Academy of Neuropsychology], INS [International Neuropsychological Society]) that requires training and experience in a relevant area of assessment; or (b) a master's degree in psychology, education, occupational therapy, speech-language pathology, social work, or in a field closely related to the intended use of the assessment, and formal training in the ethical administration, scoring, and interpretation of clinical assessments.
- Level C: Tests with a C qualification require a high level of expertise in test interpretation and can be purchased by individuals with (a) licensure or certification to practice in your state in a field related to the purchase; or (b) a doctorate degree in psychology, education, or closely related field with formal training in the ethical administration, scoring, and interpretation of clinical assessments related to the intended use of the assessment.
- Level Q: Tests can be purchased by individuals with one of the following backgrounds as determined by the particular purchase, along with formal training in the ethical use, administration, and interpretation of standardized assessment tools and psychometrics: (a) Q1: a degree or license to practice in the healthcare or allied healthcare field; or (b) Q2: formal supervised mental health, speech/language, and/or educational training specific to working with parents and assessing children, or formal supervised training in infant and child development.

The fourth step in the process involves identifying the possible factors in the environment, tester, subject, or test instrument that can potentially distort the test results. These factors are outlined in Figure 10-1. The researcher will want to eliminate as many of these factors as possible.

Once the researcher has identified the variable to be measured, the tests to be used, and the potential error factors that need to be eliminated or reduced, he or she must identify the target population for which the test is intended and for which norms have been established. Sometimes this will seem unclear. For example, a clinical researcher may want to examine the psychological effect and impact or behavior that a child with disabilities has on a parent. The target population may, at first, appear to be the parent; however, the question being asked is how the child with disabilities impacts the parent. Although a questionnaire will be given to the parents, items on the instrument will relate to the child with disabilities. Therefore, the target population is, in reality, the child.

Whether the clinical researcher is administering a standardized test or one that he or she developed, the instrument must be administered the same way every time. An alteration in the test directions or administration will confound the results and make them unreliable. When the directions or procedures are altered or modified, this must be stated in the final report. Keep in mind that the alteration or modification of administering a test will make the norms invalid.

The final step is to interpret the results based on either the typical performance as determined by the norms from a general population or a standard set prior to administration of the test. For example, a researcher wants to see the effect of treatment on reduction of anxiety. The researcher has a choice of measurements: (a) a standardized test that measures the level of anxiety (e.g., *State-Trait Anxiety Inventor* [Spielberger, Gorsuch, Lushene, Vagg, & Jacobs, 1983]) and compares the results with the expected level based on the norms for the general population, or (b) a custom-designed self-evaluation administered before and after treatment.

10.4 Characteristics of a Good Test in Clinical Research

The accuracy and precision in evaluating a client's performance or improvement in a clinical research study depend on the quality of the test instrument. What are the characteristics of a good test instrument? What are some essential questions in evaluating the purposes and "goodness" of a test?

- What is the population for whom the test is targeted (e.g., children with learning difficulties, individuals with schizophrenia, persons with muscular dystrophy)?
- What are the specific purposes of the test (e.g., planning treatment goals, determining prognosis, establishing baseline data, documenting progress)?
- What are the areas of function identified in the test (e.g., social development, pre-vocational, personality, leisure interests, perceptual-motor abilities, ADL skills, live independently, cognitive level)?
- What are the methods used to evaluate a client? Primary sources for evaluating a client include:
  - *Medical records*: Demographics, previous treatment, and outcomes
  - *Educational records*: Educational attainment, achievement scores
  - *Clinical observation of performance*: Therapists and teacher observations

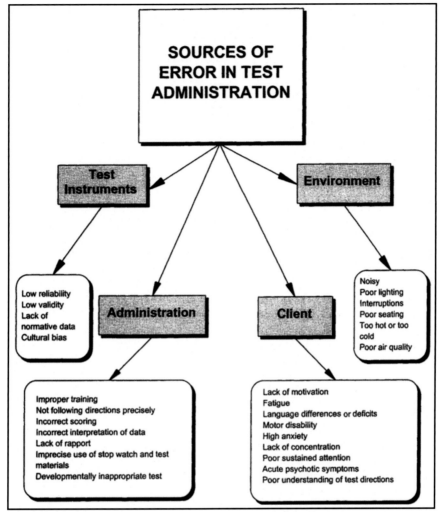

Figure 10-1. Potential sources of error in test administration. Errors come from four main areas: the instrument itself, the administration of the test, the client or subject, and the environment.

- ○ *Interviews*: Formal or unstructured individual interviews
- ○ *Objective tests*: Objectively scored paper-and-pencil tests, performance scales, and verbal tests
- ○ *Survey questionnaires*: Group tests, forced choice, or open-ended questions or items
- ○ *Self-reports*: Evaluation of treatment effectiveness through client's perspective
- ○ *Reports from peers, teacher/therapist, or family*: Informal reports or observations
- ○ *Biomechanical or physiological measurement of human factors*: Machine monitoring, test procedures
- Is there a standardized procedure or manual of instructions in administering the test and interpreting results? Are there tables of normative data?
- Are there special skills or certifications that are necessary to administer, score, and interpret results of the test?

- Is the scale of measurement used in collecting data identifiable (i.e., continuous, such as interval or ratio, or discrete, such as nominal or ordinal)?
- Are error factors controlled that can potentially interfere with obtaining reliable test results?
- Are research data reported (e.g., those derived from previous studies, including reliability, validity, and normative scores)?

10.5 Assumptions in Clinical Evaluation

What are some of the assumptions in clinical evaluation that guide a clinician in assessment? The major assumptions follow:

- Evaluation is an essential factor in the treatment process. It is used to determine the client's abilities, interests, potentials, and work traits.

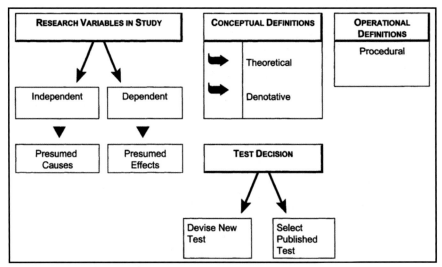

Figure 10-2. Critical steps in determining an appropriate test instrument.

- Evaluation is used to establish baseline data so as to compare with outcome results.
- Evaluation is based on reliable and valid instrumentation. The degree of accuracy in measurement depends on the degree of reliability (consistency) and validity (accuracy).
- Error is always present to a degree in evaluation, owing to anomalies in the examiner's presentation of test materials, degree of anxiety or fatigue, client's motivation, less-than-perfect reliability of test, and a less-than-ideal testing environment. Test scores obtained are a sample of the client's performance and represent an approximation of abilities within a given time frame.
- The reliability of the test score is increased by eliminating potential error factors that could endanger or distort the test results.
- Evaluation can provide data for documentation and the basis for establishing clinical efficacy and quality assurance. Evaluation is an excellent method for objectively determining client progress.

10.6 MAJOR PURPOSES OF TESTING IN CLINICAL RESEARCH

The major purposes of testing are as follows:
- Establish baseline data (experimental research, pre-test)
- Evaluate outcome or effectiveness of treatment procedure (experimental research, post-test)
- Assess the degree of relationship between two variables (correlational research)
- Evaluate quality of health care or education progress for accreditation (evaluative research)
- Assess developmental landmarks (developmental research)
- Assess individual values, interests, or attitudes (survey research)
- Evaluate differences between groups (correlational, experimental research)
- Evaluate functional assessment (screening target population)

10.7 CONCEPTUAL MODEL FOR SELECTING A TEST INSTRUMENT FOR CLINICAL RESEARCH

The decision to select a test from a published source or to construct a new test to measure a defined variable is a frequent dilemma. The measuring instrument is an essential part of a research study and represents the operational definition of a variable. Figure 10-2 shows this process.

The conceptual definition of a variable should lead the investigator to a specific test that is the most appropriate for operationally defining a variable. In clinical research, it is crucial that the investigator select a measuring instrument that has a high reliability and is a valid measurement of outcome. Measuring improvement in such areas as personality, physical capacity, cognitive functions, independent living skills, vocational skills, and perceptual-motor abilities depends directly on the adequacy and sensitivity of the instrument to measure changes. A crude measuring device that does not have the capacity to record subtle changes in an individual's functioning or behavior is of either limited or no value to the researcher.

When deciding on the instrument to use for the outcome measure, the researcher must ask the following questions:

- *What is the target population?* Examples include:
  - Typical children, adolescents, adults, elderly
  - Intellectual deficit
  - Psychiatric diagnosis
  - People with physical challenges (specify diagnosis)
  - Social, economic variables
  - Demographic variables
- *What are the specific areas of function to be measured?* Examples of these areas include:
  - Manual dexterity
  - Intellectual aptitude
  - Vocational interests
  - Independent living
  - Personality
  - Job readiness
  - Attitudes toward work
  - Work experiences
  - Work tolerance
  - Social skills
  - Self-care
  - Communication
  - Mobility and transportation
  - Educational level
- *Where will the client be assessed?* Some places for assessment include:
  - Home
  - Sheltered workshop
  - Clinical environment
  - School
  - Office
  - Hospital
- *What are the methods for evaluating function and how will the individual be assessed?* Some methods include:
  - Observation of performance
  - Paper-and-pencil test
  - Interview
  - Self-report and self-evaluation
  - Direct measure of function through standardized test instrument
  - Evaluation by teacher, therapist, or parent
  - Work samples
  - Parent, therapist, or teacher report
  - Computerized test
- *Is the test reliable and valid?*
  - Are there standardized directions for administration?
  - Are norm scores available for comparison purposes?
  - How many subjects were used in collecting norm values?
  - How was reliability of the test established (e.g., test-retest, split half, equivalent forms)?
  - How was the validity of the test established (e.g., concurrent, construct, predictive)?
- *Are the test results easily interpreted?*
- *What is the scale of measurement (i.e., ordinal, nominal, interval, or ratio)?*
- *How will the individual be tested?*
  - In a single session (summative evaluation) or over several sessions (formative evaluation)?
  - In a large group, small group, or individually?

10.8 BIBLIOGRAPHIC SOURCES

Another consideration for testing involves asking the following question: Where can I find the most appropriate test instrument? Examples and names of test instruments can be found in several sources, including:

Books on psychological testing, such as the following:

- Anastasi, A., & Urbina, S. (1997). *Psychological testing* (7th ed.). Englewood Cliffs, NJ: Prentice Hall.
- Asher, I. E. (Ed.) (2007). *Occupational therapy assessment tools: An annotated index* (3rd ed.). Rockville, MD: American Occupational Therapy Association.
- Bowling, A. (2005). *Measuring health: A review of quality of life measurement scales* (3rd ed.). Buckingham, United Kingdom: Open University Press/McGraw Hill.
- Dittmar, S. S., & Gresham, G. E. (2000). *Functional assessment and outcome measures for the rehabilitation health professional.* Gaithersburg, MD: Aspen/Canadianphysio.
- Finch, E., Brooks, D., Stratford, P., & Mayo, N. (2002). *Physical rehabilitation outcome measures* (2nd ed). Toronto, Ontario: Canadian Physiotherapy Association. (This text includes outcome measures categorized into areas of practice [e.g., general rehabilitation, geriatrics, chronic respiratory problems, back, pediatrics, stroke, and rheumatology].)
- Fischer, J., & Corcoran, K. (2007). *Measures for clinical practice: A sourcebook. Volume 1: Couples, family and children* (4th ed.). New York, NY: Free Press.
- Hemphill-Pearson, B. J. (Ed.) (2008). *Assessments in occupational therapy mental health: An integrative approach* (2nd ed). Thorofare, NJ: SLACK Incorporated.
- Lewis, C. B., & McNerney, T. (1994). *The functional tool box: Clinical measures of functional outcomes.* Washington, DC: GREAT Seminars and Books.

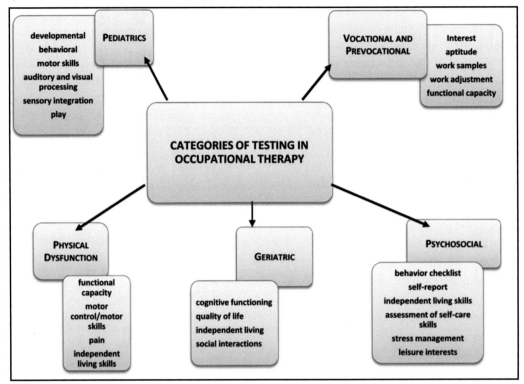

Figure 10-3. Categories of tests used in occupational therapy assessment.

- Lezak, M. D., Howieson, D. B., & Loring, D. W. (2004). *Neuropsychological assessment* (4th ed.). New York, NY: Oxford University Press.
- *Mental measurements yearbook (MMY), Mental measurements supplement, or Tests in print.* Published by The University of Nebraska Press. In 1989, the MMY began an alternate-year publication schedule with the Supplement to the Mental Measurements Yearbook or MMY-S. The 20th edition was published in 2017 (https://buros.org/mental-measurements-yearbook)
- Neistadt, M. E. (2000). *Occupational therapy evaluation for adults: A pocket guide.* Baltimore, MD: Lippincott.
- Paul, S., & Orchanian, D. (2003). *Pocketguide to assessment in occupational therapy.* Clifton Park, NY: Delmar, Cengage Learning.
- Power, P. (2006). *A guide to vocational assessment* (4th ed.). Austin, TX: Pro-Ed.
- Sattler, J. M. (2008). *Assessment of children: Cognitive foundations* (5th ed.). San Diego, CA: Author.
- Stein, F., & Cutler, S. K. (2002). *Psychosocial occupational therapy: A holistic approach* (2nd ed.). Clifton Park, NY: Delmar, Cengage Learning.
- Van Deusen, J., & Brunk, D. (1997). *Assessment in occupational therapy and physical therapy.* Philadelphia, PA: Saunders.

There are also numerous databases that can be searched and accessed through the internet. The web addresses of which frequently change, so a published list of examples here would likely be obsolete by the time of publication. As such, a good strategy to find the most recent iteration of any given database is to use a web browser to search for and access the desired database.

10.9 TEST INSTRUMENTS

Testing instruments and procedures can be found for almost every functional area that health professionals might want to assess. Figure 10-3 diagrams the major categories of tests used in occupational therapy, while the following paragraphs and sections describe the major tests. We have tried to select tests that are commonly used or are important for specific reasons (e.g., they have normative data for populations of individuals with special needs; they are used more frequently by occupational therapists; they have high validity and reliability). We recognize that not all tests are listed. For a more complete list, the reader should refer to one of the books on assessment and testing listed in the previous section or to a publisher's catalog (listed at the end of the chapter in Section 10.12). As a caution, tests are developed or revised yearly, and even the most up-to-date book may not have a description of the test. In case of doubt, it is wise to contact the publisher directly.

10.9.1 Psychosocial Tests

Assessment of psychosocial functioning occurs in several different ways. Observation of a client may occur in a hospital or residential setting. Professionals and paraprofessionals may complete checklists or rating scales as part of the evaluation. Self-report scales used for assessment of self-concept, role identity, stress management, and leisure activities are valuable in the assessment of a client's perceptions. Some of the more widely used psychosocial scales are described in Table 10-4 (checklists and self-report scales), Table 10-5 (cognitive and general assessments), Table 10-6 (independent living skills), Table 10-7 (stress management), and Table 10-8 (leisure interests). Additional tests are described in the following paragraphs. Other examples can be found in the publishers' catalogs.

10.9.1.1 Behavior Rating Scales

Behavior rating scales are used by therapists, teachers, and clinicians to obtain information about a client's behavior. Usually, the rating scales are paper-and-pencil instruments filled out by the client's parents or family. Occasionally, rating scales may be completed by a member of the peer group (e.g., another student in the classroom) or as a self-report measure.

Although rating scales are widely used, there are some disadvantages and cautions to be considered when using them. Because the rating scale is a subjective measurement, response bias is possible. For example, the responder may rate the individual either too harshly or too positively (e.g., Halo effect) than is realistic or the respondent may restrict the scores to the central range of the scale, leaving the impression that the individual being rated has few strengths or weaknesses. Second, results from rating scales obtained from different settings (e.g., individual therapy and large classroom setting) may show very different scores. This is frequently attributable to the client's varied behavior in different settings. Finally, differences obtained on the scales may occur because of the day on which the rating scale was completed (Martin, Hooper, & Snow, 1986), thereby reflecting the behavioral variability of either the respondent or the client. For these reasons, more than one informant should be used to complete the rating scale. If possible, each informant should complete a couple of rating scales over a short period of time.

10.9.1.2 Objective Personality Tests

Measurement of personality variables through paper-and-pencil tests are widely used in research studies of treatment outcome in psychiatry. The Minnesota Multiphasic Personality Inventory (MMPI), first published in 1942, is the most extensively used test for diagnosing psychological maladjustment. The researcher using objective personality tests should use caution in interpreting results. The methods of administering the tests and the subject's attitude toward the tests can potentially affect the results. Factors such as noise distractions, unmotivated and uncooperative subjects, and subject faking (sometimes referred to as *malingering*) are some of the problems encountered in personality testing. The ethical consideration in personality testing is another major consideration. The researcher should make efforts to ensure the anonymity and confidentiality of the subject. Most of the tests can only be given by evaluators trained in personality assessment. Some of the more common tests are described in the following paragraphs.

- *Minnesota Multiphasic Personality Inventory-2* (MMPI-2; Hathaway & McKinley, 1989; PsychCorp/Pearson Assessments) consists of 550 true-false items used for measuring adjustment on 10 psychiatric diagnostic scales. The test takes from 2 to 3 hours and is given to adults.

- *Million Adolescent Personality Inventory* (MAPI; Million, Green, & Meagher, 1982; PsychCorp/Pearson Assessments) is a personality test for adolescents ages 13 years and older. The test is written in language understood by adolescents and is based on a model of personality development rather than clinical pathology. The paper-and-pencil test must be scored by computer through the National Computer Systems.

- *Personality Inventory for Children-2* (PIC-2; Lachar & Gruber, 2001; Western Psychological Services) is a questionnaire containing true-false items completed by an informant (usually the parent). The scale consists of three broad scales covering categories such as behaviors at home and school, family interactions, educational achievement, and possible diagnoses. Results can be compared with 12 clinical types for use in differential diagnosis. The scale can be used with children ages 3 through 16 years.

- *Children's Depression Inventory* (CDI; Kovacs, 1992; Pearson Assessment) consists of 27 self-rating items in which the client must choose between one of three sentences that best describes his or her experience in the past 2 weeks. The test is sensitive to changes in mood and provides a valid severity level of depression. The test is designed for ages 7 to 17 years and takes about 15 minutes to complete.

- *Sixteen Personality Factor Questionnaire, Fifth Edition* (16PF; Cattell, Cattell, & Cattell, 1993; PsychCorp/Pearson Assessments) is a forced choice test used for measuring 16 independent factors of personality. It is designed for high school, college, and adult subjects and takes about 1 hour to administer.

Table 10-4

Psychosocial Assessment in Occupational Therapy: Checklists and Self-Reports

TEST	TARGET POPULATION	PURPOSE	VARIABLES ASSESSED	PUBLISHER/SOURCE
Behavior Assessment System for Children (3rd ed; BASC-3; Reynolds, Kamphaus, & Vannest, 2015)	Ages 2-0 to 21-11	Teacher, parent, and self-rating scales designed to examine maladaptive and adaptive behavior.	Categories: • Academic problems • Adaptability • Aggression • Anxiety • Attention problems • Conduct problems • Depression • Functional communication • Hyperactivity • Leadership/social skills • Somatization	Pearson Assessment/Psych Corp http://psychcorp.pearsonassessments.com/haiweb/cultures/en-us/productdetail.htm?pid=PAa30000&Community=CA_Psych_AI_Behavior
Devereaux Scales of Mental Disorders (DSMD; Naglieri, LeBuffe, & Pfeiffer, 1994), Behavior Rating Scales–School Form (Naglieri, LeBuffe, & Pfeiffer, 1992)	Ages 5 through 12 years (Child), and 13 through 18 years (Adolescent)	Allow teachers and other professionals to identify behavioral or emotional problems	Behaviors associated with psychopathology, including conduct, attention, anxiety, depression, autism, and acute problems	Pearson Assessment/Psych Corp http://psychcorp.pearsonassessments.com/HAIWEB/Cultures/en-us/Productdetail.htm?Pid=015-8048-008&Mode=summary
Reynolds Child Depression Scale (2nd ed; RCDS-2; 2014); Reynolds Adolescent Depression Scale (2nd ed.; RADS-2; 1987) Reynolds Depression Screening Inventory (1998)	Children Adolescents Adults	Self-report measures designed to screen for symptoms of depression	Symptoms of depression as defined by the *Diagnostic and Statistical Manual of Mental Disorders, Fourth Edition*. An overall score defines the level of depression.	PAR, Inc. https://www.parinc.com/products/pkey/354

(continued)

TABLE 10-4 (CONTINUED)

PSYCHOSOCIAL ASSESSMENT IN OCCUPATIONAL THERAPY: CHECKLISTS AND SELF-REPORTS

TEST	TARGET POPULATION	PURPOSE	VARIABLES ASSESSED	PUBLISHER/SOURCE
Health Status Questionnaire 2.0 (HSQ 2.0; Radosevich, Wetzler, & Wilson, 1994)	Age 14 years to adults	Designed as a general outcomes measure to be used in all settings that provide primary or mental health care services, it captures aspects of both physical and emotional health	Overall health attributes, health status change, and risk for the presence of a depressive disorder. This instrument is designed to be easily administered via self-report, personal interview, or telephone interview.	Statistics Solutions https://www.statisticssolutions.com/health-status-questionnaire-2-0-hsq
The Model of Human Occupation (MOHO), developed by Gary Kielhofner at the University of Illinois in Chicago. Many developed assessment tools were based on the MOHO model.	Children, adolescents, and adults	Self-inventory of daily activities and volitional issues for those activities	Activity patterns, classification of activities and ranking of activities according to value, interest, and personal causation	University of Illinois at Chicago College Of Applied Health Sciences http://www.moho.uic.edu Kramer, J., Kielhofner, G., & Forsyth, K. (2008). Assessments used with the Model of Human Occupation. In B. J. Hemphill-Pearson (Ed.), *Assessments in occupational therapy mental health: An integrative approach* (2nd ed., pp. 159-184). Thorofare, NJ: SLACK Incorporated.
State-Trait Anger Expression Inventory-2: Adolescents/Child (STAXI-2 C/A; Brunner & Spielberger, 2009)	Children and adolescents, ages 9 to 18 years	Assess both state and trait anger along with anger expression and control	State anger (feelings, expression); trait anger (temperament, reactions), anger expression (out), anger expression (in), anger control	PAR, Inc. http://www4.parinc.com/Products/Product.aspx?ProductID=STAXI-2C/A

TABLE 10-5

PSYCHOSOCIAL ASSESSMENT IN OCCUPATIONAL THERAPY: COGNITIVE AND GENERAL ASSESSMENT

TEST	TARGET POPULATION	PURPOSE	VARIABLES ASSESSED	PUBLISHER/SOURCE
Adolescent Role Assessment (Black, 1976; Huebner, Emery, & Shordike, 2002)	Adolescents with psychosocial dysfunction	To assess past history and present role development in home, school, and community	Six areas, including childhood play, adolescent socialization, school performance, occupational choice, and work	Black, M. M. Adolescent role assessment. (1976). *American Journal of Occupational Therapy, 30,* 73-79.
Allen Cognitive Level Screen (Allen, 1985; Allen, Earhart, & Blue, 1992; Allen et al., 2007; Earhart & Allen, 1988)	Clients with psychiatric or cognitive impairment	Screening tool to classify people into one of six cognitive levels based on Allen's theory	Six cognitive levels: 1. Automatic actions 2. Postural actions 3. Manual actions 4. Goal-directed actions 5. Exploratory actions 6. Planned actions	S & S Arts http://www.ssww.com/therapy-and-rehab/allen-diagnostic-module/ http://www.allen-cognitive-network.org/
B. H. Battery (Hemphill-Pearson, 1999)	Children and adolescents	Structured instrument to assess the psychological area of human function	Cognitive and psychosocial factors, including problem-solving and abstraction, frustration tolerance, organization and internal structure, and self-awareness	Hemphill-Pearson, B. J. (Ed.). (1999). B. H. Battery. In *Assessments in occupational therapy mental health: An integrative approach* (pp. 139-152). Thorofare, NJ: SLACK Incorporated.
Build A City (Clark, 1999)	Adults with psychosocial dysfunction who are in group therapy	Group task or activity that evaluates interactions within a standardized situation and utilizes the constructive, doing process valued in occupational therapy	Communication and work skills within a group; positive and negative interactions between group members	Clark, E. N. (1999). Build A City. In B. J. Hemphill-Pearson (Ed.), *Assessments in occupational therapy mental health: An integrative approach* (pp. 155-170). Thorofare, NJ: SLACK Incorporated.

(continued)

TABLE 10-5 (CONTINUED)

PSYCHOSOCIAL ASSESSMENT IN OCCUPATIONAL THERAPY: COGNITIVE AND GENERAL ASSESSMENT

TEST	TARGET POPULATION	PURPOSE	VARIABLES ASSESSED	PUBLISHER/SOURCE
Burns Cognitive Performance Test (Burns, Mortimer, & Merchak, 1994)	Adults with Alzheimer's disease	Assesses cognitive function in daily activities. Based on the Allen Cognitive Disability Theory	Uses performance on six ADLs to predict function in context and assess safety needs	Burns, T., Mortimer, J. A., & Merchak, P. Cognitive Performance Test: A new approach to functional assessment in Alzheimer's disease. *Journal of Geriatric Psychiatry Neurology*, (1994), 7(1), 46-54.
Canadian Occupational Performance Measure (COPM; Bowman & Llewellyn, 2002; Law et al., 1991, 1994)	Individuals age 7 years through adults; individuals with disabilities	Outcome measure designed to detect changes in client's perception of occupational performance. Based on the Model of Occupational Performance	Three subareas (self-care, productivity, and leisure) are measured with total scores obtained for performance and satisfaction. Based on the Canadian Model of Occupational Performance	Canadian Association of Occupational Therapists http://www.thecopm.ca/about
Cognitive Adaptive Skills Evaluation (CASE; Masagatani, 1994, 1999)	Clients with psychosocial dysfunction; can be used with adults and adolescents with developmental delays or cognitive dysfunction	Survey functional skills to examine individual's cognitive skills while performing a task and responding to interview questions	Performance summary using defined behavioral criteria based on analysis of task completion and responses to interview questions	Masagatani, G. N. (1999). The Cognitive Adaptive Skills Evaluation. In B. J. Hemphill-Pearson (Ed.), *Assessments in occupational therapy mental health: An integrative approach* (pp. 367-376). Thorofare, NJ: SLACK Incorporated.

(continued)

Table 10-5 (continued)

Psychosocial Assessment in Occupational Therapy: Cognitive and General Assessment

TEST	TARGET POPULATION	PURPOSE	VARIABLES ASSESSED	PUBLISHER/SOURCE
Functional Life Scale (FLS; Dittmar & Gresham, 1997; Sarno, Sarno, & Levita, 1973; Sapountzi-Krepia, et al., 1998)	Adults in the community	Assessment of an individual's ability to participate in ADLs performed by most people	Forty-four items in five categories: 1. Cognition 2. ADLs 3. Activities in the home 4. Outside activities 5. Social interaction	Sarno, J. E., Sarno, M. T., & Levita, E. (1973). The functional life scale. *Archives of Physical Medicine and Rehabilitation, 54,* 214-220.
Goal Attainment Scaling (GAS; Cott & Finch, 1991; Ottenbacher & Cusick, 1990; Rockwood, Joyce, & Stolee, 1997; Stolee, Kockwood, Fox, & Streiner, 1992)	Adolescents through adults	Assess changes in performance self-care goals	Range of change from expected change (0) to below average (-2, - 1) and above average (+2, + 1)	Cott, C., & Finch, E. (1991). Goal-setting in physical therapy practice. *Physiotherapy Canada 43,* 19-22. Ottenbacher, K., & Cusick, A. (1990). Goal attainment scaling as a method of clinical service evaluation. *American Journal of Occupational Therapy, 44,* 519-525. Stolee, P., Rockwood, K., Fox, R. A., & Streiner, D.L. (1992). The use of goal attainment scaling in a geriatric care setting. *Journal of the American Geriatrics Society, 4,* 575-578.

TABLE 10-6

PSYCHOSOCIAL ASSESSMENT OF INDEPENDENT LIVING SKILLS

TEST	TARGET POPULATION	PURPOSE	VARIABLES ASSESSED	PUBLISHER/SOURCE
Bay Area Functional Performance Evaluation (2nd ed.; BaFPE.; Williams & Bloomer, 1987; Williams et al., 2004; Klyczek & Stanton, 2008)	Adults with psychosocial dysfunction	Two components: TOA assesses goal-directed abilities, as well as cognitive, performance, and affective areas of function. SIS assesses social behaviors observed in five different settings.	Twelve functional parameters (e.g., memory, organization, attention, abstraction, task completion, affective and behavioral impression) and seven categories of verbal and nonverbal social interaction	Allegro Medical http://www.allegromedical.com/patient-care-c530/bafpe-bay-area-functional-performance-evaluation-p192719.html
COPM (4th ed.; Baptiste, 2008; Law et al., 1991, 1994, 2004)	Clients with disabilities; can be used with children as young as age 7 years	Outcome measure designed to detect changes in client's perception of occupational performance	Self-care, productivity, leisure, performance and satisfaction; based on the Canadian Model of Occupational Performance	Canadian Association of Occupational Therapists http://www.thecopm.ca/about
Comprehensive Occupational Therapy Evaluation (COTE; Brayman, 2008; Brayman, Kirby, Meisenheimer, & Short, 1976; Kunz & Brayman, 1999)	Adults with acute psychosocial dysfunction who are hospitalized	Provides standard, objective means of rating behaviors of hospitalized patients on a frequent basis	General, interpersonal, and task behaviors	Brayman, S. J. (2008). The Comprehensive Occupational Therapy Evaluation (COTE). In B. J. Hemphill-Pearson (Ed.), *Assessments in occupational therapy mental health: An integrative approach* (2nd ed., pp. 113-124). Thorofare, NJ: SLACK Incorporated.
Functional Independence Measure (FIM; Granger, Sherwood, & Greer, 1977; Keith, Granger, Hamilton, & Sherwin, 1987)	Adults	Developed as part of the Uniform Data System for Medical Rehabilitation to assess independent performance in self-care, toileting, transfers, locomotion, communication, and social cognition	Eighteen activities: 13 with motor emphasis related to self-care; 5 with a cognitive emphasis involving communication	Uniform Data System for Medical Rehabilitation http://www.udsmr.org/ http://www.scireproject.com/outcome-measures/functional-independence-measure-fim

	TABLE 10-6 (CONTINUED)			
	PSYCHOSOCIAL ASSESSMENT OF INDEPENDENT LIVING SKILLS			
TEST	TARGET POPULATION	PURPOSE	VARIABLES ASSESSED	PUBLISHER/SOURCE
Independent Living Skills Evaluation (ILSE; Johnson, Vinnicombe, & Merrill, 1981).	Adults (aged 18 years and older) with chronic psychosocial dysfunction who are living in independent living arrangements or living independently	Assess levels of living skills in areas necessary for independent community living	Ten major categories of independent living in home, community, and personal areas	Community Living Experiences, Inc. The Independent Living Project http://www.informaworld.com/smpp/content~db=all~content=a904375711
Kohlman Evaluation of Living Skills (4th ed.; KELS; 2016) (McGourty, 1988; Pickens et al., 2007; Thomson, 1992, 1999)	Clients with acute psychiatric disorders, elderly patients in acute care hospitals; adolescent through elderly; must be used cautiously with individuals hospitalized for more than 1 month	Quick assessment to provide information about a person's ability in everyday functioning in daily living skills, independent living, and work/leisure	Seventeen living skills in areas of self-care, safety/health, money management, transportation/telephone, work/leisure	American Occupational Therapy Association https://myaota.aota.org/shop_aota/prodview.aspx?TYPE=D&PID=27716288&SKU=900374
Milwaukee Evaluation of Daily Living Skills (MEDLS; Leonardelli Haertlein, 1999; Leonardelli, 1988a, 1988b)	Adults with chronic mental illness who are inpatients or outpatients in a CMHC	Assessment of behavior and skills needed for adequate functioning in the client's living situation	Twenty subtests measuring basic living skills, safety, communication, and transportation	Leonardelli Haertlein, C. (1999). The Milwaukee Evaluation of Daily Living Skills. In B. J. Hemphill-Pearson, (Ed.). Assessments in occupational therapy mental health: An integrative approach (pp. 245-257). Thorofare, NJ: SLACK Incorporated
Performance Assessment of Self-Care Skill: Version 3.1 (PASS; Holm & Rogers, 2008)	Adults	Assess the types of assistance needed to stay in or remain in the community	ADL and IADL from perspectives of independence, safety, and task outcome	Holm, M. B., & Rogers, J. C. (2008). The Performance Assessment of Self-Care Skills (PASS). In B. J. Hemphill-Pearson (Ed.), Assessments in occupational therapy mental health: An integrative approach (2nd ed., pp. 259-274). Thorofare, NJ: SLACK Incorporated.

(continued)

TABLE 10-6 (CONTINUED)

PSYCHOSOCIAL ASSESSMENT OF INDEPENDENT LIVING SKILLS

TEST	TARGET POPULATION	PURPOSE	VARIABLES ASSESSED	PUBLISHER/SOURCE
Street Survival Skills Questionnaire (SSSQ; Linkenhoker & McCarron, 1979, 1993)	Adolescents and adults with developmental disabilities, including psychosocial dysfunction	Assessment of specific aspects of adaptive behavior needed for independent living	Nine areas of adaptive behavior, including functional signs, tools, health and safety, time, and money	McCarron-Dial Systems, Inc. http://www.mccarrondial.com/index.html#anchor556866

CMHC = community mental health clinic; IADL = instrumental activities of daily living; SIS = Social Interaction Scale; TOA = Task-Oriented Assessment.

TABLE 10-7

PSYCHOSOCIAL ASSESSMENT OF STRESS

TEST	TARGET POPULATION	PURPOSE	VARIABLES ASSESSED	PUBLISHER/SOURCE
Occupational Stress Inventory–Revised (OSI-R; Osipow & Spokane, 1987)	Employed adults (age 18 to 70 years)	Generic occupational stress inventory that applies across different occupations, built on a theoretical model	Occupational adjustment, stress, psychological strain, and coping resources	PAR, Inc. http://www4.parinc.com/Products/Product.aspx?ProductID=OSI-R
Stress Management Questionnaire (SMQ; Stein, 1987, 2008; Stein, Bentley, & Natz, 1999; Stein & Cutler, 2002)	Typical adults and adults (18 years and above) with disabilities	Assess symptoms precipitated by stress, stressors that cause a stress response, and coping activities used to manage stress	Symptoms of stress, stressors, and copers	Stein, F. (2008). Stress Management Questionnaire. In B. J. Hemphill-Pearson (Ed.), *Assessments in occupational therapy mental health: An integrative approach* (2nd ed., pp. 293-307). Thorofare, NJ: SLACK Incorporated.
Survey of Recent Life Experiences (SLRE; Kohn & McDonald, 1992)	Adults	Measure of daily hassles in the lives of adults over the past month	Social and cultural difficulties, work, time pressure, finances, social acceptability, and social victimization	Kohn, P. M., & McDonald, J. E. (1992). The Survey of Recent Life Experiences: A decontaminated hassles scale for adults. *Journal of Behavioral Medicine 15,* 221-236.

TABLE 10-8

PSYCHOSOCIAL ASSESSMENT OF LEISURE SKILLS

TEST	TARGET POPULATION	PURPOSE	VARIABLES ASSESSED	PUBLISHER/SOURCE
Leisure Activities Finder (Holmberg, Rosen, & Holland, 1997)	Adults	Identify leisure time activities	Identification of leisure time activities using the self-directed search summary codes	PAR, Inc. Lutz, FL
Occupational Performance History Interview-II (OPHI-II; Kielhofner et al., 2004)	Adolescents and adults who can respond to a life-history questionnaire	Gather history of work, play, and self-care performance to determine the impact of disability and future goals	Five content areas of occupational performance, based on the MOHO	University of Illinois at Chicago College of Applied Health Sciences https://www.moho.uic.edu/resources/findTheAssessment/domain/occPerformance.aspx
Role Activity Performance Scale (RAPS; Good-Ellis, Fine, Spencer, & Divittis, 1987; Good-Ellis, 1999)	Adults with acute or chronic psychiatric disorders	Measure range of past and present role functioning as basis for treatment planning	Twelve role domains in the home, community, or interpersonal relationships up to an 18-month period	Good-Ellis, M. A. (1999). The Role Activity Performance Scale. In B. J. Hemphill-Pearson (Ed.), *Assessments in occupational therapy mental health: An integrative approach*, (pp. 205-226). Thorofare, NJ: SLACK Incorporated.
Role Checklist (Dickerson, 1999, 2008; Oakley, 1988; Oakley, Kielhofner, Barris, & Reichler, 1986)	Adults, adolescents, and elderly people with psychosocial or physical dysfunction	Assess individual's perception of and identification with roles	Continuous, disrupted changes in past, present, and future roles, and the degree of value for each role	University of Illinois at Chicago College of Applied Health Sciences https://www.moho.uic.edu/resources/findTheAssessment/domain/occPerformance.aspx Dickerson, A. E. (2008). The Role Checklist. In B. J. Hemphill-Pearson (Ed.), *Assessments in occupational therapy mental health: An integrative approach* (2nd ed., pp. 252-258). Thorofare, NJ: SLACK Incorporated.

(continued)

TABLE 10-8 (CONTINUED)

PSYCHOSOCIAL ASSESSMENT OF LEISURE SKILLS

TEST	TARGET POPULATION	PURPOSE	VARIABLES ASSESSED	PUBLISHER/SOURCE
Volitional Questionnaire–Version 4.1. (VQ; Chern, Kielhofner, de las Heras, & Magalhaes, 1996; de las Heras, Geist, Kielhofner, & Li, 2007)	Adults, adolescents, and children who can participate in a variety of occupations across different environmental settings	Provide insight into an individual's inner motives and how the environment affects volition		University of Illinois at Chicago College of Applied Health Sciences https://www.moho.uic.edu/resources/findTheAssessment/domain/occPerformance.aspx Chern, J.-S., Kielhofner, G., de las Heras, C. G., & Magalhaes, L. C. (1996). The Volitional Questionnaire: Psychometric development and practical use. *American Journal of Occupational Therapy, 50,* 516-525

10.9.2 Physical Dysfunction, Motor Control, Pain, and Independent Living

Tests of functional capacity, vocational aptitude, pain, and independent living assess the degree to which an individual can live and work independently in the community. They assess an individual's ability to perform physical movements as they relate to work, vocational activities, and ADLs. These measures are extremely important to rehabilitation research in determining whether an individual can return to work or live in independent housing.

Functional capacity evaluations are comprehensive and systematic approaches that measure the client's overall physical ability such as muscle strength, endurance, joint range of motion, ambulation, sitting, standing, and lifting. According to the American Physical Therapy Association (2008) guidelines for evaluating functional capacity:

A Functional Capacity Evaluation (FCE) is a comprehensive battery of performance based tests that is used commonly to determine ability for work, ADLs, or leisure activities. … The Functional Capacity Evaluation today quantifies safe functional abilities, and is a pivotal resource for

1.1 Return-to-work and job-placement decisions

1.2 Disability evaluation

1.3 Determination of how non-work-related illness and injuries impact work performance

1.4 Determination of functioning in non-occupational setting

1.5 Intervention and treatment planning

1.6 Case management and case closure. (p. 1)

Work samples are well-defined activities that are similar to actual jobs. They can be used to assess an individual's vocational aptitudes, worker characteristics, and vocational interests. *Independent living measures* test the degree to which an individual can perform the ADLs. They include self-care, communication, leisure, shopping, mobility, and related areas. Table 10-9 summarizes information about each of these areas and gives examples of evaluation instruments.

10.9.2.1 Outcome Measures and Functional Assessment

There is a rising trend in health care to demonstrate effectiveness and client satisfaction. Outcome measures have been designed to evaluate the overall functional status of clients who have received treatment and rehabilitation services in hospitals, outpatient clinics, rehabilitation centers and home environments. These outcome measures (Keith, 1984) are usually designed for specific populations such as individuals with stroke, brain injury, spinal cord injury, low back pain, psychological diagnoses, and developmental disabilities. The outcome measures evaluate the client's ability to perform functional ADLs, the degree of pain intensity, ability to work, to engage in leisure activities, to have restful sleep, to drive, to be mobile in the community, to communicate, to ambulate, to academically achieve, and to perform other activities related to functional abilities. Following is a list of some commonly used outcome measures for rehabilitation (also see Applegate, Blass, & Williams, 1990).

- *Levels of Rehabilitation Scale* (LORS-II; Carey & Posavac, 1980, 1982): Designed to obtain functional ratings from individuals who are in hospital-based rehabilitation programs
- *Katz Index of Independence in ADL* (Katz, Ford, Moskowitz, Jackson, & Jaffe, 1963): Developed for use with rehabilitation in patients
- *Functional Assessment Screening Questionnaire* (Granger & Wright, 1993): Used with patients who have undergone rehabilitation
- *Global Assessment of Functioning* (American Psychiatric Association, 2000): Used with individuals with psychosocial diagnoses
- *The Multilevel Assessment Instrument* (Lawton, Moss, Fulcomer, & Kleban, 1982): Designed for older individuals
- *Unified ADL Evaluation Form* (Donaldson, Wagner, & Gresham, 1973): Used to evaluate performance when performing activities of daily living
- *Functional Life Scale* (Sarno, Sarno, & Levita, 1973)
- *Community Integration Questionnaire* (Wilier, Ottenbacher, & Coad, 1994): Used with individuals with traumatic brain injury
- *Barthel Index* (Mahoney & Barthel, 1965): Designed to evaluate the degree of assistance required by an individual on 10 items of self-care and mobility
- *Health Status Questionnaire* 2.0 (HSQ 2.0) Pearson Assessments): Used to assess the functional status of adults with chronic illnesses
- The *Sickness Impact Profile* (Bergner, Bobbitt, Carter, & Gilson, 1981; Gilson et al., 1975): Used to assess a patient's function in such areas as sleep and rest, work, social interactions, leisure, and emotional behavior
- *FIM* (previously called Functional Independence Measure; Keith, Granger, Hamilton, & Sherwins, 1987): Designed as a tool to evaluate the patient's ability to complete ADLs

TABLE 10-9

FUNCTIONAL ASSESSMENT OF PHYSICAL DYSFUNCTION

	FUNCTIONAL CAPACITY EVALUATIONS	MOTOR CONTROL/MOTOR SKILLS	PAIN	INDEPENDENT LIVING SKILLS
PURPOSE	To evaluate a person's functional physical abilities as they relate to work performance (Lechner, Roth, & Straaton, 1991)	To evaluate a person's functional motor activities	To evaluate a client's pain to determine effectiveness of treatment (Ross & LaStayo, 1997)	To assess ADL and IADL skills needed to function successfully in the community (Power, 2000)
SAMPLE OF VARIABLES ASSESSED	• ROM • Muscle strength • Coordination • Manual dexterity • Muscle endurance • Position tolerance	• Muscle tone • Postural control • Gross mobility • Somatosensory function • Functional hand skills • Ambulation • Balance	• Pain intensity • Pain tolerance • Pain location http://www.soundideas.pugetsound.edu (Search for "Clinical Pain Scale Compendium" by Crow, Pilch, & Aiken, 2015) or http://painconsortium.nih.gov	• Social skills • Self-care • Safety and health • Communication • Transportation • Money management • Home making • Leisure activities • Fall risk
EXAMPLES OF WIDELY USED INSTRUMENTS	• BTE Technologies (formerly Baltimore Therapeutic Equipment, 2010) http://www.btetech.com	• Assessment of Motor and Process Skills (AMPS; Fisher, 1994; Center for Innovative OT Solutions, 2018) http://www.innovativeotsolutions.com • Bruininks-Oseretsky Test of Motor Proficiency, 2nd ed. (BOT–2; Bruininks, 1978; Bruininks & Bruininks, 2005)	• McGill Pain Questionnaire (MPQ; Melzack, 1975) https://www.gem-measures.org (National Cancer Institute) ◦ See also Short-Form McGill	• Barthel Index (Collin, Wade, Davies, & Horne, 1988; Mahoney & Barthel, 1965; Sainsbury Seebass, Bansal, & Young, 2005) http://www.strokecenter.org/wp-content/uploads/2011/08/barthel.pdf

(continued)

TABLE 10-9 (CONTINUED)

FUNCTIONAL ASSESSMENT OF PHYSICAL DYSFUNCTION

	FUNCTIONAL CAPACITY EVALUATIONS	MOTOR CONTROL/MOTOR SKILLS	PAIN	INDEPENDENT LIVING SKILLS

EXAMPLES OF WIDELY USED INSTRUMENTS	• Goniometric Range of Motion (Gilliam & Barstow, 1997)
	  ○ Rehabilitation Outlet http://www.rehaboutlet.com/goniometers.htm or
	  ○ Performance Health https://www.performancehealth.com/catalogsearch/result/?q=goniometer
	• Grip Dynamometers (Bohannon, Peolsson, Massy-Westropp, Desrosiers, & Bear-Lehman, 2006; Gilliam & Barstow, 1997)
	  ○ Rehabilitation Outlet http://www.rehaboutlet.com/grip_hand_dynamometer.htm or
	  ○ Performance Health https://www.performancehealth.com/catalogsearch/result/?q=dynamometer
	• Jebsen Hand Function Test (Jebsen, Taylor, Trieschmann, Trotter, & Howard, 1969)
		• Carr & Shepherd Motor Assessment Scale for Stroke Patients (Carr, Shepherd, Nordholm, & Lynn, 1985; Gillen, 2015)
		• Fugl-Meyer Assessment (Fugl-Meyer, Jääskö, Leyman, Olsson, & Steglind, 1975; Gladstone, Danells, & Black, 2002)
		• Rivermead Mobility Index (Collen, Wade, Robb, & Bradshaw, 1991; Wade, Collen, Robb, & Warlow, 1992) http://www.scireproject.com/outcome-measures/rivermead-mobility-index-rmi http://www.medicaleducation.co.uk/resources/Rivmob.pdf
			• Medical Rehabilitation Follow Along (MRFA; Granger, Ottenbacher, Baker, & Sehgal, 1995)
			• Numerical Pain Rating Scale (Childs, Piva, & Fritz, 2005; Jensen, Karoly, & Braver, 1986)
			• Oswestry Disability Index (Davidson, & Keating, 2002; Fairbank & Pynsent, 2000a, 2000b)
			• Pain Drawing (Bertilson, Grunnesjö, Johansson, & Strender, 2007; Ransford, Cairns, & Mooney, 1976). https://painconsortium.nih.gov
			• Short-Form McGill Pain Questionnaire–2 (SFMPQ–2; Dworkin et al., 2009; Melzack, 1987)
			• Standardized Evaluation of Pain (StEP; Scholtz et al., 2009) http://www.plosmedicine.org/article/info%3Adoi%62F10.1371%2Fjournal.pmed.1000047
				• FIM (Granger, Sherwood, & Greer, 1977; Keith, Granger, Hamilton, & Sherwins, 1987 http://www.scireproject.com/outcome-measures/functional-independence-measure-fim
				• Katz Index of Activities of Daily Living (KATZ-ADL; Katz, Ford, Moskowitz, Jackson, & Jaffe, 1963; Wallace & Shelkey, 2006)
				• Klein-Bell Activities of Daily Living Scale (Klein-Bell ADL Scale) (Dahlgren Karlsson, Lundgren Nilsson, Fridén, & Claesson, 2007; Klein & Bell, 1982, 1993)
				• Level of Rehabilitation Scale-III (LORS-III; Carey & Posavac, 1980; Velozo, Magalhaes, Pan, & Weeks, 1993)

(continued)

TABLE 10-9 (CONTINUED)			
FUNCTIONAL ASSESSMENT OF PHYSICAL DYSFUNCTION			
	FUNCTIONAL CAPACITY EVALUATIONS	**MOTOR CONTROL/MOTOR SKILLS**	**PAIN**	**INDEPENDENT LIVING SKILLS**

EXAMPLES OF WIDELY USED INSTRUMENTS	• Manual muscle tests (MMTs; Daniels & Daniels, 2013, 9th ed., by Hislop, Avers, & Brown, 2013; Kendall, McCreary, Provance, Rodgers, & Romani, 2005; Radomski & Trombly-Latham, 2014)
	• MRFA (Granger, Ottenbacher, Baker, & Sehgal, 1995)
	• Pinch meters and gauges:
	  ◦ Performance Health https://www.performancehealth.com/catalogsearch/result/?q=pinch%20gauges
	  ◦ Abledata https://abledata.acl.gov/products?search_api_views_fulltext=pinch+gauge&field_product_status=All&items_per_page=20
	• EPIC Lift Capacity + Matheson Dexterity & Range of Motion Panel System (Matheson & Ogden, 1987) https://www.mathesondevelopment.com/products/epic-lift-plus-dexterity
			• Visual Analog Scale (VAS; Carlsson, 1983; Cork et al, 2008)	• Patient Evaluation Conference System (PECS; Fisher, Harvey, & Kilgore, 1995; Harvey & Jellinek, 1981)
				• Performance of Self-Care Skills (PASS; Holm & Rogers, 2008; Rogers & Holm, 1989) www.shrs.pitt.edu/ot/about/performance-assessment-self-care-skills-pass
				• Safety Assessment of Function and the Environment for Rehabilitation (SAFER; Chiu, Oliver, Marshall, & Letts, 2001; Oliver, Bathwayt, Brackley, & Tamaki, 1993)
				• SAFER-HOME (Chiu & Oliver, 2006)
				• Measures fall risk
				  ◦ Activities-Specific Balance Confidence Scale (ABC; Powell & Myers, 1995)

(continued)

TABLE 10-9 (CONTINUED)

FUNCTIONAL ASSESSMENT OF PHYSICAL DYSFUNCTION

	FUNCTIONAL CAPACITY EVALUATIONS	MOTOR CONTROL/MOTOR SKILLS	PAIN	INDEPENDENT LIVING SKILLS

EXAMPLES OF WIDELY USED INSTRUMENTS				• Measures fear of falling, mobility confidence
				  ○ Berg Balance Scale (Berg, Wood-Dauphinee, Williams, & Maki, 1992)
				• Measures mobility and balance
				  ○ Comprehensive Falls Risk Screening Instrument (Fabre, Ellis, Kosma, Moore, McCarter, & Wood, 2010)
				• Measures history of falls, medication management, vision, mobility, and home environment
				  ○ Tinetti Performance-Oriented Mobility Assessment (POMA; Tinetti, 1986)
				• Measures mobility and balance and in-home fall hazards
				  ○ Westmead Home Safety Assessment (Cooper et al., 2002).

10.9.3 Vocational and Prevocational

In assessing an individual's prevocational ability, an evaluator seeks information on basic ability levels required for specific occupations. Most prevocational tests involve some aspect of motor coordination. Tests such as the Bennett Mechanical Comprehension Test (Bennett & Fry, 1969), Crawford Small Parts Dexterity Test (Crawford & Crawford, 1949), Strömberg Dexterity Test, and O'Conner Tweezer Dexterity Test (Table 10-10) require the subject to perform tasks using small tools in an assembly operation. Work samples are used to assess an individual's vocational aptitudes, worker characteristics, and vocational interests (Nadolsky, 1974) in areas of vocational potential in various fields, gross and fine manual dexterity, visual and tactile discrimination, and work habits. The tests purport to measure skill proficiencies related to industrial work. Tests, such as the McCarron-Dial Systems (McCarron & Dial, 1986), have been devised to evaluate work behavior at a sheltered workshop as indicative of vocational aptitude. Other work sampling tests include the Micro Tower System of Vocational Evaluation (Backman, 1977) and the VITAS (Vocational Interest, Temperament and Aptitude System; Vocational Research Institute, 1980). More elaborate methods for assessing vocational aptitude in various industrial occupations are available through the Valpar International Corporation (http://www.valparint.com) and Stout University.

There are many self-devised, unpublished, prevocational tests that are used in sheltered workshops, occupational therapy clinics, and special schools. Table 10-10 lists some of the more common prevocational tests, and Table 10-11 provides examples of the more common work sample systems and their addresses.

10.9.3.1 Vocational Interest Tests

Most investigators constructing vocational interest tests assume that the following occurs:

- Vocational interests are stable characteristics.
- Vocational interests can be measured by paper-and-pencil tests.
- Vocational interests are grouped around clusters of interest.
- Individuals in occupations share common interests and characteristics.
- There is a positive relationship between vocational interests and choice of occupation.
- Job satisfaction is related to vocational interest and aptitude.

The Strong Vocational Interest Test (Campbell, 1987) and the Kuder Occupational Interest Survey (Kuder & Findley, 1966) are the two tests most widely used by clinical psychologists and social researchers. Table 10-12 lists the most widely used tests available for measuring vocational interest.

10.9.4 Geriatrics

Several tests have been developed specifically for the geriatric population. Many of these tests can be administered in a hospital, nursing home, or home setting. Table 10-13 describes some of the most commonly used tests administered by occupational therapists.

10.9.5 Pediatrics

The basic assumption underlying all child development scales is that development is vertical, sequential, and hierarchical. Arnold Gesell and associates in the Children's Development Laboratories at Yale University during the 1920s and 1930s used observational analysis of children's behavior to develop norms. Gesell provided the earliest data correlating age with task attainment in such areas as perceptual-motor, language, and personal-social. Since Gesell, other developmental researchers have provided data demonstrating that the growth of human abilities are linked to a biological clock that determines when behavior unfolds at certain critical periods along an age continuum. Differences among child development tests are based on the factors identified and the methods used for assessment. These tests also vary in the time involved in administering a test and in the requirements needed to validly interpret results. For example, the Denver Developmental Screening *Test* (Frankenburg, Dodds, Archer, Shapiro, & Bresnick, 1992) takes about 15 minutes to administer by nonprofessional health aides, whereas the Gesell Developmental Scale requires at least 2 hours to administer by a professionally trained psychometrician. Examples of the most widely used child development scales are described in Table 10-14.

10.9.6 Special Populations

In addition to general tests in psychosocial function and physical disabilities, assessments have been developed for specific populations, such as individuals with arthritis or stroke. These tests have been standardized with these specific populations and should not be used with typical individuals. Table 10-15 provides information about many of these tests.

10.9.7 Neuropsychological Batteries

Clinical neuropsychology is a relatively new field that attempts to relate behavior to brain functioning. Neuropsychological testing is requested by clinicians, therapists, and educators in special cases. For example, neuropsychological testing is usually requested when a client has sustained a traumatic or acquired brain injury.

Table 10-10

Vocational and Prevocational Tests

TEST	TARGET POPULATION	PURPOSE	VARIABLES ASSESSED	PUBLISHER/SOURCE
Lafayette Hand Tool Dexterity Test Formerly Minnesota (Bennett) Hand Tool Dexterity Test (Bennett, 1946, 1985)	Adolescents through adults	Assesses basic skills necessary for any job requiring hand tools	• Fine motor coordination • Manual dexterity	Lafayette Instrument Company http://lafayetteevaluation.com/ products/hand-tool-dexterity
Bennett Mechanical Comprehension Test-II (Bennett, 2014)	Adolescents through adults	Online test that measures the understanding of mechanical principles or general physical concepts in practical situations	• Mechanical comprehension	Pearson Assessment/Psych Corp. https://www. pearsonclinical.com/talent/ products/100001282/bennett-mechanical-comprehension-testsupsup--ii.html
O'Connor Finger Dexterity Test (O'Connor, circa 1920a)	Adolescents through adults	Assess rapid manipulation of small objects	• Finger dexterity • Speed	Lafayette Instrument Company http://www.lafayetteevaluation. com/product_detail. asp?ItemID=161
O'Connor Tweezer Dexterity Test (O'Connor, circa 1920b)	Adolescents through adults	Assess aptitude for work involving precision with small tool usage	• Fine motor coordination • Speed	Lafayette Instrument Company http://www.lafayetteevaluation. com/product_detail. asp?ItemID=162

(continued)

Table 10-10 (continued)

Vocational and Prevocational Tests

TEST	TARGET POPULATION	PURPOSE	VARIABLES ASSESSED	PUBLISHER/SOURCE
Purdue Pegboard Test (Tiffin, 1948)	Adults	Assess fine motor dexterity	• Gross movements of hands, fingers, and arms • Fingertip dexterity necessary for assembly tasks	Lafayette Instrument Company http://www.lafayetteevaluation. com/product_detail. asp?ItemID=159
Roeder Manipulative Aptitude Test (Roeder, 1970)	Adults	Assess fine motor dexterity	• Speed and accuracy for hand-eye coordination • Finger dexterity	Lafayette Instrument Company http://www.lafayetteevaluation. com/product_detail. asp?ItemID=169
EPIC Lift Capacity + Matheson Dexterity & Range of Motion Panel System (Matheson & Ogden, 1987).	Adults	Assess safe lifting, ROM	• Lift capacity • Dexterity • ROM	Matheson Development LLC https://www. mathesondevelopment.com/ products/epic-lift-plus-dexterity

TABLE 10-11

EXAMPLES OF WORK SAMPLE SYSTEMS

MCCARRON-DIAL SYSTEMS, INC.

http://www.mccarrondial.com/

An assessment system that assesses strengths and weaknesses in verbal-cognitive-language, sensory, motor, emotional, and integration-coping. Information from these factors "may be used to estimate the appropriate program level for serving individuals in a preschool, transitional planning, prevocational or vocational setting" (McCarron-Dial, n. d., p. 1). Used with individuals ages 4 years through adult.

MICRO-TOWER SYSTEM OF VOCATIONAL EDUCATION (BACKMAN, 1977)

Work sample tests used to measure aptitudes (e.g., motor clerical skill, spatial perception, verbal, numerical) required for semiskilled and unskilled jobs. Appropriate for adolescents through adults.

MOBILE VOCATIONAL EVALUATION (MVE; HESTER, 1994)

http://lafayetteevaluation.com/product_detail.asp?ItemID=239

Normed on over 1500 individuals and linked to the *Dictionary of Occupational Titles*, this system is composed of several tests used in vocational assessment (e.g., Minnesota Manual Dexterity Test, Lafayette Pegboard Test, Hester Reaction Time Test) and designed to assist any individual with a disability to obtain a suitable vocation. For use with adolescents and adults in secondary and postsecondary schools, rehabilitation agencies, hospitals, and clinics. A Windows-compatible computer-assisted testing system is used to analyze the data and present a listing of specific vocations based on client interests and abilities.

PHYSICAL WORK CAPACITY FITNESS EVALUATION SYSTEM (PWC-FES)

http://www.lafayetteevaluation.com/product_detail.asp?ItemID=223

Well-researched and comprehensive evaluation using the Physical Work Capacity and Functional Capacity, which allows objective worker baseline physical information for physically demanding jobs. Evaluation provides data to develop treatment protocols for clients in rehabilitation. Application software is required for scoring and analyzing the results. The report can be used to make decisions about clients returning to work or new employees.

TALENT ASSESSMENT PROGRAMS (TAP; NIGHSWONGER, 1981)

http://www.talentassessment.com/TAP.html

Comprehensive assessment program measuring visualization and retention, discrimination, and dexterity through 10 manual tests related to production level capacities and vocational aptitudes of individuals in areas applicable for occupations in trade, industrial, technical, and professional. A computer program is used to analyze the results and link abilities to occupations listed in the *Dictionary of Occupational Titles* and occupational data from the Department of Labor. The test is appropriately used with adolescents through adults.

VALPAR COMPONENT WORK SAMPLES (VALPAR INTERNATIONAL CORPORATION, 1973)

http://www.valparint.com/

A comprehensive work evaluation system designed to assess vocational abilities through 23 different work samples. The original samples were developed in 1973, but have been updated as needed. Tasks include mechanical, size, discrimination, range of motion and physical capacity, clerical abilities, assembly, coordination and motor dexterity, drafting skill, and electronic skills. Scores are obtained through computer-based programs, with the criterion-referenced scores linked to the *Revised Handbook for Analyzing Jobs* (Valpar International Corporation, n.d.b.) and the *Dictionary of Occupational Titles* (Valpar International Corporation, n.d.a.).

Additional information about work sample assessment and systems can be found in *A Guide to Vocational Assessment* (4th ed.) by P. W. Power, 2006, published by Pro-Ed in Austin, TX, or by contacting the Stout Vocational Rehabilitation Institute at the University of Wisconsin-Stout (http://www3.uwstout.edu/svri/index.cfm).

TABLE 10-12

VOCATIONAL INTEREST TESTS

TEST	TARGET POPULATION	PURPOSE	VARIABLES ASSESSED	PUBLISHER/SOURCE
COPSystem (Knapp & Knapp, 1982; Knapp & Knapp-Lee, 1995; Knapp-Lee & Best, 1982)	Adolescents through adults	Identify occupational choices based on 14 occupational clusters through interests (Career Occupational Preference System Interest Inventory), abilities (Career Ability Placement Survey), and values (Career Orientation Placement and Evaluation Survey)	Self-administered inventory measures interests and values; paper-and-pencil tests in eight abilities measure aptitude	Educational & Industrial Testing Service, (EdITS) http://www.edits.net/products/copsystem.html
Geist Picture Interest Inventory-Revised (Geist, 1975)	Grade 8 through adult	Identify vocational and avocational interests using a minimum of language	Picture selection test measures occupational interest. Spanish and hearing-impaired forms available	Western Psychological Services http://portal.wpspublish.com/portal/page?_pageid=53,69273&_dad=portal&_schema=PORTAL
Kuder Career Search with Person Match (KCS; Zytowki, n.d.). Takes the place of the Kuder Occupational Interest Survey (Kuder & Zytowski, 1991).	Middle school, high school, and adults. Not recommended for career choice at middle school level.	Forced choice interest inventory using triads in which individual marks "most," "next most," and "least" preferred. Use of the Kuder Skills Assessment (Luzzo & Zytowski, 2001) and Super Work Values (Zytowski, 2001) provides comprehensive career assessment.	Pattern of interests similar to groups of people in six career clusters: 1. Outdoor/mechanical 2. Science/technical 3. Arts/communication 4. Social/personal services 5. Sales/management 6. Business detail	Kuder Inc. http://www.kuder.com/solutions/kuder-assessments.html#kuder_career_search
Reading-Free Vocational Interest Inventory (Becker, 1981, 2000)	Adolescents and older adults who are learning disabled, intellectually disabled, and disadvantaged	Measure vocational interests with special populations	Picture format measuring occupational interests. Specifically designed for individuals who cannot read	Pro-Ed http://www.proedinc.com/customer/productView.aspx?ID=3052

(continued)

TABLE 10-12 (CONTINUED)

VOCATIONAL INTEREST TESTS

TEST	TARGET POPULATION	PURPOSE	VARIABLES ASSESSED	PUBLISHER/SOURCE
Self-Directed Search Form R (4th ed.; SDS-R; Holland, 1994) and Self-Directed Search Form E (4th ed.; SDS-E; Holland, 1994)	Form R: Ages 11 to 72 Form E: Ages 15 to 72	Assess career interests using Holland's RIASEC (Realistic, Investigative, Artistic, Social, Enterprising, and Conventional) theory. Form R is for typical individuals; Form E is for those with poor reading skills.	Yields three letter summary code related to one's personality, using these factors: Realistic, Investigative, Artistic, Social, Enterprising, and Conventional	PAR, Inc. http://www4.parinc. com/Products/Product. aspx?ProductID=SDS_R http://www4.parinc. com/Products/Product. aspx?ProductID=SDS_E
Strong Interest Inventory and Skills Confidence Inventory (SCII; Betz, Borgen, & Harmon, 2004; Strong, Campbell, & Hansen, 1985)	Adolescents through adults	Assess occupational and leisure interests for individuals oriented toward college graduation and professional occupations	GOT, BIS, PSS, and OS. Computerized scoring required (disk available through Consulting Psychologist Press)	Consulting Psychologist Press https://www.cpp.com/products/ strong/strong_info.aspx
Wide Range Interest and Occupation Test (2nd ed.; WRIOT-2; Glutting & Wilkinson, 2003)	Junior high school through adult	Assess occupational interests	Picture format measuring occupational interest. Adaptations for individuals who are blind. Computer format is available, to take in two sessions.	Pearson Assessment/Psych Corp http://psychcorp. pearsonassessments.com/ HAIWEB/Cultures/en-us/ Productdetail.htm?Pid=WRIOT-2&Mode=summary

BIS = Basic Interest Scale; GOT = General Occupational Themes; OS = Occupational Scales; PSS = Personal Style Scales.

TABLE 10-13

GERIATRIC SCALES

TEST	TARGET POPULATION	PURPOSE	VARIABLES ASSESSED	PUBLISHER/SOURCE
Cognitive Function				
Contextual Memory Test (Toglia, 1996)	Measure awareness and strategy use	• Awareness of memory • Recall of drawn items • Strategy use	Interview/questionnaire	Therapy Skill Builders
Executive Function Performance Test (EFPT; Baum et al., 2008)	Executive function	• Initiation • Organization • Sequencing	Performance of real-world tasks	Washington University St. Louis, MO
Mini-Mental State Examination (2nd ed.; MMSE-2; Folstein, Folstein, White, & Messer, 2010)	Obtain a quantitative measure of cognitive performance for elderly with neurological dysfunction quickly Standard version (MMSE-2:SV) and Expanded version (MMSE-2:EV) Screening for cognitive impairment	• Safety • Task completion • Orientation • Memory • Attention and calculation • Recall • Following oral and written instructions	Oral questionnaire administered by examiner	PAR, Inc. http://www4.parinc.com/Products/Product.aspx?ProductID=MMSE-2 Folstein, M. F., Folstein, S. E., & McHugh, P. R. (1975). "Mini-mental state". A practical method for grading the cognitive state of patients for the clinician. *Journal of Psychiatric Research, 12,* 189-198.
Montreal Cognitive Assessment (MOCA; Nasreddine et al., 2005)	Adults who may be suspected of having some form of cognitive impairment	• Memory • Visuospatial • Executive function • Attention/concentration • Language • Orientation to time and place	Oral questionnaire administered by examiner; performance tasks	MOCA https://www.mocatest.org/splash/
Multiple Errands Test-Revised (MET-R, Morrison et al., 2013)	Executive function	• Cooking • Medication management • Using telephone • Bill paying	Performance of real-world tasks	Canadian Partnership for Stroke Recovery https://www.strokengine.ca/en/family/met_family/

(continued)

TABLE 10-13 (CONTINUED)

GERIATRIC SCALES

TEST	TARGET POPULATION	PURPOSE	VARIABLES ASSESSED	PUBLISHER/SOURCE
Rivermead Behavioral Memory Test (3rd ed.; RBMT3; Wilson, Baddley, Cockburn, & Hiorns, n.d.; Wilson et al., 2008)	Assess problems in memory and provide means for monitoring treatment outcomes	• Immediate memory • Short-delay in memory • Long-term memory • Overall memory function	Visual or verbal presentation of questions with verbal response	Pearson Clinical Corp https://www.pearsonclinical.com/psychology/products/100000644/rivermead-behavioural-memory-test-third-edition-rbmt3.html?Pid=978-074-9134-761&Mode=summary
Independent Living				
Assessment of Living Skills and Resources–Revised-2 (ALSAR-R2; Williams et al., 1991; Clemson, Bundy Unsworth, & Fiatarone Singh, 2008)	Assess the living skills and resources in a community-dwelling of elderly residents to determine treatment protocol and assist in problem solving	Assesses areas of IADL including: • Use of community resources • Leisure time • Medication • Finances • Home management	Rating scale, with scores combined to determine risk	University of Sydney http://www.sydney.edu.au/health-sciences/documents/assessment-living-skills.pdf
Instrumental Activities of Daily Living (IADL) Scale (Lawton & Brody, 1969; Graf, 2007)	Assess skills needed by elderly individuals to live independently	• Eight categories of IADL (e.g., housekeeping, food preparation, finances) rated according to level of independence	Rating scale, with higher scores indicating need for more assistance	Lawton, M. P., & Brody, E. M. (1969). Assessment of Older People: Self-maintaining and instrumental activities of daily living. *Gerontologist, 9*, 179-186.
Older Adults Resources and Services (OARS; Duke University Center for the Study of Aging and Human Development, 1978)	Multidimensional instrument to obtain information in basic and instrumental ADLs for elderly clients living in the community	• Social resources • Economic resources • Mental health • Physical health • ADLs	Structured interview, now available online exclusively.	Duke University Center for the Study of Aging and Human Development

(continued)

TABLE 10-13 (CONTINUED)

GERIATRIC SCALES

TEST	TARGET POPULATION	PURPOSE	VARIABLES ASSESSED	PUBLISHER/SOURCE
Quality of Life				
Life Satisfaction Index (Neugarten, Havinghurst & Tobin, 1961; Barrett & Murk, 2006)	Measure of self-perception of well-being in elderly clients	• Cognitive/short-term • Cognitive/long-term • Emotional/short-term well-being	Self-administered questionnaire	Indiana University http://hdl.handle.net/1805/1160 Neugarten, B. L., Havingurst, R. J., & Tobin, S. S. (1961). The Measurement of Life Satisfaction. *Journal of Gerontology, 16,* 134-143. Guigoz, Y., Vellas, B., Garry, P. J., & Albarede, J. L. (1994). *Facts and research in gerontology.* (Suppl.) 2, 56-62. Paris, France: Sendi Publishing Company.
World Health Organization Quality of Life-BREF (Power, Bullinger, & Harper, 1999)	Measure of quality of life across world cultures	• Physical • Psychological • Social • Environmental	Self-administered questionnaire	The WHOQOL Group, Programme on Mental Health, http://www.who.int/mental_health/media/en/76.pdf
Quality of Life Scale (QOLS; Burckhardt & Anderson 2003)	Quality of life measure for those with chronic illness	• Physical well-being • Relationships • Social/civic activities • Personal development • Recreation	Self-administered questionnaire	Oregon Health Sciences University http://www.contentedits.com/img.asp?id=13179

Fall Risk Assessment

See Table 10-9.

TABLE 10-14

PEDIATRIC ASSESSMENTS

DEVELOPMENTAL	BEHAVIOR	MOTOR AND SENSORY INTEGRATION	VISUAL, AUDITORY, AND MOTOR PROCESSING	PLAY
• Assessment of Preterm Infants' Behavior (ABIP; Als, 1984; Als, Duffy, & McAnulty, 1988a, 1988b; Als, Butler, Kosta, & McAnulty, 2005) • Bayley Scales of Infant and Toddler Development (3rd ed.; Bayley-III; Pearson, 2005) https://www.pearsonclinical.com/childhood/products/100000123/bayley-scales-of-infant-and-toddler-development-third-edition-bayley-iii.html • Denver Developmental Screening Test-II (DDST-II; Frankenburg, Dodds, Archer, Shapiro, & Bresnick, 1992) http://denverii.com	• Achenbach System of Empirically Based Assessment (ASEBA; Achenbach, 1991; Achenbach & Rescorla, 2001, 2007, 2010, 2018) http://www.aseba.org/ • Attention Deficit Disorder Evaluation Scale (4th ed.; ADDES-4; McCarney & Arthaud, 2013) http://www.hawthorne-ed.com/pages/adhd/ad1.html • Behavior Assessment System for Children-3 (BASC-3; Reynolds & Kamphaus & Vannest, 2015) https://www.pearsonclinical.com/education/products/100000658/behavior-assessment-system-for-children-second-edition-basc-2.html	• Alberta Infant Motor Scales (AIMS; Piper & Darrah, 1994; Piper, Pinnell, Darrah, Macquire, & Byrne, 1992) • Erhardt Developmental Prehension Assessment (3rd ed.; Erhardt, 1994) http://www.erhardtproducts.com/hand.html • Miller Assessment for Preschoolers (Miller, 1988) https://www.wpspublish.com/store/p/2861/map-miller-assessment-for-preschoolers • Quality of Upper Extremity Skills Test (QUEST; DeMatteo, et al., 1992, 1993) https://www.canchild.ca/en/shop/19-quality-of-upper-extremity-skills-test-quest	• Bender Visual-Motor Gestalt II (Bender, 1938; revised by Branningan & Decker, 2003) https://www.hmhco.com/search?term=Bender-Gestalt • Bruininks-Oseretsky Test of Motor Proficiency (2nd ed.; BOT-2; Bruininks & Bruininks, 2005) https://www.pearsonclinical.com/therapy/products/100000648/bruininks-oseretsky-test-of-motor-proficiency-second-edition-bot2.	• Revised Knox Preschool Play Scale (RKPPS; Knox, 1974, 1997) • Transdisciplinary Play-Based Assessment-2 (Linder, 2008) http://products.brookespublishing.com/Transdisciplinary-Play-Based-Assessment-Second-Edition-TPBA2-P215.aspx • Revised Concise Symbolic Play Scale (Westby, 2000). https://www.smartspeechtherapy.com/wp-content/uploads/2017/07/Revised-Concise-Symbolic-Play-Scale.pdf

(continued)

TABLE 10-14 (CONTINUED)

PEDIATRIC ASSESSMENTS

DEVELOPMENTAL	BEHAVIOR	MOTOR AND SENSORY INTEGRATION	VISUAL, AUDITORY, AND MOTOR PROCESSING	PLAY
• Developmental Profile-3 (DP-3; Alpern, 2007) https://www.wpspublish.com/store/p/2743/dp-3-developmental-profile-3 • Pediatric Evaluation of Disability Inventory (PEDI; Haley, Coster, Ludlow, Haltiwanger, & Andrellos, 1992) https://www.pearsonclinical.com/childhood/products/100000505/pediatric-evaluation-of-disability-inventory-pedi.html?Pid=076-1617-647&Mode=summary • Pediatric Evaluation of Disability Inventory-Computer Adaptive Test (PEDI-CAT; Haley et al., 2011) http://www.pedicat.com	• Burks Behavior Rating Scales (2nd ed.; BBRS-2; Burks, 2006) https://https://www.wpspublish.com/store/p/2673/bbrs-2-burks-behavior-rating-scales-second-edition • Children's Depression Inventory-2 (CDI-2; Kovacs, 2011) https://www.pearsonclinical.com/psychology/products/100000636/childrens-depression-inventory-2-cdi2.html?Pid=015-8044-762	• Test of Handwriting Skills-Revised (THWS-R; Milone, 2007) https://www.wpspublish.com/store/p/3042/ths-r-test-of-handwriting-skills-revised • Sensory Integration and Praxis Tests (SIPT; Ayres, 1989) https://www.wpspublish.com/store/p/2971/sipt-sensory-integration-and-praxis-tests • Sensory Processing Measure 2 (SPM-2; Miller-Kuhaneck, Henry, Glennon, 2008) https://www.researchgate.net/publication/320474683_The_New_Sensory_Processing_Measure_SPM-2 • Sensory Profile-2 (Dunn, 2014) https://www.pearsonclinical.com/therapy/products/100000822/sensory-profile-2.html	• Beery-Buktenica Developmental Test of Visual-Motor Integration, (6th ed.; BEERY VMI; Beery, Buktenica, & Beery, 2010) http://www.therapro.com/Browse-Category/Visual-Perception-and-Visual-Skills/6th-Ed-Starter-Kit.html Motor-Free Visual Perception Test-4 (MVPT-4; Colarusso & Hammill, 2015) https://www.wpspublish.com/store/p/3303/mvpt-4-motor-free-visual-perception-test-4 • Peabody Developmental Motor Scales-2 (PDMS-2; Folio & Fewell, 2000) http://www.therapro.com/Browse-Category/Gross-Motor-Fine-Motor/Complete-TEST.html • Test of Visual-Motor Skills-3 (TVMS-3; Martin, 2006) http://www.therapro.com/Welcome/?search=TVMS-3	• Pediatric Interest Profiles (Henry, 2000) https://www.moho.uic.edu/productDetails.aspx?aid=43

(continued)

TABLE 10-14 (CONTINUED)

PEDIATRIC ASSESSMENTS

DEVELOPMENTAL	BEHAVIOR	MOTOR AND SENSORY INTEGRATION	VISUAL, AUDITORY, AND MOTOR PROCESSING	PLAY
	• Adaptive Behavior Assessment System-3 (ABAS-3; Harrison & Oakland, 2015) https://www.pearsonclinical.com/psychology/products/100001262/adaptive-behavior-assessment-system-third-edition-abas-3.html • Conners 3 (Conners, 2008) https://www.mhs.com/MHS-Assessment?prodname=conners3		• Test of Visual-Perceptual Skills (nonmotor)–4 (TVPS-4; Martin, 2006, 2016) http://www.therapro.com/Tests/TVPS-4 • Miller Function & Participation Scales (M-FUN; Miller, 2006) https://www.pearsonclinical.com/therapy/products/100000557/miller-function-participation-scales.html • Goal-Oriented Assessment of Lifeskills (GOAL; Miller & Oakland, 2013) https://www.wpspublish.com/store/p/2787/goal-goal-oriented-assessment-of-lifeskills • Test of Visual-Motor Skills–3 (TVPS–3; Martin, 2006) http://www.academictherapy.com/detailATP.tpl?action=search&eqskudatarq=8519-5	

TABLE 10-15

ASSESSMENTS FOR SPECIAL POPULATIONS

ARTHRITIS	*Arthritis Impact Measurement Scales (AIMS)* **Purpose**: To measure changes in pain, mobility, social function, and global health in patients with arthritis **Versions**: An original version (AIMS); an expanded version (AIMS2; Meenan, Mason, Anderson, Guccione, & Kazis, 1992); a short-form of the AIMS2 (AIMS2-SF; Ren, Kazis, & Meenan, 1999); Haavardsholm, Kvien, Uhlig, Smedstad, & Guillemin, 2000); a child version; and a version for the elderly (Geri-AIMS) **Available From**: https://www.rheumatology.org/I-Am-A/Rheumatologist/Research/Clinician-Researchers/Arthritis-Impact-Measurement-Scales-AIMS
	Edinburgh Rehabilitation Status Scale (ERSS; Affleck, Aitken, Hunter, McGuire, & Roy, 1988) **Purpose**: To measure levels of performance and changes during rehabilitation in independence, activity, social integration, and effects of symptoms on lifestyles areas **Available From**: http://www.scientificspine.com/spine-scores/edinburgh-rehabilitation-status-scale_%28erss%29.html
	Functional Status Index (FSI; Jette, 1980, 1987) **Purpose**: To assess adult patients with arthritis living in the community. **References** • Jette, A. M. (1980). Functional Status Index: Reliability of a chronic disease evaluation instrument. *Archives of Physical Medicine and Rehabilitation, 61*, 395-401. • Jette, A. M. (1987). Functional Status Index: Reliability of a chronic disease evaluation instrument. *Journal of Rheumatology, 14*(Suppl. 15), 15-19.
	Standardized Test of Patient Mobility (Jebsen et al., 1970; Mikulic, Griffith, & Jebsen, 1976) **Purpose**: To assess patient mobility in categories of bed mobility, wheelchair activities, transfers, and ambulation **Reference** • Jebsen, R. H., Trieschmann, R. B., Mikulic, M. A., Hartley, R. B., McMillan, J. A., & Snook, M. E. (1970). Measurement of time in a standardized test of patient mobility. *Archives of Physical Medicine & Rehabilitation, 51*(3), 170-175.
LOW BACK PAIN	*Oswestry Low Back Pain Disability Questionnaire (Fairbank, Couper, Davies, & O'Brien, 1980)* **Purpose**: Self-rating questionnaire used to assess patients with low back pain by determining its impact on ADLs **Limitations**: Because this is a self-rating questionnaire, the response may be subjective and items may be left out. **Versions**: Several versions are available on the internet, including an electronic form. **Available From**: http://www.rehab.msu.edu/_files/_docs/oswestry_low_back_disability.pdf
	Sickness Impact Profile (SIP; Bergnen, Bobbitt, Carter, & Gilson, 1981; Gilson et al., 1975) **Purpose**: To provide a descriptive profile of changes in a person's behavior due to sickness. **Available From**: http://ajph.aphapublications.org/doi/abs/10.2105/AJPH.65.12.1304 **Research Study**: "Pain Measurement in Elders With Chronic Low Back Pain: Traditional And Alternative Approaches" (Weiner, Pieper, McConnell, Martinez, & Keefe, 1996)

(continued)

TABLE 10-15 (CONTINUED)

ASSESSMENTS FOR SPECIAL POPULATIONS

OSTEOARTHRITIS	**Purpose**: To analyze and compare the content of questionnaires that have been used to assess functioning in patients with hand osteoarthritis (OA) based on the ICF. The authors concluded that a "comprehensive measurements of functioning in hand OA, . . . [should] include both one instrument with a low diversity ratio (for disease-specific aspects) and another instrument with a high diversity ratio (for broader aspects of functioning including some aspects of participation). **Research Study**: "Measuring Functioning in Patients With Hand Osteoarthritis—Content Comparison of Questionnaires Based on the *International Classification of Functioning, Disability and Health* (ICF)" (Stamm et al., 2006)
SPINAL CORD INJURY	*Spinal Cord Injury-Functional Index/Assistive Technology (Slavin et al., 2016)* **Purpose**: To assess basic mobility, self-care, fine motor function, and ambulation **References** • Slavin, M. D., Ni, P., Tulsky, D. S., Kisala, P. A., Heinemann, A. W., Charlifue, S., . . . Jette, A. M. (2016). Spinal Cord Injury-Functional Index/Assistive Technology Short Forms. *Archives Physical Medicine Rehabilitation., 97*, 1745-1752
STROKE	*Frenchay Activities Index (FAI; Holbrook & Skilbeck, 1983)* **Purpose**: To assess the frequency of doing instrumental activities of daily living (IADL) through a survey or interview format. **References** • Holbrook, M., & Skilbeck, C. E. (1983). An activities index for use with stroke patients. *Age and Ageing, 12*, 166-170. • Schuling, J., deHaan, R., Limburg, M., & Groenier, K. (1993). The Frenchay Activities Index: Assessment of functional status in stroke patients. *Stroke, 13*, 1173-1177. • Singam, A., Ytterberg, C., Tham, K., & von Koch, L. (2015). Participation in complex and social everyday activities six years after stroke: Predictors for return to pre-stroke level. *PLoS One, 10*, e0144344. **Available From**: https://www.strokengine.ca/family/fai_family/
	Fugl-Meyer Assessment (Fugl-Meyer, Jääskö, Leyman, Olsson, & Steglind, 1975; Gladstone, Danells, & Black, 2002) **Purpose**: To assess motor functioning, balance, sensation, and joint functioning in patients with post-stroke hemiplegia. **Contact**: Institute of Rehabilitation Medicine, University of Gotheberg, Gotheberg, Sweden. A version of the measure is available in Fugl-Meyer et al. (1975) and Dittmar & Gresham (1997) **Available From**: http://neurophys.gu.se/digitalAssets/1520/1520603_fma-ue-protocol-english-updated-20150311.pdf
	Time Care Profile (Halstead & Hartley, 1975) **Purpose**: To describe the use of a diary method to record the amount of time the patient receives assistance during the course of a normal day as an index of dependency in ADLs. **Reference** • Halstead, L., & Hartley, R. B. (1975). Time care profile: An evaluation of a new method of assessing ADL dependence. *Archives of Physical Medicine and Rehabilitation, 56*, 110-115.

(continued)

TABLE 10-15 (CONTINUED)

ASSESSMENTS FOR SPECIAL POPULATIONS

TRAUMATIC BRAIN INJURY	*Agitated Behavior Scale (ABS)*

Purpose: To assess the nature and extent of agitation during the acute phase of recovery from acquired brain injury. Its primary purpose is to allow serial assessment of agitation by treatment professionals who want objective feedback about the course of a patient's agitation. Serial assessments are particularly important when treatment interventions are being attempted. This instrument may be useful with populations other than patients recovering from acquired brain injury. Tabloski, McKinnon-Howe, and Remington (1995) and Corrigan, Bogner, and Tabloski (1996) demonstrated the utility of the ABS for measuring agitation in nursing home residents with progressive dementias, primarily Alzheimer's disease.

Information regarding the ABS was contributed by the Ohio Regional TBI Model System. The Center for Outcome Measurement in Brain Injury.

Available From: http://www.tbims.org/combi/abs

Community Integration Questionnaire (CIQ; Corrigan & Deming, 1995; Willer, Ottenbacher, & Coad, 1994)

Purpose: To provide an objective measure for community integration after traumatic brain injury by measuring frequency of performance of activities in home integration, social integration, and productive activities

Reference

- Kratz, A. L., Chadd, E., Jensen, M. P., Kehn, M., & Kroll, T. (2015). An examination of the psychometric properties of the community integration questionnaire (CIQ) in spinal cord injury. *Journal of Spinal Cord Medicine, 38*, 446-455.

Available From: http://tbims.org/combi/ciq/index.html (including description, rating forms, directions for scoring, references and a forum for discussion)

Disability Rating Scale (Rappaport, 2005; Rappaport, Hall, Hopkins, Belleza, & Cope, 1982)

Purpose: To measure accurately general functional changes over the course of recovery.

Available From: https://www.neuroskills.com/resources/disability-rating-scale.php

---

Rabideau Kitchen Evaluation-Revised: An Assessment of Meal Preparation Skill (RKE-R; Neistadt, 1992, 1994, 2000b)

Purpose: To evaluate functional sequencing abilities of individuals with traumatic or anoxic brain trauma by the use of a meal preparation treatment protocol.

References

- Neistadt, M. E. (1992). The Rabideau kitchen evaluation, revised: An assessment of meal preparation skill. *Occupational Therapy Journal of Research, 12*, 242-255.
- Neistadt, M. E. (1993). The relationship between constructional and meal preparation skills. *Archives of Physical Medicine and Rehabilitation, 74*, 144-148.
- Neistadt, M. E. (1994). A meal preparation treatment protocol for adults with brain injury. *American Journal of Occupational Therapy, 48*, 431-438.
- Neistadt, M. E. (2000b). Rabideau Kitchen Evaluation-Revised: An assessment of meal preparation skill. In M. E. Neistadt, *Occupational therapy evaluation for adults: A pocket guide* (pp. 136-137). Baltimore, MD: Lippincott, Williams & Wilkins.

Rivermead Perceptual Assessment Battery-III (RPAB-III; Whiting, Lincoln, Cockburn, & Bhavnani, 1985; revised)

Purpose: To evaluate visual perceptual ability using 16 sub-tests in clients across a wide age range

Available From: https://www.gl-assessment.co.uk/products/rivermead-perceptual-assessment-battery

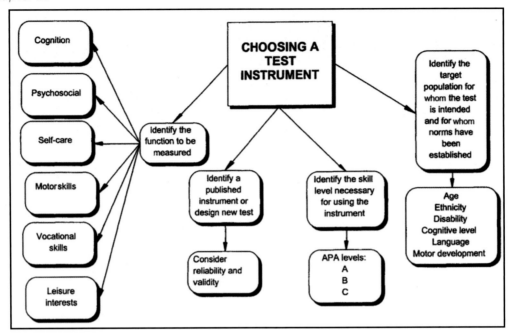

Figure 10-4. Factors in choosing a test instrument.

Neuropsychological testing may also be requested when a more specific understanding of an individual's strengths and weaknesses is desired. Although individual neuropsychological tests can be given, frequently neuropsychologists use a specific battery of tests generated by their particular philosophical stance.

The Halsted-Reitan Neuropsychological Test Battery is an adult test that consists of up to 37 individual tests, each of which must be administered to obtain a complete profile of an individual's brain functioning. Diagnosis is dependent on (a) comparing the client's score with a comparison group, (b) comparing scores between individual tests, and (c) comparing differences between scores performed on the right or left side of the body. Based on the profile of scores, treatment for deficits are suggested.

Luria (2012) developed a second approach to neuropsychological testing by developing specific test items that would allow the clinician to identify the way in which a person approached a task. The Luria-Nebraska Neuropsychological Battery (Golden & Freshwater, 2001) is an outgrowth of Luria's work. Although this battery is not frequently used, it does provide information for the clinician regarding brain-behavior relationships.

Edith Kaplan, using the philosophy and work of Luria, has proposed a third approach to neuropsychological testing: an evaluation should result in an understanding of the way in which a person approaches a task, regardless of which tests are used. This method, called the *Boston process approach*, relies less on specific instruments and more on observation of behavior during the evaluation. All neurological functioning (e.g., cognitive, perceptual, memory, language, organization, personality) is evaluated in this approach. The Wechsler Adult Intelligence Scale-IV

(Wechsler, 2014) and the Wechsler Intelligence Scale for Children–Fourth Edition, Integrated (Wechsler, 2003), are examples of instruments that incorporate the Boston process approach.

Clinical researchers may not, at first, be involved in neuropsychological testing as part of their research. Nonetheless, information obtained from these tests, as well as use of pre- and post-test data can be useful as outcome measures in examining the relationship between changes in behavior and interventions.

10.10 Reviewing and Evaluating Tests

For the researcher, the selection of a valid and reliable instrument is critical. Knowledge in assessing the adequacy of a measuring instrument is extremely important in view of the literally thousands of tests that are published by test corporations. Before the clinical researcher chooses a test to use in research, the purpose for the test must be determined. Does the researcher need to screen participants for normal intelligence or average achievement? Is adaptive behavior a concern? If the purpose of the investigation is to evaluate the effect of a treatment on reducing low back pain, the researcher will want to make sure that all subjects have clinically significant low back pain (Figure 10-4).

The next step in determining which test to use is to review the appropriate tests that are available, taking into account the psychometric properties, including the reliability, validity, and measurement scales of each test. If there are special qualifications in administering the test, the researcher must know who is able to administer the test and how long it will take to administer. The following outline and examples of reviews of tests will illustrate the manner in which tests are analyzed (Stein, 1988).

10.10.1 Outline for Reviewing Tests

1. *Title*
2. *Date published, date revised*
3. *Authors*
4. *Publisher*: Distributor of test or where test is available
5. *Target population*: What was the original sample from which data were collected in terms of age, diagnostic group, and geographical location? Is there a specific target population for which the test is appropriate?
6. *Variables assessed*: What are the specific areas of function, behavior, or personality that are being assessed? What are the major stated purposes of the test?
7. *Measurement scales*: What is the level of measurement in the test?
   a. Qualitative (subjective judgment)
      i. *Nominal scale of measurement* refers to evaluating variables using independent categories such as can or cannot perform a specific task.
      ii. *Ordinal scale of measurement* refers to evaluating variables using magnitude and ranking, such as completely dependent in task, needs assistance, or independent functioning. Variables can also be rated on a numerical scale from 1 to 5, for example, where 1 indicates no self-care and 5 indicates cares for self independently.
   b. Quantitative (objective evaluation)
      i. *Interval scale of measurement* refers to scoring variables on a continuous scale with equal distances between score values. Pulse rate, blood pressure, height, and weight are usually measured on interval scales using tests that produce mathematical data.
      ii. *Ratio scale of measurement* incorporates the concept of an absolute zero.
8. *Administration of instrument*: Who administers the test and when is it administered? How long does it take to administer? Is there special training to administer the test? Are special materials or environments required?
9. *Scoring and interpretation of results*: Are there overall scores or subtest scores derived from the test results? Are there norms available to interpret raw scores? How are the results used in treatment planning, documentation of progress, and discharge recommendations?
10. *Test reliability and validity*
11. *Other comments*: Included in this section are miscellaneous comments such as the theoretical orientation or conceptual framework of the test and its appropriateness for the clinical researcher.

12. *References*: Includes books, journals, test manuals, and other sources where the test has been published or critically evaluated.

10.10.2 Example of Test Review

1. Kohlman Evaluation of Living Skills (KELS; Gary, 2011)
2. Originally published in 1978, revised in 2011
3. Linda Kohlman Thomson, MOT, OTR, OT(C), CAPS, FAOTA
4. American Occupational Therapy Association
5. Clients with acute psychiatric disorders, elderly patients in acute care hospitals; adolescent through elderly. Must be used cautiously with individuals hospitalized for more than 1 month.
6. Seventeen living skills categorized into five main domains that are measured: self-care, safety and health, money management, transportation and telephone, and work and leisure.
7. Measurement Scales: Nominal and ordinal scales.
8. The test can be given by an occupational therapist or occupational therapist assistant when supervised by the occupational therapist.
9. Each of the 17 living skills are scored for either "independent" or "needs assistance" with a score of 1 (Vi for the work and leisure category) given if the client needs assistance. Items scored as independent are given a score of 0. Individuals obtaining an overall score of 5Vi or less are considered able to live independently; scores above 51/i suggest the client needs assistance to live in the community.
10. Interrater reliability ranges from $r = .84$ to 1.00. Concurrent validity has been measured at $r = .78$ to .89 with Global Assessment Scale; -.84 with Bay Area Functional Performance Evaluation. The test has successfully predicted which elderly patients could live independently.
11. The test provides a quick assessment to provide information about a person's ability in everyday functioning in daily living skills, independent living, and work/leisure.
12. Burnett, J., Dyer, C. M., & Naik, A. D. (2009). Convergent validation of the Kohlman Evaluation of Living Skills as a screening tool of older adults' ability to live safely and independently in the community. *Archives of Physical Medicine and Rehabilitation, 90,* 1948-1952.
13. McGourty, L. K. (1988). Kohlman Evaluation of Living Skills (KELS). In B. J. Hemphill, *Mental health assessment in occupational therapy: A integrative approach to the evaluative process* (pp. 133-146). Thorofare, NJ: SLACK Incorporated.

14. Pickens, S. Naik, A. D., Burnett, J., Kelly, P. A., Gleason, M., & Dyer, C. B. (2007). The utility of the KELS test in substantiated cases of elder self-neglect. *Journal of the American Academy of Nurse Practitioners, 19,* 137-142.

15. Thomson, L. K. (1992). *The Kohlman Evaluation of Living Skills* (KELS; 3rd ed.). Rockville, MD: American Occupational Therapy Association.

16. Thomson, L. K. (1999). The Kohlman Evaluation of Living Skills. In B. J. Hemphill-Pearson (Ed.), *Assessment in occupational therapy mental health: An integrative approach* (pp. 231-244). Thorofare, NJ: SLACK.

10.11 Criterion- and Norm-Referenced Tests

Until recently, most tests were NRTs. These tests, described previously, were developed to classify individuals into levels of instructional groups. The scores obtained by the normative sample on an NRT are distributed along a normal curve. Raw scores obtained by individuals taking an NRT are compared with the normative sample and can be converted into standard scores and percentiles.

There are several advantages to NRTs. Individuals taking the test are compared with the general population, thus the performance of a student or patient can be judged to be typical or atypical. Because NRTs are usually commercially published, psychometric characteristics, such as reliability and item analysis, are carefully considered in the development. Additionally, standardization of an NRT includes administering the test to large samples of individuals stratified across many socioeconomic groups, ages, ethnic backgrounds, and educational levels. In this way, raw scores obtained from a given individual can be compared to the raw score obtained by most of the population having the same characteristics.

At the same time, there are disadvantages to an NRT. Because the tests are broad measures of a subject and contain a limited number of items from many areas within that subject, they are often referred to as *survey tests*. It is not uncommon for an NRT designed to be used in Grades 1 through 12 to include only 100 sight words. Because there is no national or state curriculum, the content found on the test may not match the curriculum of a particular school or community. Finally, because the number of items in each area is limited, the test results cannot be used to measure small gains in progress. Likewise, there is limited value for using the results of an NRT in determining an instructional or therapeutic program.

The purposes of NRTs are (a) to compare an individual's achievement or performance with other individuals of the same age, educational level, and socioeconomic status, and (b) to obtain information regarding the normal population.

When these tests are used with atypical populations, there may be a bias, which results in systematic error. Despite these disadvantages, NRTs are useful in clinical research.

In testing circles during the last 30 years, there has been a growing interest in devising CRTs in lieu of NRTs (Deno, 1985). CRTs, first proposed by Glaser (1963), use content or curricular domains to set the standard of performance. They compare the performance of an individual with a specified level of mastery or achievement rather than with a normative population. Because the performance is compared with a criterion, performance on these tests allows the therapist or teacher to suggest specific classroom goals and objectives to use in program planning. Progress can be monitored more effectively and more discretely.

CRTs are based on a comprehensive theory that generates ideas for a specific content domain. In CRTs, items are selected systematically to represent the content domain. For example, if an investigator is interested in determining the visual perceptual skills of individuals, the first task would be to determine the dimensions of visual perception from the theoretical and experiential perspectives. The investigator would use the theoretical framework to guide the writing of test items, making sure that each aspect of the framework is covered by test items in the CRT. Operational performance standards, obtained by surveying a representational sample of the general population, are used in writing test items. For example, a survey of 10-year-olds would reveal that most of them have no difficulty with activities involving visual closure or visual figure ground. The operational performance standard, therefore, might be set at a criterion level of 90% accuracy for recognition of figures in tasks involving visual figure ground or visual closure.

One example of criterion-referenced testing occurs when measuring an individual's independent living skills. For instance, in the criteria of dressing completely, we might include the act of putting on all clothes right-side out and frontwards, tying shoes, and fastening all fasteners. The individual's ability to perform this activity is measured by a given standard. Until the individual has mastered the expected standard, the individual is not considered to have reached competency. Social skills and self-help skills are often evaluated by CRTs.

CRTs are sometimes referred to as *curriculum-based measures* (CBMs) or *curriculum-based assessments* (CBAs). CBAs and CBMs establish a student's instructional needs in relationship to the requirements of the actual curriculum being used. Just as with CRTs, the CBAs and CBMs assess mastery of learning by providing an operational performance criterion as a necessary standard for passing. Although commercial CRTs are available, teachers and occupational therapists frequently develop the measurement instrument based on their own criteria.

In summary, a CRT is constructed to obtain measurements that can be interpreted in terms of specific criteria or performance standards; however, scores obtained on NRTs are interpreted in terms of comparison to a population. The choice of which test to use depends on the outcome desired. If a researcher is interested in the progress of a particular student over time, a CRT is more appropriate; however, if the researcher is interested in the differences between two groups of subjects, then an NRT may be more appropriate.

A summary of the differences between CRTs and NRTs is given in Table 10-16. This summary may help in deciding which type of test to use.

10.11.1 Applying Criterion-Referenced Concepts to Research

The major content areas for clinical researchers in evaluation include basic living skills, interests, work behavior, and skill attainment. If one uses a criterion-referenced approach to these areas, one should look for the following factors:

- The theory underlying these concepts is identified.
- Research evidence supporting any assumptions of the test are stated.
- The content domain of the test that considers a comprehensive view of skills, interests, and behavior is discussed.
- The specific target population is operationally defined in terms of age, intelligence, education, and degree of disability.
- The test items are generated by selecting representative samples of behavior.
- Performance standards in the test are based on systematically collected data from representative samples of the target population.
- Test items are pilot-tested for clarity and ease of administration.
- Scoring methods are devised that are operationally defined.
- Reliability and validity data are documented.
- A test manual for administering, scoring, and interpreting data is provided.
- The degree of competency in the administration of the test is included in test descriptions.

TABLE 10-16

COMPARISON OF CRITERION- AND NORM-REFERENCED TESTS

CRITERION-REFERENCED TESTS	NORM-REFERENCED TESTS
Absolute standards of competence or mastery are established based on theory	Relative standards are based on normal standards
Scores are derived from standards or behaviors or competency	Scores are compared to established norms
Scores are interpreted based on what the student can or cannot do and then used diagnostically	Scores are interpreted by percentile ranks, standard scores, and organized along a normal curve
Content or items are comprehensive of domain	Content of items are a sample of domain
Cutoff score for passing is based on minimal standards of competency	Cutoff score for passing is based on preestablished percentile rank
Theoretically, all can pass or all can fail	The number of failures is predicted before the test is administered

10.12 TEST PUBLISHERS

The development of new tests and measuring instruments is a relatively recent event in the occupational therapy professions. The clinical nature of these fields and the service-oriented process of treatment have led to the emphasis in the past on developing new treatment techniques rather than measuring outcome variables. However, as the need for accountability and validation for treatment continue on federal and state governmental levels (e.g., through laws such as Individuals with Disabilities Improvement Education Act [IDEIA-2004] and Americans with Disabilities Act [ADA]), the use of tests and measuring instruments to justify therapeutic and educational intervention has become more important. Many tests have been developed for use by occupational therapists in the past 10 years. In addition to publishing their own tests, most test corporations distribute the most widely used tests. Thus, in general, a researcher is not limited to one corporation to obtain a specific test.

The following list includes test publishers that are frequently used by occupational therapists and other clinicians.

- AOTA: http:// www.aota.org/

- Consulting Psychologists Press, Inc.: http://www.cpp-db.com

- Curriculum Associates, Inc.: http://www.curriculumassociates.com

- Educational Testing Service: http://www.ets.org

- EdITS: http://www.edits.net

- Flaghouse Rehabilitation: http://www.flaghouse.com

- Institute for Personality and Ability Testing (IPAT): http://www.ipat.com/pages/home.aspx

- Lafayette Instrument: http://www.licmcf.com

- McGraw Hill: http://www.mcgraw-hill.com/

- MHS Assessments: http://www.mhs.com

- PAR, Inc.: http://www4.parinc.com/

- Pearson Assessments: http://www.pearsonassessments.com/pai/

- Pro-Ed: http://www.proedinc.com/Customer/default.aspx

- Riverside Publishing: http://www.riversidepublishing.com/

- Western Psychological Services (WPS): http://portal.wpspublish.com/portal/page?_pageid=53,53086&_dad=portal&_schema=PORTAL

- Stoelting Publishing: https://www.stoeltingco.com/stoelting/templates/99/Default

- Stout Vocational Rehabilitation Institute: http://www3.uwstout.edu/scri/index.cfm

- Trace Research and Development Center: http://trace.wisc.edu/

- Valpar International Corporation: http://www.valparint.com/

10.13 ETHICAL CONSIDERATIONS IN TESTING

"Competence in test use is a combination of knowledge of psychometric principles, knowledge of the problem situation in which the testing is to be done, technical skill and some wisdom" (AERA, APA, & NCME, 1974, p. 6). To protect psychological tests from abuse, standards fall into three areas: guidelines for devising a new psychological test, qualifications for administering tests, and the guidelines for interpreting results. The following guidelines should be adhered to in using tests:

- The researcher publishing a new test should provide reliability, validity, normative data, scoring procedure, and qualifications for using the test in an accompanying manual.

- A standardized test procedure should be carefully followed by the tester.

- Results should be reported that can be compared to specified populations.

- The researcher using psychological tests should obtain informed consent for the subject and assure the subject's confidentiality.

10.14 SUMMARY

In the last 20 years, hundreds of tests have been developed for use with individuals with disabilities. In this chapter, the authors have presented descriptions of tests that are the most commonly used in clinical practice. These tests are available to use by occupational therapists knowledgeable in the administration, scoring, and interpretation of test results. These tests can be used as outcome or descriptive measures in clinical research. The use of a specific test is a key component in the research process and could affect the results if the test selected is not sensitive to changes in individuals or is not reliable or valid; therefore, the researcher should have knowledge of reliability and validity of the test before using it. When using a test in research, the researcher must be aware of the level of qualification needed to administer it.

As new tests are developed frequently, the researcher should keep informed of newly published tests. Annual catalogs obtained from the test publishers listed in Section 10.12 are helpful in locating new tests. Before developing a new test, occupational therapists should search the literature, references in testing, textbooks, publishers' catalogs, and websites for locating new tests.

11

Scientific Writing and Thesis Preparation

Vigorous writing is concise. A sentence should contain no unnecessary words, a paragraph no unnecessary sentences, for the same reason that a drawing should have no unnecessary lines and a machine no unnecessary parts. This requires not that the writer make all his sentences short, or that he avoid all detail and treat his subjects only in outline, but that every word tell.

—Strunk & White (1979, p. 23)

OPERATIONAL LEARNING OBJECTIVES

By the end of this chapter the learner will be able to:

- State ways to prepare for writing a research paper.
- Name the important divisions of a research paper.
- Identify and correct sexist and racist language in the research paper.
- Use people-first language.
- Recognize reasons for revising the original draft.
- Write a bibliography using American Psychological Association (APA) format.
- Proof for errors in language mechanics and style.
- Critically evaluate one's own writing.
- Identify the major parts of the final format.
- Design a research proposal.
- Communicate results of research study.

Rice, M. S., Stein, F., & Tomlin, G.
Clinical Research in Occupational Therapy, Sixth Edition (pp. 339-370).
© 2019 Taylor & Francis Group.

11.1 PREPARATION FOR WRITING

It is as important to prepare oneself for writing as it is to complete the review of literature and collect the data for the research project. Prior to writing the research paper, many processes that facilitate writing should be taken into consideration.

One hindrance to the completion of the writing task is the failure to actually sit down and write; however, allowing frequent interruptions during the actual writing period is equally problematic. The first task in the preparation for writing is to get oneself into the proper frame of mind. This includes taking care of as many "settling activities" that might lead to interruptions. This can be likened to an animal preparing to go to sleep: The animal roughs up the bed, circles the bed several times, grooms, and finally settles down. Similarly, settling activities for writers include planning a large block of time, getting one's coffee or drink, assembling all the materials needed, finding a quiet and comfortable place (preferably away from a phone), arranging for child care, putting the dog or cat outside, and taking care of any needed personal toiletries. Once one has completed those tasks and is settled, writing is made easier.

Effective writing is a skill that becomes more refined as it is practiced. Clear and simple language is the hallmark of good scientific writing, and its most important quality is objective self-criticism. For some individuals, a major block to the task of writing is the initial step of organizing their ideas on paper. The desire to write as if whatever one first put on paper is chipped forever in granite sometimes prevents the flow of ideas.

The place and time in which one writes are important initial considerations. Some individuals do their best writing during the morning in a quiet, sunny room with a large table where they can spread out reference books, scrap paper, and notes filed in manila folders. Others work better in the late evening. Some individuals can work 12 to 14 hours for several days, followed by several days of complete rest. Some students do their best work in a college library or cafeteria, despite visual and auditory distractions. Some can write using paper and pencil, while others prefer writing on a computer or word processor or dictating by using speech recognition software, such as Dragon NaturallySpeaking (Nuance Communications). Whatever the method and place, one must be aware of the environment that best facilitates creative writing.

Another consideration for writers is a time schedule. Some writers report that they compose in spurts of creative inspiration, while others work daily whether or not they feel inspired. However, setting aside enough time is important, so that the writer does not feel rushed or under time constraints, allowing the writer to feel that something can be accomplished. Writing a research paper or article is unlike casual writing in which an individual can use spare minutes throughout the day to complete the task. Scientific writing takes mental energy and therefore requires concentrated effort.

A third consideration consists of assembling the materials to be used before beginning any writing task. Writing materials (e.g., pens, paper, computer), note cards prepared during the literature review, statistical analyses, and other references should be available and at hand. Just as one would not consider doing therapy without having all the tools and equipment available, one cannot expect to write adequately without having the proper tools and materials.

Writing a book, journal article, or thesis requires self-discipline. In a way, the individual should prepare for writing much as an athlete trains for a sporting event. A period of conditioning and mental rigor prior to writing is important. Some individuals take long walks, ride bicycles for miles, climb mountains, or take part in physical sports in preparation for writing. Others prepare mentally by playing chess, doing crossword puzzles, solving arithmetic problems, reading prolifically, or doing intricate manual work. Sleeping on an idea or letting it brew beneath the surface for a while also may be helpful. After the first draft, there will be ample time for revision, which in most cases will involve excision. For the author or research investigator, the completed document is analogous to giving birth. Writing is a continuous process with much editing and revision, but one should be careful not to abandon the initial efforts prematurely.

The purpose of the research paper includes an explanation of why the question was formulated and how the research methodology serves to answer the question. In the final project, that is, the research paper, the writer summarizes the literature, discusses the findings, and makes specific recommendations based on these findings. In this way, the final scientific paper becomes a part of the body of literature, placing the research findings within the context of previous works (Locke, Spirduso, & Silverman, 2013).

A well-conceived research paper requires active contemplation by the writer. The conceptual relationships between previous research and present findings must be considered. The hypothesis or guiding question(s) proposed by the researcher must be concisely and clearly stated and should cover all the points covered in the paper (Slade, 2003). The summary and arguments used in the paper to advance one's theory must be compared with viewpoints held by established researchers. On the other hand, a researcher may present findings that are contradictory to accepted beliefs in the scientific community. Under attack, the researcher must be able to defend the validity of the research findings. For example, despite a common belief that dyslexia is a result of visual-perceptual deficits, such as seeing and writing letters backward, researchers such as Libernan (1973), Shaywitz and Shaywitz (2008), and Kamhi and Catts (1998) have espoused the underlying deficit in dyslexia to be language related.

Another essential component for writing a research paper is to understand the literature encompassing the topic as fully as possible. This is accomplished by completing an exhaustive literature review as described in Chapter 6. The researcher will discover quickly, however, that much more literature has been reviewed than will be discussed in the paper. This fact does not minimize the need for an extensive literature review; rather, it emphasizes the need for the researcher to understand and master the relationship of a specific literature within the context of a body of knowledge. For example, for an understanding of the occupational therapy methods used to treat individuals with a stroke, the researcher would identify the most up-to-date research on the topic through a Cochrane Review that evaluates the effectiveness of the treatment methods and by using PubMed. It is not uncommon to revise the initial hypothesis or guiding question several times as one's knowledge base increases through reading and reviewing the literature.

Writing and reviewing literature is like an organic process that helps researchers to modify their thinking while extending their knowledge base. It is a creative process that allows one to be objective and self-critical. This process is sometimes referred to as *cognitive dissonance* (i.e., the state in which there is conflict between one's attitudes and one's behavior, generally resulting in changing one's thinking so that there is equilibrium between the two), *reflective decision making* (i.e., the process of making decisions by critically examining all sides of the issue), or the *Socratic method* (i.e., learning by raising questions). All these methods rely on the individual's ability to critically question and rethink a body of knowledge.

11.2 OUTLINING THE RESEARCH STUDY

The overall organization of the research study, outlined in Table 11-1, is dictated by tradition. Each of the major sections within the research paper contains specific issues and topics.

11.2.1 Introduction to the Research Paper

The first part of the research paper contains a brief introduction to the present study, including the purpose, the research or guiding question(s), and the significance when examined beside findings from landmark studies (Best & Kahn, 2016). A pivotal part of this portion of the research paper, article, or manuscript is a clear statement of the hypotheses or guiding questions such that they are (a) well understood, (b) lead the reader to anticipate the major sections of the paper, and (c) indicate the direction or argument in which the paper will be written (Winkler & McCuen-Metherell, 2011). Finally, this part of the research

TABLE 11-1
MAJOR PARTS OF A RESEARCH PAPER

I. Introduction to the research paper
    a. Statement of the research problem or guiding question
    b. Significance of the research problem
    c. Purposes of the study
    d. Specific definitions or terms
II. Review of the literature
    a. Major studies
    b. Critical analysis of key studies
III. Methods
    a. Research design
        1. Subjects (number; demographic data)
        2. Procedures (tests, collection of data)
        3. Statistical analyses
IV. Results
    a. Presentation and analysis of data
    b. Relevant tables and figures
V. Discussion, summary, conclusions, and implications of the findings
    a. Limitations of the study
    b. Significance of study related to prior research
    c. Future research
VI. Reference list and appendices
VII. Abstract (placed after the title page)

paper should include definitions for any terminology that are uncommon or might not be understood by the reader (Best & Kahn, 2016).

11.2.2 Review of the Literature

The second part of the research paper, which contains the literature review, is to some extent a measure of what the student knows about the subject (Best & Kahn, 2016; Krathwohl, 1988). In some papers, this section and the previous section are written as a single part. In a thesis or dissertation, this section is traditionally identified as Chapter 2 or, if written with the introduction, as Chapter 1.

The purpose of this section is to further introduce the reason for the study by reviewing previous research in the same area and by building a background for the study. Although it is not necessary to cite or review every article or book in the subject, as the researcher must presume that the reader has some knowledge in this area, the major studies must be discussed (APA, 2011). For example, a student is interested in investigating the effectiveness of constraint-induced therapy with children diagnosed with cerebral palsy. In a preliminary literature review, the student will have read and identified many research studies through PubMed using the key words *constraint induced therapy* and *cerebral palsy*. One way to outline this portion of the research paper is to organize the articles reviewed in computer files. The abstracts and citations obtained from databases such as PubMed can be used to compose the literature review. Some articles will be especially important to build a strong argument for the research design, and a critical analysis of these articles will be an integral part of the literature review. Research literature and theory need to be reviewed and discussed objectively, citing both positive and negative research findings that relate to the present research question. In this way, one can avoid researcher bias, as shown in the following example from literature on treating depression.

A student is interested in the relationship between depression and use of cognitive behavioral therapy. A review of literature identifies the following categories of studies involving the use of cognitive behavioral therapy to treat individuals with depression: (a) those in which there was no improvement (e.g., Jacobson et al., 1996; Twisk & Maes, 2009); (b) those in which there was improvement (e.g., Clarke, Rohde, Lewinsohn, Hops, & Seeley, 1999; Pinninti, Rissmiller, & Steer, 2010); and (c) those in which there was mixed success (e.g., McIntosh, Carter, Bulik, Frampton, & Joyce, 2011). Each of these articles should be critically analyzed and critiqued, with special attention given to the methodology used in the studies and the relationship of the findings to the present research question. The student should present studies in which both favorable and unfavorable results were found. In doing this, the student demonstrates objectivity in reviewing the literature and avoids research bias.

11.2.3 Methods

The third section of an experimental research paper includes a discussion of the methodology used in the study. This portion of the research paper should be written in a concise and succinct manner, with enough information available so that others can replicate the study.

Traditionally, there are three subdivisions in the methods section: (a) participants; (b) the apparatus or tests; and (c) the procedures used for data collection and analysis. Demographic information, such as the number of participants, ages, gender, and ethnicity, is critical. Other additional demographic information that may be essential for the study might include education level, socioeconomic level, handedness, disabilities, prior testing, and previous need for therapies, especially occupational therapy. If a control group is used, the demographics of the control group must be contrasted with the experimental group. The manner in which subjects were chosen (e.g., stratified random sample, voluntary response to a newspaper ad) is also described in this section.

A description of the tests or apparatus includes the names of the tests or surveys used, any laboratory equipment needed, and any specific directions or adaptations to the test or procedure that might not be found in a test manual. For example, if only part of a perceptual motor test is used, one must name the subtests chosen and justify the modification. When a standardized test is used, the reliability and validity of the test (or test portions) used must be indicated. If a survey or questionnaire has been developed for the study, a copy is put into the appendix following the major divisions of the paper.

Finally, the researcher describes the methods of data collection and the statistical procedures used to analyze it (Best & Kahn, 2016). For example, did the researcher collect data alone, in person, or by telephone? Were others trained to collect the data? If a questionnaire was used, was it mailed or left in a public place for people to fill out as desired? Was a second letter sent as a follow-up? How long did data collection occur? Was it collected in one or two sessions? Was it collected by outcome measures (pre- and post-testing)? What types of statistical procedures were used to analyze the data?

11.2.4 Results

The fourth section of the research paper presents the results and statistical findings from the study without attempting to interpret them. Each hypothesis is discussed separately, with statistical interactions and main effects reported. Tables and figures depicting significant relationships between variables often make the text more understandable; however, they should be self-explanatory and add to the information in the text rather than add new information.

11.2.5 Discussion, Summary, Conclusions, and Implications of the Findings

In the final section, the writer summarizes the findings and attempts to interpret them in the context of previous studies in the same field. Conclusions regarding acceptance or rejection of hypotheses are stated in this section. Although statements of generalization can be made here, one must be careful not to over generalize or overstate the significance of the findings. The writer should be aware of the limitations of the study and state them, expressing any cautions research regarding generalization to populations not included in the sample. Implications for further research, present practice, or policy changes are advanced, along with the arguments for these changes. The internal and external validity of the study should be discussed.

According to Best and Kahn (2016), the discussion section of the research paper is the most difficult part to write. Inexperienced authors tend to over or under generalize, thinking their results less or more important than the data would support (Winkler & McCuen-Metherell, 2011). The discussion section should be a critical and analytical summary of the findings rather than a superficial overview of the results. Because this part of the research paper is the most frequently read (Best & Kahn, 2016), it is crucial that the researchers summarize the results and critically review these findings in the context of prior studies. The usefulness of the research paper, despite the findings, can be determined by the way in which the discussion section is written.

11.2.6 Reference List and Appendices

In the last section of the research paper, the writer lists all of the cited references. The writer must be careful not to leave out any reference, to include all information in the citation, and to check for accuracy and correct spelling of information. There is nothing more frustrating than an incomplete or inaccurate citation when one wishes to obtain further information from the original article. Refer to Section 11.5 for further information.

Sometimes a writer wishes to place a bibliography and a reference list into the research paper. A bibliography contains any article, book, or chapter that might clarify the topic. A reference list, on the other hand, includes journal articles, books, or other sources used in the research and preparation of the paper and cited within the article (APA, 2011). Any additional information (e.g., copy of the survey or test protocol, drawing of specific apparatus) can be placed in an appendix following the list of references.

11.2.7 Abstract

The abstract of a research study, which is written last and then placed at the beginning of the study, contains summary statements of each independent unit or section (i.e., the problem, literature review, research design, methods, results, discussion, conclusions, limitations of the study, and recommendations for further research). The abstract should contain enough information so that the reader will know the purposes of the study, the specific variables or groups investigated, the number of participants, the measuring instruments used, the results, and the conclusions presented. An abstract of a research study is usually limited to between 150 and 300 words. When preparing an abstract, it is useful to extract key sentences from each part of the study and then integrate the sentences through transitional phrases. Abstracts are extremely important to investigators reviewing literature; therefore, it is vital to present as complete a summary of the total study as possible within the number of words permitted. Abstracts are not merely a summary or discussion of the results as perceived by some investigators. An abstract should be a complete statement representative of the total study. Key words or key phrases are usually placed below the abstract. These key words are very important for researchers in identifying relevant studies when using in data retrieval systems (see Chapter 6).

11.3 WRITING THE FIRST DRAFT

Writers begin the first draft after completing the outline. As stated previously, the outline aids in organizing the literature review, but the outline is not set in stone. After the first draft has been written, the organization may need to be revised. Nonetheless, having an outline allows the writer to have a sense of the direction in which the paper is going.

Perhaps the hardest part of writing is putting initial thoughts on paper. Writers should compose these initial thoughts with the expectation of revising them later. There will be plenty of time for revision after the first draft has been written, and writers should expect to revise their first work several times.

A difficult skill for inexperienced writers is the ability to use notes effectively. There is a tendency to quote extensively rather than paraphrase the author's words. Frequently, this is caused by a lack of understanding about what the author meant. If this is the case, researchers must do additional reading and studying until they completely understand the material. Although quotes from the original source can be an effective means of relating information, too many quotations make the research paper difficult to read and leave "the impression that students have done [no more than] 'cut and paste' from books and articles they have read" (Winkler & McCuen, 1979, p. 114). It is better to use quotations sparingly, intermixing the quotations with summaries and paraphrases of the original sources. When quoting or paraphrasing, one must document the source (see Section 11.5).

The literary and scientific styles used for citations often are determined by a particular discipline. The four most commonly used systems are *The Chicago Manual of Style, Seventeenth Edition* (University of Chicago, 2017), the *MLA Handbook, Eighth Edition* (Modern Language Association of America, 2016), the *AMA Manual of Style, Tenth Edition* (JAMA Network Editors, 2010), and the *Publication Manual of the American Psychological Association, Sixth Edition* (APA, 2011). The latter style is used most frequently in psychology, education, and social and health sciences and will be discussed in this book.

The essential reference book for APA style is the sixth edition of the *Publication Manual of the American Psychological Association* (APA, 2011), generally available in university or college bookstores. If the university or local technical bookstore does not have one, it can be obtained from the APA in Washington, D.C. Because of the extensiveness of the APA style, one will need to refer to this manual frequently. It is wise to get into the habit of referring to the APA Manual whenever there is a question about style, language mechanics, or format of the paper. Major highlights of the APA Manual will be discussed in the following sections of this chapter; however, because of space limitations, not all topics will be covered in detail.

11.4 Making Revisions

Once the research paper has been written, revisions will be necessary. Revising the research paper five or six times is not uncommon. Each time the writer reviews the research paper for accuracy and cohesiveness, he or she may discover additional ways for revision or clarity.

The function of revision is to make sure that specific editing requirements have been followed. These editing requirements are summarized in Table 11-2.

11.4.1 Bias

First, the writer will want to make sure that no type of bias (e.g., gender, sexual orientation, racial, ethnic, disability, age, or historical and interpretive inaccuracies) has been introduced into the paper or study. Several guidelines have been established by the APA for avoiding bias in one's writing. "Part of writing without bias is recognizing that differences should be mentioned only when relevant. Marital status, sexual orientation, racial and ethnic identity, or the fact that a person has a disability should not be mentioned gratuitously" (APA, 2011, p. 71).

Gender refers to role (APA, 2011, p. 73), whereas *sex* is biological (APA, 2011, p. 71). Both gender and sexual bias can be avoided by specifically describing participants, rather than using a general term to describe the population. For example, bias occurs when the writer uses the term *man* to mean the human race rather than using a less ambiguous term such as *person*, *people*, or *individual*. Additionally, use of specific gender words (e.g., his, her) or using terms that end in *man* or *men* (e.g., postman, chairman, policemen) must be avoided. Stereotyping (e.g., the psychologist … he; mothering) can be avoided by using specific language (e.g., boys enjoyed playing with Legos while girls enjoyed reading), by using parallel language (e.g., *men and women* rather than *men and girls*), or by changing the term to a plural (e.g., *their* instead of *his* or *her*). Compounds, such as his/her, or (s)he should be avoided (APA, 2011). The term *sexual orientation* is preferred over *sexual preference*.

Bias involving disabilities occurs when the writer attributes to a specific group something that has no supporting data (American Psychiatric Association, 1994). An example of this stereotyping occurs when someone writes "In general, all individuals with traumatic brain injury tend to have psychosocial difficulties."

Ethnic or racial bias can be avoided by using commonly accepted designations, such as the census categories, while being sensitive to the preferred designations. For example, some persons of Hispanic background in New Mexico might prefer to be called Hispanic or Spanish, while some persons of Hispanic background in southern California or southern Texas might consider themselves Mexicans. Avoid terms that are either dated or derogatory. Finally, terms used to refer to racial or ethnic groups are proper nouns, and therefore should be capitalized. By asking the participants their preference, ethnic or racial bias can be avoided. APA suggests that an informal test can be completed by substituting another group (e.g., your own) for the group being discussed. If the writer perceives offense in the revised statement, then bias is probably present.

When referring to individuals by age, specific ranges should be used. APA suggests that individuals aged 12 years and younger should be referred to as girls or boys, whereas young men or young women is used for individuals between 13 and 18 years. Individuals older than age 18 years are referred to as women or men. Terms such as elderly or senior are generally not acceptable, as some participants will find these terms pejorative. Other guidelines can be found in the APA manual, beginning on page 76 (APA, 2011).

11.4.2 People-First Language

A second reason for revision is to make sure that the writing is in *people-first language*. Because of the Individuals with Disabilities Education Act (1990), all references to disabilities must be written with the individual placed first. Thus, *child with autism* is correct, whereas *the autistic child* is incorrect. This convention emphasizes the value of the human being and delegates the disability to secondary importance.

The writer must distinguish also between the terms *handicap* and *disability*. A handicap can be thought of as a disadvantage imposed on an individual by the environment or by another person, whereas a disability is something that an individual is unable to do, a lack of a body part, or physical or psychosocial impairment. For example, an individual with a spinal cord injury may not be able to walk; the inability to walk is a disability. However, this disability becomes a handicap if there is no wheelchair access. The presence of a disability does not make an individual handicapped.

11.4.3 Mechanics of Writing

Clear writing requires use of a formal writing style and using grammatically correct language. A third reason to revise the manuscript is to make sure that there are no grammatical errors. Errors such as subject-verb agreement (e.g., using *data is* rather than *data are*), punctuation and capitalization, run-on sentences, and sentence fragments are common for inexperienced writers. Run-on sentences and sentence fragments are an indication that either the writer is careless and has not proofread the research paper or that the writer needs help with writing skills. Other common errors include (a) failing to use parallel structure for grammatical units (e.g., using different parts of speech in a series or in connecting phrases), (b) having dangling modifiers (e.g., sentences in which the modifier is misplaced, such as "it is however believed," rather than "However, it is believed"), (c) splitting infinitives (e.g., "to swiftly complete

TABLE 11-2
CHECKLIST FOR PROOFING ONE'S ARTICLE

1. GENDER AND ETHNIC BIAS

- Is the article free of language that might be ambiguous or stereotypical?

2. PEOPLE-FIRST LANGUAGE

- Is the manuscript written with the individual emphasized rather than the disability?
- Have all references to a disability been written in the form "individual with . . ." ?

3. GRAMMAR

- Are there run-on sentences or sentence fragments?
- Are there split infinitives, dangling modifiers, or errors in subject-verb agreement?
- Is the writing in parallel structure?
- Are relative pronouns used appropriately?
- Has a grammar program been used to check the language?
- Has past tense been used rather than presence tense (e.g., the author said)

4. SPELLING AND PUNCTUATION

- Has a spell check been used to check spelling?
- Has the article been reviewed for commas, quotation marks, hyphens, and apostrophes?

5. ABBREVIATIONS

- Is the abbreviation placed in parentheses following the full term the first time it is used?
- Are the Latin abbreviations used correctly and according to APA style?
- Are abbreviations invented by the author kept to a minimum?

6. TRANSITIONAL WORDS, PHRASES, AND SENTENCES

- Are there transitional statements or words between ideas?
- Is there a sense of unity and integration in the paper?
- Do words such as "however," "although," or "nevertheless" need to be added?

7. CLARITY

- Is the language clear and simple?
- Do any unusual terms need to be explained or defined?
- Would a figure or table help explain the information?
- Has the material been reviewed by a second reader?

8. ORGANIZATION

- Do the hypotheses or guiding question(s) drive the content of the research paper?
- Is there consistency between sections?
- Are unnecessary repetitions removed?
- Is the sequence of the research paper logical and coherent?

the task" rather than "to complete the task swiftly"), (d) improperly using relative pronouns (e.g., "an individual must keep their head" rather than, "an individual must keep his head"), (e) using the passive tense rather than the active tense (e.g., "There were seven subjects" instead of "Seven subjects"), and (f) placing prepositions at the end of sentences (e.g., "ethical and legal obligations that occupational therapists are faced with" rather than "ethical and legal obligations that occupational therapists face"). If one is unsure about the proper grammatical structure, a basic grammar book is indispensable. Additional examples of these errors, as well as the correct usages, are illustrated in Table 11-3.

Many excellent sources are available to help writers avoid grammatical errors and improve their writing. The following list provides major references and online programs:

TABLE 11-3			
COMMON ERRORS OF WRITING STYLE			
TYPE	RULES	INCORRECT EXAMPLE	CORRECT EXAMPLE
Dangling or misplaced modifier or participles	• Modifiers and participles should be put as close as possible to the word they are to modify to prevent ambiguity or missing referents. • Place "only" next to the word it modifies.	• ... would first determine • ... local issues in that particular clinic that affect job satisfaction • The participants were screened only ...	• ... would determine first • ... local issues that affect job satisfaction in that particular clinic • The participants only were screened ...
Split infinitives	• Place adverbs that modify the verb after the phrase "to ... " rather than between the "to" and the verb.	• Occupational therapists need to carefully observe behaviors ...	• Occupational therapists need to observe carefully behaviors ...

Parallel structure	• Expressions similar in function or content should be in the same grammatical construction.
	• With coordinating conjunctions (i.e., "and," "but," "or," "nor"), make sure to use all elements of the parallel structure.
		• Identification and clarification of ...
		• Assessing to ...
		• Determine whether ...
		  ◦ The children wanted both to run and play.
		  ◦ Neither the directions or the examples were ...
			• Identification and clarification of ...
			• Assessment of ...
			• Determination of...
			  ◦ The children wanted both to run and to play.
			  ◦ Neither the directions nor the examples were ...

Relative pronoun	• Use *that* with a restrictive clause (i.e., is essential to the passage). • Use *which* with an nonrestrictive clause surrounded by commas (i.e., adds information, but is not essential to the sentence). • Use *who* in nonrestrictive clauses in reference to people. • Use *since* when you mean "after that," and *while* when you mean "during."		• The chimps that participated in the study were all kept unrestrained in an open testing area. • The glasses, which were on top of the container, belonged to the patient. • The students, who all had attention deficit disorder, won ribbons at the races. • Since the development of the Wechsler Intelligence Scale for Children–Fourth Edition ... • While the music was playing, the participants ...

(continued)

TABLE 11-3 (CONTINUED)

COMMON ERRORS OF WRITING STYLE

TYPE	RULES	INCORRECT EXAMPLE	CORRECT EXAMPLE
Voice (active/passive)	• Use the active voice whenever possible.	• The information examined by the authors . . .	• The authors examined. . .
Tense	• Use past tense to report something that occurred in the past, such as discussion of another author or reporting your results.	• Jones and Smith (2005) state . . .	• Jones and Smith (2005) stated . . .
Possessives	• Place an apostrophe after the noun or pronoun to show possession. Exception: do not use an apostrophe after the word "it" when showing possession.	• The subjects score . . . • It's major strengths . . .	• The subject's score. . . • Its major strengths . . . • But: It's cold (it is cold).
Seriation	• Place elements in a series in parallel form ◦ See Table 11-4 for correct punctuation. • When the series of items is written in one sentence, use letters in parentheses to separate each item. Use commas to separate the items, unless there are internal commas. Use semicolons to separate items of major categories. • When each item in the series is placed into separate sentences or separate paragraphs, use numbers to separate the items.	• . . . asked to read the directions, fill out the information, and then to turn in the form. • The subjects were administered four tests: clinical observations, Stress Management Questionnaire, Crawford Small Parts Dexterity Test, and Strong Vocational Interest Test • The subjects were administered three outcome measures: Stress Management Questionnaire to examine coping skills, Crawford Small Parts Dexterity Test to assess dexterity, Strong Vocational Interest Test to determine interests	• . . . asked to read the directions, fill out the information, and turn in the form. • The subjects were administered four tests: (a) clinical observations, (b) Stress Management Questionnaire, (c) Crawford Small Parts Dexterity Test, and (d) Strong Vocational Interest Test. • The subjects were administered three outcome measures: 1. Stress Management Questionnaire to examine coping skills 2. Crawford Small Parts Dexterity Test to assess dexterity 3. Strong Vocational Interest Test to determine interests

(continued)

TABLE 11-3 (CONTINUED)

COMMON ERRORS OF WRITING STYLE			
TYPE	**RULES**	**INCORRECT EXAMPLE**	**CORRECT EXAMPLE**
Pronouns	• Make sure that the reference for the pronoun is clear. • Make sure that the pronoun agrees in number with the noun it replaces and/or modifies the noun.	• This was completed. • Those were put over there. • His chart was placed in their folder. • The group took their packages.	• This self-report scale was completed. • Those books were put over there, on the bottom shelf. • His chart was placed in his folder. • The group took its packages.
Subject-verb agreement	• Verbs must agree with the subject, regardless of intervening phrases and/or use of pronouns.	• Data is . . . • Phenomena is . . . • The articles that were taken from a single journal was . . .	• Data are . . . ["Data" is plural] • Phenomena are . . . [Phenomenon is the singular form] • The articles that were taken from a single journal were . . . [articles were]
Misplaced prepositions	• Avoid placing prepositions at the end of sentences.	• . . . the next area the clinicians were questions in . . .	• . . . the next area in which the clinicians were questions . . .

- Strunk, W., & White, E. B. (1999). *The elements of style* (4th ed.). Boston, MA: Allyn & Bacon.

  A classic containing a gold mine of writing ideas, including rules of usage, principles of composition form, and writing style. The epitome of concise, effective writing.

- American Psychological Association. (2011). *Publication manual of the American Psychological Association* (6th ed.). Washington, DC: Author.

  An exhaustive guide to organizing a journal article for publication. Includes content areas, such as headings, quotations, references, tables, figures, and graphs, and other matters of style that can keep a writer up all night.

- Turabian, K. L. (2013). *A manual for writers of research papers, theses, and dissertations* (W. C. Booth, G. G. Colomb, J. M. Williams, Eds.; 8th ed.). Chicago: University of Chicago Press.

  See www.chicagomanualofstyle.org/turabian/citation-guide.html for further information.

- Kipfer, B. A., (2010). *Roget's international thesaurus* (7th ed.), New York, NY: Collins.

  An invaluable guide to the writer for selecting the most appropriate word. It is helpful both in locating a specific word and in varying one's language. There are many different versions of this reference, as well as many formats.

- Venes, D. (2017). *Taber's cyclopedic medical dictionary* (21st ed.). Philadelphia, PA: F. A. Davis.

  An essential guide for those researchers needing medical terms defined and clarified. Taber's also has an online version at https://www.tabers.com/tabersonline/

- *Merriam-Webster's Collegiate Dictionary* (11th ed.). (2003). Springfield, MA: Merriam-Webster, Inc.

  Having a dictionary is a must, both for finding meanings of words or using correct spelling. This is also available online at http://www.merriam-webstercollegiate.com and is available as an eBook.

- Purdue Online Writing Lab (OWLS), available at https://owl.english.purdue.edu.

  This online resource provides over 200 resources for writing, including format and style guides for MLA and APA, help with writing and grammar, English as a Second Language, and ways to avoid plagiarism.

A fourth reason for revision is to check for spelling and punctuation errors. It is critical to check one's spelling with a spell checker to ensure that there are no errors. However, one must be careful to read the article and proof for errors, rather than relying on the computerized speller to find all the errors. It cannot find errors when the words are spelled correctly but misused. For example, if the words *to* and *too* are used incorrectly, the speller will not identify the errors.

Punctuation errors must be found and corrected. Table 11-4, adapted from the APA Manual (2011), summarizes common punctuation rules. Reading the paper aloud is one method to revise the paper and find errors in punctuation and grammar.

In scientific articles, it is common practice to abbreviate terms used repeatedly (e.g., proprioceptive facilitation as PF, neurodevelopmental therapy as NDT, learning disability as LD or SLD, perceptual-motor training as PMT, and quality food index as QFI). Abbreviations invented by the writer should be kept to a minimum and used only for terms that are long and frequently repeated. Tables of statistical data containing abbreviations should contain a footnote defining the abbreviations.

Latin abbreviations are useful for shortening sentences. The following are the most commonly used abbreviations in scientific articles. Notice that they are not italicized.

- ca. (circa): about a certain time (e.g., ca. BC 130)
- e.g. (exempli grata): for example
- et al. (et alii): and others
- et seq. (et sequens): and the following
- ibid, (ibidem): in the same place
- i.e. (id est): that is to say
- viz. (videlicet): namely, used to introduce lists

Be sure to refer to the APA manual for the proper way to use abbreviations. For example, many abbreviations (including i.e. and e.g.) must be used only within parentheses.

11.4.4 Transitional Words, Phrases, and Sentences

A fifth reason for revision is to make sure that transitional statements are present so that the flow of ideas is smooth. Writing a well-organized, integrated manuscript requires the use of words and phrases that connect ideas and summarize a section of a paper. In reviewing scientific literature, it is important to integrate the studies under topical areas and to develop a logical sequence. Writing should be coherent. The use of transitional words such as *however*, *although*, or *nevertheless*, can be used to make the transition smoother and the paper unified. (Note that many style guides frown on beginning a sentence with *however*.) In addition, sentences can be used to permit the smooth transition from one idea to another. The reader should have no

difficulty following the train of thought or the arguments used to build a case. Additionally, reading the research paper as a whole will uncover any inconsistencies or repetitions between sections (Slade & Perrin, 2007). Often, having someone unacquainted with the topic read the work serves to ensure clarity, understanding, and consistency.

11.4.5 Clarity of Thought

The scientific writer should try to communicate ideas simply and rigorously. Some of the most profound ideas can be expressed in clear, direct language. It is not a sign of intellectual prowess to present ideas so that they are difficult to understand. Therefore, a sixth reason for revision is to ensure that the paper is written clearly. Scientific writing is particularly prone to abstruseness and ambiguity, especially in clinical areas where language is used loosely without precise operational definitions. One method of ensuring clarity is to include a conceptual or operational definition for unusual terms or for terms specific to a certain discipline. Even if the writer chooses not to create a glossary, uncommon terms must be defined operationally. Use of well-thought-out charts, tables, or figures can facilitate the clarity of the research paper. It is not unusual for readers to look at charts, tables, or figures before reading the text, especially when these visual aids provide an overall summary of the principle finding.

11.4.6 Organization

Finally, the author should examine whether the background information is represented accurately, whether ideas unrelated to the topic have been introduced, and whether the hypothesis or guiding statement(s) have directed the writing (Slade & Perrin, 2007). Each statement of results should be supported by data. Differences or contradictions in findings compared with previous studies need to be discussed and, when possible, explained. The whole research paper should be reviewed for sequence of ideas. Eventually, even though additional changes are possible, the writer must accept the paper as it is.

> [T]he secret of good writing is to strip every sentence to its cleanest components. Every word that serves no function, every long word that could be a short word, every adverb which carries the same meaning that is already in the verb, every passive construction that leaves the reader unsure of who is doing what—these are the thousand and one adulterants that weaken the strength of a sentence. (Zinsser, 1990, pp. 7-8)

TABLE 11-4		
COMMON ERRORS OF PUNCTUATION		
TYPE	RULE	EXAMPLE
Spacing — With all punctuation marks	• In final copies, use one space in most instances after all punctuation marks. Do not put a space in abbreviations. In a draft copy, double spacing makes it easier to read.	• The research was completed by 10 a.m. By 11 a.m., . . . • Mathews, R. J. • . . . for the participants. Results. . .
Comma — Seriation	• Use a comma after each word in a series of three or more items.	• . . . equipment, apparatus, and tools . . .
Parenthetical expression	• Use a comma before and after a phrase that adds information but is not essential.	• Collaboration can be an informal process, where two individuals meet to discuss a problem, or . . .
Independent clause	• Use a comma to separate independent clauses, but do not use to separate the two parts of a compound predicate.	• Five of the participants were Black, and seven of the subjects were White. (But notice: Six students were in seventh grade and were taking history.)
Essential or restrictive clauses	• Do not use a comma when the modifying phrase is used to identify, limit, or define a word and is essential to the meaning.	• The subjects that were used for the control group included seven occupational therapists.
Dependent clauses	• Use a comma rather than a semicolon to separate a dependent and independent phrase.	• Although the participants with developmental disabilities were separated from the rest of the participants, all the subjects were placed into a single group for evaluation.
Semicolon — Independent clauses	• Use a semicolon when the independent clauses are not separated by a coordinating conjunction or when the clauses are separated by a conjunctive adverb.	• The apparatus was put on the shelves; the writing materials were put into the desk. • The client was interviewed . . .; however . . .
Seriation	• Use a semicolon when there is a comma contained in any part of the seriation.	• . . . (a) red box, which contained 3 balls; (b) blue box, which contained 2 balls; and (c) yellow box, which contained 6 balls.

(continued)

TABLE 11-4 (CONTINUED)			
COMMON ERRORS OF PUNCTUATION			
TYPE		**RULE**	**EXAMPLE**
Colon	References	• Use a colon after the place of publication and before the publisher.	• Boston: NY: Pearson/Allyn & Bacon.
		• Use a colon before a phrase or example of explanatory material with an introductory phrase. If the example is a complete sentence, start it with a capital letter.	• The recorded scores were in the following order: 37, 50, 24, 70. • The material was made up of the following parts: two blue boxes, each contained four toys.
Quotation marks	Direct quote (less than 40 words)	• Put quotations marks around any direct quote of 40 words or fewer. Cite the reference with the author, date, and page, or just the page, in parentheses following the quote.	• Lock, Spirduso, and Silverman (1987) caution that "[t]he problem in writing a proposal is essentially the same as in writing the final report" (p. 19). • "The problem in writing a proposal is essentially the same as in writing the final report" (Locke, Spirduso, & Silverman, 1987, p. 19).
	Direct quote (more than 40 words)	• If the direct quote is more than 40 words, offset it in a paragraph and indent on both right and left margins. Cite the reference with the author, date, and page, or just the page, in parentheses following the quote. Do not put a period at the end of the quotation.	
	With other punctuation	• Period and commas should be placed inside closing single or double quotation marks, while other punctuation marks are placed outside of the quotations, unless they are part of the quote.	• Smith stated, "General educators look at the forest, while special educators look at the trees."
	Titles	• Put quotation marks around any title of a chapter or article cited in the text. Do not put around any title in the reference list.	• John's review discussed Chapter 2, "The Scientific Method."

	Terms	• Use quotation marks when introducing a word or phrase used as slang, irony, or invented term. Use italics to introduce a technical or key term. Do not use quotation marks or italics when the word or phrase is used a second time. Do not use quotations (or italics) with commonly used foreign terms.	• Ninja coined the term "normalization" . . .
			• Removing a previously given reinforcement is called *cost response*.
			• But:
			    ○ Per se
			    ○ Vis a vis

(continued)

TABLE 11-4 (CONTINUED)

COMMON ERRORS OF PUNCTUATION

TYPE		RULE	EXAMPLE
Parentheses	Parenthetical information	• Use parentheses to set off material that is independent of the rest of the information. Put punctuation marks inside the parentheses if the material is a sentence and outside the parentheses if the material is a phrase.	• The subjects (15 boys and 2 girls) were . . . • (The subjects consisted of 15 boys and 2 girls.)
	References	• Enclose reference citations in text with parentheses.	• (Jones & Smith, 1994) • Jones and Smith (1994)
	Abbreviations	• Abbreviations should be put in parentheses the first time the full term is used. Thereafter, the abbreviation can be used instead of the full term.	• Sensory therapy (SI) . . .. SI . . .
	Seriation	• Enclose the letters used in seriation within a sentence or paragraph in parentheses. • Use periods if each item in the series is placed in a different paragraph.	• (a). . . , (b). . . , and (c). . . • 1. . . . • 2. . . . • 3. . . .
Brackets	Parenthetical material	• Enclose parenthetical material that is within parentheses in brackets unless the use of the commas will not confuse the reader.	• (Miller Assessment for Preschoolers [MAP], 1988) • (Johns, 1998; Smith, 2009).
	References	• Enclose material inserted into a quotation with brackets.	• ". . . [the participants in the study] were asked to come . . ." • "[T]he study showed . . ."

Adapted from American Psychological Association. (2011). *Publication manual of the American Psychological Association* (6th ed.). Washington, DC: Author.

11.5 QUOTATIONS, REFERENCED MATERIAL, AND BIBLIOGRAPHIC CITATIONS

Whenever one uses material written by another person, whether the material is directly quoted or only paraphrased, one must make reference to the original author(s). Failure to do so is plagiarism. Some authors (Winkler & McCuen, 1998) have suggested that plagiarism is common in everyday language. For example, one might use in speech an example stated in a lecture by a professor and fail to give that professor the credit. In another case, one may use a proverb such as "A stitch in time saves nine" and fail to give Benjamin Franklin the credit. Although these examples are not routinely considered plagiarism and are generally acceptable in everyday speech, plagiarism is not accepted in a research or scholarly paper.

Plagiarism occurs when a researcher deliberately takes another person's ideas and incorporates them into his or her own writing without giving any credit to the original author. Examples of plagiarism include the following: (a) taking another's research ideas and submitting them as one's own, (b) paraphrasing an article without giving credit to the author, or (c) directly copying part of an article without citing the authors. Any copyrighted material used without giving credit to the original author is considered plagiarism (Winkler & McCuen, 1998).

If the material used is a direct quote from another author or authors, the writer must cite the author(s), year of publication, and page number of the quotation in the text. There must be no change in spelling, phrasing, capitalization, or punctuation from the original. The exception to this rule is when the first word of a quotation needs to be capitalized or placed in lower case to make the statement grammatically correct. When it is necessary to make changes (e.g., when a pronoun must be clarified or a word added to make the content more understandable), the change must be put in square brackets ([ ]). When a word is misspelled or the grammar is incorrect in the original, "[sic]" follows the misspelling or grammatical error to show that the quotation is reproduced exactly. For example, "The article was written by an england *[sic]* author."

A quote can be introduced as part of a grammatical sentence, or it may stand alone as a sentence. When material is omitted from the quotation, then an ellipsis (…) replaces the material that is left out. When the quote is more than 40 words, it should stand alone as a separate paragraph. In this case, the quoted material is punctuated, and the reference for the quoted material is placed after the paragraph, in parenthesis and with no punctuation. Examine the following:

> Slang, hackneyed or flippant phrases, and folksy style should be avoided. Since objectivity is the primary goal, there should be no element of exhortation or persuasion. The research report should describe and explain, rather than try to convince or move to action. In this respect, the research report differs from the essay or the feature article. (Best, 1977, p. 317)

When the material has fewer than 40 words, it is placed within the paragraph. The reference is placed in parentheses at the end of the quote. For example: According to Best (1977), "The research report should be presented in a style that is creative, clear, and concise" (p. 317).

When the writer wishes to paraphrase another author's material, then the writer must cite the author(s) and date of publication. Examine the following two examples:

1. Best and Kahn (2016) suggested that when writing a research article, one must be careful to write concisely and clearly.

2. When writing a research article, one must be careful to write concisely and clearly (Best & Kahn, 2016; Winkler & McCuen, 1998).

Notice that no page numbers are used in either reference and that the author's name is put within parentheses at the end of the sentence if it has not been used as part of the sentence structure. Additional information regarding common citations of authors in the text is summarized in Table 11-5.

Whether the writer has quoted the source directly or paraphrased the material, a complete reference must be placed in the reference list at the end of the research paper. Table 11-6 summarizes the different styles for common reference citations, and Table 11-7 shows some examples of these citations. Further information regarding the appropriate style for dissertations, secondary sources, movies, or films can be found in the APA manual. Regardless of the type of publication, all citations must include enough information so that the reader can locate the original source.

11.6 FORMAT OF A PAPER

The format of the research paper is dictated by the style of writing used. For journal publications using the APA style, the size of the margins, line spacing, and size of print are specified. Individual professors and non-APA style journals may have different requirements. In a thesis or dissertation, additional sections are required. A typical organization of the sequence for a thesis or dissertation is listed below.

1. Title page (Figure 11-1)
2. Approval page indicating names and titles of thesis readers (required for a thesis or dissertation only)
3. Acknowledgments, including individuals who aided in the study and any grant support accepted
4. Table of contents, including chapter and section headings, appendix, and bibliography
5. List of statistical tables
6. List of illustrations, photographs, and figures
7. Abstract
8. The content of the text
   a. Introduction
   b. Review of the literature
   c. Methods
   d. Results
   e. Discussion, including clinical implications of findings and limitations of study
   f. Conclusions and further research
9. Bibliography and references
10. Appendix
11. Vita, listing professional education, work history, and previous publications

A running title, consisting of no more than 50 words, is placed in capital letters in the upper left-hand corner of each page. One-inch margins are used for the top, bottom, and both sides. APA style dictates the position of page numbers (usually below the running title), the use of Roman and Arabic numbers, the type of paper, the levels of headings, spacing, and use of quotations.

Table 11-5

Using Citations in Text Using APA Style

TYPE OF CITATION	FIRST CITATION	ADDITIONAL CITATIONS IN THE TEXT
One author, citation with page numbers	• Last name, year, page (when applicable): ◦ Sanchez (2010) . . . (p. 94); (Sanchez, 2010, p. 94)	• Same as the first citation.

One author, citation with no page numbers	• Last name, year, paragraph (when applicable):
	  ◦ Miller (2009) . . . (para. 4.)
	• When there are short headings in the article use the heading and paragraph following the heading:
	  ◦ Miller (2010) . . . (Results, para. 1).
	• If the heading is too long, shorten the title and put in quotations marks:
	  ◦ Miller (2010) . . . ("Covering Schools with no AYP", para. 2). [The original heading was Covering Urban Schools which have not received AYP]
		• Same as the first citation

Two authors	• Last names, "and" or "&": ◦ Smith and Miller (2011); (Smith & Miller, 2011)	• Same as the first citation.

Three to five authors	• Last name of all authors. "and" or "&" placed before the last author:
	  ◦ Rasmussen, Miller, Sanchez, Rogers, and Thomas (2011) . . .
	  ◦ (Rasmussen, Miller, Sanchez, Rogers, & Thomas, 2011) . . .
	• When two or more references would shorten to the same citation, cite as many authors as necessary to distinguish between the two citations and follow with (comma) et al.
	  ◦ DeWitt, Sherer, Johnson, and Smith (2011) vs. De Witt, Sherer, Jones, Johnson, and Dennis, (2011).
		• List the first author and replace the rest of the authors with et al.
		  ◦ Rasmussen et al., (2011); (Rasmussen et al., 2011)
		• Shorten to DeWitt, Sherer, Johnson, et al. (2011) and (De Witt, Sherer, Jones, et al., 2011)

(continued)

TABLE 11-5 (CONTINUED)		
USING CITATIONS IN TEXT USING APA STYLE		
TYPE OF CITATION	FIRST CITATION	ADDITIONAL CITATIONS IN THE TEXT
Six or more authors	• Last name of first author followed by et al. (year) ○ Steinberg et al. (2009) • When two or more references would shorten to the same citation, cite as many authors as necessary to distinguish between the two citations, and follow with (comma) et al. • (See Three to Five authors.)	• Same as the first citation.
Two or more citations	• List citations alphabetically by first author's name, followed by a semicolon: ○ (James, Smith, & Johnson, 2009; Marley & Barnett, 2008)	• Same as the first citation.
The sequence of authors is determined by the sequence in the article. When the citation is used a second time in the same paragraph, leave out the date unless there are two citations by the same author or the citation can be confused with another citation.		

11.6.1 Outline of a Research Proposal

1. Title of study
2. Investigator
3. Date
4. The research problem
   a. Statement of problem in question form
   b. Justification and need for the study
   c. Implications of anticipated results in relation to clinical treatment, professional, education, or administrative problems
5. The literature review
   a. Outline of major areas to be reviewed
   b. Plan for search of related literature
   c. Annotated bibliographical notation organized under major areas reviewed
6. Research design
   a. Research model, (e.g., experimental, correlational, methodological)
   b. Operational definitions of variables
   c. Statement of hypotheses or guiding questions
   d. Identification of presumed independent or dependent variables
   e. Theoretical explanation underlying study

7. Methods
   a. Procedure for selecting sample and screening criteria for subject inclusion
   b. Setting for study and procedure for collecting data
   c. Tests, questionnaires, or instruments applied to study
   d. Methodological studies to include evaluation of
      i. Reliability
      ii. Validity
   e. Tentative time schedule for study
      i. Time period for literature review
      ii. Collection of data: number of hours required
      iii. Date for completion of research
   f. Projected costs for study
      i. Clerical
      ii. Instrumentation
      iii. Other

11.7 SAMPLE PROPOSAL OF A GRADUATE RESEARCH PROJECT

An example of a graduate research project is listed at the end of this chapter. The project has been reprinted with the permission of the author. Additionally, this work was subsequently submitted to and published in a peer-reviewed journal (Applegate, Rice, Stein, & Maitra, 2008).

TABLE 11-6

COMMON BIBLIOGRAPHIC REFERENCES

	BOOK	JOURNAL	CHAPTER IN A BOOK

AUTHOR(S)	• Last name, initials. . . . & last name, initials; no additional punctuation at the end.
	  ◦ Jones, M. J., & Smith, J. C.
		• Last name, initials. . . . & last name, initials; no additional punctuation at the end.
		  ◦ Jones, M. J., Johnson, P. G., & Smith, J. C.
			• Last name, initials. . . . & last name, initials; no additional punctuation at the end.
			  ◦ Johnson, M. J., & James, P. G.

YEAR	• Place the year in parentheses, and put period after the parentheses.
	  ◦ (1994).
		• Place the year in parentheses, and put period after the parentheses. For weekly issues, put the month, date, and year in parentheses.
		  ◦ (1977, October 15).
			• Place the year in parentheses, and put period after the parentheses.
			  ◦ (1994).

TITLE OF BOOK, ARTICLE, CHAPTER	• Capitalize the first word of the book and first word after a colon. End with a period unless there is an edition number. Underline title of book or put in italics.
	  ◦ Evaluation of therapeutic progress
		• Capitalize the first word of the journal article and first word after a colon. End with a period. Do not underline the article title or put it in quotations.
		• Evaluation of classroom procedures
			• Capitalize first word of the chapter from a book and first word after a colon. End the chapter title with a period.
			  ◦ Evaluation of classroom procedures.

TITLE OF JOURNAL		• Capitalize the important words in the journal title and underline it. Put a comma after the title. ◦ Journal of Aging,	

Note: Additional information regarding the appropriate style of dissertations, secondary sources, movies, or films or other sources can be found in the APA manual.

Adapted from the American Psychological Association. (2011). *Publication manual of the American Psychological Association* (6th ed.). Washington, DC: Author; Slade, C., Campbell, W. G., & Ballou, S. V. (1997). *Form and style: Research papers, reports, theses* (10th ed.). Boston, MA: Houghton Mifflin.

11.8 PREPARATION FOR PRESENTATION

11.8.1 Poster Session

A poster display is an opportunity for researchers to present their research in an informal environment. At many conferences, a portion of the conference area is set aside for poster displays. Usually the researcher stays with the poster and discusses the data analysis and procedures with the conference participants. This is an opportunity for the participants to ask questions related to the research.

The poster should be presented in a clear and comprehensive manner. Components of the poster itself include (a) an abstract written in 25 to 50 words, (b) the purpose or aim of the study, (c) the methodology including subject selection, measurements, procedures, or treatment techniques, (d) results presented in graphic form, and (e) a summary of the conclusions. In addition to the poster, a handout is usually available that may include all the components, plus a summary of literature review and a means of contacting the researchers.

TABLE 11-7	
EXAMPLES OF BIBLIOGRAPHIC REFERENCES USING APA STYLE	
BOOK	Locke, L. F., Spirduso, W. W., & Silverman, S. J. (1997). *Proposals that work* (3rd ed.). Newbury Park: Sage.
JOURNAL ARTICLE	Smith, J. G, & Jones, J. M. (1993). Reconstructing the facial features. *Journal of Paleontology, 17,* 339-431.
CHAPTER IN A BOOK	Rutter, M., Chadwick, O., & Shaffer, D. (1983). Head injury. In M. Rutter (Ed.), *Developmental neuropsychiatry* (pp. 83-111). New York, NY: Guilford.
ELECTRONIC SOURCES	ClickArt 10,000. (No Date). [CD-ROM] Broderbund. Available: CLT844AE–CD. [1999, August 3]
	Crane, N. (1997). *Bibliographic formats for citing electronic information.* Retrieved from http://www.uvm.edu/~ncrane/estyles

Note. Additional information regarding the appropriate style for dissertations, secondary sources, and movies or films can be found in the APA manual.

Adapted from the American Psychological Association. (2011). *Publication manual of the American Psychological Association* (6th ed.). Washington, DC: Author; Slade, C., Campbell, W. G., & Ballou, S. V. (1997). *Form and style: Research papers, reports, theses* (10th ed.). Boston, MA: Houghton Mifflin.

Boston University: Sargent College
College of Health and Rehabilitation Sciences

The Effect of Sensory Integration
on a 10-Year-Old Child with Learning Disabilities

By
Barbara Stein, B. S.

Submitted in partial fulfillment
of the requirements for the degree of
Master of Occupational Therapy (MOT)
September, 2010

Figure 11-1. Example of a title page for a research paper, thesis, or dissertation.

11.8.1.1 Key Points of Preparing a Poster

- *Size of print*: The print size should be large enough for participants to read it at a distance of 4 feet, generally a font size of 18- to 24-points.
- *Layout*: The layout is determined by the space provided at the conference and directions from the conference committee. Try different layouts designs. The material should be arranged to facilitate understanding of the material, generally top to bottom in a left-to-right sequence (Figure 11-2).
- *Amount of information*: Information should be written in bullets (three- to four-word phrases) rather than in sentences. Include essential information about the design, procedure, and results. Figures, charts, and photographs are helpful in displaying results. Additional information can be included in the handout.

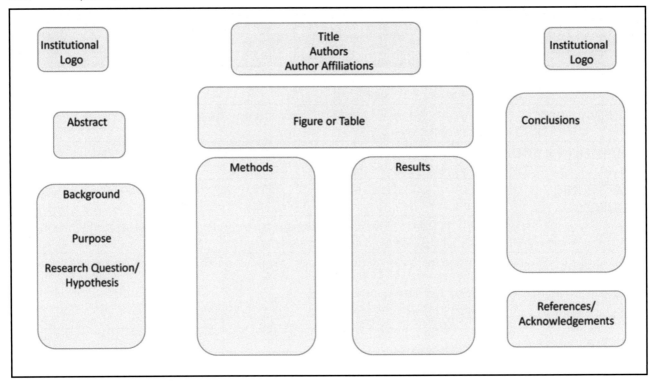

Figure 11-2. Sample of the layout of a poster session.

- *Color*: Use color in highlighting the results and conclusions. A light color (e.g., yellow) printed on a dark paper is frequently easier to read.
- *Background*: Use of contrasting color or border behind the individual components will make the poster visually attractive.

11.8.2 Conference Paper

Researchers are encouraged to present the results of their findings at local, state, national, and international conferences. A call for papers is issued in *OT Practice*. When presenting a paper, it is important to recognize that those in attendance are adult learners with a heterogeneous knowledge base.

11.8.2.1 Key Points of Presenting a Paper

- Rehearse the presentation, considering time available for the presentation.
- Consider the number of people and the size of the room when preparing the paper. If a presenter has only 10 to 15 minutes, discussing one or two major points is more feasible than if the presentation is a 90-minute workshop.
- Consider who will be in the audience (e.g., parents, professionals, new graduates, experienced clinicians) and plan your presentation accordingly.
- If the paper must be read verbatim, use conversational expression and eye contact with members of the audience.

- When presentations are more than 15 minutes long, prepare a visual presentation, such as a Microsoft PowerPoint presentation, that can be used to discuss the paper rather than reading it verbatim.
- Use 3-x-5 cards to organize and remember the key points to present.
- Allow 5 to 10 minutes for questions from the audience.
- Speak loudly enough for everyone in the audience to hear.
- Prepare the visual presentation so that people in the last row can see them. If possible, provide handouts of the overheads (in smaller fonts).
- When preparing PowerPoint presentations, be sure that the print is large (fonts of 36 points or above) and that students have handouts of the presentations. A light print with a dark background (e.g., dark blue background with yellow print) is easier to read. A sans serif font (e.g., Arial) is also preferable. Although adding animations can be entertaining, they may distract from the presentation.
- Be sure that equipment works prior to the presentation. Go to the room at least 10 minutes before the presentation and try out the equipment.
- Include a beginning, middle, and end in your presentation. The beginning should establish rapport and set the purpose of the presentation with the audience. The ending should summarize the presentation. Make your conclusion memorable.

- Generally, the audience will be adult learners. Adult learners are pragmatic, eager to apply what they learn, have a variety of experiences, and often challenge the presenter.
- Include a one-page handout with references.

11.8.2.2 Audiovisual Aids

- *PowerPoint*: This is a useful tool for the organization of material. Individual points can be displayed as they are discussed, rather than all at once, as they would be on a transparency or slide. Sequencing and timing are easier than when using slides or overheads. Handouts should be used to help the audience follow the program. In addition, speaker notes can be scripted to remind the speaker of specific points. Because PowerPoint is updated frequently, the speaker should verify that the software and hardware are compatible. This is particularly true if the PowerPoint presentation has embedded video or audio within the presentation.
- *Document Monitors*: Document monitors will project items (e.g., printed material or other physical objects) onto a projection screen. In general, prepare items with a word-processing program rather than free-hand print. Use contrasting colors if possible. Pictures can be scanned into a document and printed. The print should be large enough for those in the back to see. Graphics should be clear without distracting material.
- *Flip Charts*: Use dark-colored markers, write in large lettering, and place the easel on a platform above the audience so those in the back can see the chart.

11.8.3 Publication

Numerous opportunities exist for students and clinicians to publish their research in occupational therapy journals. The following outline lists the steps in selecting a journal and preparing the research study for publication. In addition, based on the first author's experience as an editor, questions used to evaluate a submitted manuscript to a referred journal have been included.

11.8.3.1 Selecting the Appropriate Journal

An extensive list of all occupational therapy journals is found in Chapter 6. The researcher should obtain the instructions for submission of a paper before submission. The style (e.g., APA, Turabian), margins, page length, manuscript length, number of copies, and the arrangement of the manuscript are specific to each journal. Most journals require work to be submitted electronically, either through email or directly through the publisher's website.

11.8.3.2 Classifying the Manuscript

- Research paper, presenting original data (quantitative and qualitative)
- The position paper (e.g., advocating change in health care system)
- Review article (integration of research studies)
- Description of clinical program
- Description of clinical device
- Book review
- Letter to the editor

11.8.3.3 Components of the Manuscript

- Title: Include variables, subjects, settings
- Author(s): Include degrees, affiliation, email address, and corresponding address
- Abstract: 100- to 175-word summary of article
- Key words: 4 to 5 descriptive words
- Literature review and introduction
- Methods
- Results
- Discussion
- Conclusions
- Recommendations for further research and limitations of study
- Acknowledgments
- References
- Tables and figures

11.8.3.4 Process of Getting Into Print

- Rewriting and multiple drafts are necessary.
- Keep in mind that approximately 60% of manuscripts are rejected.
- The lag between submitting an article and seeing it in print is often up to 1 year.
- Refereed journals: The types of decisions made include (a) accept with minor revisions, (b) accept with major revisions, (c) resubmit for additional review, and (d) reject.

11.8.3.5 The Journal Review Process (Questions Posed for the Reviewer)

- Is the title representative of the article?
- Is the abstract a summary of the main points of the study?
- Does the author justify the need and significance of research?
- Is the literature review comprehensive and up to date?
- Is the research design rigorous (internal validity)?
- Is generalization to target population valid (external validity)?
- Does the investigator use the appropriate statistical tests?
- Are results consistent with statistical findings?
- Are the conclusions justified?
- Are the references up to date and from a variety of sources?

- Does the author recommend further research and state limitations of study?
- Are the figures and graphs labeled correctly?
- Do the figures and graphs add to the information presented?

11.9 SUMMARY

One of the important purposes of this book is to help the student and practitioner generate clinical research studies that validate practice. The authors have presented the research process in a systematic method. The research process presented incorporates both qualitative and quantitative research models. For the clinical researcher, these models can be used to validate practice. Research does not exist in a vacuum. There is a strong historical background for research that has led to the progress in medicine, rehabilitation, and habilitation. Occupational therapists are part of the behavioral medicine tradition that applies nonsurgical and nonpharmaceutical methods. Occupational therapists employing behavioral techniques and assistive technology, such as sensory integration therapy, neurodevelopmental theory, creative arts, relaxation therapy, splinting, and prescriptive exercise can use the clinical research methods described to establish evidence-based practice for the 21st century. It is the authors' intention that the development of treatment protocols can be useful in the establishment of a scientific foundation for occupational therapy.

Knowledge of Results and Learning to Tell Time in Persons with Cognitive Developmental Disabilities

Samantha Meng

The University of Toledo

June, 2006

Table of Contents

1.0 The Research Problem

1.1 Statement of Research Problem in Question Form

- What is developmental delay (DD)?

- What is the cause of DD?

- How is mental retardation/DD categorized?

- How do people with DD acquire skill?

- What are effective strategies for teaching people with DD new skills?

- What type of services do people with DD typically receive?

- What is occupational therapy's typical focus when treating a person with DD?

- What is Knowledge of Results (KR)?

- What are effective strategies employed using KR?

- Is the use of KR effective in teaching people with DD?

1.2 Justification and Need for Study

The Arc (2004) defines developmental delay (DD) as a substantial limitation in present functioning that is characterized by significantly sub average intellectual functioning, along with related limitations in two of ten areas, including communication, self-care, home living, social skills, and safety. The American Psychiatric Association (1994) also states that the age of onset must occur before age 18 years. DD is in the category of developmental disabilities (Dirckx & Stedman, 1997). Developmental disabilities can occur prenatal, perinatal, or in early childhood (Merrill & Mulligan, 2003).

There is no cure for DD, but those who have DD can learn to do many things, it may just take them more time and effort than others, depending on the severity of involvement. One way of categorizing DD, is in four distinct levels. These levels have been established based upon intelligence quotient (IQ) scores; however these levels are not universally used. The highest level of DD, mild DD, is associated with the highest IQ range. For instance individual over the age of 21 years with an IQ ranging from 52 to 68, are considers to have mild DD. These individuals usually have achieved enough social and vocational skills for self support, however they do need support under social or economical stress (dealing with relationship or financial needs). The moderate level of DD involves an IQ range of 36 to 51. Individuals in this range may achieve self support by performing in assisted conditions and need support in mildly stressful social and economic situations. The third level of DD, referred to as severe, involves an IQ range of 20 to 35. Individuals in this category need complete supervision but are able to contribute partially to their own self care. Profound is the lowest level of DD. The IQ range for a person who is profoundly mentally retarded is 19 or below. As an adult, a person in this category may achieve very little independent self care and usually requires nursing assistance (Porter, 2018). One way to understand the levels of classification are to associate how the level of IQ relates to the abilities of the individual with DD. The relationship is proportional in that the higher the IQ, the greater the ability. Conversely needing support or complete supervision is often associated with a reduced ability to meet self-care, household, community interaction, social interaction, leisure time, and vocational needs and goals.

The care and treatment of those with DD has changed greatly as societal attitudes have evolved through the past century and beyond. Most recently, the shift has involved deinstitutionalization resulting in placing those with DD into family or group homes. Some individuals with DD are even living independently while requiring minimal assistance. There are several advantages for community-based group homes compared to institutional life. One advantage to those who move to group settings is that they have increased contact with their families and are provided more time in a wider variety of activities outside the house (Firth & Short, 1987). They also provide opportunities for clients to learn both basic and advanced living skills. This is important for two reasons. First, it is a "real life" living situation. For instance, household chores need to be done or more self care is done by individuals with DD due to the fact that there is less staff available to them.

They also learn skills in real life situations that might be hard to simulate in institutions, like going grocery shopping or taking care of a dog (Neistadt, 1987). Secondly, the social structure of the group home provides a ready-made peer support network. Peer support can increase their social skills. They will also learn to offer emotional and physical assistance as needed (Neistadt, 1987). It has been shown that individuals living in institutions are also less active, mobile, social, and independent compared to a nondisabled reference group (O'Neill, Brown, Gordon, & Schonhorn, 1985). Individuals placed in communities also have a greater level of cognitive and social skills than those not placed in community living (Eastwood & Fisher, 1988). However, adults with developmental disabilities residing in group homes generally have not yet reached the peak of their functional abilities in spite of being placed in a more naturalistic community setting (Neistadt, 1987). Occupational therapy has the opportunity to help those with DD fulfill some of those cognitive and psychosocial abilities given the right interventions.

Although there is great variability among individuals with DD, many higher functioning individuals may want to enter the work environment or socialize outside the group home. A basic skill that is essential for being able to hold a job or engage in social events in the community is the skill of telling time. This is a very important instrumental activity of daily living (IADL) because telling time is an essential precursor for knowing when to leave for a job or social gathering, how long they have to get to their destination, and when they need to leave to return home. Therefore the purpose of the present study is to see if there is an effect on learning to tell time when KR is present in a population with DD who is residing in a group home. Telling time is an important IADL that can lead to increased independence in the home and work settings. This is an important skill to any subpopulation of DD, but it is especially important to those interested in prevocational opportunities.

2.0 The Literature Review

2.1 How the Literature Was Searched

- PubMed

- MEDLINE

- CINAHL (Cumulative Index to Nursing and Allied Health)

- Google Scholar

- Internet Resources

- American Occupational Therapy Association (AOTA)

- American Occupational Therapy Foundation

2.2 Underlying Theoretical Assumptions

- There is variability in the cognitive abilities of people with cognitive developmental delay (Porter, 2018).

- Learning ADLs and IADLs is possible in people with cognitive developmental delay (Porter, 2018).

- Providing a reduced frequency of KR is an effective strategy for teaching motor skills (Schmidt & Lee, 2005).

- People with cognitive DD can learn a skill through using reduced frequency of KR (Rice & Hernandez, 2006).

2.3 Target Population

The target population is adult-aged people with cognitive DD.

2.4 Literature Review Summary

Occupational therapists work with a broad range of clientele, helping them develop useful life skills that will permit them to be more independent, successful, and to improve their quality of life. One population occupational therapist work directly with is the mentally retarded/developmentally disabled population. As many as 3 out of every 100 people in the United States have DD (The Arc, 2004). As occupational therapists, we have the responsibility to ensure the most appropriate and efficacious intervention programs are provided to all populations. Evidence based practice is needed in occupational therapy to establish important strategies for assessment and treatment. By giving those with DD the best possible treatment, the occupational therapist can help these individuals reach their maximum potential in life. This population has a wide array of characteristics and abilities.

There are many different causes of developmental disabilities. Some are genetic, where developmental disability results from the abnormality of genes inherited from parents during conception. The use of drugs and alcohol by the mother while pregnant can also cause developmental disabilities. Malnutrition, rubella, granular disorders and diabetes, cytomegalovirus, HIV, and many other illnesses of the mother during pregnancy can also cause developmental disabilities. An unusual amount of stress during birth can also injure the baby's brain, as can insufficient oxygen, and extreme premature birth. Other causes of developmental disabilities include childhood diseases, such as whooping cough, chicken pox, measles, and haemophilus influenzae type B disease,which may lead to meningitis and encephalitis, all of which can damage the brain. Accidents that affect the brain similar to a blow to the head or a near drowning accident can also cause developmental disabilities. Toxic substances, such as mercury or lead, can cause permanent damage to the brain and nervous system. Children in deprived families may become mentally retarded because of malnutrition or inadequate medical care. Overall, damage to the brain occurs resulting in cognitive mental retardation (Porter, 2018).

A study done by Eastwood and Fisher (1988) compared skill acquisition among those institutionalized to those who had been moved from an institution to a community setting. They found that clients who were in the community setting had a significantly greater level of cognitive and social skills after placement than did a matched group of control clients who were still residing in institutions. The community group scored higher than the institution group on seven of eight skill areas, including reading/writing, quantitative, independent living, community orientation, recreation/leisure time, vocational, and social interaction.

O'Neill et al. (1985) evaluated the change in activity pattern and skills of severely and profoundly DD individuals after they moved from an institution to community living. They found that when compared to a nondisabled reference group the individuals with DD become much more similar to the reference group in their activity patterns after being deinstitutionalized. They also improved in 4 of 16 skill areas within 3 months of leaving the institutions. The skill areas they improved in were expressive communication; eating; serving meals/washing dishes; and meal preparation, all of which are occupations of daily living (ODL).

Poole et al. (1991) stated: "The overall goal of occupational therapy for the person with cognitive impairments is to enhance performance in daily living." Occupational therapists also focus on improving instrumental occupations of daily living (IODL) skills with their clients. An IODL is a complex occupation or task that a person does to maintain independence in the home and community (Law, 2002). This could include meal planning, taking care of pets, cleaning the house, or telling time. Increasing these skills in an individual with DD can drastically improve his or her quality of life, independence level, and social functioning.

One of the main objectives of occupational therapy is to enhance the learning process (Flinn & Radomski, 2002). Unfortunately group homes can also make it very difficult for clients to learn, due to the high turnover rate of staff and the stresses that are associated with the turnover rates (Neistadt, 1987). The hope is that occupational therapists facilitate learning processes in ways that enhance the probability that their clients will remember the learned information.

A strategy that has been shown to be effective in motor learning uses a certain type of augmented feedback known as *Knowledge of Results*. KR is extrinsic, or external, information presented after the task is completed (Flinn & Radomski, 2002). It is a type of feedback given to the client so that he or she can change his or her responses or behaviors on subsequent trials to increase the likelihood of reaching a desired goal. KR is not feedback about the movement itself ("Your wrist was locked") but it is about movement outcome in terms of an environmental goal ("You missed your target") (Schmidt & Lee, 2005). This type of feedback has shown to increase the chances of learning fine and gross motor skills in "normal" populations. KR has typically been used with motor learning tasks. Motor learning, as defined by Schmidt and Lee (2005), is a process of how movements are produced and learned as a direct result of practice and experience by the individual.

A large number of recent studies using "normal" participants investigated whether KR works better at 100% or at a reduced frequency. Giving 100% KR involves providing feedback after every trial, giving KR at 50% or 75%, involves providing feedback after every other or after every three trials, respectively. Overall these studies found that when given 100% KR individuals perform better in the acquisition phase and those given KR at a reduced frequency performed better in the retention phase. One reason behind this thought, explained by Sidaway, Fairweather, Powell, and Hall (1992), is that KR functions to guide performance rather than enhance the learning process. Another suggestion is that the individual becomes reliant on the KR and does not use environmental and task cues to encode the skills to long-term memory (Schmidt, Lange, & Young, 1990). Shea and Wulf (2005) stated that when compared with constant practice (trial-to-trial practice), variable practice generally resulted in more effective retention and transfer. Little is known about the applicability of using KR strategies with individuals with DD. The few studies that have been completed with participants with DD focused more on whether 100% KR was more effective than when KR is given less than 100% of the time.

Gillespie (2003) recruited 32 individuals with mild intellectual disabilities and found that participants in the 100% KR performed better in the acquisition phase than those with 50% KR. Conversely participants with 50% KR performed better in the retention phase than the 100% KR group did. The task involved in this study was putting a golf ball. They performed 50 acquisition trial, 25 1-day retention trials, and 25 1-week retention trials.

In a more recent study, Rice and Hernandez (2006) investigated the effect of 100% KR vs. 50% KR in a group of individuals with DD and a group of age-matched average individuals. The task involved matching a yellow bar to a blue target bar on a computer screen by moving the access device (i.e., a knob). Participants received KR in the form of a green bar that indicated the level of success in matching the blue bar to the position of the yellow bar on the computer screen. There were 30 trials in the first phase where KR was provided (acquisition), and 5 in the second phase (retention) where KR was not provided. KR was provided directly after each trial. The results show that participants with DD who were assigned to the 100% KR group performed better during the acquisition phase than the participants assigned to the 50% KR group. Similar to the results in the Gillespie (2003) study, the 50% KR group performed better than the 100% KR group in the retention phase. This was the case for both the individuals with DD and the age matched individuals without DD.

Presently, a large number of individuals with DD reside in group homes, which some might say is a more conductive environment for learning. It appears that KR may facilitate the individual's ability to perform a motor task; unfortunately the tasks involved in these KR studies did not indicate any type of ODL or IODL training. Consequently no research has been done to investigate this strategy using a task where the individual learns an ODL or an IODL. Learning ODLs or IODLs can help any individual reach his or her full potential.

One of the advantages to working in a group home is that the client gets more individualized attention from all health care providers, due to the fact that the ratio of health care providers to residents is higher. Leaning an IODL is very specific to every individual. How one individual learns to tell time may be completely different than from how another individual learns that same skill. Single-case research studies are focused on providing individualized treatment to a certain individual, producing changes that are specifically designed and appropriate for that individual (AOTA, 1985). One advantage of single-case research studies is that the researcher does not need to obtain a group that is homogenous, especially within the special population where there is often great variability person to person. It is often difficult to attain a homogenous group for a study when certain conditions vary extensively depending on the individual and his or her deficits and needs (Payton, 1988). A second reason single-case research designs are important is that they focus on the individual's abilities and what treatments are particularly effective for him or her (Payton, 1988). Single-case research designs let the therapist focus directly on the individual and allow the therapist to tailor the intervention to the individual's needs and situation (Ottenbacher & York, 1984). Another reason single-case research designs are useful is that they can be used as a precursor to investigating a phenomenon using a large number of individuals. For instance, a case study using a few individuals can be used as a pilot study to see if the phenomenon exists. Therefore, a single-case study involving participants with DD, who will be learning an IODL (telling time), is particularly suited and needed at this point in time. Single-case research designs show the difference between one treatment (A) and another type of treatment (B) (Payton, 1988). In most situations, treatment A is a non-treatment control (Payton, 1988). The A phase is also called a *baseline* or *no treatment condition* (Ottenbacher & York, 1984). B phase is called the *treatment condition* (Payton, 1988). It is during this phase that acquisition of the task should take place. Some single-case studies will repeat the A phase after the treatment is withdrawn to strengthen their findings and to see if the patient was able to obtain the information learned (Ottenbacher & York, 1984). This phase can also be termed as the *retention phase*.

KR may provide, and, hopefully, improve task performance for a long-term result, it may, however, only elicit short term or temporary results. Some studies report that participants were more interested and put more effort into the task when KR was present (Arps, 1920; Crawley, 1926; Elwell & Grindley, 1938). Salmoni, Schmidt, and Walter (1984) noted this as a temporary phenomenon, which can dissipate with a brief rest or alter in condition from the original task. Similar to that, KR can also provide a strong guidance function for future performance. It may provide the participant with the information needed to change his or her performance before the next performance occurs. This too could be a temporary effect in which performance deteriorates quickly (Salmoni et al., 1984).

3.0 Research Design

This study will use an ABAB single-case experimental design. The A phases will represent no treatment and the B phases will represent when treatment is present. Each phase will consist of six trials per time period given. The times given on the clock will be six on the hour and six on the half hour. The task will last approximately 20 minutes each day for 4 consecutive weeks.

3.1 Research Design Questions

- How will persons with DD be found?

- Where will data be collected?

- How will the independent variable be administered?

- How can compliance be ensured during the data collection process?

- How will the data be collected?

- How will the data be analyzed?

3.2 Guiding Question

We first hypothesize that performance during intervention phases (B1 and B2) will be significantly better than during the baseline performance (A1 and A2). We also hypothesize that performance during post phases (A2 and B2) will be significantly better than during the initial phases (A1 and B1 respectively).

3.3 Diagrammatical Relationship Between Variables

Target Population	Adults with cognitive DD
Representative Sample	Adults with cognitive DD located in Northwest Ohio
Method	ABAB single subject research design
Guiding Question	We first hypothesize that performance during intervention phases (B1 and B2) will be significantly better than during the baseline performance (A1 and A2). We also hypothesize that performance during post phases (A2 and B2) will be significantly better than during the initial phases (A1 and B1 respectively).
Statistical Test	Visual observation of celebration lines and Wilcoxon Signed-Rank test

3.4 Possible Limitations of the Study

There will be several possible limitations to the study. As this is a single subject research design, which by design employs a small sample size, the ability to generalize the study's results to a larger population is limited. Another potential limitation will be the lack of control over participant compliance during the data collection process. Lastly, the researcher is aware of the hypothesis and could therefore influence the study by introducing bias.

4.0 Methods

4.1 Target Population

Participants will consist of four to eight individuals with DD. Participants will be selected from a large group of individuals with DD who reside in community-based housing. Each participant will be classified as an individual with mild to moderate DD. Inclusion criteria includes that individuals have mild to moderate DD, be over 18 years of age, and currently have not demonstrated the ability to consistently tell time accurately. Participant's age, gender, diagnosis, and years of schooling will be recorded. The identities of the participants will be kept confidential.

4.2 Apparatus

A Pentium IV laptop computer with custom software will be used to deliver the independent variable.

4.3 Data Collection Procedure

Prior to any data collection, informed consent will be obtained. To ensure participants understand their rights and the study's procedures, the participants will state back their understanding of their rights and the study's procedures. Each participant will complete the task independently of each other. Participants will be given the directions of the task and will be given a chance to become familiar with all of the equipment. Each participant will be given three practice trials each day to ensure they understand the task and how to use the equipment. These practice trials will not be used in the results.

During the explanation of the task, the participants will each be shown the face clock on the computer screen and will be told that they are to match the correct digital time with what is being shown on the face clock. Demonstration will be provided to show the participants how to select their desired digital time using the computer mouse.

During the treatment trials (B1 and B2), it will then be explained to the participant that if he or she chooses the correct digital time, balloons will be shown on the screen and "great job" will be heard along with the time that the participant chose. If the participant chooses the wrong digital time, one that does not match what was shown on the face clock, the phrase "sorry" will be heard along with the time that was chosen and the desired time. A new face clock will also appear on the computer screen displaying the correct time and the time chosen by the participant, the hands of the clock will be in red to show the difference between the two times. Each time will be repeated six times to increase the chance that learning will occur in the individual. This will give the participant verbal and visual feedback on their performance. The feedback will be provided directly after each trial.

During the A phases, the same procedure will be followed as in the B phases, only no feedback of any kind will be given. That is, after the participant selects a time, the next trial will appear.

4.4 Projected Time Schedule for Completing Study

Selection of Topic ....3 hours
Literature Review .... 50 hours
Research Proposal .... 45 hours
Recruitment Activity..10 hours
Software Development and Testing... 80 hours
Travel .... 20 hours
Data Analysis .... 30 hours
Write Discussion ....10 hours
Complete Research ....10 hours
Total Time to Complete Study... Approximately 12 months

4.5 Research and Statistical Design

This study will use an A1B1A2B2 single case experimental design. The A phases will represent no treatment and the B phases will represent when treatment is present. Each phase will consist of six trials per time period given, the times given will be six on the hour and six on the half hour, lasting approximately 20 minutes each day for 4 weeks straight.

Visual observation through a celeration line will be used to see if the slopes differed over the four phases. Observation of the slopes will also include an analysis to test if the slopes are different from zero during each phase. If the slopes differ from zero in each phase then all phases will be combined to see if slope made any differences across all phases. A positive slope for number of correct responses indicates an improvement in the participant's performance. When analyzing time differences, if a negative slope is observed, that also indicates improvement in the participant's performance. A Wilcoxon Signed-Rank Test will compare the performance between each subject for each block of time, and to distinguish any significant differences between the blocks of time, particularly between phases B1 and B2, and between A1 and A2. Finally the B phases will be compared to the A phases for both correct responses and time.

4.6 Projected Costs of Study

Travel $100

Photo Copies $20

Computer Thumb Drive.. $20

Binder for Study $5

Total Cost of Study .... Approximately $145

4.7 Definition of Terms

Mental Retardation: A generalized term referring to an impairment in adaptive functioning and cognition that occurs prior to the age of 18 years and has an intelligent quotient score of 70.

Developmental Delay (DD): A term to describe a chronic condition of either physical or cognitive impairments lasting throughout one's life and whose manifestation of symptoms occurs prior to the age of 8 years.

Cognitive Impairment: Lack of cognitive development and adaptive behavior often manifesting itself during the developmental years. Persons with cognitive impairment are diagnosed with a psychiatric disorder, organic impairment, or a developmental disorder where cognitive abilities including judgment and reasoning are diminished.

Motor Learning: "A set of [internal] processes associated with practice or experience leading to relatively permanent changes in the capability for responding" (Schmidt, 1988, p. 346).

Knowledge of Results (KR): A type of extrinsic feedback provided after a task is completed that gives information regarding how accurate the performance was based upon a desired goal.

Instrumental Activities of Daily Living (IADLs): Personal tasks beyond fundamental tasks associated with ADLs. IADLs involve those tasks often associated with maintaining one's independence and can include activities such as, but not limited to, time management, money management, and grocery shopping.

Activities of Daily Living (ADLs): Fundamental and personal tasks required on a daily basis to maintain personal hygiene, adaptive functioning and cognitive, physical, and emotional health.

Single-Subject Research Design: A general term for research that involves a small sample size and is not intended for external validity, rather it is intended for comparing behavior on an individual basis.

Intelligence Quotient (IQ): A number, based upon standardized testing ,that purports to assign a value to intelligence.

5.0 References

American Occupational Therapy Association. (1985). *Standards of Practice for Occupational Therapy*. Rockville, MD.

American Psychiatric Association. (1994). *Diagnostic and statistical manual of mental disorders* (4th ed.). Washington, DC: Author.

The Arc (2004, October). Introduction to mental retardation. Retrieved from http://www.thearc.org/faqs/intromr.pdf

Arps, G. F. (1920). Work with KR versus work without KR. *Psychological Monographs, 28*.

Crawley, S. L. (1926). An experimental investigation of recovery from work. *Archives of Psychology, 13*, 26.

Dirckx, J. H., & Stedman, T. L. (Eds.). (1997). *Stedman's concise medical dictionary for the health professions* (3rd ed.) Philadelphia, PA: Lippincott Williams & Wilkins.

Eastwood, E. A., & Fisher, G. A. (1988). Skills acquisition among matched samples of institutionalized and community-based persons with mental retardation. *American Journal of Mental Retardation, 93*, 75-83.

Elwell, J. L., & Grindley, G. S. (1938). The effects of knowledge of results on learning and performance. *British Journal of Psychology, 29*, 39-53.

Firth, H. & Short, D. (1987). A move from hospital to community: Evaluation of community contacts. *Child: Care, Health, and Development, 13*, 341-354.

Flinn, N. A., & Radomski, M. V. (2002). Learning. In C. A. Trombly & M. V. Radomski (Eds.), *Occupational therapy for physical dysfunction* (5th ed.). Baltimore, MD: Lippincott Williams & Wilkins.

Gillespie, M. (2003). Summary versus every-trial knowledge of results for individuals with intellectual disabilities. *Adapted Physical Activity Quarterly, 20*, 46-57.

Law, M. (2002). Assessing roles and competence. In C. A. Trombly & M. V. Radomski (Eds.), *Occupational therapy for physical dysfunction* (5th ed.). Baltimore: Lippincott Williams &Wilkins.

Merrill, S.C., & Mulligan, S. E. (2003). Neurological dysfunction in children. In E. B. Crepeau, E. S. Cohn, & B.A. Boyt Schell (Eds.), *Willard & Spackman's occupational therapy* (10th ed.). Baltimore, MD: Lippincott Williams & Wilkins.

Porter, R. S. (Ed.). (2018). *The Merck manual of medical information* (20th ed.). Hoboken, NJ: John Wiley & Sons.

Neistadt, M. E. (1987). An occupational therapy program for adults with developmental disabilities. *American Journal of Occupational Therapy, 41,* 433-438.

O'Neil, J., Brown, M., Gordon, W., & Schonhern, R. (1985). The impact of deinstitutionalization on activities and skills of severely/profoundly mentally retarded multiply-handicapped adults. *Applied Research in Mental Retardation, 6,* 361-371.

Ottenbacher, K., & York, J. (1984). Strategies for evaluating clinical change: Implications for practice and change. *American Journal of Occupational Therapy, 38* 647-659.

Payton, O. (1994). *Research: The validation of clinical research* (3rd ed.). Philadelphia, PA: F.A. Davis.

Poole, J., Dunn, W., Schell, B., Tiernam, K., McKay Barnhart, J., & Abreu, B. (1991). Statement: Occupational therapy services management of persons with cognitive impairments. *American Journal of Occupational Therapy, 45,* 1067-1068.

Rice, M.S., & Hernandez, H. G. (2006). Frequency of knowledge of results and motor learning in persons with developmental delay. *Occupational Therapy International, 13*(1), 35-48.

Salmoni, A. W., Schmidt, R. A., & Walter, C. B. (1984). Knowledge of results and motor learning: A review and critical reappraisal. *Psychological Bulletin, 95,* 355-386.

Schmidt, R. A., Lange, C. J., & Young, D. E. (1990). Optimizing summary knowledge of results for skill learning. *Human Movement Science, 9,* 325-348.

Schmidt, R. A., & Lee, T. D. (2005) *Motor control and learning: A behavioral emphasis* (4th ed.). Champaign, IL: Human Kinetics.

Shea, C. H., & Wulf, G. (2005). Schema theory: A critical appraisal and reevaluation. *Journal of Motor Behavior, 37,* 85-101.

Sidaway, B., Fairweather, M., Powell, J., & Hall, G. (1992). The acquisition and retention of a timing task: Effects of summary KR and movement time. *Research Quarterly for Exercise and Sport, 63,* 328-334.

6.0 Annotated Bibliography

Firth, H. (1987). A move from hospital to community: Evaluation of community contacts. *Child: Care, Health, and Development, 13,* 341-354.

> *Abstract*: A small-scale evaluation was made of the activities and social contacts of a group of young mentally handicapped people in one project, leaving hospital to a house in the community. The results are consistent with other recent work in suggesting that residential provision in small homes for people with severe or profound intellectual or multiple handicaps is likely to lead to increased family contact, increased participation in activities outside of the residence, and an increased frequency and duration of contact with non-handicapped people. The study suggests that many of these benefits of life in the community are dependent in various ways upon the staff employed. The nature of the young people's social contacts is examined and conclusions are drawn about specific issues, including staff selection and training, and attention to the maintenance as well as the provision of social contact.

Gillespie, M. (2003). Summary versus every-trial knowledge of results for individuals with intellectual disabilities. *Adapted Physical Activity Quarterly, 20,* 46-57.

> *Abstract*: The purpose of this study was to examine the effect of a summary KR feedback schedule (KR after every fifth trial) vs. every-trial KR on the acquisition and retention of a golf putting task for individuals with intellectual disabilities. Thirty-two individuals with mild intellectual disabilities were randomly assigned to either a summary or every-trial KR group. Participants performed 50 acquisition trials, 25 1-day retention trials, and 25 1-week retention trials. Participants in the every-trial KR group scored significantly better during acquisition, while the summary KR group performed significantly better for both retention intervals. Because of the absence of an acquisition block effect, results relative to learning must be viewed with caution. Findings partially support the guidance hypothesis.

Rice, M. S., & Hernandez, H. G. (2006). Frequency of knowledge of results and motor learning in persons with developmental delay. *Occupational Therapy International, 13,* 35-48.

> *Abstract*: The purpose of this study was to investigate the effect of high vs. low frequency KR in a group of 16 individuals with DD and in gender and age-matched average individuals learning a motor skill on a laptop computer. Participants were randomly assigned to either a 100% or a 50% KR group. KR was provided during the acquisition phase according to group assignment as participants learned the motor skill, whereas no KR was provided during the retention phase. Results indicated both populations who received 50% KR in the acquisition phase demonstrated better performance in the retention phase than those who received 100% KR. The results of this study suggest that, as has been found in the average population, feedback that is too frequent can interfere with learning and retention of tasks for individuals with developmental disabilities. Limitations involved the small sample size along with the task potentially being artificial in nature. Future research is needed to study further the effects of frequency of KR on skill acquisition, particularly in IADLs in this population.

Shea, C. H., & Wulf, G. (2005). Schema theory: A critical appraisal and reevaluation. *Journal of Motor Behavior, 37,* 85-101.

Abstract: The authors critically review a number of the constructs and associated predictions proposed in schema theory (Schmidt, 1975). The authors propose that new control and learning theories should include a reformulated (a) notion of a generalized motor program that is not based on motor program but still accounts for the strong tendency for responses to maintain their relative characteristics; (b) mechanism or processes whereby an abstract movement structure based on proportional principles (e.g., relative timing, relative force) is developed through practice; and (c) explanation for parameter learning that accounts for the benefits of parameter variability but also considers how variability is scheduled. Furthermore, they also propose that new theories of motor learning must be able to account for the consistent findings spawned as a result of the schema theory proposal and must not be simply discounted because of some disfavor with the motor program notion, in general, or schema theory, more specifically.

7.0 Informed Consent

See Chapter 7 for an example.

Commonly Used Abbreviations in Occupational Therapy

A

a	of each
AAC	augmentative and alternative communication
AAOx3	awake, alert, oriented to person, place
AAROM	active assisted range of motion
ABI	acquired brain injury
a.c.	before a meal
ACTH	adrenocorticotropic hormone
ad lib.	freely
ADA	Americans with Disabilities Act
ADD	attention-deficit disorder
ADHD	attention-deficit/hyperactivity disorder
adm	admission
admov.	apply
AFO	ankle foot orthosis
AIDS	acquired immunodeficiency syndrome
AK	above knee amputation
ALS	amyotrophic lateral sclerosis
alt. dieb	every other day
AMA	against medical advice
amb	ambulation or ambulate
ap	before dinner
AROM	active range of motion
as tol	as tolerated
ASAP	as soon as possible
AT	assistive technology

B

bal	balance
BE	below elbow amputation
bib.	drink
b.i.d.	twice per day
bilat	bilateral
BK	below knee amputation
BMI	body mass index
bol.	pill
BP	blood pressure
BRP	bathroom privileges
BSC	bedside commode

C

c̄	with
CA	cancer
CABG	coronary artery bypass graft
CBC	complete blood count
Cc	cubic centimeters
CHF	congestive heart failure
CMC	carpometacarpal joint
CMV	cytomegalovirus
CNS	central nervous system
c/o	complains of
COPD	chronic obstructive pulmonary disease
CP	cerebral palsy
CPR	cardiopulmonary resuscitation
CRPS	complex regional pain syndrome

Rice, M. S., Stein, F., & Tomlin, G.
Clinical Research in Occupational Therapy, Sixth Edition (pp. 371-374).
© 2019 Taylor & Francis Group.

CSF	cerebrospinal fluid
CT	computed tomography, also referred to as *CAT* (computed axial tomography)
CTLSO	cervical thoracic lumbar sacral orthosis
CTS	carpal tunnel syndrome
CVA	cerebrovascular accident

D

/d	per day
d	daily
D and C	dilatation and curettage
DIP	distal interphalangeal
DM	diabetes mellitus
DME	durable medical equipment
DNR	do not resuscitate
DO	Doctor of Osteopathic Medicine
DOB	date of birth
DOE	dyspnea on exertion
DTR	deep tendon reflex
DUI	driving under the influence
DV	domestic violence
DVT	deep vein thrombosis
Dx	diagnosis

E

ECG	electrocardiogram
ECT	electroconvulsive therapy
ED	emergency departure
EEG	electroencephalogram
EMG	electromyogram
EOB	edge of bed
ER	emergency room

F

FAE	fetal alcohol effects
FAS	fetal alcohol syndrome
FASD	fetal alcohol spectrum disorder
FWB	full weightbearing
FWW	front wheeled walker
fx	fracture

G

GBS	Guillain-Barre syndrome
GI	gastrointestinal

H

H$_2$0	water
H&P	history and physical
H/A	headache
Hct	hematocrit
Hgb	hemoglobin
HIV	human immunodeficiency virus
HR	heart rate
HTN	hypertension
Hx	history

I

ICU	intensive care unit
IDEIA	Individuals with Disabilities Education Improvement Act of 2004, also referred to as *IDEA-2004*
IEP	individualized education program
IFSP	individualized family service plan
IM	intramuscular
IP	interphalangeal
IQ	intelligence quotient
ITP	individualized transition plan
IV	intravenous

K

kg	kilogram
KVO	keep vein open

L

lb	pound
LBP	low back pain
LOB	loss of balance
LOC	loss of consciousness
LOS	length of stay
LP	lumbar puncture
LTC	long-term care

M

MCA	middle cerebral artery
MCP	metacarpophalangeal
MD	muscular dystrophy
MED	minimum effective dose
MET	metabolic equivalent

MI	myocardial infarction		p.r.n.	as needed
MMR	measles-mumps-rubella vaccine		PTSD	post-traumatic stress disorder
MP	metacarpophalangeal		PVD	peripheral vascular disease
MR	mental retardation		PWB	partial weight bearing
MRI	magnetic resonance imaging			
MRSA	methicillin resistant *Staphylococcus aureus*			
MS	multiple sclerosis			
MVA	motor vehicle accident			
MVR	mitral valve replacement			

Q

			q2h, q3h, …	every 2 hours, every 3 hours, etc.
			q.h.	every hour
			q.i.d.	four times per day
			quotid	everyday

N

R

NG	nasogastric			
NICU	neonatal intensive care unit			
NKA	no known allergies		RA	rheumatoid arthritis
NP	nurse practitioner		RBC	red blood cells
NPO	nothing by mouth; nothing to eat or drink usually within a defined time frame		RC	rotator cuff
			REM	rapid eye movement
NSAID	nonsteroidal anti-inflammatory drug		RESNA	Rehabilitation Engineering and Assistive Technology Society of North America
NWB	non-weightbearing			
			R/O or r/o	rule out
			ROM	range of motion
			RR or R/R	respiratory rate
			RTW	return to work
			Rx	prescription, treatment, or therapy

O

S

OA	osteoarthritis			
OB/GYN	obstetrics and gynecology			
OD	Doctor of Osteopathic Medicine		SCI	spinal cord injury
ODA	operating day admission		sine	without
OOB	out of bed		SLP	speech-language pathologist
OR	operating room		SNF	skilled nursing facility
ORIF	open reduction, internal fixation		SOB	shortness of breath
Ox3	oriented to person, place, time		S/P or s/p	status post
			STD	sexually transmitted disease
			Strep	streptococcus
			Sx	symptoms

P

T

p̄	after			
PA	physician's assistant			
PAC	premature atrial contraction		TBI	traumatic brain injury
p.c.	after meals		THR or THA	total hip replacement (arthroplasty)
PDD	pervasive developmental disorder		TIA	transient ischemia attacks
PE	physical examination		t.i.d.	three times per day
per	by		TTWB	toe-touch weightbearing
per os	by mouth			
PET	positron emission tomography			
PICC Line	peripherally inserted central catheter for delivery of medication			
PIP	proximal interphalangeal			
p.o.	by mouth or orally			
PROM	passive range of motion			

U

U.S.P.	United States Pharmacopoeia
URI	upper respiratory infection
UTI	urinary tract infection

V

VS	vital signs
VSD	ventricular septal defect

W

w/	with
WB	weightbearing
WBC	white blood cells
W/C	wheel chair
WNL	within normal limits
w/o	without

B

Landmarks in the History of Occupational Therapy

1752 Pennsylvania Hospital in Philadelphia was established. Psychiatric patients were prescribed manual labor to counteract disease process.

1780 Clement-Joseph Tissot, a French physician in the cavalry, published a book prescribing the use of crafts and recreational activities for individuals with muscle and joint injuries.

1786 Philippe Pinel, a French psychiatrist in the Bicetre Asylum for the Insane, prescribed humane treatment in the care of the mentally ill, including physical exercises, manual occupation, and music.

1803 Johanann Christian Reil, a German psychiatrist, advocated that activities such as swimming, dancing, gymnastics, arts and crafts, music, and theater be part of the everyday routine for patients.

1812 Benjamin Rush, the father of American psychiatry, prescribed work, leisure activities, chess and other board games, exercise, and theater for treatment of mental illness.

1813 Samuel Tuke, an English Quaker, founded the Retreat Asylum for the Insane in York, England. Tuke introduced the term *moral treatment*, which was the application of humane practices—including exercise, recreation, arts and crafts, gardening, and regular employment—in the maintenance of the hospital.

1833 Samuel Woodard, a physician at the Worcester State Lunatic Hospital in Massachusetts, introduced the term *occupational therapy* as a therapeutic method to keep inmates active in varied tasks and leisure activities in regular routines. The therapeutic program was clinically effective and produced a significant recovery rate.

1838 Jean Etienne Esquirol, a French psychiatrist, described the importance of corporal exercise, horseback riding, tennis, fencing, swimming, and travel for the treatment of depression.

1840 Francois Leuret, a French psychiatrist, advised that moral treatment, including arts and crafts and work, are effective in treating individuals with mental illness and intellectual disabilities.

1843 Dorothea Dix, a social reformer, worked diligently in the United States for humanistic care for individuals with mental illness, which included the use of therapeutic activities.

1854 Thomas Kirkbride, one of the founders of the American Psychiatric Association, advocated a highly structured regimen for patients that included exercise, lectures, music, arts and crafts, and entertainment.

1895 William Rush Dunton, a psychiatrist and innovator in applying occupational therapy, used arts and crafts activities at Sheppard and Pratt Asylum in Baltimore, Maryland.

Rice, M. S., Stein, F., & Tomlin, G.
Clinical Research in Occupational Therapy, Sixth Edition (pp. 375-379).
© 2019 Taylor & Francis Group.

1895/1922   Adolf Meyer, a strong advocate of occupation, believed in a holistic approach to treatment centering on sleep habits, nutrition, work, play, and socialization.

1895   Mary Potter Meyer, a social worker and the wife of Adolf Meyer, used arts and crafts activities in the State Hospital in Worcester, Massachusetts.

1904   Herbert Hall, a physician, prescribed occupation as a medicine to regulate the life and direct interests of the patient. He called this the *work cure*.

1905   Susan Tracy, a nurse, applied occupational therapy activities in working with individuals with mental illness while she was director of the Training School for Nurses at the Adams Nervine Asylum in Boston, Massachusetts.

1906   Herbert Hall was awarded a grant of $1000 by Harvard University to study the application of activities and graded manual occupation in the treatment of psychiatric disorders.

1908   Training courses in occupations for hospital attendants were initiated at Chicago School of Civics and Philanthropy.

1909   Clifford Beers, founder of the National Committee for Mental Hygiene, described his emotional illness in the book, *A Mind that Found Itself* (Beers, 1908). Beers reinforced the application of therapeutic activities in treating individuals with mental illness.

1910   Susan Tracy authored the first book on occupation studies, *Studies in Invalid Occupations: A Manual for Nurses and Attendants* (Tracy, 1910).

1911   Susan Tracy initiated the first course on occupation in a general hospital at Massachusetts General Hospital in Boston.

1911   Eleanor Clark Slagle, a social worker, established an occupation department at Phipps Psychiatric Clinic at Johns Hopkins University in Baltimore.

1914   George Edward Barton, an architect who had contracted tuberculosis, introduced the term *occupational therapy* at a meeting of hospital workers in Boston, Massachusetts.

1917   The National Society for the Promotion of Occupational Therapy was founded in Consolation House in Clifton Springs, New York. The charter members included George Barton, an architect; Eleanor Clark Slagle, a social worker at Hull House in Chicago, Illinois; Thomas Kidner, a vocational specialist from Canada; William Rush Dunton, a psychiatrist at Sheppard and Pratt Hospital in Baltimore, Maryland; Susan Cox Johnson, an arts and crafts instructor from New York City; Isabel Gladwin (Newton) Barton, first Secretary of the Society ; and Susan E. Tracy, a nurse at the Adams Nervine Asylum in Boston, Massachusetts. This meeting led to the occupational therapy profession in the United States.

1917   Reconstruction aides were recruited to serve in army hospitals during World War I, applying arts and crafts and exercises in the treatment of physical and mental disorders.

1918   Formal educational training programs in occupational therapy were established at the Henry B. Favil School in Chicago, Teachers College of Columbia University, and the Boston School of Occupational Therapy.

1919   Bird T. Baldwin authored the *U.S. Army Manual on Occupational Therapy* (Baldwin, 1919) that included information on evaluation and treatment procedures for the restoration of physical function.

1919   George Barton (1919) wrote the book *Teaching the Sick: A Manual of Occupational Therapy as Reeducation*.

1922   The *Archives of Occupational Therapy* was published and became the official journal of the American Association of Occupational Therapy.

1925   *Occupational Therapy and Rehabilitation* was first published.

1928   Six programs were available to prepare occupational therapists: Boston School, Philadelphia School, St. Louis School, Milwaukee-Downer College, University of Minnesota, and the University of Toronto.

1931   National registry for the American Occupational Therapy Association was established.

1933 The American Medical Association (AMA) began the accreditation of occupational therapy education programs.

1934 Essentials of an acceptable education curriculum in occupational therapy was adopted by the American Medical Education Council on Medical Education and Hospitals.

1939 Among all AMA-approved hospitals, 13% employed occupational therapists.

1943 The Barden-LaFollette Vocational Rehabilitation Act was passed by Congress providing coverage of medical services including occupational therapy for individuals in vocational rehabilitation programs.

1945 Eighteen approved occupational therapy programs were available in the United States, compared with five in 1940.

1947 First national registration examination for U.S. occupational therapists was given.

1947 Advanced master's degree in occupational therapy was offered at the University of Southern California and New York University.

1947 Helen Willard and Clare S. Spackman, occupational therapy educators, authored the first textbook in occupational therapy.

1952 The World Federation of Occupational Therapy (WFOT) was established. The 10 founding member countries were Australia, Canada, Denmark, Great Britain, India, Israel, New Zealand, South Africa, Sweden, and the United States.

1958 Essentials and Guidelines for an approved Educational Program for Occupational Therapy Assistant in the U.S. adopted.

1964 Certified occupational therapy assistant (COTA) certifications were available in the United States.

1964 The first entry-level master's program in occupational therapy was established at the University of Southern California. Shortly thereafter, basic master's programs were begun at Boston University and Virginia Commonwealth University.

1965 The American Occupational Therapy Foundation (AOTF) established as philanthropic organization for advancing the science of occupational therapy.

1965 Lyndon B. Johnson signed Medicare into law on July 30, 1965.

1973 The Rehabilitation Act passed by Congress protecting the rights of persons with disabilities. Section 504 of the Rehabilitation Act of 1973 prohibits discrimination based on disability in programs or activities receiving federal financial assistance. (See http://www.access.gpo.gov/nara/cfr/waisidx_99/34cfr104_99.html and http://www2.ed.gov/policy/speced/reg/narrative.html)

1974 New York University developed the first doctoral program in occupational therapy.

1975 Education for All Handicapped Children Act (EHA; PL 94–142) facilitated free appropriate public education services for students with disabilities at all levels and provided funding for these services. The concept of least restrictive environment, inherent in the law, specifies that students with disabilities are educated with typical students "to the maximum extent possible."

1976 Support was given to students for development of their organization on a national level, which was later named the American Student Occupational Therapy Alliance.

1979 "Uniform Terminology System for Reporting Occupational Therapy Services" developed and adopted by the Representative Assembly (RA).

1980 AOTF published the *Occupational Therapy Journal of Research*.

1981 Entry-level role delineation for OTRs and COTAs adopted by the RA.

1986 Medicare amendments expanded coverage for occupational therapy services under Part B in the United States.

1990 The Americans with Disabilities Act (ADA; PL 101–336; [42 USC 12101]) was passed by Congress and signed by President George H. W. Bush. The ADA guarantees equal opportunity for individuals with disabilities in employment, public accommodations, transportation, governmental services and telecommunications (Family Center on Technology and Disability, 2010). (See also http://www.usdoj.gov/crt/ada/cguide.htm#anchor62335 and http://www.ada.gov)

1990 PL 94–142 was reauthorized and renamed the Individuals with Disabilities Education Act (IDEA). This law continued federal funding from PL 94–142 and increased services by adding related services, transition from school to work, and parental involvement. Under this act, occupational therapy is considered a related service in helping students with disabilities in public schools.

1991 The AOTA RA approved a physical agent modalities (PAMs) position paper that recommended the use of PAMs as an adjunct to purposeful activity to enhance occupational performance.

1994   *Occupational Therapy International* is founded as the first refereed journal, publishing manuscripts by occupational therapists throughout the world.

1997   The Balanced Budget Act (BBA; PL 105–33) significantly changed the procedures for payment of services for rehabilitation personnel affecting the quality of care, especially in home health.

1998   The Assistive Technology Act (PL105–394 [29 USC 2201]) passed. This legislation provides funds to the States to support the establishment of assistive technology (AT) demonstration centers, information centers, facilities, referral services, and advocacy services to help people with disabilities access AT services. The act also provides low-interest loans to purchase AT (FCTD, 2010). (See also http://www.ataporg.org/atap/index.php and http://www.assistivetech.net/webresources/stateTechActProjects.php for information regarding State projects)

1998   Carl D. Perkins Vocational and Technical Education Act Amendments of 1998 (PL105–332 Section 1 (b) [20 USC 2302]). This act requires schools to integrate academic, vocational, and technical training; increase technology use; provide professional development opportunities; develop, implement, and expand quality programs; and link secondary and post-secondary vocational education (FCTD, 2010). (See also http://www.ed.gov/offices/OVAE/CTE/legis.html)

1999   The AOTA RA passes a resolution to mandate that entry-level education in occupational therapy should be at the post-baccalaureate level.

2001   The *International Classification of Functioning, Disability and Health*, known more commonly as ICF, is a classification of health and health-related domains. These domains are classified from body, individual, and societal perspectives by means of two lists: a list of body functions and structures, and a list of domains of activity and participation. As an individual's functioning and disability occur in a context, the ICF also includes a list of environmental factors. The ICF is the World Health Organization's framework for measuring health and disability at both individual and population levels.

2002   No Child Left Behind (NCLB; PL 107–110; http://www2.ed.gov/policy/elsec/leg/esea02/index.html) enacted. As part of the need to improve education, the law focused on requiring each state to develop and implement a statewide accountability system that insured adequate yearly gain for all schools in reading and math. It is based on the concept that setting standards and measurable educational goals can improve academic performance in the classroom.

2002   *The Occupational Therapy Practice Framework: Domain and Process* was developed in response to current practice needs, intended to "more clearly affirm and articulate occupational therapy's unique focus on occupation and daily life activities and the application of an intervention process that facilitates engagement in occupation to support participation in life" (AOTA, 2002, p. 609).

2004   The Individuals with Disabilities Education Improvement Act of 2004 (IDEIA; PL108–556; http://idea.ed.gov/) is the reauthorization of PL 94–142 enacted in 1975. The law ensures that services to more than 6.5 million eligible infants, toddlers, children, and youths with disabilities throughout the nation. With this reauthorization, IDEA-2000 was aligned with NCLB. In addition to funding, IDEIA governs how states and public agencies provide early intervention, special education, and related services.

2004   The fourth edition of the *Canadian Occupational Performance Measure* (COPM; Law et al., 2004) is published. It is an individualized, client-centered measure designed for use by occupational therapists to detect change in a client's self-perception of occupational performance over time. It is designed to be used as an outcome measure. The COPM is designed for use with clients with a variety of disabilities and across all developmental stages. The COPM has been used in more than 35 countries and has been translated into over 20 languages.

2008   *Occupational Therapy Practice Framework: Domain and Process, Second Edition* is published (AOTA, 2008; Roley et al., 2008).

2009 New emerging areas of occupational therapy practice in the United States identified by the AOTA: psychosocial needs of children and youth, health and wellness, driver rehabilitation, low-vision services, ergonomics, community health, welfare to work, and technology and assistive device development and consulting.

2009 Americans with Disabilities Act Amendment (PL 110–325; http://www.judiciary.state.nj.us/legis/110-325_Law.pdf), signed on September 25, 2008 by President George W. Bush and went into effect on January 1, 2009. Under the Amendment, millions more Americans qualify as disabled and fall under the Act's protections. Under the Amendment, the definition of disability was modified so that the individual may be regarded as having an impairment, without regard to whether it substantially limits a major life activity. The Amendment also expands the phrase "major life activities" as "caring for oneself, performing manual tasks, seeing, hearing, eating, sleeping, walking, standing, lifting, bending, speaking, breathing, learning, reading, concentrating, thinking, communicating, and working." Another important change requires that impairments that are episodic or in remission qualify as a disability if they would qualify in their active stage.

2010 WFOT meets in Santiago, Chile for its 15th Congress. There are 70 member countries of the WFOT.

2010 On March 23, President Barack Obama signed the Affordable Health Care for America Act (PL 111–148; http://democrats.senate.gov/reform/patient-protection-affordable-care-act-as-passed.pdf). The general principle is to ensure that all Americans have access to quality, affordable health care. It is projected that the Act will provide health care coverage to 95% of Americans. (See http://www.aota.org/Practitioners/Advocacy/Federal/Highlights/Reform.aspx for the impact of the Act on occupational therapy)

2014 The third edition of the *Occupational Therapy Practice Framework: Domain and Process* is published by the AOTA (2014).

2014 WFOT meets in Yokohama, Japan for its 16th Congress.

2014 The fifth edition of the *Canadian Occupational Performance Measure* is published (Law et al., 2014). The COPM is now used in over 40 countries and has been translated into more than 35 languages.

2017 AOTA celebrates its 100th Anniversary in Philadelphia, Pennsylvania, during the Annual Conference.

2018 WFOT meets in Cape Town, South Africa. There are now over 92 member organizations and approximately 400,000 occupational therapists internationally.

Statistical Tables

Rice, M. S., Stein, F., & Tomlin, G.
Clinical Research in Occupational Therapy, Sixth Edition (pp. 381-414).
© 2019 Taylor & Francis Group.

TABLE C-1

RANDOM NUMBERS

427	8168	6022	1839	7551	7267	564	64	4222	1950
1885	7999	4901	722	5651	8026	4538	2708	7452	7185
5645	1859	5837	3622	7633	6679	9463	1294	4654	1751
7272	6252	8537	7784	4123	3723	7284	1009	7751	7957
6603	8698	9063	8612	7935	6835	4364	7568	171	359
1933	4688	8046	7018	5698	4972	4696	345	7031	3179
428	9076	7159	1140	8954	282	7156	3069	377	2840
5491	2932	7401	3914	9995	6403	9741	4253	5871	3239
7865	4053	6181	7053	9354	5612	4695	7449	3608	9309
1696	4956	3296	244	6718	5004	8328	1376	6646	420
6179	1046	3714	810	9147	2692	6401	6099	669	8070
4385	6107	2097	7800	9436	969	8948	215	7896	5162
3005	2849	1387	5231	9834	5303	6140	3450	4357	2246
1645	8446	6072	9321	6452	8687	6807	9294	9384	427
4352	5114	3458	557	4203	953	4706	9187	1881	4197
8097	6886	6117	3612	5835	6029	9914	2690	9935	4020
4319	9787	8537	442	5920	8919	6542	8858	3186	5251
534	422	2504	3190	5592	5344	9150	4082	869	6470
2699	234	82	924	9748	8198	8789	8730	7687	2632
8867	2771	1589	9630	5033	8720	9067	9478	8867	4530
2304	9779	9008	5321	5668	4491	7197	7064	9148	4923
888	6251	2110	506	9504	3517	2131	1564	2691	2627
2563	380	8805	6190	1595	7281	4167	5632	7715	2688
1786	3293	3752	7526	5646	6807	6694	9449	7124	5329
4712	3580	7627	4029	7676	7655	3567	1122	1874	3335
9882	9208	1618	5801	8704	7508	228	4341	5369	2478
8544	4571	7681	6847	2311	1801	1476	3521	8780	7339
6719	4638	8527	7588	551	6291	531	2090	1837	7324
8709	8569	9953	378	8475	905	9591	1728	9705	9611
8652	1830	505	9129	5314	4766	5920	2332	3008	4333

(continued)

TABLE C-1 (CONTINUED)

RANDOM NUMBERS

1595	143	5277	8354	9102	5071	8807	9340	9972	3130
8777	1096	7081	2112	712	8941	4650	742	9205	6917
8126	1021	1162	5014	8803	7157	8410	9875	7513	2531
4490	8445	9244	7937	1673	8441	7297	3349	5619	2608
5323	7144	5045	7122	4784	368	6908	7499	5399	4083
1107	5926	5966	2489	7955	5832	720	1504	932	8389
5241	2417	4227	4850	4047	4723	7251	9534	5538	253
1938	2683	4457	7591	7971	6626	4025	6117	8421	5663
9097	2967	6611	9832	5372	3222	833	5015	3778	5350
5499	4836	7250	5446	1007	1281	7239	6918	5068	3711

Source: The table was generated using Microsoft Office Excel 2013.

TABLE C-2

PROPORTION OF AREAS UNDER THE NORMAL CURVE (PERCENTILE RANK)

Z	0	0.01	0.02	0.03	0.04	0.05	0.06	0.07	0.08	0.09
0.0	.50000	.50399	.50798	.51197	.51595	.51994	.52392	.52790	.53188	.53586
0.1	.53983	.54380	.54776	.55172	.55567	.55962	.56356	.56749	.57142	.57535
0.2	.57926	.58317	.58706	.59095	.59483	.59871	.60257	.60642	.61026	.61409
0.3	.61791	.62172	.62552	.62930	.63307	.63683	.64058	.64431	.64803	.65173
0.4	.65542	.65910	.66276	.66640	.67003	.67364	.67724	.68082	.68439	.68793
0.5	.69146	.69497	.69847	.70194	.70540	.70884	.71226	.71566	.71904	.72240
0.6	.72575	.72907	.73237	.73565	.73891	.74215	.74537	.74857	.75175	.75490
0.7	.75804	.76115	.76424	.76730	.77035	.77337	.77637	.77935	.78230	.78524
0.8	.78814	.79103	.79389	.79673	.79955	.80234	.80511	.80785	.81057	.81327
0.9	.81594	.81859	.82121	.82381	.82639	.82894	.83147	.83398	.83646	.83891
1.0	.84134	.84375	.84614	.84849	.85083	.85314	.85543	.85769	.85993	.86214
1.1	.86433	.86650	.86864	.87076	.87286	.87493	.87698	.87900	.88100	.88298
1.2	.88493	.88686	.88877	.89065	.89251	.89435	.89617	.89796	.89973	.90147
1.3	.90320	.90490	.90658	.90824	.90988	.91149	.91309	.91466	.91621	.91774
1.4	.91924	.92073	.92220	.92364	.92507	.92647	.92785	.92922	.93056	.93189
1.5	.93319	.93448	.93574	.93699	.93822	.93943	.94062	.94179	.94295	.94408
1.6	.94520	.94630	.94738	.94845	.94950	.95053	.95154	.95254	.95352	.95449
1.7	.95543	.95637	.95728	.95818	.95907	.95994	.96080	.96164	.96246	.96327
1.8	.96407	.96485	.96562	.96638	.96712	.96784	.96856	.96926	.96995	.97062
1.9	.97128	.97193	.97257	.97320	.97381	.97441	.97500	.97558	.97615	.97670
2.0	.97725	.97778	.97831	.97882	.97932	.97982	.98030	.98077	.98124	.98169
2.1	.98214	.98257	.98300	.98341	.98382	.98422	.98461	.98500	.98537	.98574
2.2	.98610	.98645	.98679	.98713	.98745	.98778	.98809	.98840	.98870	.98899
2.3	.98928	.98956	.98983	.99010	.99036	.99061	.99086	.99111	.99134	.99158
2.4	.99180	.99202	.99224	.99245	.99266	.99286	.99305	.99324	.99343	.99361
2.5	.99379	.99396	.99413	.99430	.99446	.99461	.99477	.99492	.99506	.99520
2.6	.99534	.99547	.99560	.99573	.99585	.99598	.99609	.99621	.99632	.99643
2.7	.99653	.99664	.99674	.99683	.99693	.99702	.99711	.99720	.99728	.99736
2.8	.99744	.99752	.99760	.99767	.99774	.99781	.99788	.99795	.99801	.99807
2.9	.99813	.99819	.99825	.99831	.99836	.99841	.99846	.99851	.99856	.99861
3.0	.99865	.99869	.99874	.99878	.99882	.99886	.99889	.99893	.99896	.99900
3.1	.99903	.99906	.99910	.99913	.99916	.99918	.99921	.99924	.99926	.99929
3.2	.99931	.99934	.99936	.99938	.99940	.99942	.99944	.99946	.99948	.99950
3.3	.99952	.99953	.99955	.99957	.99958	.99960	.99961	.99962	.99964	.99965
3.4	.99966	.99968	.99969	.99970	.99971	.99972	.99973	.99974	.99975	.99976
3.5	.99977	.99978	.99978	.99979	.99980	.99981	.99981	.99982	.99983	.99983

(continued)

				TABLE C-2 (CONTINUED)					

PROPORTION OF AREAS UNDER THE NORMAL CURVE (PERCENTILE RANK)

Z	0	0.01	0.02	0.03	0.04	0.05	0.06	0.07	0.08	0.09
3.6	.99984	.99985	.99985	.99986	.99986	.99987	.99987	.99988	.99988	.99989
3.7	.99989	.99990	.99990	.99990	.99991	.99991	.99992	.99992	.99992	.99992
3.8	.99993	.99993	.99993	.99994	.99994	.99994	.99994	.99995	.99995	.99995
3.9	.99995	.99995	.99996	.99996	.99996	.99996	.99996	.99996	.99997	.99997
4.0	.99997	.99997	.99997	.99997	.99997	.99997	.99998	.99998	.99998	.99998
4.1	.99998	.99998	.99998	.99998	.99998	.99998	.99998	.99998	.99999	.99999
4.2	.99999	.99999	.99999	.99999	.99999	.99999	.99999	.99999	.99999	.99999
4.3	.99999	.99999	.99999	.99999	.99999	.99999	.99999	.99999	.99999	.99999
4.4	.99999	.99999	>.99999	>.99999	>.99999	>.99999	>.99999	>.99999	>.99999	>.99999

Note: z-score values are provided at two decimal places. For example, a z-score of 1.27 represents .89796 proportion of the normal curve or percentile rank.

Source: The table was generated using Microsoft Office Excel 2013.

TABLE C-3

CRITICAL VALUES FOR *T*-TEST

LEVEL OF SIGNIFICANCE FOR ONE-TAILED TEST

	0.1	0.05	0.025	0.01	0.005	0.0005

LEVEL OF SIGNIFICANCE FOR TWO-TAILED TEST

df	0.2	0.1	0.05	0.02	0.01	0.001
1	3.0777	6.3138	12.7062	31.8205	63.6567	636.6192
2	1.8856	2.9200	4.3027	6.9646	9.9248	31.5991
3	1.6377	2.3534	3.1824	4.5407	5.8409	12.9240
4	1.5332	2.1318	2.7764	3.7469	4.6041	8.6103
5	1.4759	2.0150	2.5706	3.3649	4.0321	6.8688
6	1.4398	1.9432	2.4469	3.1427	3.7074	5.9588
7	1.4149	1.8946	2.3646	2.9980	3.4995	5.4079
8	1.3968	1.8595	2.3060	2.8965	3.3554	5.0413
9	1.3830	1.8331	2.2622	2.8214	3.2498	4.7809
10	1.3722	1.8125	2.2281	2.7638	3.1693	4.5869
11	1.3634	1.7959	2.2010	2.7181	3.1058	4.4370
12	1.3562	1.7823	2.1788	2.6810	3.0545	4.3178
13	1.3502	1.7709	2.1604	2.6503	3.0123	4.2208
14	1.3450	1.7613	2.1448	2.6245	2.9768	4.1405
15	1.3406	1.7531	2.1314	2.6025	2.9467	4.0728
16	1.3368	1.7459	2.1199	2.5835	2.9208	4.0150
17	1.3334	1.7396	2.1098	2.5669	2.8982	3.9651
18	1.3304	1.7341	2.1009	2.5524	2.8784	3.9216
19	1.3277	1.7291	2.0930	2.5395	2.8609	3.8834
20	1.3253	1.7247	2.0860	2.5280	2.8453	3.8495
21	1.3232	1.7207	2.0796	2.5176	2.8314	3.8193
22	1.3212	1.7171	2.0739	2.5083	2.8188	3.7921
23	1.3195	1.7139	2.0687	2.4999	2.8073	3.7676
24	1.3178	1.7109	2.0639	2.4922	2.7969	3.7454
25	1.3163	1.7081	2.0595	2.4851	2.7874	3.7251
26	1.3150	1.7056	2.0555	2.4786	2.7787	3.7066
27	1.3137	1.7033	2.0518	2.4727	2.7707	3.6896
28	1.3125	1.7011	2.0484	2.4671	2.7633	3.6739
29	1.3114	1.6991	2.0452	2.4620	2.7564	3.6594
30	1.3104	1.6973	2.0423	2.4573	2.7500	3.6460

(continued)

TABLE C-3 (CONTINUED)

CRITICAL VALUES FOR *T*-TEST

	LEVEL OF SIGNIFICANCE FOR ONE-TAILED TEST					
	0.1	*0.05*	*0.025*	*0.01*	*0.005*	*0.0005*
	LEVEL OF SIGNIFICANCE FOR TWO-TAILED TEST					
df	*0.2*	*0.1*	*0.05*	*0.02*	*0.01*	*0.001*
31	1.3095	1.6955	2.0395	2.4528	2.7440	3.6335
32	1.3086	1.6939	2.0369	2.4487	2.7385	3.6218
33	1.3077	1.6924	2.0345	2.4448	2.7333	3.6109
34	1.3070	1.6909	2.0322	2.4411	2.7284	3.6007
35	1.3062	1.6896	2.0301	2.4377	2.7238	3.5911
36	1.3055	1.6883	2.0281	2.4345	2.7195	3.5821
37	1.3049	1.6871	2.0262	2.4314	2.7154	3.5737
38	1.3042	1.6860	2.0244	2.4286	2.7116	3.5657
39	1.3036	1.6849	2.0227	2.4258	2.7079	3.5581
40	1.3031	1.6839	2.0211	2.4233	2.7045	3.5510
41	1.3025	1.6829	2.0195	2.4208	2.7012	3.5442
42	1.3020	1.6820	2.0181	2.4185	2.6981	3.5377
43	1.3016	1.6811	2.0167	2.4163	2.6951	3.5316
44	1.3011	1.6802	2.0154	2.4141	2.6923	3.5258
45	1.3006	1.6794	2.0141	2.4121	2.6896	3.5203
46	1.3002	1.6787	2.0129	2.4102	2.6870	3.5150
47	1.2998	1.6779	2.0117	2.4083	2.6846	3.5099
48	1.2994	1.6772	2.0106	2.4066	2.6822	3.5051
49	1.2991	1.6766	2.0096	2.4049	2.6800	3.5004
50	1.2987	1.6759	2.0086	2.4033	2.6778	3.4960
51	1.2984	1.6753	2.0076	2.4017	2.6757	3.4918
52	1.2980	1.6747	2.0066	2.4002	2.6737	3.4877
53	1.2977	1.6741	2.0057	2.3988	2.6718	3.4838
54	1.2974	1.6736	2.0049	2.3974	2.6700	3.4800
55	1.2971	1.6730	2.0040	2.3961	2.6682	3.4764
56	1.2969	1.6725	2.0032	2.3948	2.6665	3.4729
57	1.2966	1.6720	2.0025	2.3936	2.6649	3.4696
58	1.2963	1.6716	2.0017	2.3924	2.6633	3.4663
59	1.2961	1.6711	2.0010	2.3912	2.6618	3.4632
60	1.2958	1.6706	2.0003	2.3901	2.6603	3.4602

(continued)

TABLE C-3 (CONTINUED)

CRITICAL VALUES FOR *T*-TEST

LEVEL OF SIGNIFICANCE FOR ONE-TAILED TEST

	0.1	0.05	0.025	0.01	0.005	0.0005

LEVEL OF SIGNIFICANCE FOR TWO-TAILED TEST

df	0.2	0.1	0.05	0.02	0.01	0.001
61	1.2956	1.6702	1.9996	2.3890	2.6589	3.4573
62	1.2954	1.6698	1.9990	2.3880	2.6575	3.4545
63	1.2951	1.6694	1.9983	2.3870	2.6561	3.4518
64	1.2949	1.6690	1.9977	2.3860	2.6549	3.4491
65	1.2947	1.6686	1.9971	2.3851	2.6536	3.4466
66	1.2945	1.6683	1.9966	2.3842	2.6524	3.4441
67	1.2943	1.6679	1.9960	2.3833	2.6512	3.4417
68	1.2941	1.6676	1.9955	2.3824	2.6501	3.4394
69	1.2939	1.6672	1.9949	2.3816	2.6490	3.4372
70	1.2938	1.6669	1.9944	2.3808	2.6479	3.4350
71	1.2936	1.6666	1.9939	2.3800	2.6469	3.4329
72	1.2934	1.6663	1.9935	2.3793	2.6459	3.4308
73	1.2933	1.6660	1.9930	2.3785	2.6449	3.4289
74	1.2931	1.6657	1.9925	2.3778	2.6439	3.4269
75	1.2929	1.6654	1.9921	2.3771	2.6430	3.4250
76	1.2928	1.6652	1.9917	2.3764	2.6421	3.4232
77	1.2926	1.6649	1.9913	2.3758	2.6412	3.4214
78	1.2925	1.6646	1.9908	2.3751	2.6403	3.4197
79	1.2924	1.6644	1.9905	2.3745	2.6395	3.4180
80	1.2922	1.6641	1.9901	2.3739	2.6387	3.4163
81	1.2921	1.6639	1.9897	2.3733	2.6379	3.4147
82	1.2920	1.6636	1.9893	2.3727	2.6371	3.4132
83	1.2918	1.6634	1.9890	2.3721	2.6364	3.4116
84	1.2917	1.6632	1.9886	2.3716	2.6356	3.4102
85	1.2916	1.6630	1.9883	2.3710	2.6349	3.4087
86	1.2915	1.6628	1.9879	2.3705	2.6342	3.4073
87	1.2914	1.6626	1.9876	2.3700	2.6335	3.4059
88	1.2912	1.6624	1.9873	2.3695	2.6329	3.4045
89	1.2911	1.6622	1.9870	2.3690	2.6322	3.4032
90	1.2910	1.6620	1.9867	2.3685	2.6316	3.4019

(continued)

			TABLE C-3 (CONTINUED)			

CRITICAL VALUES FOR *T*-TEST

	LEVEL OF SIGNIFICANCE FOR ONE-TAILED TEST					
	0.1	*0.05*	*0.025*	*0.01*	*0.005*	*0.0005*
	LEVEL OF SIGNIFICANCE FOR TWO-TAILED TEST					
df	*0.2*	*0.1*	*0.05*	*0.02*	*0.01*	*0.001*
91	1.2909	1.6618	1.9864	2.3680	2.6309	3.4007
92	1.2908	1.6616	1.9861	2.3676	2.6303	3.3994
93	1.2907	1.6614	1.9858	2.3671	2.6297	3.3982
94	1.2906	1.6612	1.9855	2.3667	2.6291	3.3971
95	1.2905	1.6611	1.9853	2.3662	2.6286	3.3959
96	1.2904	1.6609	1.9850	2.3658	2.6280	3.3948
97	1.2903	1.6607	1.9847	2.3654	2.6275	3.3937
98	1.2902	1.6606	1.9845	2.3650	2.6269	3.3926
99	1.2902	1.6604	1.9842	2.3646	2.6264	3.3915
100	1.2901	1.6602	1.9840	2.3642	2.6259	3.3905
101	1.2900	1.6601	1.9837	2.3638	2.6254	3.3895
102	1.2899	1.6599	1.9835	2.3635	2.6249	3.3885
103	1.2898	1.6598	1.9833	2.3631	2.6244	3.3875
104	1.2897	1.6596	1.9830	2.3627	2.6239	3.3865
105	1.2897	1.6595	1.9828	2.3624	2.6235	3.3856
106	1.2896	1.6594	1.9826	2.3620	2.6230	3.3847
107	1.2895	1.6592	1.9824	2.3617	2.6226	3.3838
108	1.2894	1.6591	1.9822	2.3614	2.6221	3.3829
109	1.2894	1.6590	1.9820	2.3610	2.6217	3.3820
110	1.2893	1.6588	1.9818	2.3607	2.6213	3.3812
111	1.2892	1.6587	1.9816	2.3604	2.6208	3.3803
112	1.2892	1.6586	1.9814	2.3601	2.6204	3.3795
113	1.2891	1.6585	1.9812	2.3598	2.6200	3.3787
114	1.2890	1.6583	1.9810	2.3595	2.6196	3.3779
115	1.2890	1.6582	1.9808	2.3592	2.6193	3.3771
116	1.2889	1.6581	1.9806	2.3589	2.6189	3.3764
117	1.2888	1.6580	1.9804	2.3586	2.6185	3.3756
118	1.2888	1.6579	1.9803	2.3584	2.6181	3.3749
119	1.2887	1.6578	1.9801	2.3581	2.6178	3.3742
120	1.2886	1.6577	1.9799	2.3578	2.6174	3.3735
						(continued)

TABLE C-3 (CONTINUED)

CRITICAL VALUES FOR T-TEST

	LEVEL OF SIGNIFICANCE FOR ONE-TAILED TEST					
	0.1	0.05	0.025	0.01	0.005	0.0005
	LEVEL OF SIGNIFICANCE FOR TWO-TAILED TEST					
df	0.2	0.1	0.05	0.02	0.01	0.001
121	1.2886	1.6575	1.9798	2.3576	2.6171	3.3728
122	1.2885	1.6574	1.9796	2.3573	2.6167	3.3721
123	1.2885	1.6573	1.9794	2.3570	2.6164	3.3714
124	1.2884	1.6572	1.9793	2.3568	2.6161	3.3707
125	1.2884	1.6571	1.9791	2.3565	2.6157	3.3701
126	1.2883	1.6570	1.9790	2.3563	2.6154	3.3694
127	1.2883	1.6569	1.9788	2.3561	2.6151	3.3688
128	1.2882	1.6568	1.9787	2.3558	2.6148	3.3682
129	1.2881	1.6568	1.9785	2.3556	2.6145	3.3675
130	1.2881	1.6567	1.9784	2.3554	2.6142	3.3669
131	1.2880	1.6566	1.9782	2.3552	2.6139	3.3663
132	1.2880	1.6565	1.9781	2.3549	2.6136	3.3658
133	1.2879	1.6564	1.9780	2.3547	2.6133	3.3652
134	1.2879	1.6563	1.9778	2.3545	2.6130	3.3646
135	1.2879	1.6562	1.9777	2.3543	2.6127	3.3641
136	1.2878	1.6561	1.9776	2.3541	2.6125	3.3635
137	1.2878	1.6561	1.9774	2.3539	2.6122	3.3630
138	1.2877	1.6560	1.9773	2.3537	2.6119	3.3624
139	1.2877	1.6559	1.9772	2.3535	2.6117	3.3619
140	1.2876	1.6558	1.9771	2.3533	2.6114	3.3614

(continued)

TABLE C-3 (CONTINUED)

CRITICAL VALUES FOR *T*-TEST

LEVEL OF SIGNIFICANCE FOR ONE-TAILED TEST

	0.1	0.05	0.025	0.01	0.005	0.0005

LEVEL OF SIGNIFICANCE FOR TWO-TAILED TEST

df	0.2	0.1	0.05	0.02	0.01	0.001
141	1.2876	1.6557	1.9769	2.3531	2.6111	3.3609
142	1.2875	1.6557	1.9768	2.3529	2.6109	3.3604
143	1.2875	1.6556	1.9767	2.3527	2.6106	3.3599
144	1.2875	1.6555	1.9766	2.3525	2.6104	3.3594
145	1.2874	1.6554	1.9765	2.3523	2.6102	3.3589
146	1.2874	1.6554	1.9763	2.3522	2.6099	3.3584
147	1.2873	1.6553	1.9762	2.3520	2.6097	3.3579
148	1.2873	1.6552	1.9761	2.3518	2.6095	3.3575
149	1.2873	1.6551	1.9760	2.3516	2.6092	3.3570
150	1.2872	1.6551	1.9759	2.3515	2.6090	3.3566

STEPS IN DETERMINING CRITICAL VALUES FOR *T* FOR TABLE C-3

1. Calculate the degrees of freedom (*df*):
   a. In a one-sample *t*-test, it is the number of cases of the sample minus 1.
   b. In a paired-data of correlated *t*-test, it is the number of pairs minus 1.
   c. In an independent *t*-test, it is the number of cases in N1 + N2 minus 2.
2. Determine if hypothesis requires a one-tailed or two-tailed test.
3. Establish level of significance (α) (e.g., .05 or .01)
4. Locate *t* critical (t_{crit}) value. For example, if *df* is 10, using a two-tailed test with a $\alpha = .05$, then $t_{crit} = 2.2281$.
5. Note that these critical values are the same for negative or positive numbers.
6. Calculate *t* observed (t_{obs}) using an appropriate *t*-test formula (i.e., one-sample, paired, or independent t-test).
7. Decision rule:
   a. If t_{obs} is equal to or above t_{crit}, then reject the null hypothesis.
   b. If t_{obs} is below t_{crit}, then do not reject the null hypothesis.

Source: The table was generated using Microsoft Office Excel 2013.

Table C-4

Critical Values for F (Analysis of Variance)

Denominator DF	a	\multicolumn{10}{c}{Numerator DF}									
		1	2	3	4	5	6	7	8	9	10
1	0.01	4052	4999	5403	5625	5764	5859	5928	5981	6022	6056
	0.05	161.4	199.5	215.7	224.6	230.2	234.0	236.8	238.9	240.5	241.9
2	0.01	98.50	99.00	99.17	99.25	99.30	99.33	99.36	99.37	99.39	99.40
	0.05	18.513	19.000	19.164	19.247	19.296	19.330	19.353	19.371	19.385	19.396
3	0.01	34.116	30.817	29.457	28.710	28.237	27.911	27.672	27.489	27.345	27.229
	0.05	10.1280	9.5521	9.2766	9.1172	9.0135	8.9406	8.8867	8.8452	8.8123	8.7855
4	0.01	21.198	18.000	16.694	15.977	15.522	15.207	14.976	14.799	14.659	14.546
	0.05	7.7086	6.9443	6.5914	6.3882	6.2561	6.1631	6.0942	6.0410	5.9988	5.9644
5	0.01	16.258	13.274	12.060	11.392	10.967	10.672	10.456	10.289	10.158	10.051
	0.05	6.6079	5.7861	5.4095	5.1922	5.0503	4.9503	4.8759	4.8183	4.7725	4.7351
6	0.01	13.7450	10.9248	9.7795	9.1483	8.7459	8.4661	8.2600	8.1017	7.9761	7.8741
	0.05	5.9874	5.1433	4.7571	4.5337	4.3874	4.2839	4.2067	4.1468	4.0990	4.0600
7	0.01	12.2464	9.5466	8.4513	7.8466	7.4604	7.1914	6.9928	6.8400	6.7188	6.6201
	0.05	5.5914	4.7374	4.3468	4.1203	3.9715	3.8660	3.7870	3.7257	3.6767	3.6365
8	0.01	11.2586	8.6491	7.5910	7.0061	6.6318	6.3707	6.1776	6.0289	5.9106	5.8143
	0.05	5.3177	4.4590	4.0662	3.8379	3.6875	3.5806	3.5005	3.4381	3.3881	3.3472
9	0.01	10.5614	8.0215	6.9919	6.4221	6.0569	5.8018	5.6129	5.4671	5.3511	5.2565
	0.05	5.1174	4.2565	3.8625	3.6331	3.4817	3.3738	3.2927	3.2296	3.1789	3.1373
10	0.01	10.0443	7.5594	6.5523	5.9943	5.6363	5.3858	5.2001	5.0567	4.9424	4.8491
	0.05	4.9646	4.1028	3.7083	3.4780	3.3258	3.2172	3.1355	3.0717	3.0204	2.9782
11	0.01	9.6460	7.2057	6.2167	5.6683	5.3160	5.0692	4.8861	4.7445	4.6315	4.5393
	0.05	4.8443	3.9823	3.5874	3.3567	3.2039	3.0946	3.0123	2.9480	2.8962	2.8536
12	0.01	9.3302	6.9266	5.9525	5.4120	5.0643	4.8206	4.6395	4.4994	4.3875	4.2961
	0.05	4.7472	3.8853	3.4903	3.2592	3.1059	2.9961	2.9134	2.8486	2.7964	2.7534

(continued)

TABLE C-4 (CONTINUED)

CRITICAL VALUES FOR F (ANALYSIS OF VARIANCE)

DENOMINATOR DF	a	NUMERATOR DF 1	2	3	4	5	6	7	8	9	10
13	0.01	9.0738	6.7010	5.7394	5.2053	4.8616	4.6204	4.4410	4.3021	4.1911	4.1003
	0.05	4.6672	3.8056	3.4105	3.1791	3.0254	2.9153	2.8321	2.7669	2.7144	2.6710
14	0.01	8.8616	6.5149	5.5639	5.0354	4.6950	4.4558	4.2779	4.1399	4.0297	3.9394
	0.05	4.6001	3.7389	3.3439	3.1122	2.9582	2.8477	2.7642	2.6987	2.6458	2.6022
15	0.01	8.6831	6.3589	5.4170	4.8932	4.5556	4.3183	4.1415	4.0045	3.8948	3.8049
	0.05	4.5431	3.6823	3.2874	3.0556	2.9013	2.7905	2.7066	2.6408	2.5876	2.5437
16	0.01	8.5310	6.2262	5.2922	4.7726	4.4374	4.2016	4.0259	3.8896	3.7804	3.6909
	0.05	4.4940	3.6337	3.2389	3.0069	2.8524	2.7413	2.6572	2.5911	2.5377	2.4935
17	0.01	8.3997	6.1121	5.1850	4.6690	4.3359	4.1015	3.9267	3.7910	3.6822	3.5931
	0.05	4.4513	3.5915	3.1968	2.9647	2.8100	2.6987	2.6143	2.5480	2.4943	2.4499
18	0.01	8.2854	6.0129	5.0919	4.5790	4.2479	4.0146	3.8406	3.7054	3.5971	3.5082
	0.05	4.4139	3.5546	3.1599	2.9277	2.7729	2.6613	2.5767	2.5102	2.4563	2.4117
19	0.01	8.1849	5.9259	5.0103	4.5003	4.1708	3.9386	3.7653	3.6305	3.5225	3.4338
	0.05	4.3807	3.5219	3.1274	2.8951	2.7401	2.6283	2.5435	2.4768	2.4227	2.3779
20	0.01	8.0960	5.8489	4.9382	4.4307	4.1027	3.8714	3.6987	3.5644	3.4567	3.3682
	0.05	4.3512	3.4928	3.0984	2.8661	2.7109	2.5990	2.5140	2.4471	2.3928	2.3479
21	0.01	8.0166	5.7804	4.8740	4.3688	4.0421	3.8117	3.6396	3.5056	3.3981	3.3098
	0.05	4.3248	3.4668	3.0725	2.8401	2.6848	2.5727	2.4876	2.4205	2.3660	2.3210
22	0.01	7.9454	5.7190	4.8166	4.3134	3.9880	3.7583	3.5867	3.4530	3.3458	3.2576
	0.05	4.3009	3.4434	3.0491	2.8167	2.6613	2.5491	2.4638	2.3965	2.3419	2.2967
23	0.01	7.8811	5.6637	4.7649	4.2636	3.9392	3.7102	3.5390	3.4057	3.2986	3.2106
	0.05	4.2793	3.4221	3.0280	2.7955	2.6400	2.5277	2.4422	2.3748	2.3201	2.2747
24	0.01	7.8229	5.6136	4.7181	4.2184	3.8951	3.6667	3.4959	3.3629	3.2560	3.1681
	0.05	4.2597	3.4028	3.0088	2.7763	2.6207	2.5082	2.4226	2.3551	2.3002	2.2547

(continued)

TABLE C-4 (CONTINUED)
CRITICAL VALUES FOR F (ANALYSIS OF VARIANCE)

| DENOMINATOR DF | α | \multicolumn{10}{c}{NUMERATOR DF} |
		1	2	3	4	5	6	7	8	9	10
25	0.01	7.7698	5.5680	4.6755	4.1774	3.8550	3.6272	3.4568	3.3239	3.2172	3.1294
	0.05	4.2417	3.3852	2.9912	2.7587	2.6030	2.4904	2.4047	2.3371	2.2821	2.2365
26	0.01	7.7213	5.5263	4.6366	4.1400	3.8183	3.5911	3.4210	3.2884	3.1818	3.0941
	0.05	4.2252	3.3690	2.9752	2.7426	2.5868	2.4741	2.3883	2.3205	2.2655	2.2197
27	0.01	7.6767	5.4881	4.6009	4.1056	3.7848	3.5580	3.3882	3.2558	3.1494	3.0618
	0.05	4.2100	3.3541	2.9604	2.7278	2.5719	2.4591	2.3732	2.3053	2.2501	2.2043
28	0.01	7.6356	5.4529	4.5681	4.0740	3.7539	3.5276	3.3581	3.2259	3.1195	3.0320
	0.05	4.1960	3.3404	2.9467	2.7141	2.5581	2.4453	2.3593	2.2913	2.2360	2.1900
29	0.01	7.5977	5.4204	4.5378	4.0449	3.7254	3.4995	3.3303	3.1982	3.0920	3.0045
	0.05	4.1830	3.3277	2.9340	2.7014	2.5454	2.4324	2.3463	2.2783	2.2229	2.1768
30	0.01	7.5625	5.3903	4.5097	4.0179	3.6990	3.4735	3.3045	3.1726	3.0665	2.9791
	0.05	4.1709	3.3158	2.9223	2.6896	2.5336	2.4205	2.3343	2.2662	2.2107	2.1646
35	0.01	7.4191	5.2679	4.3957	3.9082	3.5919	3.3679	3.2000	3.0687	2.9630	2.8758
	0.05	4.1213	3.2674	2.8742	2.6415	2.4851	2.3718	2.2852	2.2167	2.1608	2.1143
40	0.01	7.3141	5.1785	4.3126	3.8283	3.5138	3.2910	3.1238	2.9930	2.8876	2.8005
	0.05	4.0847	3.2317	2.8387	2.6060	2.4495	2.3359	2.2490	2.1802	2.1240	2.0772
45	0.01	7.2339	5.1103	4.2492	3.7674	3.4544	3.2325	3.0658	2.9353	2.8301	2.7432
	0.05	4.0566	3.2043	2.8115	2.5787	2.4221	2.3083	2.2212	2.1521	2.0958	2.0487
50	0.01	7.1706	5.0566	4.1993	3.7195	3.4077	3.1864	3.0202	2.8900	2.7850	2.6981
	0.05	4.0343	3.1826	2.7900	2.5572	2.4004	2.2864	2.1992	2.1299	2.0734	2.0261
55	0.01	7.1194	5.0132	4.1591	3.6809	3.3700	3.1493	2.9834	2.8534	2.7485	2.6617
	0.05	4.0162	3.1650	2.7725	2.5397	2.3828	2.2687	2.1813	2.1119	2.0552	2.0078
60	0.01	7.0771	4.9774	4.1259	3.6490	3.3389	3.1187	2.9530	2.8233	2.7185	2.6318
	0.05	4.0012	3.1504	2.7581	2.5252	2.3683	2.2541	2.1665	2.0970	2.0401	1.9926

(continued)

TABLE C-4 (CONTINUED)

CRITICAL VALUES FOR *F* (ANALYSIS OF VARIANCE)

DENOMINATOR *DF*	α	NUMERATOR *DF*								
		1	2	3	4	5	6	7	8	9	10
80	0.01	6.9627	4.8807	4.0363	3.5631	3.2550	3.0361	2.8713	2.7420	2.6374	2.5508
	0.05	3.9604	3.1108	2.7188	2.4859	2.3287	2.2142	2.1263	2.0564	1.9991	1.9512
100	0.01	6.8953	4.8239	3.9837	3.5127	3.2059	2.9877	2.8233	2.6943	2.5898	2.5033
	0.05	3.9361	3.0873	2.6955	2.4626	2.3053	2.1906	2.1025	2.0323	1.9748	1.9267
120	0.01	6.8509	4.7865	3.9491	3.4795	3.1735	2.9559	2.7918	2.6629	2.5586	2.4721
	0.05	3.9201	3.0718	2.6802	2.4472	2.2899	2.1750	2.0868	2.0164	1.9588	1.9105

STEPS IN DETERMINING CRITICAL VALUES FOR *F* FOR TABLE C-4

1. Calculate the degrees of freedom (*df*) for numerator and denominator:

   a. The *df* for numerator is derived from the number of groups in the study minus 1. For example, if three treatment methods are being compared, then df equals 3 - 1, or 2 *df* for numerator.

   b. The *df* for denominator is derived from the total number of subjects in all groups being compared minus the number of groups. For example, for three treatment methods with 6 subjects in each group, the *df* for the denominator will equal 18 - 3, or 15 *df*.

2. Apply the level of significance (α) (e.g., .05, .01).

3. Locate critical value of *F*. For example, a numerator *df* of 2, a denominator *df* of 15 with α = .05, the F_{crit} = 6.3589.

4. Calculate F_{obs} for data.

5. Decision rule:

   a. If F_{obs} is equal to or above F_{crit}, then reject the null hypothesis.

   b. If F_{obs} is below F_{crit}, then do not reject the null hypothesis.

Source: The table was generated using Microsoft Office Excel 2013.

Table C-5

Critical Values for the Pearson Product-Moment Correlation Coefficient (*R*)

	LEVEL OF SIGNIFICANCE FOR ONE-TAILED TEST					
	0.1	*0.05*	*0.025*	*0.01*	*0.005*	*0.0005*
	LEVEL OF SIGNIFICANCE FOR TWO-TAILED TEST					
df	*0.2*	*0.1*	*0.05*	*0.02*	*0.01*	*0.001*
1	0.951057	0.987688	0.996917	0.999507	0.999877	0.999999
2	0.8	0.9	0.95	0.98	0.99	0.999
3	0.687049	0.805384	0.878339	0.934333	0.958735	0.991139
4	0.6084	0.729299	0.811401	0.882194	0.9172	0.974068
5	0.550863	0.669439	0.754492	0.832874	0.874526	0.950883
6	0.506727	0.621489	0.706734	0.78872	0.834342	0.924904
7	0.471589	0.582206	0.666384	0.749776	0.797681	0.89826
8	0.442796	0.549357	0.631897	0.715459	0.764592	0.872115
9	0.418662	0.521404	0.602069	0.685095	0.734786	0.847047
10	0.398062	0.497265	0.575983	0.65807	0.707888	0.823305
11	0.380216	0.476156	0.552943	0.633863	0.683528	0.800962
12	0.364562	0.4575	0.532413	0.612047	0.661376	0.779998
13	0.350688	0.440861	0.513977	0.59227	0.641145	0.760351
14	0.338282	0.425902	0.497309	0.574245	0.622591	0.741934
15	0.327101	0.41236	0.482146	0.557737	0.605506	0.724657
16	0.316958	0.400027	0.468277	0.542548	0.589714	0.708429
17	0.307702	0.388733	0.455531	0.528517	0.575067	0.693163
18	0.29921	0.378341	0.443763	0.515505	0.561435	0.678781
19	0.291384	0.368737	0.432858	0.503397	0.548711	0.665208
20	0.28414	0.359827	0.422714	0.492094	0.5368	0.652378
21	0.277411	0.351531	0.413247	0.481512	0.52562	0.64023
22	0.271137	0.343783	0.404386	0.471579	0.515101	0.62871
23	0.26527	0.336524	0.39607	0.462231	0.505182	0.617768
24	0.259768	0.329705	0.388244	0.453413	0.495808	0.60736
25	0.254594	0.323283	0.380863	0.445078	0.486932	0.597446
26	0.249717	0.317223	0.373886	0.437184	0.478511	0.587988
27	0.24511	0.31149	0.367278	0.429693	0.470509	0.578956
28	0.240749	0.306057	0.361007	0.422572	0.462892	0.570317
29	0.236612	0.300898	0.355046	0.415792	0.455631	0.562047
30	0.232681	0.295991	0.34937	0.409327	0.448699	0.554119

(continued)

TABLE C-5 (CONTINUED)

CRITICAL VALUES FOR THE PEARSON PRODUCT-MOMENT CORRELATION COEFFICIENT (*R*)

LEVEL OF SIGNIFICANCE FOR ONE-TAILED TEST

	0.1	0.05	0.025	0.01	0.005	0.0005

LEVEL OF SIGNIFICANCE FOR TWO-TAILED TEST

df	0.2	0.1	0.05	0.02	0.01	0.001
35	0.215598	0.274611	0.324573	0.380976	0.418211	0.518898
40	0.201796	0.257278	0.304396	0.357787	0.393174	0.48957
45	0.190345	0.242859	0.287563	0.338367	0.372142	0.464673
50	0.180644	0.23062	0.273243	0.321796	0.354153	0.443201
60	0.164997	0.210832	0.250035	0.294846	0.324818	0.407865
65	0.158558	0.202673	0.240447	0.283682	0.31264	0.393085
70	0.152818	0.195394	0.231883	0.273695	0.301734	0.379799
75	0.147659	0.188847	0.224174	0.264694	0.291895	0.367771
80	0.14299	0.182916	0.217185	0.256525	0.282958	0.356816
85	0.138738	0.177511	0.210811	0.249069	0.274794	0.346782
90	0.134844	0.172558	0.204968	0.242227	0.267298	0.337549
95	0.13126	0.167998	0.199584	0.235919	0.260383	0.329014
100	0.127947	0.163782	0.194604	0.230079	0.253979	0.321095

STEPS IN DETERMINING CRITICAL VALUES FOR PEARSON *R* FOR TABLE C-5

1. Determine the number of variables being correlated. For example, if x = 20 and y = 20, then n = 20.
2. Determine if hypothesis calls for a one-tailed or two-tailed test. Usually a null hypothesis indicates a one-tailed test and a directional hypothesis indicates a two-tailed test of significance.
3. Apply level of significance (a) (e.g., .05, .01).
4. Locate critical value of *r* from statistical table. For example, with n = 20, two-tailed test, a = .05, then r_{crit} = .4438l; *df* = 18.
5. Calculate r_{obs} from data.
6. Decision rule:
   a. If r_{obs} is equal to or greater than r_{crit}, then reject null hypothesis.
   b. If r_{obs} is below r_{crit}, then do not reject the null hypothesis.

Source: The table was generated using Microsoft Office Excel 2013.

TABLE C-6

SPEARMAN RANK ORDER CORRELATION COEFFICIENT (R)

LEVEL OF SIGNIFICANCE FOR ONE-TAILED TEST

	.05	.025	.01	.005

LEVEL OF SIGNIFICANCE FOR TWO-TAILED TEST

n*	.10	.05	.02	.01
5	.900	1.000	1.000	—
6	.829	.886	.943	1.000
7	.714	.786	.893	.929
8	.643	.738	.833	.881
9	.600	.683	.783	.833
10	.564	.648	.746	.794
12	.506	.591	.712	.777
14	.456	.544	.645	.715
16	.425	.506	.601	.665
18	.399	.475	.564	.625
20	.377	.450	.534	.591
22	.359	.428	.508	.562
24	.343	.409	.485	.537
26	.329	.392	.465	.515
28	.317	.377	.448	.496
30	.306	.364	.432	.478

STEPS IN DETERMINING CRITICAL VALUES FOR SPEARMAN R_S (FORMERLY RHO) FOR TABLE C-6

1. Determine the number of pairs of variables being correlated.
2. Determine if hypothesis calls for a one-tailed or two-tailed test.
3. Apply level of significance (a) (e.g., .05, .01).
4. Locate critical value of r_s from statistical table. For example, with n = 12, two-tailed test, a = .05, then $r_{s\text{-crit}}$ = .591.
5. Calculate $r_{s\text{-obs}}$ from data.
6. Decision rule:
   a. If $r_{s\text{-obs}}$ is equal to or greater than $r_{s\text{-crit}}$, then reject the null hypothesis.
   b. If $r_{s\text{-obs}}$ is below $r_{s\text{-crit}}$, then do not reject the null hypothesis.

*n = number of pairs

Adapted from Olds, E. G. (1949). The 5 percent significance levels of sums of squares of rank differences and a correction. *Annals of Mathematical Statistics, 20,*117-118; Olds, E. G. (1938). Distribution of the sum of squares of rank differences for small numbers of individuals. *Annals of Mathematical Statistics, 9,* 133-148; Runyon, R. P., & Haber, A. (1967). *Fundamentals of Behavioral Statistics.* Reading, MA: Addison-Wesley.

TABLE C-7A
CRITICAL VALUES FOR THE MANN–WHITNEY U TEST[a]

n_A

n_B	1	2	3	4	5	6	7	8	9	10	11	12	13	14	15	16	17	18	19	20	21	22	23	24	25
1																									
1																									
2								_16_	_18_	_20_	_22_	_23_	_25_	_27_	_29_	_31_	_32_	_34_	_36_	_38_	_39_	_41_	_43_	_45_	_47_
2								0	0	0	0	1	1	1	1	1	2	2	2	2	3	3	3	3	3
3					_15_	_17_	_20_	_22_	_25_	_27_	_30_	_32_	_35_	_37_	_40_	_42_	_45_	_47_	_50_	_52_	_55_	_57_	_60_	_62_	_65_
3					0	1	1	2	2	3	3	4	4	5	5	6	6	7	7	8	8	9	9	10	10
4				_16_	_19_	_22_	_25_	_28_	_32_	_35_	_38_	_41_	_44_	_47_	_50_	_53_	_57_	_60_	_63_	_66_	_69_	_72_	_75_	_79_	_82_
4				0	1	2	3	4	4	5	6	7	8	9	10	11	11	12	13	14	15	16	17	17	18
5			_15_	_19_	_23_	_27_	_30_	_34_	_38_	_42_	_46_	_49_	_53_	_57_	_61_	_65_	_68_	_72_	_76_	_80_	_83_	_87_	_91_	_95_	_98_
5			0	1	2	3	5	6	7	8	9	11	12	13	14	15	17	18	19	20	22	23	24	25	27
6			_17_	_22_	_27_	_31_	_36_	_40_	_44_	_49_	_53_	_58_	_62_	_67_	_71_	_75_	_80_	_84_	_89_	_93_	_97_	_102_	_106_	_111_	_115_
6			1	2	3	5	6	8	10	11	13	14	16	17	19	21	22	24	25	27	29	30	32	33	35
7			_20_	_25_	_30_	_36_	_41_	_46_	_51_	_56_	_61_	_66_	_71_	_76_	_81_	_86_	_91_	_96_	_101_	_106_	_111_	_116_	_121_	_126_	_131_
7			1	3	5	6	8	10	12	14	16	18	20	22	24	26	28	30	32	34	36	38	40	42	44
8		_16_	_22_	_28_	_34_	_40_	_46_	_51_	_57_	_63_	_69_	_74_	_80_	_86_	_91_	_97_	_102_	_108_	_114_	_119_	_125_	_131_	_136_	_142_	_147_
8		0	2	4	6	8	10	13	15	17	19	22	24	26	29	31	34	36	38	41	43	45	48	50	53
9		_18_	_25_	_32_	_38_	_44_	_51_	_57_	_64_	_70_	_76_	_82_	_89_	_95_	_101_	_107_	_114_	_120_	_126_	_132_	_139_	_145_	_151_	_157_	_163_
9		0	2	4	7	10	12	15	17	20	23	26	28	31	34	37	39	42	45	48	50	53	56	59	62
10		_20_	_27_	_35_	_42_	_49_	_56_	_63_	_70_	_77_	_84_	_91_	_97_	_104_	_111_	_118_	_125_	_132_	_138_	_145_	_152_	_159_	_166_	_173_	_179_
10		0	3	5	8	11	14	17	20	23	26	29	33	36	39	42	45	48	52	55	58	61	64	67	71
11		_22_	_30_	_38_	_46_	_53_	_61_	_69_	_76_	_84_	_91_	_99_	_106_	_114_	_121_	_129_	_136_	_143_	_151_	_158_	_166_	_173_	_180_	_188_	_195_
11		0	3	6	9	13	16	19	23	26	30	33	37	40	44	47	51	55	58	62	65	69	73	76	80
12		_23_	_32_	_41_	_49_	_58_	_66_	_74_	_82_	_91_	_99_	_107_	_115_	_123_	_131_	_139_	_147_	_155_	_163_	_171_	_179_	_187_	_195_	_203_	_211_
12		1	4	7	11	14	18	22	26	29	33	37	41	45	49	53	57	61	65	69	73	77	81	85	89

(continued)

Table C-7A (continued)

Critical Values for the Mann—Whitney U Test[a]

n_A

n_B	1	2	3	4	5	6	7	8	9	10	11	12	13	14	15	16	17	18	19	20	21	22	23	24	25
13		1	4	8	12	16	20	24	28	33	37	41	45	50	54	59	63	67	72	76	80	85	89	94	98
13		25	35	44	53	62	71	80	89	97	106	115	124	132	141	149	158	167	175	184	193	201	210	218	227
14		1	5	9	13	17	22	26	31	36	40	45	50	55	59	64	69	74	78	83	88	93	98	102	107
14		27	37	47	57	67	76	86	95	104	114	123	132	141	151	160	169	178	188	197	206	215	224	234	243
15		1	5	10	14	19	24	29	34	39	44	49	54	59	64	70	75	80	85	90	96	101	106	111	117
15		29	40	50	61	71	81	91	101	111	121	131	141	151	161	170	180	190	200	210	219	229	239	249	258
16		1	6	11	15	21	26	31	37	42	47	53	59	64	70	75	81	86	92	98	103	109	115	120	126
16		31	42	53	65	75	86	97	107	118	129	139	149	160	170	181	191	202	212	222	233	243	253	264	274
17		2	6	11	17	22	28	34	39	45	51	57	63	69	75	81	87	93	99	105	111	117	123	129	135
17		32	45	57	68	80	91	102	114	125	136	147	158	169	180	191	202	213	224	235	246	257	268	279	290
18		2	7	12	18	24	30	36	42	48	55	61	67	74	80	86	93	99	106	112	119	125	132	138	145
18		34	47	60	72	84	96	108	120	132	143	155	167	178	190	202	213	225	236	248	259	271	282	294	305
19		2	7	13	19	25	32	38	45	52	58	65	72	78	85	92	99	106	113	119	126	133	140	147	154
19		36	50	63	76	89	101	114	126	138	151	163	175	188	200	212	224	236	248	261	273	285	297	309	321

(continued)

TABLE C-7A (CONTINUED)

CRITICAL VALUES FOR THE MANN—WHITNEY U TEST[a]

n_A

n_B	1	2	3	4	5	6	7	8	9	10	11	12	13	14	15	16	17	18	19	20	21	22	23	24	25
20		2	8	14	20	27	34	41	48	55	62	69	76	83	90	98	105	112	119	127	134	141	149	156	163
20		38	52	66	80	93	106	119	132	145	158	171	184	197	210	222	235	248	261	273	286	299	311	324	337
21		3	8	15	22	29	36	43	50	58	65	73	80	88	96	103	111	119	126	134	142	150	157	165	173
21		39	55	69	83	97	111	125	139	152	166	179	193	206	219	233	246	259	273	286	299	312	326	339	352
22		3	9	16	23	30	38	45	53	61	69	77	85	93	101	109	117	125	133	141	150	158	166	174	182
22		41	57	72	87	102	116	131	145	159	173	187	201	215	229	243	257	271	285	299	312	326	340	354	368
23		3	9	17	24	32	40	48	56	64	73	81	89	98	106	115	123	132	140	149	157	166	175	183	192
23		43	60	75	91	106	121	136	151	166	180	195	210	224	239	253	268	282	297	311	326	340	354	369	383
24		3	10	17	25	33	42	50	59	67	76	85	94	102	111	120	129	138	147	156	165	174	183	192	201
24		45	62	79	95	111	126	142	157	173	188	203	218	234	249	264	279	294	309	324	339	354	369	384	399
25		3	10	18	27	35	44	53	62	71	80	89	98	107	117	126	135	145	154	163	173	182	192	201	211
25		47	65	82	98	115	131	147	163	179	195	211	227	243	258	274	290	305	321	337	352	368	383	399	414

[a]Test for a one-tailed test at .025 or a two-tailed test at .05. If the U_{obs} value falls within the two values in the table for n_A and n_B, then do not reject the null hypothesis. If the U_{obs} is less than or equal to the lower value in the table or greater than or equal to the larger value in the table, then reject the null hypothesis.

TABLE C-7B

CRITICAL VALUES FOR THE MANN—WHITNEY U TEST[b]

n_A

n_B	1	2	3	4	5	6	7	8	9	10	11	12	13	14	15	16	17	18	19	20	21	22	23	24	25
1																				0	0	0	0	0	0
1																				20	21	22	23	24	25
2					0	0	0	1	1	1	1	2	2	2	3	3	3	4	4	4	5	5	5	6	6
2					10	12	14	15	17	19	21	22	24	25	27	29	31	32	34	36	37	39	41	42	44
3				0	1	2	2	3	3	4	5	5	6	7	7	8	9	9	10	11	11	12	13	13	14
3				12	14	16	19	21	23	26	28	31	33	35	38	40	42	45	47	49	52	54	56	59	61
4			0	1	2	3	4	5	6	7	8	9	10	11	12	14	15	16	17	18	19	20	21	22	23
4			12	15	18	21	24	27	30	33	36	39	42	45	48	50	53	56	59	62	65	68	71	74	77
5		0	1	2	4	5	6	8	9	11	12	13	15	16	18	19	20	22	23	25	26	28	29	30	32
5		10	14	18	21	25	29	32	36	39	43	47	50	54	57	61	65	68	72	75	79	82	86	90	93
6		0	2	3	5	7	8	10	12	14	16	17	19	21	23	25	26	28	30	32	34	36	37	39	41
6		12	16	21	25	29	34	38	42	46	50	55	59	63	67	71	76	80	84	88	92	96	101	105	109
7		0	2	4	6	8	11	13	15	17	19	21	24	26	28	30	33	35	37	39	41	44	46	48	50
7		14	19	24	29	34	38	43	48	53	58	63	67	72	77	82	86	91	96	101	106	110	115	120	125
8		1	3	5	8	10	13	15	18	20	23	26	28	31	33	36	39	41	44	47	49	52	54	57	60
8		15	21	27	32	38	43	49	54	60	65	70	76	81	87	92	97	103	108	113	119	124	130	135	140
9		1	3	6	9	12	15	18	21	24	27	30	33	36	39	42	45	48	51	54	57	60	63	66	69
9		17	23	30	36	42	48	54	60	66	72	78	84	90	96	102	108	114	120	126	132	138	144	150	156
10		1	4	7	11	14	17	20	24	27	31	34	37	41	44	48	51	55	58	62	65	68	72	75	79
10		19	26	33	39	46	53	60	66	73	79	86	93	99	106	112	119	125	132	138	145	152	158	165	171
11		1	5	8	12	16	19	23	27	31	34	38	42	46	50	54	57	61	65	69	73	77	81	85	89
11		21	28	36	43	50	58	65	72	79	87	94	101	108	115	122	130	137	144	151	158	165	172	179	186
12		2	5	9	13	17	21	26	30	34	38	42	47	51	55	60	64	68	72	77	81	85	90	94	98
12		22	31	39	47	55	63	70	78	86	94	102	109	117	125	132	140	148	156	163	171	179	186	194	202

(continued)

TABLE C-7B (CONTINUED)

CRITICAL VALUES FOR THE MANN—WHITNEY U TEST[b]

n_A

n_B	1	2	3	4	5	6	7	8	9	10	11	12	13	14	15	16	17	18	19	20	21	22	23	24	25
13		2	6	10	15	19	24	28	33	37	42	47	51	56	61	65	70	75	80	84	89	94	98	103	108
13		24	33	42	50	59	67	76	84	93	101	109	118	126	134	143	151	159	167	176	184	192	201	209	217
14		2	7	11	16	21	26	31	36	41	46	51	56	61	66	71	77	82	87	92	97	102	107	113	118
14		25	35	45	54	63	72	81	90	99	108	117	126	135	144	153	161	170	179	188	197	206	215	223	232
15		3	7	12	18	23	28	33	39	44	50	55	61	66	72	77	83	88	94	100	105	111	116	122	128
15		27	38	48	57	67	77	87	96	106	115	125	134	144	153	163	172	182	191	200	210	219	229	238	247
16		3	8	14	19	25	30	36	42	48	54	60	65	71	77	83	89	95	100	107	113	119	125	131	137
16		29	40	50	61	71	82	92	102	112	122	132	143	153	163	173	183	193	203	213	223	233	243	253	263
17		3	9	15	20	26	33	39	45	51	57	64	70	77	83	89	96	102	109	115	121	128	134	141	147
17		31	42	53	65	76	86	97	108	119	130	140	151	161	172	183	193	204	214	225	236	246	257	267	278
18		4	9	16	22	28	35	41	48	55	61	68	75	82	88	95	102	109	116	123	130	136	143	150	157
18		32	45	56	68	80	91	103	114	125	137	148	159	170	182	193	204	215	226	237	248	260	271	282	293
19		4	10	17	23	30	37	44	51	58	65	72	80	87	94	101	109	116	123	130	138	145	152	160	167
19		34	47	59	72	84	96	108	120	132	144	156	167	179	191	203	214	226	238	250	261	273	285	296	308

(continued)

TABLE C-7B (CONTINUED)
CRITICAL VALUES FOR THE MANN–WHITNEY U TEST[b]

n_B	1	2	3	4	5	6	7	8	9	10	11	12	13	14	15	16	17	18	19	20	21	22	23	24	25
20	0	4	11	18	25	32	39	47	54	62	69	77	84	92	100	107	115	123	130	138	146	154	161	169	177
20	20	36	49	62	75	88	101	113	126	138	151	163	176	188	200	213	225	237	250	262	274	286	299	311	323
21	0	5	11	19	26	34	41	49	57	65	73	81	89	97	105	113	121	130	138	146	154	162	170	179	187
21	21	37	52	65	79	92	106	119	132	145	158	171	184	197	210	223	236	248	261	274	287	300	313	325	338
22	0	5	12	20	28	36	44	52	60	68	77	85	94	102	111	119	128	136	145	154	162	171	179	188	197
22	22	39	54	68	82	96	110	124	138	152	165	179	192	206	219	233	246	260	273	286	300	313	327	340	353
23	0	5	13	21	29	37	46	54	63	72	81	90	98	107	116	125	134	143	152	161	170	179	189	198	207
23	23	41	56	71	86	101	115	130	144	158	172	186	201	215	229	243	257	271	285	299	313	327	340	354	368
24	0	6	13	22	30	39	48	57	66	75	85	94	103	113	122	131	141	150	160	169	179	188	198	207	217
24	24	42	59	74	90	105	120	135	150	165	179	194	209	223	238	253	267	282	296	311	325	340	354	369	383
25	0	6	14	23	32	41	50	60	69	79	89	98	108	118	128	137	147	157	167	177	187	197	207	217	227
25	25	44	61	77	93	109	125	140	156	171	186	202	217	232	247	263	278	293	308	323	338	353	368	383	398

n_A

bTest for a one-tailed test at .05 or a two-tailed test at .10. If the U_{obs} value falls within the two values in the table for n_A and n_B, then do not reject the null hypothesis. If the U_{obs} is less than or equal to the lower value in the table or greater than or equal to the larger value in the table, then reject the null hypothesis.

TABLE C-7C

CRITICAL VALUES FOR THE MANN–WHITNEY U TEST[c]

Within each n_B block, the upper (underlined) value is the upper critical value and the lower value is the lower critical value.

n_B		n_A=1	2	3	4	5	6	7	8	9	10	11	12	13	14	15	16	17	18	19	20	21	22	23	24	25
1	upper																									
1	lower																									
2	upper													26	28	30	32	34	36	37	39	41	43	45	47	49
2	lower													0	0	0	0	0	0	1	1	1	1	1	1	1
3	upper							21	24	26	29	32	34	37	40	42	45	47	50	53	55	58	60	63	66	68
3	lower							0	0	1	1	1	2	2	2	3	3	4	4	4	5	5	6	6	6	7
4	upper					20	23	27	30	33	37	40	43	47	50	53	57	60	63	67	70	73	77	80	83	87
4	lower					0	1	1	2	3	3	4	5	5	6	7	7	8	9	9	10	11	11	12	13	13
5	upper				20	24	28	32	36	40	44	48	52	56	60	64	68	72	76	80	84	88	92	96	100	104
5	lower				0	1	2	3	4	5	6	7	8	9	10	11	12	13	14	15	16	17	18	19	20	21
6	upper				23	28	33	38	42	47	52	57	61	66	71	75	80	84	89	94	98	103	108	112	117	121
6	lower				1	2	3	4	6	7	8	9	11	12	13	15	16	18	19	20	22	23	24	26	27	29
7	upper			21	27	32	38	43	49	54	59	65	70	75	81	86	91	96	102	107	112	117	123	128	133	139
7	lower			0	1	3	4	6	7	9	11	12	14	16	17	19	21	23	24	26	28	30	31	33	35	36
8	upper			24	30	36	42	49	55	61	67	73	79	84	90	96	102	108	114	120	126	132	138	144	150	155
8	lower			0	2	4	6	7	9	11	13	15	17	20	22	24	26	28	30	32	34	36	38	40	42	45
9	upper			26	33	40	47	54	61	67	74	81	87	94	100	107	113	120	126	133	140	146	153	159	166	172
9	lower			1	3	5	7	9	11	14	16	18	21	23	26	28	31	33	36	38	40	43	45	48	50	53
10	upper			29	37	44	52	59	67	74	81	88	96	103	110	117	124	132	139	146	153	160	167	175	182	189
10	lower			1	3	6	8	11	13	16	19	22	24	27	30	33	36	38	41	44	47	50	53	55	58	61
11	upper			32	40	48	57	65	73	81	88	96	104	112	120	128	135	143	151	159	167	174	182	190	198	205
11	lower			1	4	7	9	12	15	18	22	25	28	31	34	37	41	44	47	50	53	57	60	63	66	70
12	upper			34	43	52	61	70	79	87	96	104	113	121	130	138	146	155	163	172	180	188	197	205	213	222
12	lower			2	5	8	11	14	17	21	24	28	31	35	38	42	46	49	53	56	60	64	67	71	75	78

(continued)

TABLE C-7C (CONTINUED)

CRITICAL VALUES FOR THE MANN–WHITNEY U TESTᶜ

n_B	1	2	3	4	5	6	7	8	9	10	11	12	13	14	15	16	17	18	19	20	21	22	23	24	25
13		0	2	5	9	12	16	20	23	27	31	35	39	43	47	51	55	59	63	67	71	75	79	83	87
13		26	37	47	56	66	75	84	94	103	112	121	130	139	148	157	166	175	184	193	202	211	220	229	238
14		0	2	6	10	13	17	22	26	30	34	38	43	47	51	56	60	65	69	73	78	82	87	91	95
14		28	40	50	60	71	81	90	100	110	120	130	139	149	159	168	178	187	197	207	216	226	235	245	255
15		0	3	7	11	15	19	24	28	33	37	42	47	51	56	61	66	70	75	80	85	90	94	99	104
15		30	42	53	64	75	86	96	107	117	128	138	148	159	169	179	189	200	210	220	230	240	251	261	271
16		0	3	7	12	16	21	26	31	36	41	46	51	56	61	66	71	76	82	87	92	97	102	108	113
16		32	45	57	68	80	91	102	113	124	135	146	157	168	179	190	201	212	222	233	244	255	266	276	287
17		0	4	8	13	18	23	28	33	38	44	49	55	60	66	71	77	82	88	93	99	105	110	116	122
17		34	47	60	72	84	96	108	120	132	143	155	166	178	189	201	212	224	235	247	258	269	281	292	303
18		0	4	9	14	19	24	30	36	41	47	53	59	65	70	76	82	88	94	100	106	112	118	124	130
18		36	50	63	76	89	102	114	126	139	151	163	175	187	200	212	224	236	248	260	272	284	296	308	320
19		1	4	9	15	20	26	32	38	44	50	56	63	69	75	82	88	94	101	107	113	120	126	133	139
19		37	53	67	80	94	107	120	133	146	159	172	184	197	210	222	235	248	260	273	286	298	311	323	336

n_A

(continued)

TABLE C-7C (CONTINUED)
CRITICAL VALUES FOR THE MANN–WHITNEY U TEST[c]

n_B	1	2	3	4	5	6	7	8	9	10	11	12	13	14	15	16	17	18	19	20	21	22	23	24	25
20		1	5	10	16	22	28	34	40	47	53	60	67	73	80	87	93	100	107	114	121	127	134	141	148
20		39	55	70	84	98	112	126	140	153	167	180	193	207	220	233	247	260	273	286	299	313	326	339	352
21		1	5	11	17	23	30	36	43	50	57	64	71	78	85	92	99	106	113	121	128	135	142	150	157
21		41	58	73	88	103	117	132	146	160	174	188	202	216	230	244	258	272	286	299	313	327	341	354	368
22		1	5	11	18	24	31	38	45	53	60	67	75	82	90	97	105	112	120	127	135	143	150	158	166
22		43	60	77	92	108	123	138	153	167	182	197	211	226	240	255	269	284	298	313	327	341	356	370	384
23		1	6	12	19	26	33	40	48	55	63	71	79	87	94	102	110	118	126	134	142	150	158	167	175
23		45	63	80	96	112	128	144	159	175	190	205	220	235	251	266	281	296	311	326	341	356	371	385	400
24		1	6	13	20	27	35	42	50	58	66	75	83	91	99	108	116	124	133	141	150	158	167	175	184
24		47	66	83	100	117	133	150	166	182	198	213	229	245	261	276	292	308	323	339	354	370	385	401	416
25		1	7	13	21	29	36	45	53	61	70	78	87	95	104	113	122	130	139	148	157	166	175	184	192
25		49	68	87	104	121	139	155	172	189	205	222	238	255	271	287	303	320	336	352	368	384	400	416	433

n_A

cTest for a one-tailed test at .01 or a two-tailed test at .02. If the U_{obs} value falls within the two values in the table for n_A and n_B, then do not reject the null hypothesis. If the U_{obs} is less than or equal to the lower value in the table or greater than or equal to the larger value in the table, then reject the null hypothesis.

Source: The table was generated using R, version 3.43.

TABLE C-8

CRITICAL VALUES OF *T* FOR THE WILCOX SIGNED-RANK TEST

SIGNIFICANCE LEVELS FOR ONE-TAILED TEST				SIGNIFICANCE LEVELS FOR ONE-TAILED TEST				
	.05	.025	.01	.005		.05	.025	.01	.005
SIGNIFICANCE LEVELS FOR TWO-TAILED TEST				SIGNIFICANCE LEVELS FOR TWO-TAILED TEST				
N	.10	.05	.02	.01	N	.10	.05	.02	.01
5	0				33	187	170	151	138
6	2	0			34	200	182	162	148
7	3	2	0		35	213	195	173	159
8	5	3	1	0	36	227	208	185	171
9	8	5	3	1	37	241	221	198	182
10	10	8	5	3	38	256	235	211	194
11	13	10	7	5	39	271	249	224	207
12	17	13	9	7	40	286	264	238	220
13	21	17	12	9	41	302	279	252	233
14	25	21	15	12	42	319	294	266	247
15	30	25	19	15	43	336	310	281	261
16	35	29	23	19	44	353	327	296	276
17	41	34	27	23	45	371	343	312	291
18	47	40	32	27	46	389	361	328	307
19	53	46	37	32	47	407	378	345	322
20	60	52	43	37	48	426	396	362	339
21	67	58	49	42	49	446	415	379	355
22	75	65	55	48	50	466	434	397	373
23	83	73	62	54	51	486	453	416	390
24	91	81	69	61	52	507	473	434	408
25	100	89	76	68	53	529	494	454	427
26	110	98	84	75	54	550	514	473	445
27	119	107	92	83	55	573	536	493	465
28	130	116	101	91	56	595	557	514	484
29	140	126	110	100	57	618	579	535	504
30	151	137	120	109	58	642	602	556	525
31	163	147	130	118	59	666	625	578	546
32	175	159	140	128	60	690	648	600	567

Note: The T_{crit} value indicates the smaller sum of ranks associated with differences that are all of the same sign. For any given N (number of ranked differences), the T_{obs} is significant at a given level if it is equal to or less than the critical value in the table.

Source: The table was generated using R, version 3.43.

TABLE C-9

STUDENT RANGE STATISTIC FOR TUKEY'S HONESTLY SIGNIFICANTLY DIFFERENCE TEST

K=NUMBER OF TREATMENTS

DF FOR ERROR TERM	2	3	4	5	6	7	8	9	10	11	12
4	**3.927**	**5.040**	**5.757**	**6.287**	**6.706**	**7.053**	**7.347**	**7.602**	**7.826**	**8.027**	**8.208**
4	6.511	8.120	9.173	9.958	10.583	11.101	11.542	11.925	12.263	12.565	12.839
5	**3.635**	**4.602**	**5.218**	**5.673**	**6.033**	**6.330**	**6.582**	**6.801**	**6.995**	**7.167**	**7.323**
5	5.702	6.976	7.804	8.421	8.913	9.321	9.669	9.971	10.239	10.479	10.696
6	**3.460**	**4.339**	**4.896**	**5.305**	**5.628**	**5.895**	**6.122**	**6.319**	**6.493**	**6.649**	**6.789**
6	5.243	6.331	7.033	7.556	7.972	8.318	8.612	8.869	9.097	9.300	9.485
7	**3.344**	**4.165**	**4.681**	**5.060**	**5.359**	**5.606**	**5.815**	**5.997**	**6.158**	**6.302**	**6.431**
7	4.949	5.919	6.542	7.005	7.373	7.678	7.939	8.166	8.367	8.548	8.711
8	**3.261**	**4.041**	**4.529**	**4.886**	**5.167**	**5.399**	**5.596**	**5.767**	**5.918**	**6.053**	**6.175**
8	4.745	5.635	6.204	6.625	6.959	7.237	7.474	7.680	7.863	8.027	8.176
9	**3.199**	**3.948**	**4.415**	**4.755**	**5.024**	**5.244**	**5.432**	**5.595**	**5.738**	**5.867**	**5.983**
9	4.596	5.428	5.957	6.347	6.657	6.915	7.134	7.325	7.494	7.646	7.784
10	**3.151**	**3.877**	**4.327**	**4.654**	**4.912**	**5.124**	**5.304**	**5.460**	**5.598**	**5.722**	**5.833**
10	4.482	5.270	5.769	6.136	6.428	6.669	6.875	7.054	7.213	7.356	7.485
11	**3.113**	**3.820**	**4.256**	**4.574**	**4.823**	**5.028**	**5.202**	**5.353**	**5.486**	**5.605**	**5.713**
11	4.392	5.146	5.621	5.970	6.247	6.476	6.671	6.841	6.992	7.127	7.250
12	**3.081**	**3.773**	**4.199**	**4.508**	**4.750**	**4.950**	**5.119**	**5.265**	**5.395**	**5.510**	**5.615**
12	4.320	5.046	5.502	5.836	6.101	6.320	6.507	6.670	6.814	6.943	7.060
13	**3.055**	**3.734**	**4.151**	**4.453**	**4.690**	**4.884**	**5.049**	**5.192**	**5.318**	**5.431**	**5.533**
13	4.260	4.964	5.404	5.726	5.981	6.192	6.372	6.528	6.666	6.791	6.903
14	**3.033**	**3.701**	**4.111**	**4.407**	**4.639**	**4.829**	**4.990**	**5.130**	**5.253**	**5.364**	**5.463**
14	4.210	4.895	5.322	5.634	5.881	6.085	6.258	6.409	6.543	6.663	6.772
15	**3.014**	**3.673**	**4.076**	**4.367**	**4.595**	**4.782**	**4.940**	**5.077**	**5.198**	**5.306**	**5.403**
15	4.167	4.836	5.252	5.556	5.796	5.994	6.162	6.309	6.438	6.555	6.660
16	**2.998**	**3.649**	**4.046**	**4.333**	**4.557**	**4.741**	**4.896**	**5.031**	**5.150**	**5.256**	**5.352**
16	4.131	4.786	5.192	5.489	5.722	5.915	6.079	6.222	6.348	6.461	6.564
17	**2.984**	**3.628**	**4.020**	**4.303**	**4.524**	**4.705**	**4.858**	**4.991**	**5.108**	**5.212**	**5.306**
17	4.099	4.742	5.140	5.430	5.659	5.847	6.007	6.147	6.270	6.380	6.480
18	**2.971**	**3.609**	**3.997**	**4.276**	**4.494**	**4.673**	**4.824**	**4.955**	**5.071**	**5.173**	**5.266**
18	4.071	4.703	5.094	5.379	5.603	5.787	5.944	6.081	6.201	6.309	6.407
19	**2.960**	**3.593**	**3.977**	**4.253**	**4.468**	**4.645**	**4.794**	**4.924**	**5.037**	**5.139**	**5.231**
19	4.046	4.669	5.054	5.334	5.553	5.735	5.889	6.022	6.141	6.246	6.342
20	**2.950**	**3.578**	**3.958**	**4.232**	**4.445**	**4.620**	**4.768**	**4.895**	**5.008**	**5.108**	**5.199**
20	4.024	4.639	5.018	5.293	5.510	5.688	5.839	5.970	6.086	6.190	6.285

(continued)

TABLE C-9 (CONTINUED)

STUDENT RANGE STATISTIC FOR TUKEY'S HONESTLY SIGNIFICANTLY DIFFERENCE TEST

K=NUMBER OF TREATMENTS

DF FOR ERROR TERM	2	3	4	5	6	7	8	9	10	11	12
25	**2.913**	**3.523**	**3.890**	**4.153**	**4.358**	**4.526**	**4.667**	**4.789**	**4.897**	**4.993**	**5.079**
25	3.942	4.527	4.885	5.144	5.347	5.513	5.655	5.778	5.886	5.983	6.070
30	**2.888**	**3.486**	**3.845**	**4.102**	**4.301**	**4.464**	**4.601**	**4.720**	**4.824**	**4.917**	**5.001**
30	3.889	4.455	4.799	5.048	5.242	5.401	5.536	5.653	5.756	5.848	5.932
35	**2.871**	**3.461**	**3.814**	**4.066**	**4.261**	**4.421**	**4.555**	**4.606**	**4.773**	**4.863**	**4.945**
35	3.852	4.404	4.739	4.980	5.169	5.323	5.453	5.566	5.666	5.755	5.835
40	**2.858**	**3.442**	**3.791**	**4.039**	**4.232**	**4.388**	**4.521**	**4.634**	**4.735**	**4.824**	**4.904**
40	3.825	4.367	4.695	4.931	5.114	5.265	5.392	5.502	5.599	5.685	5.764
50	**2.841**	**3.416**	**3.758**	**4.002**	**4.190**	**4.344**	**4.473**	**4.584**	**4.681**	**4.768**	**4.846**
50	3.787	4.316	4.634	4.863	5.040	5.185	5.308	5.414	5.507	5.590	5.665
60	**2.829**	**3.399**	**3.737**	**3.977**	**4.163**	**4.314**	**4.441**	**4.550**	**4.646**	**4.732**	**4.808**
60	3.762	4.282	4.594	4.818	4.991	5.133	5.253	5.356	5.447	5.528	5.601
80	**2.814**	**3.377**	**3.711**	**3.947**	**4.129**	**4.277**	**4.402**	**4.509**	**4.603**	**4.686**	**4.761**
80	3.732	4.241	4.545	4.763	4.931	5.069	5.185	5.284	5.372	5.451	5.521
100	**2.806**	**3.365**	**3.695**	**3.929**	**4.109**	**4.256**	**4.379**	**4.484**	**4.577**	**4.659**	**4.733**
100	3.714	4.216	4.516	4.730	4.896	5.031	5.144	5.242	5.328	5.405	5.474
150	**2.794**	**3.348**	**3.674**	**3.905**	**4.083**	**4.227**	**4.348**	**4.451**	**4.542**	**4.623**	**4.696**
150	3.690	4.184	4.478	4.687	4.849	4.980	5.091	5.187	5.270	5.345	5.412
200	**2.789**	**3.339**	**3.664**	**3.893**	**4.069**	**4.212**	**4.332**	**4.435**	**4.525**	**4.605**	**4.677**
200	3.678	4.168	4.459	4.666	4.826	4.956	5.065	5.159	5.242	5.315	5.381

Note: Bolded critical Q-values are at $p=.05$. Non-bolded critical Q-values are at $p=.01$.

Source: The table was generated using R, version 2.13.0.

TABLE C-10

CRITICAL VALUES FOR THE CHI-SQUARE DISTRIBUTION (x^2)

df	.25	.1	.05	.025	.01	.005	.001
				a			
1	1.3233	2.7055	3.8415	5.0239	6.6349	7.8794	10.8276
2	2.7726	4.6052	5.9915	7.3778	9.2103	10.5966	13.8155
3	4.1083	6.2514	7.8147	9.3484	11.3449	12.8382	16.2662
4	5.3853	7.7794	9.4877	11.1433	13.2767	14.8603	18.4668
5	6.6257	9.2364	11.0705	12.8325	15.0863	16.7496	20.5150
6	7.8408	10.6446	12.5916	14.4494	16.8119	18.5476	22.4577
7	9.0371	12.0170	14.0671	16.0128	18.4753	20.2777	24.3219
8	10.2189	13.3616	15.5073	17.5345	20.0902	21.9550	26.1245
9	11.3888	14.6837	16.9190	19.0228	21.6660	23.5894	27.8772
10	12.5489	15.9872	18.3070	20.4832	23.2093	25.1882	29.5883
11	13.7007	17.2750	19.6751	21.9200	24.7250	26.7568	31.2641
12	14.8454	18.5493	21.0261	23.3367	26.2170	28.2995	32.9095
13	15.9839	19.8119	22.3620	24.7356	27.6882	29.8195	34.5282
14	17.1169	21.0641	23.6848	26.1189	29.1412	31.3193	36.1233
15	18.2451	22.3071	24.9958	27.4884	30.5779	32.8013	37.6973
16	19.3689	23.5418	26.2962	28.8454	31.9999	34.2672	39.2524
17	20.4887	24.7690	27.5871	30.1910	33.4087	35.7185	40.7902
18	21.6049	25.9894	28.8693	31.5264	34.8053	37.1565	42.3124
19	22.7178	27.2036	30.1435	32.8523	36.1909	38.5823	43.8202
20	23.8277	28.4120	31.4104	34.1696	37.5662	39.9968	45.3147
21	24.9348	29.6151	32.6706	35.4789	38.9322	41.4011	46.7970
22	26.0393	30.8133	33.9244	36.7807	40.2894	42.7957	48.2679
23	27.1413	32.0069	35.1725	38.0756	41.6384	44.1813	49.7282
24	28.2412	33.1962	36.4150	39.3641	42.9798	45.5585	51.1786
25	29.3389	34.3816	37.6525	40.6465	44.3141	46.9279	52.6197
26	30.4346	35.5632	38.8851	41.9232	45.6417	48.2899	54.0520
27	31.5284	36.7412	40.1133	43.1945	46.9629	49.6449	55.4760
28	32.6205	37.9159	41.3371	44.4608	48.2782	50.9934	56.8923
29	33.7109	39.0875	42.5570	45.7223	49.5879	52.3356	58.3012
30	34.7997	40.2560	43.7730	46.9792	50.8922	53.6720	59.7031
31	35.8871	41.4217	44.9853	48.2319	52.1914	55.0027	61.0983
32	36.9730	42.5847	46.1943	49.4804	53.4858	56.3281	62.4872
33	38.0575	43.7452	47.3999	50.7251	54.7755	57.6484	63.8701
34	39.1408	44.9032	48.6024	51.9660	56.0609	58.9639	65.2472
35	40.2228	46.0588	49.8018	53.2033	57.3421	60.2748	66.6188

(continued)

TABLE C-10 (CONTINUED)

CRITICAL VALUES FOR THE CHI-SQUARE DISTRIBUTION (x^2)

df	.25	.1	.05	.025	.01	.005	.001
36	41.3036	47.2122	50.9985	54.4373	58.6192	61.5812	67.9852
37	42.3833	48.3634	52.1923	55.6680	59.8925	62.8833	69.3465
38	43.4619	49.5126	53.3835	56.8955	61.1621	64.1814	70.7029
39	44.5395	50.6598	54.5722	58.1201	62.4281	65.4756	72.0547
40	45.6160	51.8051	55.7585	59.3417	63.6907	66.7660	73.4020
41	46.6916	52.9485	56.9424	60.5606	64.9501	68.0527	74.7449
42	47.7663	54.0902	58.1240	61.7768	66.2062	69.3360	76.0838
43	48.8400	55.2302	59.3035	62.9904	67.4593	70.6159	77.4186
44	49.9129	56.3685	60.4809	64.2015	68.7095	71.8926	78.7495
45	50.9849	57.5053	61.6562	65.4102	69.9568	73.1661	80.0767
46	52.0562	58.6405	62.8296	66.6165	71.2014	74.4365	81.4003
47	53.1267	59.7743	64.0011	67.8206	72.4433	75.7041	82.7204
48	54.1964	60.9066	65.1708	69.0226	73.6826	76.9688	84.0371
49	55.2653	62.0375	66.3386	70.2224	74.9195	78.2307	85.3506
50	56.3336	63.1671	67.5048	71.4202	76.1539	79.4900	86.6608

STEPS IN DETERMINING CRITICAL VALUES FOR CHI-SQUARE (X^2) FOR TABLE C-10

1. Calculate the degrees of freedom (*df*). The formula is df = (r - 1) (c - 1), where r = number of rows in the matrix and c = number of columns in the matrix. For example, in a 2 x 3 matrix, 2 rows and 3 columns, *df* = (2 - 1) (3 - 1) = 2 *df*.

2. Apply level of significance (*a*) (e.g., .05, .01).

3. Locate critical value for chi-square from statistical table. For example, *df* = 2, *a* = .05, x^2_{crit} = 5.9915.

4. Calculate x^2_{obs} from data.

5. Decision rule:

   a. If x^2_{obs} is equal to or above x^2_{crit}, then reject the null hypothesis.

   b. If x^2_{obs} is below x^2_{crit}, then do not reject the null hypothesis.

Source: The table was generated using Microsoft Office Excel 2013.

TABLE C-11

BINOMIAL DISTRIBUTION TABLE

									X							
Y	**0**	**1**	**2**	**3**	**4**	**5**	**6**	**7**	**8**	**9**	**10**	**11**	**12**	**13**	**14**	**15**
1	0.500	1.000														
2	0.250	0.750	1.000													
3	0.125	0.500	0.875	1.000												
4	0.063	0.313	0.688	0.938	1.000											
5	**0.031**	0.188	0.500	0.813	0.969	1.000										
6	***0.016***	0.109	0.344	0.656	0.891	0.984	1.000									
7	0.008	0.063	0.227	0.500	0.773	0.938	0.992	1.000								
8	0.004	**0.035**	0.145	0.363	0.637	0.855	0.965	0.996	1.000							
9	0.002	***0.020***	0.090	0.254	0.500	0.746	0.910	0.980	0.998	1.000						
10	0.001	0.011	0.055	0.172	0.377	0.623	0.828	0.945	0.989	0.999	1.000					
11	0.000	0.006	**0.033**	0.113	0.274	0.500	0.726	0.887	0.967	0.994	1.000	1.000				
12		0.003	***0.019***	0.073	0.194	0.387	0.613	0.806	0.927	0.981	0.997	1.000	1.000			
13		0.002	0.011	**0.046**	0.133	0.291	0.500	0.709	0.867	0.954	0.989	0.998	1.000	1.000		
14		0.001	0.006	0.029	0.090	0.212	0.395	0.605	0.788	0.910	0.971	0.994	0.999	1.000	1.000	
15		0.000	0.004	***0.018***	0.059	0.151	0.304	0.500	0.696	0.849	0.941	0.982	0.996	1.000	1.000	1.000
16			0.002	0.011	**0.038**	0.105	0.227	0.402	0.598	0.773	0.895	0.962	0.989	0.998	1.000	1.000
17			0.001	0.006	***0.025****	0.072	0.166	0.315	0.500	0.685	0.834	0.928	0.975	0.994	0.999	1.000
18			0.001	0.004	0.015	**0.048**	0.119	0.240	0.407	0.593	0.760	0.881	0.952	0.985	0.996	0.999
19			0.000	0.002	0.010	0.032	0.084	0.180	0.324	0.500	0.676	0.820	0.916	0.968	0.990	0.998
20				0.001	0.006	***0.021***	0.058	0.132	0.252	0.412	0.588	0.748	0.868	0.942	0.979	0.994

(continued)

TABLE C-11 (CONTINUED)

BINOMIAL DISTRIBUTION TABLE

Y	0	1	2	3	4	5	6	7	8	9	10	11	12	13	14	15
21				0.001	0.004	0.013	*0.039*	0.095	0.192	0.332	0.500	0.668	0.808	0.905	0.961	0.987
22				0.000	0.002	0.008	0.026	0.067	0.143	0.262	0.416	0.584	0.738	0.857	0.933	0.974
23					0.001	0.005	*0.017*	*0.047*	0.105	0.202	0.339	0.500	0.661	0.798	0.895	0.953
24					0.001	0.003	0.011	0.032	0.076	0.154	0.271	0.419	0.581	0.729	0.846	0.924
25					0.000	0.002	0.007	*0.022*	0.054	0.115	0.212	0.345	0.500	0.655	0.788	0.885
26						0.001	0.005	0.014	**0.038**	0.084	0.163	0.279	0.423	0.577	0.721	0.837
27						0.001	0.003	0.010	0.026	0.061	0.124	0.221	0.351	0.500	0.649	0.779
28						0.000	0.002	0.006	*0.018*	*0.044*	0.092	0.172	0.286	0.425	0.575	0.714
29							0.001	0.004	0.012	0.031	0.068	0.132	0.229	0.356	0.500	0.644
30							0.001	0.003	0.008	*0.021*	*0.049*	0.100	0.181	0.292	0.428	0.572
31							0.000	0.002	0.005	0.015	0.035	0.075	0.141	0.237	0.360	0.500
32								0.001	0.004	0.010	0.025	0.055	0.108	0.189	0.298	0.430
33								0.001	0.002	0.007	*0.018*	*0.040*	0.081	0.148	0.243	0.364
34								0.000	0.001	0.005	0.012	0.029	0.061	0.115	0.196	0.304
35									0.001	0.003	0.008	**0.020**	**0.045**	0.088	0.155	0.250

Note: x = number of successful trials, y = number of independent trials. Values shown are for one-tailed test; double values for two-tailed test. Bolded values are probabilities for one-tailed test $p < .05$. Bolded and italicized values are probabilities for two-tailed test $p < .05$ when doubled. *$p < .05$ when doubled because of rounding (i.e., with $x = 17$, $y = 4$, $p = .0245$ carried to the fourth decimal place).

A one-tailed example would be, if you flip a coin 8 times and you expect it to land on heads all 8 times, you will have more than a 95% chance of accurately calling heads at least one time. A two-tailed example would be if a you have 9 people and you ask them to guess either heads or tails, there is more than a 95% chance that at least one person will accurately guess what they called.

Source: The table was generated using Microsoft Office Excel 2013.

Glossary

A

a priori: Reasoning from cause to effect. A priori criteria are criteria that an investigator states before collecting data.

AB research design: Single subject research where the A phase represents the collection of baseline data and the B phase represents the intervention phase. Variations of this include ABA, ABAB, and other related research designs. *See also* case study.

abscissa: The horizontal coordinate, or x-axis, in a distribution.

abstract: A summary of a published article (150 to 300 words) that contains the important points of each section, including purpose of study, literature review, methodology, results, limitations of research design, and recommendations for further research.

action research: Application of research to a site-specific environment using a problem-solving approach. It is an outgrowth of both qualitative and quantitative research. For example, an occupational therapist is interested in finding the best splint to use with a client who has a cumulative trauma injury. The methodology may be replicated in another setting to test of generalizability of the results.

alpha (α): The probability of a Type I error predetermined to be acceptable in research. It is usually set at .05 or .01 in the social sciences. It is also referred to as *significance level*. The *p*-value of a particular comparison is compared to the alpha level in order to decide to reject the null hypothesis or not.

alternative hypothesis (H): The hypothesis that is the opposite of the stated hypothesis and is not predicted to be true.

analysis of covariance (ANCOVA): A statistical test arising from an analysis of variance that adjusts for a priori differences in comparison groups.

analysis of variance (ANOVA): An inferential statistical test that is applied to data when comparing two or more independent group means. An F score is derived. The formula for F in a one-way ANOVA is:

$$F = \frac{variance\ among\ group\ means}{variance\ within\ groups}$$

annotated bibliography: Includes the bibliographical citation and the abstract, perhaps with critical commentary.

ANOVA: *See also* analysis of variance.

applied research: The direct application of research to improving the quality of life in areas such as reduction of work injuries, prevention of alcoholism, and evaluation of clinical treatment methods. *See also* problem-oriented research.

aptitude: Inherent, natural ability of an individual; underlying capacity to learn or perform in a specific area.

artifact: An unexplained result in an experiment not caused by the independent variable.

associational relationship: Degree of correlation between two variables.

attitude scale: A measure of an individual's feeling, belief, or opinion toward a subject or topic.

Average: There are three different types of average:
1. **Mean**: What one often thinks of as average—add all the values and divide by the number of values added together.
2. **Median (or midpoint)**: The value in the exact center of the list of responses.
3. **Mode**: The most commonly appearing value.

Rice, M. S., Stein, F., & Tomlin, G.
Clinical Research in Occupational Therapy, Sixth Edition (pp. 415-427).
© 2019 Taylor & Francis Group.

B

bar graph: A histogram with unattached bars.

baseline data: The results of initial testing of a subject before intervention.

basic research: Investigations in areas related to processes, functions, and attributes that can lead to applied research. An example of basic research is examining how serotonin, a neurochemical transmitter, operates in the brain. The results of basic research often have important significance for clinical researchers.

before-and-after design: An experimental research design in which performance or characteristics are measured before and after an intervention. Often referred to as a *pre- and post-test repeated measures design.*

beta (β): The probability of a Type 2 error in research. *See also* power.

bias: Any prejudicial factor in the researcher or methodology that may distort results.

biased sample: A sample that is not representative of a target population from which it is drawn. As it does not reflect the major characteristics of the target population, the results from a biased sample cannot be confidently generalized.

bibliographical citation: The exact reference for a journal, book, or article referred to in the research paper or manuscript. The citation includes the author; title of article, journal, or book; volume and page numbers; and in books, the place of publication and the publisher.

bimodal: A frequency distribution showing the two highest points.

binomial distribution: Probability distribution used to describe dichotomous outcomes in a population.

bivariate analysis: Statistical analysis in which there is one dependent variable and one independent variable.

box-and-whisker plots, box plots, box graphs: Type of exploratory data analysis that produces descriptive figures which display the maximum and minimum scores and the median and quartiles in a rectangular box. Useful in demonstrating graphically the degree of skewness of data.

C

case study: Intensive study of an individual or a defined entity through a comprehensive extraction of data from many sources, including observation, interview, and document analysis.

central tendency: A summary measure of a distribution indicated by the mean, median, or mode. Frequently referred to as *measures of central tendency.*

chi-square: A nonparametric statistical technique that tests the probability between observed and expected frequencies derived from nominal (categorical) level measurement.

clinical observation research: The systematic and objective investigation of normal development, course of a disease, or responses to an intervention.

clinical trial: In experimental medical research, refers to large-scale studies exploring the effectiveness of drugs or vaccines on populations.

closed-ended questions: Questions that can be answered by either *yes* or *no*. This type of question is not considered useful in survey research. The opposite of a closed-ended question is an open-ended question.

coding: A term in qualitative research referring to the systematic categorization of interview responses, focus group conversations, or observed documents with common characteristics (e.g., residents of a community or an occupational group).

cohort: A study sample with some common experience or characteristic.

concurrent validity: A new test's correlation with an established instrument to indicate its accuracy in measuring the variable of interest. For example, a new test for intelligence frequently will be correlated with the Wechsler Intelligence Scales because it has a high reliability and established validity. New tests are developed to update concepts and improve administration, cost, and time considerations.

confidence interval: The area in a sample distribution that most likely contains the population parameter. The width of the confidence interval is affected by the level of statistical confidence desired in the results.

confounding variable: An extraneous variable affecting research results. For example, test anxiety, fatigue, and lack of sleep may be confounding variables.

content validity: The most elementary type of validity. It is determined by a logical analysis of test items to see whether the items are consistent and measure what they purport to measure. *See also* face validity.

contingency table: A table of values that includes observed and expected frequencies, such as a chi-square table.

continuous variable: A quantitative measure that can assume an infinite number of values between any two points. Examples of continuous variables are height, weight, and heart rate.

control group: A comparative group included in a study to control for the Hawthorne effect and other extraneous variables. Both the experimental and comparative groups receive equal time or attention.

convenience sample: A sample selected that is readily available. For example, a researcher will select participants who are in a hospital where the researcher is employed.

correlation: A statistical test used to quantify the association between two (usually continuous) variables.

correlation coefficient: A statistical value that indicates the degree of relationship between two variables. It can range from +1.00 through 0 to -1.00.

correlation matrix: A statistical table describing the degree of correlation between pairs of variables, applied to many variables. The correlation matrix indicates the correlation coefficient index for each pair of correlates.

correlational research: Retrospective investigations into the relationship between variables. Variables are not manipulated by the researcher, as they would be in experimental research.

covariate: A suspected or discovered variable important in a study for its effect on the dependent variable.

Cox proportional hazard regression: Statistical test for assessing time to a dichotomous event where the independent variables are nominal or continuous.

credibility: In qualitative research, the authenticity of the results based on acceptance of the conclusions from the phenomenological evidence. Triangulation (i.e., obtaining data from different perspectives) increases the credibility of the research.

criterion: Standard of performance that is the basis or yardstick for comparisons.

criterion-referenced test: A test based on a standard of performance, competence, or mastery, rather than on a comparison with a normative group. For example, for an individual to pass a test in driver competency, he or she would have to demonstrate mastery of a specific set of criteria. The determination of the criteria is not based on the bell-shaped curve but is based on socially acceptable minimal standards for performance.

critical value: The statistical value displayed in tables that is used to judge whether or not to reject the null hypothesis.

cross-validation: A method to measure test validity by replicating the original testing in other groups.

Cronbach's alpha coefficient: A statistic that is used to measure internal consistency and reliability using continuous data. *See also* Kuder-Richardson coefficient.

culture-free test: A test that is not culturally biased and can be fairly administered across cultures.

D

data: The numerical results of a study. The term is always plural (e.g., data are …).

decile: A point in a distribution where 10% of the cases fall at or below that point.

deductive reasoning: Inference to particulars from a general principle. For example, proposing a theory and then hypothesizing specific results from an experiment.

degrees of freedom (df): A mathematically derived value that is used in reading statistical tables.

demographic variables: Related to the statistical characteristics of a target population, such as distribution of ages, gender, income, presence of disease (morbidity), death rates (mortality), occupation, accident and injury rates, health status, and nutritional input.

demography: The application of statistical methods to describe human populations regarding factors, such as mortality, morbidity, birth and marriage rates, gender differences, physical and intellectual characteristics, socioeconomic status, and religious beliefs.

dependent variable: Resultant effect of the independent variable. In clinical research, the selection of the dependent variable indicates the desired outcome, such as decrease in anxiety, increase in range of motion, or increase in reading achievement.

descriptive statistics: Statistical tests or procedures to describe a population, sample, or variable. Examples of descriptive statistics are measures of central tendency, measures of variability, frequency distribution, vital statistics, scatter diagram, polygons, and histograms.

developmental test: A measure of a child's performance in age-related areas such as language, perceptual-motor, social, emotional, and ambulation.

dichotomous variable: Variable that only has two possible values.

directional hypothesis: A statement by the researcher predicting that there will be a statistically significant difference between groups in a certain direction. For example, a clinical researcher states, "Aerobic exercise is more effective than anti-depressive medication in reducing anxiety in individuals with clinical depression."

discourse analysis: The study of communication through the forms and mechanisms of verbal interaction.

discrete variable: A variable that is distinct and does not have an infinite number of values between categories. Examples of discrete variables are gender, diagnostic categories, or eye color.

double-blind control: A research design in which neither the researcher nor the participants know whether they are in the experimental or control group.

E

effect modification (interaction): A situation in which two or more independent factors modify the effect of each other with regard to an outcome; thus, the outcome differs depending on whether or not an effect modifier is present.

effect size: A method for determining the relative size of the effect of the independent variable without regard to the degrees of freedom. It is based upon the difference in population means and the size of the population standard deviation and is usually considered to be small, medium, or large (see Cohen, 1988).

empiricism: The philosophy that advocates knowledge based on controlled observation and experiment.

error variance: Variability in measurement due to contaminating factors in the participant, researcher, test instrument, or environment that threaten internal validity. These factors include poor motivation, fatigue, and test anxiety in the participant; researcher bias; unreliability of the test instrument; and a distracting or noisy testing environment.

ethnoscience: The study of the characteristics of language as culture in terms of lexical or semantic relations.

evaluation research: The qualitative and systematic evaluation of systems and organizations such as hospitals and educational programs by applying a priori criteria or standards.

evidence-based practice: The use of research studies to inform intervention decisions. The occupational therapist translates the results of study protocols to the current practice setting.

ex post facto design: A retrospective study in which the investigator examines the relationships of variables that have already occurred.

experimental group: The group that is manipulated by the researcher; for example, the experimental group receives an innovative method of teaching.

experimental research: A prospective study in which the investigator seeks to discover cause-and-effect relationships by manipulating the independent variable and observing the effects on the dependent variable.

experimental study: Study that examines groups where an intervention has been allocated.

external validity: The degree to which the results of a study can be generalized to a target population. External validity depends on the representativeness of the sample and the rigor of the experiment. Replication of a study producing consistent results increases the external validity.

extraneous historical factors: Threats to internal validity when unexpected events take place during an experiment that affect the results. These unpredictable events in the participant are extraneous variables.

extraneous variable: A variable other than the independent variable that can potentially affect the results of a study. Extraneous variables can include factors such as gender, intelligence, severity of disability, or socioeconomic status. These variables, if they are uncontrolled, can threaten the internal validity of a study.

F

factor analysis: A statistical method to categorize data into identifiable factors. The procedure is an extension of a correlation matrix where many variables are correlated with each other, and clusters of co-variability are extracted.

factorial design: A research study exploring the interaction between variables, such as a two-factor analysis of variance.

feasible research study: A study in which the investigator has examined in detail and provided solutions for the practical aspects of implementation, such as costs, time, setting, availability of participants, ethics, selection of outcome measures, and procedure for collecting data.

Fisher's exact test: Statistical test used to compare two unpaired (independent) samples where the outcome is dichotomous or nominal and the sample size is small; alternative to the chi-square test.

forced choice test items: Items that require participants to make a choice when completing a questionnaire, rating scale, or attitude inventory. Participants select from among items generated by the researcher.

frequency distribution table: A descriptive statistic summarizing data by showing the number of times each score value occurs in a set category or interval.

frequency polygon: A line graph depicting the number of cases that fall into designated categories. It is composed of an X and a Y axis.

Frequency ratio or Fisher ratio (F): Variability among groups divided by variability within groups. A larger F value makes it more likely the null hypothesis can be rejected.

Friedman's test: Statistical test used to compare three or more paired (dependent) samples when the outcome is either ordinal or continuous with a skewed distribution.

functional capacity evaluation (FCE): A comprehensive and systematic approach to measuring a client's overall physical capacity, including muscle strength and endurance.

G

generalizable: The extent to which findings from a study sample can be applied to the entire population.

grounded theory analysis: Referring to qualitative research, the search for regularities by constantly comparing and contrasting similarities and differences in incidents to form categories or themes with distinctive properties and conceptual relationships.

Guttman scale: A cumulative attitude scale that indicates an individual's feelings toward a specific issue. The respondent usually answers *yes* or *no* to a statement.

H

halo effect: A carry-over effect from previous knowledge in an individual, resulting in a bias on the part of a tester or rater. Halo effects typically occur when raters positively prejudge a participant's performance based on the rater's previous experience with him or her. It is a bias in testing.

Hawthorne effect: A confounding variable that creates a positive result that is not caused by the independent variable. The Hawthorne effect is eliminated by introducing a control group or by using the participant as one's own control.

hermeneutics: The study and interpretation of text in which each event is understood by reference to the whole of which it is a part, especially the broader historical context.

heterogeneous: Of different origin or characteristic, such as mixed ages or educational levels.

heuristic research: Investigations that seek to discover relationships between variables through pilot studies and factor analysis. The major purpose is to generate further research.

histogram: A descriptive statistic describing a frequency distribution using attached bars.

historical research: The systematic and objective investigation, through primary sources, into the events and people that shaped history.

homogeneous: Of like origin or characteristic such as age, gender, or occupation.

honeymoon effect: A confounding variable that produces a short-term beneficial effect. It is created by the initial optimism of the researcher desiring to show the positive effects of a specific intervention and the participant wanting the intervention to work. The participant rejects the initial effects of intervention and disregards side effects or negative results. It is controlled by long-term follow-up and reducing researcher bias.

hypothesis: A statement that predicts results and that can be tested. An example of a hypothesis is "Aerobic exercise lowers blood pressure in middle-aged, sedentary men." A hypothesis can be stated in a null (no difference) or in a directional form.

I

idiographic approach: Intensive study of an individual or dynamic case study.

incidence rate: The rate of the initial occurrence or new cases of a disease over a period of time. For example, the incidence of AIDS in the United States for the year 2010 includes all the new cases of AIDS diagnosed during 2010.

independent living evaluation: An assessment tool used to measure a client's ability to perform the activities of daily living. An example is the Barthel Self Care Index.

independent variable: A variable manipulated by the researcher. In clinical research, it represents the intervention, such as sensory integration therapy, or cognitive behavioral therapy.

inductive reasoning: Inferences from particulars or experiments to the general. For example, integrating the results of research studies into a general theory or conclusion.

inferential statistics: Statistical tests for making inferences from samples and populations based on objectively derived data. They include *t*-tests, analysis of variance, chi-square, correlation coefficients, factor analysis, and multiple regression.

information retrieval systems: Automated system for storing and retrieving information. In the health fields, examples include OT Search, MEDLINE, PubMed, CINAHL, ERIC, or HealthStar.

informed consent form: A voluntary consensual agreement between the investigator and the participant detailing the procedures in the study and the possible psychological and physical risks that could result in harm.

institutional review board (IRB): An interdisciplinary committee established in a university, hospital, or private industry to protect human participants from possible harm that could occur by participating in a research study. It is required at institutions receiving federal funding that all research with human participants be screened with ethical considerations before data are collected or the research is initiated.

internal validity: The degree of rigor in an experiment in controlling for extraneous variables and error variance. Potential threats to internal validity have been identified as extraneous historical factors, maturation, instrumentation, and lack of random sampling. Internal validity is an indication of the trustworthiness of the results. Well-designed studies with good control of variables that could potentially distort the results have high internal validity. The quality of a research study is increased by eliminating the threats to internal validity.

interquartile range (IQR): Measure of spread or dispersion in the data calculated as the difference between the 25th and 75th percentile values.

inter-rater reliability: The degree of agreement and consistency between two independent raters in measuring a variable.

interval scale of measurement: Quantification of a variable in which there are infinite points between each measurement, as well as equal intervals. Examples include the measurement of systolic blood pressure or intelligence scores as measured by the Wechsler scales. An absolute zero is not assumed in measuring a variable, nor are comparative statements assumed, such as X is twice as large as Y.

intra-rater reliability: The degree of consistency over time within a single rater.

K

Kappa test (k): A statistical procedure to estimate the degree of inter-rater agreement factoring in the probability of chance agreement.

Kendall's coefficient of concordance: Statistical test used to quantify the association between two ordinal variables.

key word: An important word or concept in a study that is identified by the researcher. It is used to electronically retrieve a study when it is part of a database.

Kruskal-Wallis test: Nonparametric statistical test used to compare three or more unpaired (independent) samples where the outcome is either ordinal or continuous with a skewed distribution.

Kuder-Richardson coefficient: A statistic that is used to measure internal consistency and reliability using dichotomous data. *See also* Cronbach's alpha coefficient.

L

Likert scale: A measurement scale used in questionnaires to assess a participant's extent of agreement or disagreement with a statement. Likert scales usually include five to seven descriptors (e.g., totally agree, agree, neutral, disagree, totally disagree).

linear regression: Regression analysis used to quantify the association between one independent variable and a continuous dependent variable that is normally distributed.

logical positivism: A philosophical approach of the 1920s and 1930s. Logical positivists asserted that statements about reality must be verified by empirical data.

logistic regression: Regression analysis used to quantify the association between one independent variable and a dichotomous outcome.

M

Mann–Whitney U test: A nonparametric test that is an alternative to the independent *t*-test when testing differences between the means of two independent groups. The normality and equal variances assumptions of the *t*-test need not be satisfied in the Mann–Whitney test.

matched group: A control group selected to use as a comparison to the experimental group. Variables matched typically include age, gender, socioeconomic status, and degree of disability.

maturation: A threat to internal validity that occurs when the researcher does not account for the participant's maturity during an experiment. For example, in testing children, the researcher must consider age in measuring changes from pre- to post-test evaluation. Maturation can also refer to a practice effect and development in the participant during the experiment.

McNemar's test: Statistical test used to compare two paired (dependent) samples when the outcome of interest is dichotomous (or nominal with only two outcomes).

mean: The arithmetic average derived from all scores in a distribution. It is a measure of central tendency.

measurement error: In measuring a variable, errors in test results can occur due to participant anxiety, unreliability of test instrument, noisy setting for testing and tester's inability to follow test protocol accurately.

measures of central tendency: Mean, mode, and median.

measures of variability or dispersion: Range, variance, and standard deviation.

mechanism of change: The underlying causes of change in behavior, attitude, or physiology by an intervention. For example, exercise relieves clinical depression by increasing the neurohormone serotonin that then increases the likelihood of physical activity.

median: The score at the 50th percentile or midpoint where all the cases in a distribution are divided in half. It is a measure of central tendency.

member checking: A validation method to increase the trustworthiness of a qualitative study by providing preliminary results to the participant and receiving feedback.

meta-analysis: A quantitative analysis of a group of related research studies to determine the overall average effectiveness of an intervention. Meta-analysis is based on the effect size of studies and incorporates consideration of sample sizes and the degree of consistency among studies. (See Rosenthal & Rosnow, 1991, for a detailed discussion of meta-analysis.)

methodological research: Objective and systematic investigation for analyzing instruments, tests, procedures, curriculum, software programs, and intervention programs.

mixed method designs: Using qualitative and quantitative research methods in a study. For example, applying interview questions and standardized tests or physiological measures in the same study.

mode: The most frequent score or numerical value in a frequency distribution. A measure of central tendency.

multiple analysis of covariance (MANCOVA): A statistical technique that is based on the analysis of variance where multiple variables are being analyzed and corrected for differences in initial score statistical significance between the groups being compared.

multiple baseline designs: Used in measuring variables for more than one participant, outcome, or setting, before and after intervention.

multiple linear regression: Linear regression used to quantify the association between more than one independent variable and a continuous outcome that is normally distributed.

multiple logistic regression: Logistic regression used to quantify the association between more than one independent variable and a dichotomous outcome.

multiple regression: A statistical method that is used to predict the individual effects of independent variables on a designated dependent variable. Multiple regression has been used in medical research to identify the multiple risk factors in certain diseases, such as cardiovascular disease, stroke, or emphysema. For example, multiple regression is used to predict the effect of designated risk factors (presumed independent variables) on a dependent variable (e.g., heart disease).

multinomial logistic regression: Logistic regression used to quantify the association between one or more independent variables and a nominal outcome having more than 2 levels.

multivariable analysis: Statistical analysis in which there is one dependent variable and more than one independent variable.

N

n: Number of participants in a sub-group

N: Number of participants in the entire study.

nominal scale of measurement: Classification of the values of a variable into discrete categories, such as diagnostic groups, professions, or gender. There is no specific order in the categories; no category is more important than any other category. Likewise, each category is mutually exclusive of any other category.

nominal variable: Variable having (descriptive) categorical values.

nomothetic approach: Research leading to general laws in science or universal knowledge.

nonparametric regression: A type of regression used to quantify the association between one or more independent variables and a continuous outcome having a skewed distribution

nonparametric statistical tests: Inferential statistical procedures on samples whose data are not distributed according to the normal curve, or on small samples. These tests include, but are not limited to, the Mann-Whitney U, Kruskall-Wallis, chi-square, Spearman rho correlation, and Wilcoxon tests.

non-response bias: In survey research when those responding to a questionnaire are not representative of non-responders. The non-respondents may have significantly different knowledge, attitudes, practices, or opinions from those who responded to the survey.

normal curve: A bell-shaped curve that describes a mathematical probability distribution of a population where most scores cluster around the mean. Also known as a *Gaussian distribution*.

norm-referenced test: A test used to assess the degree of achievement, aptitude, capacity, interest, or attitude compared to established norms or standard scores based on a population.

null hypothesis (H_0): A statement by the researcher that predicts no statistically significant differences between groups or relationships between variables. For example, "There is no statistically significant difference between exercise and splinting in reducing spasticity in children with cerebral palsy."

O

objective psychological test: Standardized test that contains comparative norms for interpreting individual raw scores.

observational study: Descriptive study that examines groups at one or more points in time without allocation of an intervention.

observed statistical value: The value obtained from applying a statistical formula to the data of a study. These values, such as *t* or *F* observed, are compared to the critical value that is derived from a statistical table to allow the decision to reject the null hypothesis or not.

one-tailed test of statistical significance: Used when a researcher makes a directional hypothesis that there will be a statistically significant difference between groups or predicts the direction of a correlation.

open-ended questions: Used in survey research. The investigator elicits attitudes, beliefs, and emotions from participants by asking questions that cannot be answered by *yes* or *no*, or by the selection from a limited set of options. The opposite of an open-ended question is a closed-ended question.

operational definition of variable: Specific test, procedure, or set of criteria that defines independent or dependent variables. This definition is crucial for replicating a study or in evaluating a group of studies such as through a meta-analysis.

operationalization: The process by which a non-measurable phenomena is defined by, and its existence denoted by other phenomena. This strategy is more common in psychology, physics, and social and life sciences.

ordinal logistic regression: Logistic regression used to quantify the association between one or more independent variables and an ordinal outcome.

ordinal scale of measurement: Classification of values of a variable into rank order, such as the degree of anxiety, academic achievement, or grade level. The classification defines which group is first, second, third, and so forth; however, it does not define the distance between categories.

ordinal variable: Variable having categories with an implicit ranking.

outcome measure: The specific test or procedure to measure the dependent variable. For example, an outcome measure for pain is the McGill-Melzack Pain Inventory.

outlier: A test result or score outside the normal range of values.

P

paired *t*-test (or correlated *t*-test): Used to compare two paired (dependent) samples where the outcome measure is continuous and normally distributed.

parameter: A descriptive value assigned to a condition in a population. Parameters are set at any given point in time, such as the age characteristics of a specified population.

parametric statistical tests: Inferential statistics that are based on certain assumptions, such as a normal distribution of variable values, equal number of participants in groups, homogeneity of variance, and independence of data.

Pearson product-moment correlation: An inferential test used to determine whether there is a statistically significant linear association between two variables. The derived *r* coefficient can range from +1.00 (a perfect correlation), to 0.00 (no correlation), to -1.00 (a perfect negative or inverse correlation).

percentage: The number of cases per hundred.

percentile: Value in a distribution below which a given percentage of the cases fall. For example, the 80th percentile is the point where 80% of the cases are at that point or below.

performance test: A test of an individual's skill to enact a task, such as grip strength, range of motion, manual dexterity, or driving skills.

personal equation in measurement: The effect of the presence of the tester on the participant's performance. The tester, as the evaluator, is a variable in the test situation and, if uncontrolled, can distort the test results.

pilot study: A research study usually with a small number of participants that is innovative but that does not control for all extraneous variables. The primary advantage of a pilot study is that it generates further research.

placebo effect: A confounding variable that occurs when the participant shows signs of improvement or in the reduction of symptoms that is not caused by the intervention under study. It is instead caused by the participant 's belief that an intervention is causing improvement even though the participant is receiving a "dummy" or "sham" intervention. The placebo effect was initially observed in drug studies where an experimental drug was compared to a placebo or nonactive drug. Researchers observed that some of the subjects receiving a placebo improved.

population (N): An entire collection of people (e.g., the entire University of South Dakota student body).

positive correlation: A relationship between two variables where high scores on one variable are associated with high scores on the other, as well as low scores on one with low scores on the other.

post-testing: Testing after the intervention has taken place.

postulate: An unproven, foundational assumption.

power: The ability of a study to detect a difference when one exists; probability of rejecting the null hypothesis when it is false.

predictive validity: The degree to which a test or measuring instrument can predict future performance, functioning, or behavior. For example, a test for performance of ADLs administered during an in-patient stay has good predictive validity in its estimation of ADL performance at home after discharge.

pre-testing: Testing before intervention is applied.

prevalence rate: The number of individuals with a disability or disease divided by the total individuals in a population. For example, the prevalence rate of spinal cord injury in the United States in 2014 is the number of individuals with spinal cord injury living in the United States in 2014 divided by the total population in the United States in 2014.

primary prevention: The prevention of the initial onset of a disease, such as the prevention of polio with a vaccination.

primary source: Published article or conference proceedings that is the original report of data, such as an empirical research study or a theoretical paper.

probability: The mathematical or statistical likelihood that an event will occur.

probability distribution: A description of the probability associated with all possible observed outcomes.

Probability value (p): The probability that the results found were the result of chance and not an actual difference in value. A smaller p-value allows for greater confidence in rejecting the null hypothesis of no difference. For example, $p < .01$ allows more confidence than $p < .05$, and $p < .001$ more than $p < .01$. Also known as *significance*.

problem-oriented research: Applied research initiated by the investigator identifying a significant problem, such as a rapid increase in attention deficit disorders in children or the dramatic rise of individuals who are homeless in urban areas. The research design addresses the problem directly.

Procrustean Bed: Applying an intervention as a panacea for all patients regardless of individual differences and needs. For example, applying a paraffin bath to all patients with arthritis, without regard to the specific needs of individual patients. In this approach, the patient is fitted to the intervention rather than the intervention being selected as the best indicated for this individual.

proportion: Fraction in which the numerator consists of a subset of individuals represented in the denominator.

prospective study: Research that is future oriented and attempts to discover cause-effect relationships between variables. In prospective studies, the investigator manipulates or observes an independent variable that is predicted to affect function or performance and then collects data. Experimental or longitudinal research are examples of prospective designs.

purposive sampling: Selective or nonobjective selection of participants.

p-value: The level of significance, or the risk of making a Type I error when the null hypothesis is rejected. In the social sciences, it is usually established at the .05 or .01 (alpha) level.

Q

qualitative research: Study of people and events in their natural setting. This type of research uses multimodal methods in a naturalistic setting. The researcher using qualitative research methods seeks to explore perceptions and experiences to understand phenomena in terms of the meanings that people ascribe to them. Data sources for this type of research include interviews with open-ended questions, prolonged participant observation, and document analysis.

qualitative variable: Variable that describes attributes (ordinal or nominal).

quantitative research: The application of the scientific method to test hypotheses. The quantitative researcher begins with a testable hypothesis, collects data, and uses statistical analyses to decide whether to accept or reject the hypothesis. Objectivity of the researcher, operational definitions of the variables, and control of extraneous factors are the key points in quantitative research.

quantitative variable: Variable that describes an amount or quantity (continuous or ratio).

quartile: A point in a distribution where 25% of the cases fall at or below that point. Quartiles are values that divide a set of data into four equal parts.

quasi-experimental designs: A term defined by Campbell and Stanley (1963) to identify research studies in which participants are not randomly assigned to equivalent groups. In general, most clinical research studies are within the quasi-experimental model because it is almost impossible to truly select a random sample from a target population or to have truly equivalent experimental and control groups.

quota sampling: Non-random sampling where the researcher tries to maintain proportional groups such as in a population of 60% female vs. 40% male; in this case, the quota sample would reflect this proportion.

R

r: Pearson correlation coefficient.

r^2: A statistic that is associated with a regression model and represents the portion of the observed variance that is accounted for by the regression model. The higher the r^2 value, the better the regression model is at defining the relationship between the independent and dependent variables.

random assignment: Assigning participants to multiple groups with each participant having an equal chance of being selected for any one of the groups.

random errors: The effect of uncontrolled variables in an experiment, such as unexpected events, test procedural errors, and anxiety within the participant. These errors are unpredictable and unsystematic.

random sample: An unbiased portion of a target population that has been selected by chance, such as through random numbers.

randomization: A process that involves selecting a participant or entity for a specific assignment with no predetermined bias, that is, through chance.

randomized controlled trial (RCT): A prospective study where participants are randomly assigned to either an intervention group or a control group, thereby avoiding administrator bias.

range: A measure of variability that is the difference between the highest and lowest values in a distribution of scores.

rank order variables: Examples of ordinal scale measurement in which ranks are assigned in measuring a variable. Most personality tests, such as the Minnesota Multiphasic Personality Inventory, measure rank order variables.

rating scale: An evaluator's appraisal regarding variables such as competence, nonacademic qualities in students, or patient behavior in a psychiatric hospital.

ratio scale of measurement: Quantification of a variable that includes equal intervals and an absolute zero point, such as in measuring heart rate, height, and weight. Comparative statements using "twice as" or "half" are possible with ratio scales.

referral source: A database that lists journal articles and books (e.g., Index Medicus), and information retrieval systems accessed by computer (e.g., OT Search, ERIC, MedLine, email, news lists).

regression analysis: Statistical method used to describe the association between one dependent variable and one or more independent variables; used to adjust for confounding variables.

regression line: A figure that best describes the linear relationship between the X and Y variables. In a high correlation, the researcher is able to predict the unknown value of Y from the known value of X with a certain high level of confidence.

regression to the mean: When an initial very high or very low score usually comes closer to the group mean upon re-measurement.

relative frequency: The ratio of the number of observations having a certain characteristic or value divided by the total number of observations.

reliability: A measure of the consistency of a test instrument. For example, a test has high reliability if it produces consistent results when measuring a variable. Threats to test reliability include ambiguity in the questions and poor implementation of exact test procedures. Reliability is indicated by the correlation coefficient (r). An acceptable test reliability is usually an r of .7 or above.

repeated measures analysis of variance: Measurements are made repeatedly on each participant (e.g., before, during, and after an intervention). Repeated measures ANOVAs are suited for 2 x 2 (or larger) designs where one or both factors are repeated or where there are repeated factors in a 1 x n design.

repeated measures designs: The replication of observations of the effects of interventions over a period of time (e.g., measuring the effects of biofeedback in reducing anxiety after meditation or exercise).

replicate a research design: To carry out a research design for the second time by replicating the research methodology. The purposes are to strengthen generalizability of the findings and to confirm the internal validity of the original study.

representative sample: An unbiased portion of a target population that is representative in terms of demographic characteristics.

research: The systematic and unbiased investigation into a topic by stating a hypothesis, guiding question, or purpose and collecting primary data. It includes quantitative and qualitative designs.

research question (or purpose of the study): The central question that should be answered by the research. A good research article has this labeled clearly, either at the beginning or after reviewing some literature.

response rate: The number and proportion of responses to a researcher's questionnaire or survey. If a researcher sends surveys to 100 people, and 89 respond, then the response rate is 89%.

retrospective study: Research based on causative factors that have already occurred. For example, in a correlational study the researcher may want to examine the relationship between the onset of emphysema and previous smoking behavior. Both variables have already occurred. The researcher tries to reconstruct events and to hypothesize regarding a possible cause-effect relationship. Retrospective research can be used to justify experimental designs to further investigate cause-effect relationships.

rigor: Refers to the systematic control of variables that may affect the results of a study.

risk-benefit ratio: Estimation by the investigator of the possible risks to the research participant and the benefits accrued from the study. The researcher reveals the potential risks and benefits to prospective participants in the study through an informed consent form.

S

sample (n): A subset of a population. For example, a random sample of occupational therapy students from the University of South Dakota.

sampling error: The error that results from estimating a population value from a sample.

scales of measurement: The level at which a test or instrument measures a specific variable such as intelligence, behavior, personality, muscle strength, or academic achievement. Traditionally, scales of measurement are classified into four levels: nominal, ordinal, interval, and ratio.

scattergram, scatter diagram, scatterplot: A figure describing the relationship between the X and Y variables, where pairs of values are plotted as points on a two-dimensional graph.

scientific law: A statement of consistent and uniform occurrences that are predictable (e.g., Mendelian law of genetic determination predicts characteristics of offspring when genetic traits of parents are known).

scientific method: Non-biased, systematic investigation into a subject by stating a hypothesis, collecting empirical data, and considering alternative explanations of the results.

secondary prevention: The prevention of the recurrence of a disease, such as preventing a second stroke in an individual.

secondary source: A published article or book that reviews primary sources, such as a literature review.

selection bias: Participants selected for a research study are selected in a non-random method and may not be representative of the target population.

self-evaluation method: Participants in a clinical research study assess their own progress. Self-evaluation is an important factor in assessing intervention effectiveness. Other methods used in assessing effectiveness include objective tests, psychophysiological measures, and mechanical procedures.

self-fulfilling prophecy: The expectation by the researcher or rater that a participant will perform at a certain level based on prejudice or bias toward the group to which the participant belongs.

semantic differential: An attitude scale in which the respondent rates concepts such as good-bad, fast-slow, and hard-soft.

sensitivity: As applied to test measurement, it is the degree to which a test or assessment measures what it purports to measure. This is also known as *true positive rate*. The reliability and validity of a test instrument would impact its sensitivity to measure a variable. *See also* specificity.

significance: The probability that the results presented are a result of chance and not an actual difference in values. A smaller significance allows for greater confidence in rejecting the null hypothesis of no difference. Also known as *probability value* or *p-value*.

significance level: In testing a hypothesis, it is the predetermined level of confidence required in order to reject the null hypothesis (alpha level), usually .05 or .01.

simple linear regression: Regression analysis used to quantify the association between one independent variable and a continuous outcome that is normally distributed.

simple logistic regression: Regression analysis used to quantify the association between one independent variable and a dichotomous outcome.

single-case experimental design (SCED): Research design that systematically compares the performance of a participant under experimental and control conditions. It may include more than one participant, but comparisons are made only within each participant's performance. Common designs include ABA and ABAB, where A is the baseline condition and B is the experimental (intervention) condition. Not be confused with a case study.

skewed distribution: A distribution of values that is not symmetric (i.e., not bell-shaped).

- **positively skewed:** Data are distributed such that a greater proportion of the observations have values less than or equal to the mean (i.e., more observations with lower values).

- **negatively skewed:** Data are distributed such that a greater proportion of the observations have values greater than or equal to the mean (i.e., more observations with higher values).

skewness: An indication in a frequency polygon of the asymmetry of a distribution. A distribution can be skewed to the right or left side of the polygon.

slope: The linear direction and angle of a line. It is calculated in the regression line.

Spearman rank correlation: Nonparametric test used on two ordinal variables to determine the degree of relationship between them. It is an alternative to the Pearson product-moment correlation coefficient (*r*). Also called *Spearman rho*.

specificity: The ability of a test to accurately identify individuals without a specific disease. This is also known as a test's *true negative rate*. *See also* sensitivity.

split-half reliability: A method to estimate the degree of consistency in a test by correlating one half of the test items, such as even numbered items, with the other half of the test, the odd numbered items.

standard deviation (SD): Statistical measure of the variability of scores from the mean. This is one measure of dispersion or variability. The larger the standard deviation, the more varied the data. Standard deviation equals the square root of the variance.

standard error of measurement (SEM or SE$_m$): statistical value that indicates the band of error surrounding a test score. For example, a raw score of 90 with an SEM of 4 indicates a true score probably ranging from 86 to 94.

standard score: Calculated by subtracting a raw score from the mean and then dividing the difference by the standard deviation. The sign of the standard score is positive if above the mean or negative if below the mean.

standardized test: A test that has been administered to a target population and for which norms are available.

statistical assumptions: Conditions in research required for a specific statistical test. These assumptions relate to distribution shape of scores, variability of scores, scale of measurement, sample size, and independence of samples.

statistical pie: A descriptive statistic using the circumference of a circle to describe the percentage of cases for each category within a frequency distribution.

statistical sample: A portion of a target population selected to represent the population in an unbiased way.

statistical significance: Probability of the result of a statistical test occurring by chance. For example, a *p* level of 0.01 means that you can be 99% confident that these results did not happen due to chance. Most researchers in occupational therapy accept the .05 level of statistical significance (95% confidence interval).

stem-and-leaf display: Descriptive data analysis that orders and organizes data to display trends and patterns in a distribution. The stem contains the first digit or digits of each observation and the leaf contains the remaining digit or digits of each observation.

survey research: Systematic and objective investigation into the characteristics, attitudes, opinions, and behaviors of target populations through questionnaires or interviews.

T

target population: An identified group from which a representative or random sample of participants is selected.

tertiary prevention: The prevention of secondary problems that can result from a disability (e.g., preventing decubiti in individuals with spinal cord injury).

test battery: A group of tests selected to comprehensively measure an individual's capacity (e.g., performance, vocational interests, attitudes, cognition).

test-retest reliability: A method to estimate the degree of consistency of a test. In this method, a test is readministered to the same group of participants after a short period of time. Maturation and changes in the subjects can affect the results and must be considered by the investigator.

theory: A comprehensive model that attempts to explain, for example, how individuals contract and resist disease, learn motoric tasks, or develop cognitive and language functions.

time series research: In experimental research, time series research indicates the measurement of the dependent variable over time intervals (e.g., 2 weeks or 3 months). Its purpose is to evaluate the effect of several interventions or techniques with the same participant or group.

transformational research: The use of research as a personal-political activity whereby the research participants become empowered by active engagement in the research process.

treatment effects: In experimental research, the application of the independent variable in producing a desired or predicted outcome (e.g., the use of sensory integration therapy in reducing tactile defensiveness).

treatment protocols: Operational definitions of the methods used by practitioners. The procedure is described in enough detail so that replication is possible. Treatment protocols should be influenced by research findings and are a component of evidence-based practice.

triangulation: The use of multiple approaches in collecting data. For example, in measuring a variable such as functional independence, the investigator would use a standardized ADL scale, make observations in a naturalistic setting, and employ a self-report measure where the patient evaluates his or her performance in self-care activities.

***t*-tests:** Inferential statistics used to determine whether the difference between two means is statistically significant or is too likely to have occurred by chance. They include one-sample *t*-test, independent *t*-test, and correlated or paired-data *t*-test. For testing two independent groups with approximately the same variance, the formula is:

$$t = \frac{mean_1 - mean_2}{standard\ error\ of\ the\ difference\ between\ the\ means}$$

Type I error: The error that results when the null hypothesis is rejected when it is really true; stating there is a difference in outcome when none exists. It is analogous to a false positive in medicine when a physician diagnoses a disease when that disease is not present.

Type II error: The error that results when the null hypothesis is not rejected when it is really false; stating there is no difference in outcome when one actually exists. It is analogous to a false negative in medicine when a physician fails to detect a disease when that disease is present.

U

unobtrusive methodology: A research method in which the investigator collects data from indirect sources, such as patient records, historical documents, letters, and relics.

unpaired (independent) sample: Study design that compares the outcome of two groups where the groups are not matched on any characteristic.

V

validity: As pertaining to measurement, it refers to the degree to which a test or measuring instrument actually measures what it purports to measure. Validity can also refer to the rigor of an experiment in controlling extraneous variables (internal validity) and the generalizability of the results of a study to a target population (external validity).

variability: *See* measures of variability.

variables: Characteristics, factors, or attributes that can be measured qualitatively or quantitatively. Variables can be homogeneous groups, such as physical therapy students, individuals with stroke, or hospital administrators. Variables can also be interventions, such as exercise or biofeedback, or outcomes, such as muscle strength, spasticity, functional capacity, or academic achievement.

variance: The average of each score's deviation from the mean. Variance is an intermediate value that is used in calculating the standard deviation. The variance is the square of the standard deviation. It is a measure of variability or dispersion.

vocational interest test: A measure of an individual's preferences toward occupation-related tasks or jobs.

W

Wilcoxon signed rank test for correlated samples: Nonparametric test and alternative to the correlated *t*-test when comparing matched participants or two sets of scores from the same participants, such as in before-and-after studies.

within subjects test: The scores of participants in an experimental study that are compared (e.g., pre- and post-intervention or by repeated measures on a test). Each participant is his or her own control.

work samples: Well-defined activities that are similar to an actual job task. Examples include Valpar and Micro-Tower.

Z

z-score: A score based on standard deviation units from the mean (e.g., a *z*-score of +1 is one standard deviation unit above the mean).

References

Achenbach, T. M. (1991). *Achenbach system of empirically based assessment: Manual for the teacher's report form and 1991 profile.* Burlington, VT: University Medical Education Associates

Ackoff, R. L., & Rivett, P. (1963). *A manager's guide to operational research.* New York, NY: John Wiley & Sons.

Adger, C. (1994). *Enhancing the delivery of services to Black special education students from non-standard English backgrounds. Final Report.* College Park: Maryland University, College Park Institute for the Study of Exceptional Children and Youth. (ERIC Document Reproduction Service No ED 370-377)

Adler, P. A., & Adler, P. (1994). Observational techniques. In N. K. Denzin & Y. S. Lincoln (Eds.), *Handbook of qualitative research* (pp. 377-392). Thousand Oaks, CA: Sage Publications.

Affleck, J. W., Aitken, R. C, Hunter, J. A., McGuire, R. J., & Roy, C. W. (1988). Rehabilitation status: A measure of medicosocial dysfunction. *Lancet, 1,* 230-233.

Ahmed, M. B. (2001). Alzheimer's disease: Recent advances in etiology, diagnosis, and management. *Texas Medicine, 97*(12), 50-58.

Alberg, A. J., & Samet, J. M. (2003). Epidemiology of lung cancer. *Chest, 123*(Suppl.), 21S-49S.

Allen, C. K. (1985). *Occupational therapy for psychiatric diseases: Measurement and management of cognitive disabilities.* Boston, MA: Little, Brown.

Allen, C. K., Austin, S. L., David, S. K., Earhart, C. A., McCraith, D. B., & Riska-Williams, L. (2007). *Allen Cognitive Level Screen-5 (ACLS-5)/Large Allen Cognitive Level Screen-5 (LACLS-5).* Camarillo, CA: ACLS and LACLS Committee.

Allen, C. K., Earhart, C. A., & Blue, T. (1992). *Occupational therapy treatment goals for the physically and cognitively disabled.* Rockville, MD: American Occupational Therapy Association.

Alpern, G. D. (2007). *Developmental profile 3 (DP-3).* Los Angeles, CA: Western Psychological Services.

Als, H., Butler, S., Kosta, S., & McAnulty, G. (2005). The Assessment of Preterm Infants' Behavior (APIB): Furthering the understanding and measurement of neurodevelopmental competence in preterm and full-term infants. *Mental Retardation and Developmental Disabilities Research Reviews, 11*(1), 94-102.

American Association of Intellectual and Developmental Disabilities. (2017). Mission. Retrieved from https://aaidd.org/about-aaidd/mission#.WdL8iBNSx24

American Educational Research Association, American Psychological Association, and National Council on Measurement in Education. (1974). *Standards for educational and psychological testing.* Washington, DC: Author.

American Physical Therapy Association. (2008). *Guidelines: Occupational health physical therapy: Evaluating functional capacity.* Retrieved from https://www.orthopt.org/uploads/content_files/OHSIG_Guidelines/Occupational_Hlth_PT_Evaluating_Functional_Capacity_040610__2_.pdf

American Psychiatric Association. (1994). *Diagnostic and statistical manual of mental disorders* (4th ed.). Washington, DC: Author.

American Psychiatric Association. (2000). *Diagnostic and statistical manual of mental disorders—Text revision* (DSM–IV–TR). Arlington, VA: Author.

American Psychiatric Association. (2013). *Diagnostic and statistical manual of mental disorders* (DSM-5). Washington, DC: Author.

American Psychological Association. (2011). *Publication manual of the American Psychological Association* (6th ed.). Washington, DC: Author.

American Occupational Therapy Association. (1985). *Standards of Practice for Occupational Therapy.* Rockville, MD: Author.

American Occupational Therapy Association. (2002). *Occupational therapy practice framework: Domain and process.* Bethesda, MD: Author.

American Occupational Therapy Association. (2008). Occupational therapy practice framework: Domain and Process (2nd ed.). *American Journal of Occupational Therapy, 62,* 625-683.

American Occupational Therapy Association. (2014). Occupational therapy practice framework: Domain and process (3rd ed.). *American Journal of Occupational Therapy, 68*(Suppl. 1), S1-S48.

American Occupational Therapy Foundation. (n.d.). Resources & the Wilma L. West (WLW) library. Retrieved from http://www.aotf.org/resourceswlwlibrary

Americans with Disabilities Act of 1990 (1990). (HCUP), H. C. a. U. P. (2018). SASD Database Documentation. Rockville, MD.

AMPS Project International. (2010). *Assessment of motor and process skills.* Retrieved from http://www.innovativeotsolutions.com/tools/amps

Anastasi, A. (1988). *Psychological testing* (6th ed.). New York, NY: Macmillan.

Anastasi, A., & Urbina, S. (1997). *Psychological testing* (7th ed.). Englewood Cliffs, NJ: Prentice Hall.

Anderson, M. H., Bechtol, C. O., & Sollaris, R. E. (1959). *Clinical prosthetics for physicians and therapists: A handbook of clinical practices related to artificial limbs.* Springfield, IL: Charles C. Thomas.

Anderson, P. J., & Burnett, A. (2017). Assessing developmental delay in early childhood—concerns with the Bayley-III scales. *The Clinical Neuropsychologist, 31,* 371-381.

Annual Reviews. (2018). *Welcome to Annual Reviews.* Retrieved: https://www.annualreviews.org/.

Applegate, S. L., Rice, M. S., Stein, F., & Maitra, K. K. (2008). Knowledge of results and learning to tell the time in an adult male with an intellectual disability: A single-subject research design. *Occupational Therapy International, 15,* 32-44.

Applegate, W. B., Blass, J. P., & Williams, T. F. (1990). Instruments for the functional assessment of older patients. *New England Journal of Medicine, 322,* 1207-1214.

Arps, G. F. (1920). Work with knowledge of results versus work without knowledge of results: Awareness and partial awareness as factors conditioning efficiency. *Psychological Monographs, 28*(3), i-41.

Arthanat, S., Curtin, C., & Kontak, D. (2015). An evaluation protocol for selection of educational technologies for students with developmental disabilities: A demonstration study using iPad apps. *Journal of Occupational Therapy, Schools, & Early Intervention, 8,* 236-255.

Rice, M. S., Stein, F., & Tomlin, G.
Clinical Research in Occupational Therapy, Sixth Edition (pp. 429-445).
© 2019 Taylor & Francis Group.

Arthur, G. (1949). The Arthur adaptation of the Leiter International Performance Scale. *Journal of Clinical Psychology, 5*, 345-349.

Åsberg, M., Perris, C., Schalling, D., & Sedval, G. (1987). The CPRS—Development and applications of a psychiatric rating scale. *Acta Psychiatrica Scandinavia, 27*(Suppl.), 1-27.

Asher, I. E. (Ed.) (2007). *Occupational therapy assessment tools: An annotated index* (3rd ed.). Rockville, MD: American Occupational Therapy Association.

Atwal, A., Spiliotopoulou, G., Stradden, J., Fellows, V., Anako, E., Robinson, L., & McIntyre, A. (2014). Factors influencing occupational therapy home visit practice: A qualitative study. *Scandinavian Journal of Occupational Therapy, 21*, 40-47.

Atwater, E. C. (1973). The medical profession in a new society, Rochester, New York (1811-60). *Bulletin of the History of Medicine, 47*, 221-235.

Ayres, A. J. (1972). *Sensory integration and learning disorders.* Torrance, CA: Western Psychological Services.

Ayres, A. J. (1989). *Sensory integration and praxis tests (SIPT).* Torrance, CA: Western Psychological Services.

Babbie, E. R. (2010). *The practice of social research.* Belmont, CA: Wadsworth Cengage.

Backman, M. E. (1977). *The development of Micro-TOWER: A battery of standardized work samples for assessing vocational aptitudes.* (ERIC Document Reproduction Service No ED152834)

Baillargeon-Normand, F., Rochette, A., & Gaulin, P. (2016). Circumstances surrounding stroke onset: symbolic meaning of time factors related to numbers and days of the week. *Disability and Rehabilitation, 38*, 282-288.

Baldwin, B. T. (1919). *Occupational therapy applied to the restoration of the function of disabled joints.* Report of the Department of Occupational Therapy: (Monograph) Walter Reed General Hospital, Tacoma Park, DC: Published by the Authority of the Surgeon General of the Army.

Bamm, E. L., Rosenbaum, P., Wilkins, S., Stratford, P., & Mahlberg, N. (2015). Exploring client-centered care experiences in in-patient rehabilitation settings. *Global Qualitative Nursing Research, 2*, 2333393615582036.

Baptiste, S. (2008). Client-centered assessment: The Canadian Occupational Performance Measure. In B. J. Hemphill-Pearson (Ed.), *Assessments in occupational therapy mental health: An integrative approach* (2nd ed., pp. 35-47). Thorofare, NJ: SLACK Incorporated.

Baratchi, M., Meratnia, N., Havinga, P. J., Skidmore, A. K., & Toxopeus, B. A. (2013). Sensing solutions for collecting spatio-temporal data for wildlife monitoring applications: A review. *Sensors (Basel, Switzerland), 13*, 6054-6088.

Barnhart, R. C. (2001). Aging adult children with developmental disabilities and their families: Challenges for occupational therapists and physical therapists. *Physical and Occupational Therapy in Pediatrics, 21*(4), 69-81.

Barrett, A. J., & Murk, P. J. (2006). *Life satisfaction index for the third age (LSITA): A measurement of successful aging.* Retrieved from http://hdl.handle.net/1805/1160

Barton, G. E. (1919). *Teaching the sick: A manual of occupational therapy as reeducation.* Philadelphia, PA: W. B. Saunders Company.

Barzun, J. (1974). *Clio and the doctors: Psycho-history, quanto-history, & history.* Chicago, IL: University of Chicago Press.

Barzun, J., & Graff, H. (1970). *The modern researcher.* New York, NY: Harcourt, Brace and World.

Batool, S., Soomro, N., Amjad, F., & Fauz, R. (2015). To compare the effectiveness of constraint induced movement therapy versus motor relearning programme to improve motor function of hemiplegic upper extremity after stroke. *Pakistan Journal of Medical Sciences, 31*, 1167-1171.

Baum, C. M., Connor, L. T., Morrison, T., Hahn, M., Dromerick, A. W., & Edwards, D. F. (2008). Reliability, validity, and clinical utility of the Executive Function Performance Test: A measure of executive function in a sample of people with stroke. *American Journal of Occupational Therapy, 62*(4), 446-455.

Bayley, N. (2005). *Bayley Scales of Infant and Toddler Development* (3rd ed.). San Antonio. TX: Pearson.

Beard, J. D. (2008). Which is the best revascularization for critical limb ischemia: Endovascular or open surgery? *Journal of Vascular Surgery, 48*(6 Suppl.), 11S-16S.

Beck, A. T., Ward, C. H., Mendelson, M., Mock, J., & Erbaugh, J. (1961). An inventory for measuring depression. *Archives of General Psychiatry, 4*, 561-571.

Becker, R. L. (1981). *Reading-Free Vocational Interest Inventory.* Columbus, OH: Elbern Publications.

Becker, R. L. (2000). *Reading-Free Vocational Interest Inventory-Revised (R-FVII:2).* Columbus, OH: Elbern Publications.

Beers, C. (1908). *A mind that found itself: An autobiography.* New York, NY: Doubleday.

Beery, K. K., Buktenica, N. A., & Beery, N. A. (2010). *Beery-Buktenica Developmental Test of Visual-Motor Integration* (6th ed.; VMI-6). San Antonio, TX: Pearson.

Bellows, L. L., Gavin, W. J., Johnson, S. L., Boles, R. E., & Davies, P. (2015). Obesity prevention study: A physical activity program improved gross motor skills in preschool children. *American Journal of Occupational Therapy, 69.* doi: 10.5014/ajot.2015.69S1-RP304D.

Bender, L. (1938). *A visual motor Gestalt test and its clinical use.* Crozet, VA: American Orthopsychiatric Association

Benison, S. (1972). The history of polio research in the United States: Appraisal and lessons. In G. Holton (Ed.), *Twentieth century sciences: Studies in the biography of ideas* (pp. 306-343). New York, NY: W. W. Norton & Company.

Bennett, A. E., Power, T. J., Eiraldi, R. B., Leff, S. S., & Blum, N. J. (2009). Identifying learning problems in children evaluated for ADHD: The academic performance questionnaire. *Pediatrics, 124*(4), e633-e639.

Bennett, G. K. (1946). *Hand Tool Dexterity Test.* San Antonio, TX: Pearson/PsychCorp.

Bennett, G. K. (1994). *Bennett Mechanical Comprehension Test.* San Antonio, TX: Pearson/PsychCorp.

Bennett, G. K., & Fry, D. E. (1969). *Bennett Mechanical Comprehension Test.* New York, NY: Psychological Corporation.

Berg, K. O., Wood-Dauphinee, S. L., Williams, J. I., & Maki, B. (1992). Measuring balance in the elderly: Validation of an instrument. *Canadian Journal of Public Health, 83*, S7-S11.

Bergner, M., Bobbitt, R. A., Carter, W. B., & Gilson, B. S. (1981). The Sickness Impact Profile: Development and final revision of a health status measure. *Medical Care, 19*, 787-805.

Bernard, C. (1957). *An introduction to the study of experimental medicine* (H. C. Greene, Trans.). New York, NY: Dover. (Original work published 1865)

Bertilson, B., Grunnesjö, M., Johansson, S. E., & Strender, L. E. (2007). Pain drawing in the assessment of neurogenic pain and dysfunction in the neck/shoulder region: Inter-examiner reliability and concordance with clinical examination. *Pain Medicine, 8*(2), 134-146.

Best, J. W. (1977). *Research in education.* Englewood Cliffs, NJ: Prentice Hall.

Best, J. W., & Kahn, J. V. (2016). *Research in education* (10th ed.). India: Pearson Education.

Best, S., & Knapp-Lee, L. (1982). Relationship of interest measurement derived from the COPSystem Interest Inventory and the Kuder General Interest Survey: Construct validation of two measures of occupational activity preferences. *Educational and Psychological Measurement, 42*(4), 1289-1293.

Bettelheim, B. (1967). *The empty fortress: Infantile autism and the birth of the self.* New York, NY: Free Press.

Betz, N. E., Borgen, F. H., & Harmon, L. W. (2004). *Strong Interest Inventory*. Mountain View, CA: CPP, Inc.

Binet, A. (1899/1912). *The psychology of reasoning: based on experimental researches in hypnotism* (A. G. Whyte, Trans.; 2nd ed.). Chicago, IL: The Open Court Publishing Company.

Binet, A., & Simon, T. (1916). *The development of intelligence in children: The Binet-Simon Scale*. Baltimore, MD: Lippincott Williams & Wilkins.

Blake, J. B., & Roos, C. (1967). *Medical reference works 1679-1966: A selected bibliography*. Chicago, IL: Medical Library Association.

Blue, F. R. (1979). Aerobic running as a treatment for moderate depression. *Perceptual and Motor Skills, 48*(1), 228.

Blumberg, D. F. (1971). The city as a system. *Simulation, 17*(4), 155-167.

Bockoven, J. S. (1971). Occupational therapy—A historical perspective. Legacy of moral treatment—1800's to 1910. *American Journal of Occupational Therapy, 25*, 223-225.

Bohannon, R. W., Peolsson, A., Massy-Westropp, N., Desrosiers, J., & Bear-Lehman, J. (2006). Reference values for adult grip strength measured with a Jamar dynamometer: A descriptive meta-analysis. *Physiotherapy, 92*, 11-15. doi:10.1016/j.physio.2005.05.003

Bone, C., Cheung, G., & Wade, B. (2010). Evaluating person centred care and dementia care mapping in a psychogeriatric hospital in New Zealand: A pilot study. *New Zealand Journal of Occupational Therapy, 57*, 35-40.

Bootes, K., & Chapparo, C. J. (2002). Cognitive and behavioural assessment of people with traumatic brain injury in the work place: occupational therapists' perceptions. *Work, 19*, 255-268.

Booth, T., & Booth, W. (1994). The use of depth interviewing with vulnerable subjects: Lessons from a research study of parents with learning difficulties. *Social Science and Medicine, 39*, 415-424.

Bosscher, R. J. (1993). Running and mixed physical exercises with depressed psychiatric patients. *International Journal of Sport Psychology, 24*, 170-184.

Bowling, A. (2005). *Measuring health: A review of quality of life measurement scales* (3rd ed.). Buckingham, United Kingdom: Open University Press/McGraw-Hill.

Bowman, J., & Llewellyn, G. (2002). Clinical outcomes research from the occupational therapist's perspective. *Occupational Therapy International, 9*, 145-166.

Brannigan, G. G., & Decker, S. L. (2003). *Bender visual-motor Gestalt test-II* (2nd ed.). Itasca, IL: Riverside Publishing.

Brayman, S. J. (2008). The Comprehensive Occupational Therapy Evaluation (COTE). In B. J. Hemphill-Pearson (Ed.), *Assessments in occupational therapy mental health: An integrative approach* (2nd ed., pp. 113-124). Thorofare, NJ: SLACK Incorporated.

Brayman, S. J., Kirby, T. F., Meisenheimer, A. M., & Short, M. J. (1976). The comprehensive occupational therapy evaluation scale. *American Journal of Occupational Therapy, 30*, 94-100.

Brollier, C., Hamrick, N., & Jackson, B. (1994). Aerobic exercise: A potential occupational therapy modality for adolescents with depression. *Occupational Therapy in Mental Health, 12*, 19-29.

Bronfenbrenner, U. (1979). *The ecology of human development: Experiments by nature and design*. Cambridge, MA: Harvard University.

Bruininks, R. H. (1978). *Bruininks-Oseretsky Test of Motor Proficiency*. Circle Pines, MN: American Guidance Service.

Bruininks, R. H., & Bruininks, B. D. (2005). *Bruininks-Oseretsky Test of Motor Proficiency, Second Edition* (BOT-2). San Antonio, TX: Pearson/PsychCorp

Brunner, T. M., & Spielberger, C. D. (2009). *State-Trait Anger Expression Inventory-2™ Child and Adolescent (STAXI-2™ C/A)*. Lutz, FL: PAR, Inc.

Bryman, A., & Burgess, R. G. (Eds.). (1994). *Developments in qualitative data analysis: An introduction*. New York, NY: Routledge.

BTE Technologies. (2018). Physical therapy equipment, occupational therapy equipment, & athletic training equipment. Retrieved from http://www.btetech.com

Bulmer, M. (1982). *Social research ethics: An examination of the merits of covert participant observation*. London, United Kingdom: Macmillan.

Burckhardt, C. S., & Anderson, K. L. (2003). The Quality of Life Scale (QOLS): Reliability, validity, and utilization. *Health and Quality of Life Outcomes, 1*(1), 60.

Burke, J. P., & Gitlin, L. N. (2012). How do we change practice when we have the evidence? *American Journal of Occupational Therapy, 66*, e85-e88.

Burks, H. F., & Gruber, C. P. (2006). *Burks' Behavior Rating Scale–2 (BBRS-2)*. Los Angeles, CA: Western Psychological Services.

Burnett, J., Dyer, C. M., & Naik, A. D. (2009). Convergent validation of the Kohlman Evaluation of Living Skills as a screening tool of older adults' ability to live safely and independently in the community. *Archives of Physical Medicine and Rehabilitation, 90*, 1948-1952.

Burns, T., Mortimer, J. A., & Merchak, P. (1994). Cognitive Performance Test: A new approach to functional assessment in Alzheimer's disease. *Journal of Geriatric Psychiatry and Neurology, 7*, 46-54.

Cahill, S. M., McGuire, B., Krumdick, N. D., & Lee, M. M. (2014). National survey of occupational therapy practitioners' involvement in response to intervention. *American Journal of Occupational Therapy, 68*, e234-e240.

Callinan, N. J., & Mathiowetz, V. (1996). Soft versus hard resting hand splints in rheumatoid arthritis: Pain relief, preference, and compliance. *American Journal of Occupational Therapy, 50*, 347-353.

Campbell, D. T., & Stanley, J. C. (1963). *Experimental and quasi-experimental designs for research*. Chicago, IL: Rand McNally.

Campbell, V. L. (1987). Strong-Campbell interest inventory, fourth edition. *Journal of Counseling & Development, 66*, 53-56.

Campione, J. C., & Brown, A. L. (1978). Toward a theory of intelligence: Contributions from research with retarded children. *Intelligence, 2*, 279-304.

Cannon, W. B. (1932). *The wisdom of the body*. New York, NY: W. W. Norton & Company.

Carey, R. G., & Posavac, E. J. (1982). Rehabilitation program evaluation using a revised level of rehabilitation scale (LORS–II). *Archives of Physical Medicine and Rehabilitation, 63*, 367-370.

Carlson, J. F., Geisinger, K. F., & Jonson, J. L. (2014). *The nineteenth mental measurements yearbook*. Lincoln, NE: Buros Center for Testing.

Carlsson, A. M. (1983). Assessment of chronic pain. I. Aspects of the reliability and validity of the Visual Analogue Scale. *Pain, 16*, 87-101. doi:10.1016/0304-3959(83)90088-X

Carter, N., Bryant-Lukosius, D., DiCenso, A., Blythe, J., & Neville, A. J. (2014). The use of triangulation in qualitative research. *Oncology Nursing Forum, 41*, 545-547.

Casby, J. A., & Holm, M. B. (1994). The effect of music on repetitive disruptive vocalizations of persons with dementia. *American Journal of Occupational Therapy, 48*, 883-889.

Case-Smith, J., & O'Brien, J. C. (2015). *Occupational therapy for children and adolescents* (7th ed.). St. Louis, MO: Elsevier.

Cattell, J. M. K. (1890). Mental tests and measurements. *Mind, 15*, 373-381.

Cattell, R. B. (1950). *Culture Fair Intelligence Test*. Champaign, IL: Institute for Personality and Ability Testing.

Cattell, R. B. (1963). Theory of fluid and crystallized intelligence: A critical experiment. *Journal of Educational Psychology, 54*, 615-618.

Cattell, R. B., Cattell, A. K., & Cattell, H. E. P. (1993). *Sixteen Personality Factor Questionnaire* (5th ed.). San Antonio, TX: Pearson/Psych Corp.

Center for Innovative OT Solutions (2018). Amps overview. Retrieved from https://www.innovativeotsolutions.com/tools/amps/

Chae, G. S., & Chang, M. (2016). The correlation between occupational performance and well-being in stroke patients. *Journal of Physical Therapy Science, 28*, 1712-1715.

Chang, Y. J., Chen, S. F., & Huang, J. D. (2011). A Kinect-based system for physical rehabilitation: A pilot study for young adults with motor disabilities. *Research in Developmental Disabilities, 32*(6), 2566-2570.

Cheng, T. C. E. (1993). Operations research and higher education administration. *Journal of Educational Administration, 31*(1) 77-99.

Childs, J. D., Piva, S., R., & Fritz, J. M. (2005). Responsiveness of the numeric pain rating scale in patients with low back pain. *Spine, 30,* 1331-1334. doi: 10.1097/01.brs. 0000164099.92112.29

Chiu, T., & Oliver, R. (2006). Factor analysis and construct validity of the SAFER-HOME. *OTJR: Occupation Participation and Health, 26*(4): 132-142.

Chiu, T., Oliver, R., Marshall, L., & Letts, L. (2001). *Safety Assessment of Functional and the Environment of Rehabilitation (SAFER) tool manual.* Toronto, Ontario, Canada: COTA Comprehensive Rehabilitation and Mental Health Services.

Clandinin, D. J., & Connelly, F. M. (1994). Personal experience methods. In N. K. Denzin & Y. S. Lincoln (Eds.), *Handbook of qualitative research* (pp. 413-427). Thousand Oaks, CA: Sage.

Clark, F., Azen, S. P., Zemke R., Jackson, J., Carlson, M., Mandel, D., … Lipson, L. (1997). Occupational therapy for independent-living older adults. A randomized controlled trial. *Journal of American Medical Association, 278,* 1321-1326.

Clarke, G. N., Rohde, P., Lewinsohn, P. M., Hops, H., & Seeley, J. R. (1999). Cognitive-behavioral treatment of adolescent depression: Efficacy of acute group treatment and booster sessions. *Journal of the American Academy of Child and Adolescent Psychiatry, 38,* 272-279.

Clemson, L., Bundy, A., Unsworth, C., & Fiatarone Singh, M. (2008). *Assessment of Living Skills and Resources–Revised 2 (ALSAR-R2).* Sydney, Australia: University of Sydney. Retrieved from http://sydney.edu.au/health_sciences/ageing_ work_health/docs/Clemson_ALSAR.pdf

Cochrane Library (2018). *About the Cochrane Library.* Retrieved https://www.cochranelibrary.com/about/about-cochrane-library

Cockburn, L. (2005). Canadian occupational therapists' contributions to prisoners of war in World War II. *Canadian Journal of Occupational Therapy, 72,* 183-188.

Cohen, J. (1988). *Statistical power analysis for the behavioral sciences* (2nd ed.). Hillsdale, NJ: Lawrence Erlbaum Associates.

Colarusso, R. P., & Hammill, D. D. (2015). *Motor Free Visual Perceptual Test-4* (MFVPT-4; 4th ed.). Novato, CA: Academic Therapy Publications.

Collen, F. M., Wade, D. T., Robb, G. F., & Bradshaw, C. M. (1991). The Rivermead Mobility Index: A further development of the Rivermead Motor Assessment. *International Disability Studies, 13,* 50-54.

Collin, C., Wade, D. T., Davies, S., & Horne, V. (1988). The Barthel ADL Index: A reliability study. *International Disabilities Studies, 10,* 61-63.

Conant, J. B. (1951). *Science and common sense* (vol. 49). New Haven, CT: Yale University Press.

Consensus Report of the Working Group on: "Molecular and Biochemical Markers of Alzheimer's Disease." The Ronald and Nancy Reagan Research Institute of the Alzheimer's Association, and The National Institute on Aging Working Group. (1998). *Neurobiology of Aging, 19,* 109-116.

Cooper, B., Rigby, P., Letts, L., Stewart, D., Strong, S., & Law, M. (2002). Assessing Context: Home, community, and workplace access. *Occupational Therapy for Physical Dysfunction,* 235-256.

Cooper, C., O'Cathain, A., Hind, D., Adamson, J., Lawton, J., & Baird, W. (2014). Conducting qualitative research within Clinical Trials Units: Avoiding potential pitfalls. *Contemporary Clinical Trials, 38,* 338-343.

Cork, R. C., Isaac, I., Elsharydah, A., Saleemi, S., Zavisca, F., & Alexander, L. (2004). A comparison of the Verbal Rating Scale and the Visual Analog Scale for pain assessment. *The Internet Journal of Anesthesiology, 8*(1). Retrieved http://ispub.com/IJA/8/1/9797

Cott, C., & Finch, E. (1991). Goal-setting in physical therapy practice. *Physiotherapy Canada, 43,* 19-22.

Crawford, J. E., & Crawford, D. M. (1949). *The Crawford Small Parts Dexterity Test.* San Antonio, TX: Pearson/PsychCorp.

Crawley, S. L. (1926). An experimental investigation of recovery from work. *Archives of Psychology, 13,* 66.

Creswell, J. W. (1998). *Qualitative inquiry and research design: Choosing among five traditions.* Thousand Oak, CA: Sage.

Crocker, M. D., MacKay-Lyons, M., & McDonnell, E. (1997). Forced use of the upper extremity in cerebral palsy: A single-case design. *American Journal of Occupational Therapy, 51,* 824-833.

Crow, T. M., Pilch, N. J., & Aiken, J. P. (2015). Clinical pain scale compendium. Retrieved from https://soundideas.pugetsound.edu/ptsymposium/1/

Crowe, T., Sanchez, V., Weber, A., & Murtagh, A. (2016). The influence of a Mexican cultural immersion experience on personal and professional healthcare practices. *Occupational Therapy International, 23,* 318-327.

Crowther, J. G., & Whiddington, R. (1948). *Science at war.* New York, NY: Philosophical Library.

Cullen, K. A., Hall, M. J., & Golosinskiy, A. (2009). *Ambulatory surgery in the United States, 2006. National Health Statistics Reports, #11.* Hyattsville, MD: National Center for Health Statistics.

Dahlgren, A., Karlsson, A-K., Lundgren Nilsson Å., Fridén, J., & Claesson, L. (2007). Activity performance and upper extremity function in cervical spinal cord injury patients according to the Klein-Bell ADL Scale. *Spinal Cord, 45,* 475-484.

Daniels, H. H., & Daniels, W. C. (2013). *Worthingham's Muscle Testing: Techniques of Manual Examination and Performance Testing.* Amsterdam, Netherlands: Elsevier.

Daniels, L., Williams, M., & Worthingham, C. (1956). *Muscle testing: Techniques of manual examination.* Philadelphia, PA: W. B. Saunders.

Das, J. P., Kirby, J., & Jarman, R. F. (1975). Simultaneous and successive synthesis: An alternative model for cognitive abilities. *Psychological Bulletin, 82,* 87-103.

Davidson, M., & Keating, J. L. (2002). A comparison of five low back disability questionnaires: reliability and responsiveness. *Physical Therapy, 82*(1), 8-24.

Dawber, T. R., & Kannel, W. B. (1958). An epidemiologic study of heart disease: The Framingham study. *Nutrition Reviews, 16*(1), 1-4.

Dawber, T. R., Meadors, G. F., & Moore, F. E. (1951). Epidemiological approaches to heart disease: The Framingham study. *American Journal of Public Health, 41,* 279-286.

de las Heras, C. G., Geist, R., Kielhofner, G., & Li, Y. (2007). The Volitional Questionnaire (VQ; version 4.1). *Moho Clearing House.* Retrieved from http://www.moho.uic. edu/assess/vq.html

Dean, C., & Gadd, E. M. (1990). Home treatment for acute psychiatric illness. *British Medical Journal, 302,* 1021-1023.

DeMatteo, C., Law, M., Russell, D., Pollock, N., Rosenbaum, P., & Walter S. (1992). *QUEST: Quality of Upper Extremity Skills Test manual.* Hamilton, Ontario, Canada: CanChild Center for Childhood Disability.

DeMatteo, C., Law, M., Russell, D., Pollock, N., Rosenbaum, P., & Walter, S. (1993). The reliability and validity of Quality of Upper Extremity Skills Test. *Physical and Occupational Therapy in Pediatrics 13*(2), 1-18.

Deno, S. L. (1985). Curriculum-based measurement: The emerging alternative. *Exceptional Children, 52,* 219-232.

Denzin, N., & Lincoln, Y. (1994a). *Handbook of qualitative research.* Thousand Oaks, CA: Sage.

Denzin, N., & Lincoln, Y. (1994b). Introduction: Entering the field of qualitative research. In N. Denzin & Y. Lincoln (Eds.), *Handbook of qualitative research* (pp. 1-17). Thousand Oaks, CA: Sage.

DePoy, E., & Gitlin, L. N. (2016). *Introduction to research: Understanding and applying multiple strategies.* St. Louis, MO: Elsevier.

DeVries, R. C., Deitz, J., & Anson, D. (1998). A comparison of two computer access systems for functional text entry. *American Journal of Occupational Therapy, 52,* 656-665.

Dewey, J. (1933). *How we think: A restatement of the relation of reflective thinking to the educative process.* Chicago, IL: Henry Regnery.

Dickerson, A. E. (1999). The Role Checklist. In B. Hemphill-Pearson (Ed.), *Assessments in occupational therapy mental health: An integrative approach* (pp. 175-182). Thorofare, NJ: SLACK Incorporated.

Dickerson, A. E., & Brown, L. E. (2007). Pediatric constraint-induced movement therapy in a young child with minimal active arm movement. *American Journal of Occupational Therapy, 61,* 563-573.

Dickinson, D., Tenhula, W., Morris, S., Brown, C., Peer, J., Spencer, K., … Bellack, A. S. (2010). A randomized, controlled trial of computer-assisted cognitive remediation for schizophrenia. *American Journal of Psychiatry, 167,* 170-180.

Dirckx, J. H., & Stedman, T. L. (1997). *Stedman's concise medical dictionary for the health professions.* Baltimore, MD: Lippincott, Williams & Wilkins.

Dittmar, S. S., & Gresham, G. E. (2000). *Functional assessment and outcome measures for the rehabilitation health professional.* Gaithersburg, MD: Aspen/Canadianphysio.

Doarn, C. R., McVeigh, F., & Poropatich, R. (2010). Innovative new technologies to identify and treat traumatic brain injuries: Crossover technologies and approaches between military and civilian applications. *Telemedicine Journal and e-Health, 16,* 373-381.

Domínguez-Gerpe, L., & Araújo-Vilar, D. (2008). Prematurely aged children: molecular alterations leading to Hutchinson-Gilford progeria and Werner syndromes. *Current Ageing Science, 1,* 202-212.

Donaldson, S. W., Wagner, C. C., & Gresham, G. E. (1973). Unified ADL evaluation form. *Archives of Physical Medicine and Rehabilitation, 54,*175-179, 185.

Downer, A. H. (1970). *Physical therapy procedures: Selected techniques.* Springfield, IL: Charles C. Thomas.

Doyle, S., Bennett, S., & Gustafsson, L. (2013). Clinical decision making when addressing upper limb post-stroke sensory impairments. *British Journal of Occupational Therapy, 76,* 254-263.

Doyne, E. J., Chambless, D. L., & Beutler, L. E. (1983). Aerobic exercise as a treatment for depression in women. *Behavior Therapy, 14,* 434-440.

Doyne, E. J., Ossip-Klein, D. J., Bowman, E. D., Osborn, K. M., McDougall-Wilson, I. B., & Neimeyer, R. A. (1987). Running versus weight lifting in the treatment of depression. *Journal of Consulting and Clinical Psychology, 55,* 748-754.

Duke University Center for the Study of Aging and Human Development. (1978). *Functional assessment: The OARS methodology.* Durham, NC: Duke University.

Dukes, W. F. (1965). N=1. *Psychological Bulletin, 64,* 74-79.

Dunn, L. M. (1968). Special education for the mildly retarded: Is much of it justifiable? *Exceptional Children, 35,* 5-22.

Dunn, W. (2014). *Sensory Profile 2 Manual: Strengths based approach to assessment and planning.* Bloomington, MN: Pearson Education Inc.

Dworkin, R. H., Turk, D. C., Revicki, D. A., Harding, G., Coyne, K. S., Peirce-Sandner, S., … Melzack, R. (2009). Development and initial validation of an expanded and revised version of the Short Form McGill Pain Questionnaire (SF-MPQ-2). *Pain, 144,* 35-42.

Earhart, C. A., & Allen, C. A. (1988). *Cognitive disabilities: Expanded activity analysis.* Los Angeles, CA: University of Southern California Medical Center.

Easton, D. (1961). *A framework for political analysis.* Englewood Cliffs, NJ: Prentice-Hall.

Eastwood, E. A., & Fisher, G. A. (1988). Skills acquisition among matched samples of institutionalized and community-based persons with mental retardation. *American Journal of Mental Retardation, 93,* 75-83.

Ebbinghaus, H. (2013). Memory: A contribution to experimental psychology. *Annals of Neurosciences, 20,* 155-156.

Edgerton, R. B., & Langness, L. L. (1978). Observing mentally retarded persons in community settings: An anthropological perspective. In G. P. Sackett (Ed.), *Observing behavior: Theory and applications in mental retardation* (pp. 335-348). Baltimore, MD: University Park Press.

Edwards, D. R., & Bristol, M. M. (1991). Autism: Early identification and management in family practice. *American Family Physician, 44,* 1755-1763.

Ellis, H. (2001). *History of surgery.* Cambridge, United Kingdom: Cambridge University Press.

Elsevier.com. (n.d.) Biomedical research—Embase. Retrieved from https://www.elsevier.com/solutions/embase-biomedical-research

Elwell, J. L., & Grindley, G. C. (1938). The effect of knowledge of results on learning and performance. *British Journal of Psychology, 29,* 39-54.

Epps, S., & Tindall, G. (1987). The effectiveness of differential programming in serving students with mild handicaps: Placement options and instructional programming. In M. C. Wang, M. C. Reynolds, & H. J. Walberg (Eds.), *Handbook of special education: Research and practice* (Vol. 1, pp. 213-248). Oxford, United Kingdom: Pergamon Press.

Erhardt, R. P. (1994). *Erhardt Developmental Prehension Assessment* (3rd ed). Maplewood, MN: Erhardt Developmental Products.

Erikson, E. H. (1950). *Childhood and society.* New York, NY: W.W. Norton & Company.

Ernst, A. A., Houry, D., & Weiss, S. J. (1997). Research funding in the four major emergency medicine journals. *American Journal of Emergency Medicine, 15,* 268-270.

Esquirol, É. (1838). *Des maladies mentales considérées sous les rapports médical, hygiénique et médico-légal* (Vol. 1). Paris, France: Chez J.-B. Baillière.

Fabre, J. M., Ellis, R., Kosma, M., Moore, D. S., McCarter, K. S., & Wood, R. H. (2010). Development and validation of the comprehensive falls risk screening instrument. *Physical & Occupational Therapy in Geriatrics, 28*(2), 181-194.

Fairbank, J. C. T., Couper, J., Davies., J. B., & O'Brien, J. B. (1980). The Oswestry low back pain questionnaire. *Physiotherapy, 66,* 271-273.

Fairbank, J. C. T., & Pynsent, P. B. (2000a). The Oswestry disability index. *Spine, 25,* 2940-2953.

Fairbank, J. C. T., & Pynsent, P. B. (2000b). The Oswestry disability questionnaire. Retrieved from http://www.tac.vic.gov. au/upload/Oswestry.pdf

Falk-Ross, F. (1996). *Classroom-based language remediation programs: Roles, routines, and reflections.* Paper presented at the 36th Annual Convention of the Illinois Speech-Language-Hearing Association. (ERIC Document Reproduction Service No. ED 417-539)

Family Center on Technology and Disability. (2010). *FCTD Fact Sheets: Assistive technology laws.* Washington, DC: Office of Special Education and Rehabilitation

Feigin, G., An, C., Connors, D., & Crawford, I. (1996). Shape up, ship out: How a team of OR analysts redefined manufacturing strategy for the IBM PC Company in Europe. *ORMS Today, 23*(2), 24-31.

Ferguson, P. M., Ferguson, D. L., & Taylor, S. J. (Eds.). (1992). *Interpreting disability: A qualitative reader.* New York, NY: Teachers College Press.

Finch, E., Brooks, D., Stratford, P., & Mayo, N. (2002). *Physical rehabilitation outcome measures* (2nd ed.). Toronto, ON, Canada: Canadian Physiotherapy Association/B. C. Decker, Inc.

Findley, T. W. (1989). Research in physical medicine and rehabilitation. II. The conceptual review of the literature or how to read more articles than you ever want to see in your entire life. *American Journal of Physical Medicine Rehabilitation, 68*, 97-102.

Firth, H., & Short, D. (1987). A move from hospital to community: Evaluation of community contacts. *Child: Care Health and Development, 13*, 341-354.

Fischer, A. (1994). *Assessment of motor and process skills (AMPS)*. Unpublished manual. Chicago, IL: University of Illinois at Chicago.

Fischer, J., & Corcoran, K. (2007). *Measures for clinical practice: A sourcebook. Volume 1: Couples, family and children* (4th ed.). New York, NY: Free Press.

Fisher, B., Bhavnani, V., & Winfield, M. (2009). How patients use access to their full health records: A qualitative study of patients in general practice. *Journal of the Royal Society of Medicine, 102*, 539-544.

Fisher, W. P., Harvey, R. F., & Kilgore, K. M. (1995). New developments in functional assessment: Probabilistic models for gold standards. *NeuroRehabilitation, 5*(1), 3-25.

Fitzgerald, M. H., Mullavey-O'Byrne, C., & Clemson, L. (1997). Cultural issues from practice. *Australian Occupational Therapy Journal, 44*, 1-21.

Flegal, K. M., Kruszon-Moran, D., Carroll, M. D., Fryar, C. D., & Ogden, C. L. (2016). Trends in obesity among adults in the United States, 2005 to 2014. *Journal of the American Medical Association, 315*, 2284-2291.

Fleischman, D. A., & Gabrieli, J. D. (1998). Repetition priming in normal aging and Alzheimer's disease: A review of findings and theories. *Psychology of Aging, 13*, 88-119.

Flexner, A., Pritchett, H., & Henry, S. (1910). *Medical education in the United States and Canada bulletin number four (The Flexner Report)*. New York, NY: The Carnegie Foundation for the Advancement of Teaching.

Flinn, N. A., & Radomski, M. V. (2002). Learning. In C. A. Trombly & M. V. Radomski (Eds.), *Occupational therapy for physical dysfunction* (pp. 283-297). Baltimore, MD: Lippincott, Williams and Wilkins.

Flood, J. F., & Morley, J. E. (1998). Learning and memory in the SAMP8 mouse. *Neuroscience & Biobehavioral Review, 22*(1), 1-20.

Folan, A., Barclay, L., Cooper, C., & Robinson, M. (2015). Exploring the experience of clients with tetraplegia utilizing assistive technology for computer access. *Disability and Rehabilitation: Assistive Technology, 10*, 46-52.

Folio, M. R., & Fewell, R. R. (2000). *Peabody Developmental Motor Scales-2* (2nd ed.; PDMS-2). Austin, TX: Pro-Ed.

Folstein, M. F., Folstein, S. E., White, T., & Messer, M. A. (2010). *Mini-Mental * State Examination: User's manual* (MMSE®-2™; 2nd ed.). Lutz, FL: PAR.

Fontana, A., & Frey, J. (1994). The art of science. In N. Denzin & Y. Lincoln (Eds.), *Handbook of qualitative research* (pp. 361-376). Thousand Oaks, CA: Sage.

Forness, S. R., & Kavale, K. A. (1984). Education of the mentally retarded: A note on policy. *Education and Training of the Mentally Retarded, 19*, 239-245.

Fraenkel, J. R., & Wallen, N. E. (1990). *How to design and evaluate research in education*. New York, NY: McGraw-Hill.

Fraga, S. (2010). TABACOPanaceia no Século XVI e Patologia no Século XX [Tobacco: Panacea in the XVI century and pathology in the XX century]. *Acta Médica Portuguesa, 23*, 243-246.

Frank, G. (1992). Opening feminist histories of occupational therapy. *American Journal of Occupational Therapy, 46*, 989-999.

Frank, G., Bernardo, C. S., Tropper, S., Noguchi, F., Lipman, C., Maulhardt, B., & Weitze, L. (1997). Jewish spirituality through actions in time: Daily occupations of young Orthodox Jewish couples in Los Angeles. *American Journal of Occupational Therapy, 51*, 199-206.

Frankenburg, W., Dodds, J., Archer, P., Bresnick, B., Mashka, P., Edelman, N., & Shapiro, H. (1990). *Denver Developmental Screening Test (Denver-II)*. Denver, CO: Denver Developmental Materials: Inc.

Frankenburg, W. K., Dodds, J., Archer, P., Shapiro, H., & Bresnick, B. (1992). The Denver II: A major revision and restandardization of the Denver Developmental Screening Test. *Pediatrics, 89*, 91-97.

Frederic, M. T. (1928). *Gang, a study of 1,313 gangs in Chicago*. Chicago, IL: University of Chicago Press.

French, S. (1994). *On equal terms: Working with disabled people*. Oxford, United Kingdom: Butterworth-Heinemann.

Frey, J. J., & Fontana, A. (1995). *The group interview*. Newbury Park, CA: Sage.

Friedland, J., & Silva, J. (2008). Evolving identities: Thomas Bessell Kidner and occupational therapy in the United States. *American Journal of Occupational Therapy, 62*, 349-360.

Frost, M. H., Reeve, B. B., Liepa, A. M., Stauffer, J. W., Hays, R. D.; the Mayo/FDA Patient-Reported Outcomes Consensus Meeting Group. (2007). What is sufficient evidence for the reliability and validity of patient-reported outcome measures? *Value in Health, 10*(Suppl. 2), S94-S105.

Fuchs, D., Fuchs, L. S., & Fernstrom, P. (1993). A conservative approach to special education reform: Mainstreaming through transenvironmental programming and curriculum-based measurement. *American Educational Research Journal, 30*, 149-177.

Fugl-Meyer, A. R., Jääskö, L., Leyman, I., Olsson, S., & Steglind, S. (1975). The poststroke hémiplégie patient I. A method for evaluation of physical performance. *Scandinavian Journal of Rehabilitation Medicine, 7*, 13-31.

Fukutani, Y., Sasaki, K., Mukai, M., Matsubara, R., Isaki, K., & Cairns, N. J. (1997). Neurons and extracellular neurofibrillary tangles in the hippocampal subdivisions in early-onset familial Alzheimer's disease: A case study. *Psychiatry & Clinical Neurosciences, 51*, 227-231.

Galton, F. (1883). *Inquiries into the human faculty & its development*. New York, NY: AMS Press.

Gambrill, E. (2012). *Social work practice: A critical thinker's guide* (3rd ed.). Oxford, United Kingdom: Oxford University Press.

Gardner, H. (2011). *Frames of mind: The theory of multiple intelligences*. New York, NY: Basic Books.

Gardner, H. E. (2000). *Intelligence reframed: Multiple intelligences for the 21st century*. New York, NY: Basic Books.

Gary K. W. (2011) Kohlman Evaluation of Living Skills. In: J. S. Kreutzer, J. DeLuca, & B. Caplan (Eds.), *Encyclopedia of Clinical Neuropsychology* (pp. 1410-1411). New York, NY: Springer.

Gee, W. (1950). *Social science research methods*. New York, NY: Appleton-Century-Crofts.

Geist, H. (1988). *Geist Picture Interest Inventory* (Rev.). Torrance, CA: Western Psychological Services.

Gesell, A. (1928). *Infancy and human growth*. New York, NY: McGraw-Hill.

Gesell, A., & Thompson, H. (1923). *Infant behavior: Its genesis and growth*. New York, NY: McGraw-Hill.

Geslani, D. M., Tierney, M. C., Herrmann, N., & Szalai, J. P. (2005). Mild cognitive impairment: An operational definition and its conversion rate to Alzheimer's disease. *Dementia and Geriatric Cognitive Disorders, 19*, 383-389.

Gewurtz, R., Stergiou-Kita, M., Shaw, L., Kirsh, B., & Rappolt, S. (2008). Qualitative meta-synthesis: reflections on the utility and challenges in occupational therapy. *Canadian Journal of Occupational Therapy, 75*, 301-308.

Gillespie, M. (2003). Summary versus every-trial knowledge of results for individuals with intellectual disabilities. *Adapted Physical Activity Quarterly, 20*, 46-56.

Gilliam, J., & Barstow, I. K. (1997). Joint range of motion. In J. Van Deusen & D. Brunt (Eds.), *Assessment in occupational therapy and physical therapy* (pp. 49-77). Philadelphia, PA: W. B. Saunders.

Gilson, B. S., Gilson, J. S., Bergner, M., Bobbitt, R. A., Kressel, S., Pollard, W. E., & Vesselago, M. (1975). The Sickness Impact Profile: Development of an outcome measure of health care. *American Journal of Public Health, 65,* 1304-1310.

Gladstone, D. J., Danells, C. J., & Black, S. E. (2002). The Fugl-Meyer assessment of motor recovery after stroke: A critical review of its measurement properties. *Neurorehabilitation and Neural Repair, 16,* 232-240. doi: 10.1177/154596802401105171

Glaser, B. G., & Strauss, A. L. (1967). *The discovery of grounded theory: Strategies for qualitative research.* Chicago, IL: AldineTransaction.

Glaser, R. (1963). Instructional technology and the measurement of learning outcomes: Some questions. *American Psychologist, 18,* 519-521.

Gleason, J. J. (1990). Meaning of play: Interpreting patterns in behavior of persons with severe developmental disabilities. *Anthropology and Education Quarterly, 21,* 59-77.

Glutting, J. J., & Wilkinson, G. (2003). *Wide Range Interest and Occupation Test—Second edition* (WRIOT-2). San Antonio, TX: Pearson Assessments/PsychCorp.

Goddard, H. H. (1920). *Human efficiency and levels of intelligence.* Princeton, NJ: Princeton University Press.

Goffman, E. (1961). *Asylums: Essays on the social situation of mental patients and other inmates.* Garden City, NJ: Anchor Books.

Gold, R. L. (1958). Roles in sociological field observations. *Social Forces, 36,* 217-223.

Goldberg, R. T. (1974). Rehabilitation research, new directions. *Journal of Rehabilitation, 40*(3), 12-14.

Golden, C. J., & Freshwater, S. M. (2001). Luria-Nebraska neuropsychological battery. In W. I. Dorfman & M. Hersen (Eds.), *Understanding psychological assessment: Perspectives on individual differences* (pp. 59-75). Boston, MA: Springer.

Goleman, D. (1995). *Emotional intelligence.* New York, NY: Bantam Books.

Good-Ellis, M. A., Fine, S. B., Spencer, J. H., & Divittis, A. (1987). Developing a role activity performance scale. *American Journal of Occupational Therapy, 41,* 232-241.

Google Scholar, (2018). *About Google Scholar.* Retrieved https://scholar.google.com/intl/en/scholar/about.html.

Gordon, E. E. (1968). A view of the target population. In A. J. Tannenbaum (Ed.), *Special education programs for disadvantaged children and youth* (pp. 5-18). Washington, DC: The Council for Exceptional Children.

Gould, J., & Kolb, J. G. (Eds.). (1964). *A dictionary of the social sciences.* New York, NY: The Free Press.

Gould, S. J. (1996). *The mismeasure of man* (Rev. ed.). New York, NY: W.W. Norton & Co.

Graf, C. (2007). The Lawton Instrumental Activities of Daily Living (IADL) Scale. *Annals of Long Term Care: Clinical Care and Aging, 15*(7).

Granger, C. V., Ottenbacher, K. J., Baker, J. G., & Sehgal, A. (1995). Reliability of a brief outpatient functional outcome assessment measure. *American Journal of Physical Medicine & Rehabilitation, 74*(6), 469-475.

Granger, C. V., Sherwood, C. C., & Greer, D. S. (1977). Functional status measures in a comprehensive stroke care program. *Archives of Physical Medicine and Rehabilitation, 58,* 555-561.

Granger, C. V., & Wright, B. (1993). Looking ahead to the use of functional assessment in ambulatory physiatric and primary care. *Physical Medicine and Rehabilitation Clinics of North America, 4*(3), 1-11.

Gravetter, F. J., & Wallnau, L. B. (2009). *Statistics for the behavioral sciences.* Bellmont, CA: Cengage.

Greist, J. H., Klein, M. H., Eischens, R. R., Faris, J., Gurman, A. S., & Morgan, W. P. (1979). Running as treatment for depression. *Comprehensive Psychiatry, 20,* 41-54.

Guba, E. G. (1990). Carrying on the dialog. In E. G. Guba (Ed.), *The paradigm dialogue* (pp. 368-378). Newbury Park, CA: Sage.

Guigoz, Y., Vellas, B., Garry, P. J., & Albarede, J. L. (1994). *Facts and research in gerontology.* (Suppl.) 2, 56-62. Paris, France: Sendi Publishing Company.

Guilford, J. P. (1967). *The nature of human intelligence.* New York, NY: McGraw-Hill.

Gustafsson, L., Patterson, E., Marshall, K., Bennett, S., & Bower, K. (2016). Efficacy of compression gloves in maintaining edema reductions after application of compression bandaging to the stroke-affected upper limb. *American Journal of Occupational Therapy, 70,* 7002290030p1-9.

Gutman, S. A. (1995). Influence of the U.S. military and occupational therapy reconstruction aides in World War I on the development of occupational therapy. *American Journal of Occupational Therapy, 49,* 256-262.

Gutman, S. A., Raphael-Greenfield, E., & Rao, A. K. (2012). Effect of a motor-based role-play intervention on the social behaviors of adolescents with high-functioning autism: Multiple-baseline single-subject design. *American Journal of Occupational Therapy, 66,* 529-537.

Haavardsholm, E. A., Kvien, T. K., Uhlig, T., Smedstad, L. M., & Guillemin, F. (2000). A comparison of agreement and sensitivity to change between AIMS2 and a short form of AIMS2 (AIMS2-SF) in more than 1,000 rheumatoid arthritis patients. *Journal of Rheumatology, 27,* 2810-2816.

Haeger, K. (1988). *The illustrated history of surgery.* London, United Kingdom: Harold Starke.

Hajat, S., Fitzpatrick, R., Morris, R., Reeves, B., Rigge, M., Williams, O., ... Gregg, P. (2002). Does waiting for total hip replacement matter? Prospective cohort study. *Journal of Health Services Research & Policy, 7,* 19-25.

Haley, S. M., Coster, W. J., Dumas, H. M., Fragala-Pinkham, M. A., Kramer, J., Ni, P., ... Ludlow, L. H. (2011). Accuracy and precision of the Pediatric Evaluation of Disability Inventory computer-adaptive tests (PEDI-CAT). *Developmental Medicine & Child Neurology, 53*(12), 1100-1106.

Hall, E. T. (1966). *The hidden dimension.* New York, NY: Doubleday.

Hallahan, D. P., & Kauffman, J. M. (1994). *Teaching exceptional children: Cases for reflection and analysis for exceptional children, introduction to special education* (6th ed.). Boston, MA: Allyn & Bacon.

Halstead, L., & Hartley, R. B. (1975). Time care profile: An evaluation of a new method of assessing ADL dependence. *Archives of Physical Medicine and Rehabilitation, 56,* 110-115.

Hamilton, M. (1960). A rating scale for depression. *Journal of Neurology, Neurosurgery, and Psychiatry, 23,* 468-477.

Hamlin, R. B. (1992). Embracing our past, informing our future: A feminist re-vision of health care. *American Journal of Occupational Therapy, 46,* 1028-1035.

Harper, D. (1989). Visual sociology: Expanding sociological vision. In G. Blank, J. McCartney, & E. Brent (Eds.), *New technology in sociology: Practical applications in research and work* (pp. 81-97). New Brunswick, NJ: Transaction Books.

Harvard Medical School. (1991). *Guidelines for investigators in scientific research.* Boston, MA: Author.

Harvard Medical School. (1996). *Guidelines for investigators in clinical research.* Retrieved from https://ari.hms.harvard.edu/guidelines-investigators-clinical-research

Harvey, R. F., & Jellinek, H. M. (1981). Functional performance assessment: A program approach. *Archives of Physical Medicine and Rehabilitation, 62,* 456-460.

Harvey, W. (1938). On the motion of the heart and blood in animals (R. Willis, Trans.). In C. W. Elliot (Ed.), *The Harvard classics scientific papers* (pp. 273-274). New York, NY: P.E. Collier and Sonds.

Hathaway, S. R., McKinley, J. C., & MMPI Restandardization Committee. (1989). *MMPI-2: Minnesota Multiphasic Personality Inventory-2: Manual for administration and scoring.* Minneapolis, MN: University of Minnesota Press.

Havighurst, R. J. (1952). *Developmental tasks and education.* New York, NY: Longmans, Green.

Haynes, M. C., & Jenkins, J. R. (1986). Reading instruction in special education resource rooms. *American Educational Research Journal, 23,* 161-191.

Health Education Research. (n.d.). About the journal. Retrieved from https://academic.oup.com/her/pages/About

Health Outcomes Institute. (1995). *Health Status Questionnaire* (HSQ–12, version 2.0). San Antonio, TX: Pearson Assessment/PsychCorp.

Healthcare Cost and Utilization Project. (2019). *What is HCUP?* Retrieved from https://www.hcup-us.ahrq.gov

Hemphill-Pearson, B. J. (1999). *Assessments in occupational therapy mental health: An integrative approach.* Thorofare, NJ: SLACK Incorporated.

Hemphill-Pearson, B. J. (2008). *Assessments in occupational therapy mental health: An integrative approach* (2nd ed.). Thorofare, NJ: SLACK Incorporated.

Henry, A. D. (2000). *Pediatric interest profiles: Surveys of play for children and adolescents, kid play profile, preteen play profile, adolescent leisure interest profile.* San Antonio, TX: Psychological Corporation.

Henry, J. (1971). *Pathways to madness.* New York, NY: Random House.

Hester, P. H. (1994). *A contextual analysis of classroom interaction at the university level: An operations research approach.* Paper presented at the Annual Meeting of the Mid–South Educational Research Association, Nashville, TN. (ERIC Document Reproduction Service Number ED 382 139.)

Higgs, J. (Ed.). (1997). *Qualitative research: Discourse on methodologies.* Sydney, Australia: Hampden.

Higgs, J. (Ed.). (1998). *Writing qualitative research.* Sydney, Australia: Hampden.

Hill, A. B. (1971). *Principles of medical statistics.* New York, NY: Oxford University Press.

Hinshelwood, J. (1917). Congenital word-blindness. *Lancet, 190*(4922), 980.

Hislop, H., Avers, D., & Brown, M. (2013). *Daniels and Worthingham's muscle Testing-E-Book: Techniques of manual examination and performance testing.* Amsterdam, Netherlands: Elsevier Health Sciences.

Hoaglin, D. C., Mosteller, F., & Tukey, J. W. (1991). *Fundamentals of exploratory analysis of variance.* New York, NY: John Wiley & Sons.

Hodgetts, S., McConnell, D., Zwaigenbaum, L., & Nicholas, D. (2014). The impact of autism services on mothers' occupational balance and participation. *OTJR: Occupation, Participation and Health, 34,* 81-93.

Hoffman, H. G., Meyer, W. J. III, Ramirez, M., Roberts, L., Seibel, E. J., Atzori, B., ... Patterson, D. R. (2014). Feasibility of articulated arm mounted Oculus Rift Virtual Reality goggles for adjunctive pain control during occupational therapy in pediatric burn patients. *Cyberpsychology, Behavior, and Social Networking, 17,* 397-401.

Holbrook, M., & Skilbeck, C. E. (1983). An activities index for use with stroke patients. *Age and Ageing, 12,* 166-170.

Holland, J. L. (1994). *The self-directed search: Professional users guide.* Odessa FL: PAR, Inc.

Holm, M. B., & Rogers, J. C. (2008). The Performance Assessment of Self-Care Skills (PASS). In B. J. Hemphill-Pearson (Ed.), *Assessments in occupational therapy mental health: An integrative approach* (2nd ed., pp. 259-274). Thorofare, NJ: SLACK Incorporated.

Holmberg, K., Rosen, D., & Holland, J. L. (1999). *The Leisure Activities Finder ™ (LAF).* Odessa, FL: PAR Inc.

Holstein, J. A., & Gubrium, J. F. (1995). *The active interview.* Thousand Oaks, CA: Sage.

Horghagen, S., Josephsson, S., & Alsaker, S. (2007). The use of craft activities as an occupational therapy treatment modality in Norway during 1952-1960. *Occupational Therapy International, 14,* 42-56.

Horn, J. L. (1968). Organization of abilities and the development of intelligence. *Psychological Review, 75,* 242-259.

Howland, D. S., Trusko, S. P., Savage, M. J., Reaume, A. G., Lang, D. M., Hirsch, J. D., ... Flood, D. G. (1998). Modulation of secreted beta-amyloid precursor protein and amyloid beta-peptide in brain by cholesterol. *Journal of Biological Chemistry, 273,* 16576-16582.

Huebner, R. A., Emery, L. J., & Shordike, A. (2002). The adolescent role assessment: Psychometric properties and theoretical usefulness. *American Journal of Occupational Therapy, 56,* 202-209.

Huebsch, J. A., Kottke, T. E., McGinnis, P., Nichols, J., Parker, E. D., Tillema, J. O., & Hanson, A. M. (2015). A qualitative study of processes used to implement evidence-based care in a primary care practice. *Family Practice, 32,* 578-583.

Huezo, C. (1997). Factors to address when periodic abstinence is offered by multi-method family planning programs. *Advances in Contraception, 13,* 261-267.

Hunt, N., & Marshall, K. J. (1994). *Exceptional children and youth: An introduction to special education.* Boston, MA: Houghton Mifflin.

Hutchins, R. M. (1952). *Hippocratic writings* (F. Adams, Trans.; Vol. 10). Chicago, IL: W. Benton.

Illingworth, W. H. (1910). *History of the education of the blind.* London, United Kingdom: S. Low, Marston & Company.

Individuals with Disabilities Education Improvement Act of 2004. (2004).

Jacob, T., & Shapira, A. (2010). Quality of life and health conditions reported from two post-polio clinics in Israel. *Journal of Rehabilitation Medicine, 42,* 377-379.

Jacobson, N. S., Dobson, K. S., Truax, P. A., Addis, M. E., Koerner, K., Gollan, J. K., ... Prince, S. E. (1996). A component analysis of cognitive-behavioral treatment for depression. *Journal of Consulting and Clinical Psychology, 64,* 295-304.

Jahoda, M., Deutsch, M., & Cook, S. W. (1951). *Research methods in social relations.* New York, NY: The Dryden Press.

JAMA Network Editors. (2010). *AMA Manual of Style* (10th ed.). New York, NY: Oxford University Press.

Jebsen, R. H., Taylor, N., Trieschmann, R. B., Trotter, M. J., & Howard, L. A. (1969). An objective and standardized test of hand function. *Archives of Physical Medicine and Rehabilitation, 50,* 311-319.

Jensen, K. B. (2013). *A handbook of media and communication research: Qualitative and quantitative methodologies* (2nd ed.). Abingdon, United Kingdom: Routledge.

Jensen, M. P., Karoly, P., & Braver, S. (1986). The measurement of clinical pain intensity: A comparison of six methods. *Pain, 27,* 117-126.

Jessor, R., Colby, A., & Shweder, R. A. (1996). *Ethnography and human development: Context and meaning in social inquiry.* Chicago, IL: University of Chicago.

Jette, A. M. (1980). Functional Status Index: Reliability of a chronic disease evaluation instrument. *Archives of Physical Medicine and Rehabilitation, 61,* 395-401.

Johnson, D. (2015). Evaluative measures: Assessing the effectiveness of exhibits and programs in zoos. Unpublished thesis. Rochester, NY; Rochester Institute of Technology.

Johnson, T. P., Vinnicombe, B. J., & Merrill, G. W. (1981). Independent living skills evaluation. *Occupational Therapy in Mental Health, 1*(2), 5-18. doi: 10.1300/J004v01n02_02.

Kamhi, A. G., & Catts, H. W. (1998). *Language and reading disabilities.* Boston, MA: Allyn & Bacon.

Kaplan, K., Mendelson, L. B., & Dubroff, M. P. (1983). The effect of a jogging program on psychiatric inpatients with symptoms of depression. *OTJR: Occupation, Participation and Health, 3,* 173-175.

Katz, S., Ford, R. Q., Moskowitz, R. W., Jackson, B. A., & Jaffe, M. W. (1963). Studies of illness in the aged, the index of ADL: A standardized measure of biological and psychosocial functions. *Journal of the American Medical Association, 185,* 914-918.

Kaufman, A. S., & Kaufman, N. L. (1993). *Kaufman adolescent and adult intelligence test.* Circle Pines MN: American Guidance Service.

Ke, K. M., Blazeby, J. M., Strong, S., Carroll, F. E., Ness, A. R., & Hollingworth, W. (2013). Are multidisciplinary teams in secondary care cost-effective? A systematic review of the literature. *Cost Effectiveness and Resource Allocation, 11*, 7.

Kehoe, R., & Rice, M. (2016). Reality, virtual reality, and imagery: Quality of movement in novice dart players. *British Journal of Occupational Therapy, 79*, 244-251.

Keith, R. A. (1984). Functional assessment measures in medical rehabilitation: Current status. *Archives of Physical Medicine and Rehabilitation, 65*, 74-78.

Keith, R. A., Granger, C. V., Hamilton, B. B., & Sherwin, F. S. (1987). The Functional Independence Measure: A new tool for rehabilitation. *Advances in Clinical Rehabilitation, 1*, 6-18.

Kendall, F. P., McCreary, E. K., Provance, P. G., Rodgers, M. M., & Romani, W. A. (2005). *Muscles: Testing and function, with posture and pain (Kendall, muscles)*. Philadelphia, PA: Lippincott Williams & Wilkins.

Kendall, H. O., & Kendall, F. P. (1949). *Muscles: Testing and function*. Baltimore, MD: Lippincott, Williams & Wilkins.

Kerlinger, F. N. (1973). *Foundations of behavioral research* (2nd ed.). New York, NY: Holt, Rinehart and Winston.

Kerlinger, F. N. (1986). *Foundations of behavioral research* (3rd ed.). New York, NY: Holt, Rinehart and Winston.

Kielhofner, G., Mallinson, T., Crawfold, C., Nowak, M., Rigby, M., Henry, A., & Walens, D. (2004). *Occupational Performance History Interview II* (OPHI-II; ver. 2.1). Retrieved from http://www. moho. uic.edu/assess/ophi%202.1.html

Kipfer, B. A. (2010). *Roget's international thesaurus* (7th ed.). New York, NY: Collins.

Kirk, J., & Miller, M. L. (1986). *Reliability and validity in qualitative research*. Thousand Oaks, CA: Sage.

Kirk, S. A. (1963, April). *Behavioral diagnosis and remediation of learning disabilities*. Paper presented at the Proceedings of the Conference on Exploration Into the Problems of the Perceptually Handicapped Child: First Annual Meeting, Volume 1. Chicago, IL: Association for Children with Learning Disabilities.

Kirk, S. A., & Gallagher, J. J. (1989). *Educating exceptional children* (5th ed.). Boston, MA: Houghton Mifflin.

Klein, R. M., & Bell, B. (1982). Self-care skills: Behavior measurements with the Klein-Bell ADL Scale. *Archives of Physical Medicine and Rehabilitation, 63*, 335-338.

Klein, R. M., & Bell, B. (1993). *Klein-Bell Activities of Daily Living Scales*. Seattle, WA: University of Washington.

Kliebsch, U., Stürmer, T., Siebert, H., & Brenner, H. (1998). Risk factors of institutionalization in an elderly disabled population. *European Journal of Public Health, 8*, 106-112.

Klimidis, S., Minas, H., & Kokanovic, R. (2006). Ethnic minority community patients and the Better Outcomes in Mental Health Care initiative. *Australasian Psychiatry, 14*, 212-215.

Klyczek, J. P., & Stanton, E. (2008). The Bay Area Functional Performance Evaluation. In B. J. Hemphill-Pearson (Ed.), *Assessments in occupational therapy mental health: An integrative approach* (2nd ed.; pp. 217-237). Thorofare, NJ: SLACK Incorporated.

Knapp, L. F., & Knapp, R. R. (1982). *CAPS*. San Diego, CA: Educational & Industrial Testing Service.

Knapp, R. B., & Knapp-Lee, L. (1995). *COPSystem Interest Inventory* (Rev. ed.). San Diego, CA: Educational & Industrial Testing Service.

Knox, S. H. (1974). A play scale. In M. Reilly (Ed.), *Play as exploratory learning* (pp. 247-266). Los Angeles, CA: Sage.

Knox, S. H. (1997). Knox Preschool Play Scale (Rev. ed.). Developmental and current use of the Knox Preschool Play Scale. In L. D. Parham & L. S. Fanzio (Eds.), *Play in occupational therapy for children* (pp. 35–51). St. Louis, MO: Mosby-Year Book.

Koch, R. (1880). *Investigations into the etiology of traumatic infective diseases* (Vol. 88) [W. W. Cheyne, Trans.]. London, United Kingdom: New Sydenham Society. (Original work published 1878)

Kohlberg, L. (1981). *The philosophy of moral development, Vol. I*. San Francisco, CA: Harper & Row.

Kohs, S. (1923). *Intelligence measurements*. New York, NY: Macmillan.

Kovacs, M. (1992). *Children's depression inventory*. North Tonawanda, NY: Multi-Health Systems.

Kovacs, M. (2011). *Children's Depression Inventory–2nd edition* (CDI-2). San Antonio TX: Pearson/ PsychCorp.

Kraepelin, E. (1919). *Dementia praecox and paraphrenia* (R. M. Barclay, Trans. & G. M. Robertson, Ed.). Chicago, IL: Chicago Medical Book Co.

Kramer, J., Kielhofner, G., & Forsyth, K. (2008). Assessments used with the Model of Human Occupation. In B. J. Hemphill-Pearson (Ed.), *Assessments in occupational therapy mental health: An integrative approach* (2nd ed., pp. 159-184). Thorofare, NJ: SLACK Incorporated.

Krathwohl, D. R. (1988). *How to prepare a research proposal: Guidelines for funding and dissertations in the social and behavioral sciences* (3rd ed.). Syracuse, NY: Syracuse University Press.

Kratz, A. L., Chadd, E., Jensen, M. P., Kehn, M., & Kroll, T. (2015). An examination of the psychometric properties of the community integration questionnaire (CIQ) in spinal cord injury. *Journal of Spinal Cord Medicine, 38*, 446-455.

Krogh, J., Speyer, H., Gluud, C., & Nordentoft, M. (2015). Exercise for patients with major depression: A protocol for a systematic review with meta-analysis and trial sequential analysis. *Systematic Reviews, 4*, 40.

Kuder, F., & Zytowski, D.G. (1991). *Kuder occupational interest survey, General manual* (3rd ed.). Adel, IA: National Career Assessment Services, Inc.

Kuder, G. F., & Findley, W. G. (1966). The occupational interest survey. *Journal of Counseling & Development, 45*, 72-77.

Kunz, K. R., & Brayman, S. J. (1999). The Comprehensive Occupational Therapy Evaluation. In B. J. Hemphill-Pearson (Ed.), *Assessments in occupational therapy mental health: An integrative approach* (pp. 259-274). Thorofare, NJ: SLACK Incorporated.

Lachar, D., & Gruber, C. P. (2001). *Manual for the Personality Inventory for Children Second Edition* (PIC-2). Los Angeles, CA: Western Psychological Services.

Landsberger, H. A. (1958). *Hawthorne revisited: Management and the worker, its critics, and developments in human relations in industry*. Ithaca, NY: Cornell University Press.

Lane, H. (1976). *The wild boy of Aveyron*. Cambridge, MA: Harvard University Press.

Lane, J. D., Ledford, J. R., & Gast, D. L. (2017). Single-case experimental design: Current standards and applications in occupational therapy. *American Journal of Occupational Therapy, 71*, 7102300010p1-7102300010p9.

Law, M. (2002). Assessing roles and competence. In C. A. Trombly & M. V. Radomski (Eds.), *Occupational therapy for physical dysfunction* (5th ed., pp. 31-45). Baltimore, MD: Lippincott, Williams & Wilkins.

Law, M., Baptiste, S., Carswell, A., McColl, M., Polatajko, H., & Pollock, N. (1994). *Canadian Occupational Performance Measure* (2nd ed.). Toronto, Ontario, Canada: Canadian Association of Occupational Therapists.

Law, M., Baptiste, S., Carswell, A., McColl, M., Polatajko, H., & Pollock, N. (2004). *Canadian Occupational Performance Measure* (4th ed.) Ottawa, ON, Canada: CAOT Publications ACE.

Law, M., Baptiste, S., Carswell, A., McColl, M., Polatajko, H., & Pollock, N. (2014). *Canadian Occupational Performance Measure* (5th ed.). Ottawa, ON: CAOT Publications ACE.

Law, M., Baptiste, S., Carswell-Opzoomer, A., McColl, M., Polatajko, H., & Pollock, N. (1991). *Canadian Occupational Performance Measure manual*. Toronto, Ontario, Canada: Canadian Association of Occupational Therapists.

Lawton, E. B. (1956). *Activities of daily living: Testing, training and equipment*. New York, NY: New York Institute of Physical Medicine and Rehabilitation Medicine, NYU-Bellevue Medical Center.

Lawton, M. P., Moss, M., Fulcomer, M., & Kleban, M. H. (1982). A research and service orientated multilevel assessment instrument. *Journal of Gerontology, 37*, 91-99.

Lechner, D. E., Roth, D., & Straaton, K. (1991). Functional capacity evaluation in work disability. *Work, 1*, 37-47.

Lehman, L. A., Sindhu, B. S., Shechtman, O., Romero, S., & Velozo, C. A. (2010). A comparison of the ability of two upper extremity assessments to measure change in function. *Journal of Hand Therapy, 23*, 31-40.

Lehr, R. (1992). Sixteen S-squared over D-squared: A relation for crude sample size estimates. *Statistics in Medicine, 11*, 1099-1102.

Leiter, R. G. (1948). *Leiter International Performance Scale*. Chicago, IL: Stoelting.

Leonardelli, C. A. (1988a). The Milwaukee Evaluation of Daily Living Skills: Evaluation in long-term psychiatric care. In B. J. Hemphill (Ed.), *Mental health assessment in occupational therapy: An integrative approach to the evaluative process* (pp. 151-162). Thorofare, NJ: SLACK Incorporated.

Leonardelli, C. A. (1988b). *The Milwaukee Evaluation of Daily Living Skills: Evaluation in Long-Term Psychiatric Care (MEDLS)*. Thorofare, NJ: SLACK Incorporated.

Leung, A. Y., Bo, A., Hsiao, H. Y., Wang, S. S., & Chi, I. (2014). Health literacy issues in the care of Chinese American immigrants with diabetes: A qualitative study. *BMJ Open, 4*(11), e005294.

Lewin, K. (1939). Field theory and experiment in social psychology: Concepts and methods. *American Journal of Sociology, 44*, 868-896.

Lewis, C. B., & McNerney, T. (1994). *The functional tool box: Clinical measures of functional outcomes*. Washington, DC: Learn.

Lezak, M. D., Howieson, D. B., & Loring, D. W. (2004). *Neuropsychological assessment* (4th ed.). New York, NY: Oxford University Press.

Libernan, L. Y. (1973). Segmentation of the spoken word and reading acquisition. *Bulletin of the Orion Society, 23*, 65-77.

Lifshutz, J., & Colohan, A. (2004). A brief history of therapy for traumatic spinal cord injury. *Neurosurgical Focus, 16*, E5.

Lifton, R. J. (2017). *The Nazi doctors: Medical killing and the psychology of genocide* (2nd ed.). New York, NY: Basic Books.

Lin, K.-C., Wu, Y.-F., Chen, I. C., Tsai, P.-l., Wu, C.-Y., & Chen, C.-L. (2015). Dual-task performance involving hand dexterity and cognitive tasks and daily functioning in people with schizophrenia: A pilot study. *American Journal of Occupational Therapy, 69*, 6903250020p1-6903250020p7.

Lincoln, Y. S., & Guba, E. G. (1985). *Naturalistic inquiry*. Beverly Hills, CA: Sage.

Linder, T. W. (2008). *Transdisciplinary Play-Based Assessment-2 (TPBA2)*. Baltimore, MD: P. H. Brookes.

Linkenhoker, D., & McCarron, L. T. (1979). *Adaptive behaviors: Street Survival Skills Questionnaire (SSSQ)*. Dallas, TX: McCarron-Dial Systems.

Linkenhoker, D., & McCarron, L. T. (1993). *Adaptive behaviors: Street Survival Skills Questionnaire (SSSQ, Rev. ed.)*. Dallas, TX: McCarron-Dial Systems.

Linkov, I., Loney, D., Cormier, S., Satterstrom, F. K., & Bridges, T. (2009). Weight-of-evidence evaluation in environmental assessment: Review of qualitative and quantitative approaches. *Science of the Total Environment, 407*, 5199-5205.

Llewellyn, G. (1995). Qualitative research with people with intellectual disability. *Occupational Therapy International, 2*, 108-127.

Locke, L. F., Spirduso, W. W., & Silverman, S. J. (1987). *Proposals that work: A guide for planning dissertations and grant proposals* (2nd ed.). Newbury Park, CA: Sage.

Locke, L. F., Spirduso, W., & Silverman, S. (2000). *Proposals that work: A guide for planning dissertations and grant proposals* (4th ed.). Thousand Oaks, CA: Sage.

Locke, L. F., Spirduso, W., & Silverman, S. (2013). *Proposals that work: A guide for planning dissertations and grant proposals* (6th ed.). Thousand Oaks, CA: Sage.

Locke, L. F., Spirduso, W. W., & Silverman, S. J. (2014). *Proposals that work* (6th ed.). Thousand Oaks, CA: Sage.

Lofquist, L. H. (1957). *Vocational counseling with physically handicapped*. New York, NY: Appleton-Century-Crofts.

Longmore, D. (1970). *Machines in medicine: The medical practice of the future*. New York, NY: Doubleday.

Lorenz, K. Z. (1957). The nature of instinct. In C. H. Schiller (Ed., Trans.), *Instinctive behavior: The development of a modern concept* (pp. 129-175). New York, NY: International Universities Press. (Original work published 1937)

Lubin, B. (1981). Additional data on the reliability and validity of the brief lists of the depression adjective checklists. *Journal of Clinical Psychology, 37*, 809-811.

Luera, M. (1994). *Understanding family uniqueness through cultural diversity. Project TAKOS*. Albuquerque, NM: Alta Mira Specialized Family Services, Inc. (ERIC Document Reproduction Service No. ED 379-839)

Lundquist, T. S., & Ready, R. E. (2008). Young adult attitudes about Alzheimer's disease. *American Journal of Alzheimer's Disease & Other Dementias, 23*(3), 267-273.

Luria, A. R. (1961). *The role of speech in the regulation of normal and abnormal behaviour*. London, United Kingdom: Pergaman.

Luria, A. R. (2012). *Higher cortical functions in man*. New York, NY: Springer.

Macdonald, K. C., Epstein, C. F., & Vastano, S. (1986). Roles and functions of occupational therapy in adult day-care. *American Journal of Occupational Therapy, 40*, 817-821.

MacDonald, M., Lord, C., & Ulrich, D. (2013). The relationship of motor skills and adaptive behavior skills in young children with autism spectrum disorders. *Research in Autism Spectrum Disorders, 7*, 1383-1390.

Mahoney, F. I., & Barthel, D. W. (1965). Functional evaluation: Barthel Index. *Maryland State Medical Journal, 14*, 61-65.

Malave, L. M., & Duquette, G. (1991). *Language, culture and cognition: A collection of studies in first and second language acquisition* (Vol. 69, Multilingual Matters). (ERIC Document Reproduction Service No. ED 386-929)

Markowitz, J. D. (2007). Post-traumatic stress disorder in an elderly combat veteran: A case report. *Military Medicine, 172*(6), 659-662.

Marston, D. (1987-1988). The effectiveness of special education: A time series analysis of reading performance in regular and special education settings. *The Journal of Special Education, 27*, 466-480.

Martí-Ibáñez, F. (1962). *The epic of medicine*. New York, NY: Bramhall House.

Martin, N. A. (2006). *Test of Visual-Perceptual Skills (nonmotor)—3* (3rd ed.). Ann Arbor, MI: Academic Therapy Publications.

Martin, R. P., Hooper, S., & Snow, J. (1986). Behavior rating scale approaches to personality assessment in children and adolescents. In H. M. Knoff (Ed.), *The assessment of child and adolescent personality* (pp. 309-351). New York, NY: Guilford.

Martinsen, E. W., Hoffart, A., & Solberg, O. (1989). Comparing aerobic with nonaerobic forms of exercise in the treatment of clinical depression: A randomized trial. *Comprehensive Psychiatry, 30*, 324-331.

Martinsen, E. W., Medhus, A., & Sandvik, L. (1985). Effects of aerobic exercise on depression: a controlled study. *British Medical Journal (Clinical Research Edition), 291*, 109.

Masagatani, G. N. (1994). *Cognitive Adaptive Skills Evaluation manual* (Rev. ed.). Unpublished manuscript. Richmond, KY: Eastern Kentucky University

Maslow, A. H. (1954). *Motivation and personality*. New York, NY: Harper & Row.

Matheson, L., & Ogden, L. (1987). *Work Capacity Evaluation.* Anaheim, CA: Employment and Rehabilitation Institute of Southern California.

Mayer, J. D., Salovey, P., & Caruso, D. R. (2008). Emotional intelligence: New ability or eclectic traits? *American Psychologist, 63,* 503-517.

McBride, M. R., & Lewis, R. D. (2004). African American and Asian American elders: An ethnogeriatric perspective. *Annual Review of Nursing Research, 22,* 161-214.

McCall, R. B., & Kagan, J. (1986). *Fundamental statistics for behavioral sciences* (4th ed.). San Diego, CA: Harcourt Brace Jovanovich.

McCarney, R., Warner, J., Iliffe, S., van Haselen, R., Griffin, M., & Fisher, P. (2007). The Hawthorne Effect: A randomised, controlled trial. *BMC Medical Research Methodology, 7,* 30.

McCarney, S. B., & Arthaud, T. J., (2013). *Attention deficit disorder evaluation scale-Fourth Edition (ADDES-4).* Columbia, MO: Hawthorne Educational Services.

McCarron, L. T., & Dial, J. G. (1986). *McCarron-Dial evaluation system: A systematic approach to vocational, educational and neuropsychological assessment.* Dallas, TX: McCarron-Dial Systems.

McCarron-Dial Systems, Inc. (n.d.). Homepage, Retrieved from http://www.mccarrondial.com

McColl, M. A., & Paterson, J. (1997). A descriptive framework for community-based rehabilitation. *Canadian Journal of Rehabilitation, 10,* 297-306.

McDermott, D. (1994). Jean Itard: The first child and youth counsellor. *Journal of Child and Youth Care, 9,* 59-71.

McGourty, L. K. (1988). Kohlman Evaluation of Living Skills (KELS). In B. J. Hemphill-Pearson, *Mental health assessment in occupational therapy: A integrative approach to the evaluative process* (pp. 133-146). Thorofare, NJ: SLACK Incorporated.

McGowan, J. F. (Ed.). (1960). *An introduction to the vocational rehabilitation process.* Washington, DC: U.S. Department of Health, Education, and Welfare, Vocational Rehabilitation Administration.

McGrew, K. S. (2005). The Cattell-Horn-Carroll theory of cognitive abilities: Past, present, and future. In D. O. Flanagan & P. I. Harrison (Eds.), *Contemporary intellectual assessment: Theories, tests and issues* (2nd ed., pp. 136-181). New York, NY: Guilford.

McGrew, K. S., Flanagan, D. P., Keith, T. Z., & Vanderwood, M. (1997). Beyond g: The impact of Gf-Gc specific cognitive abilities research on the future use and interpretation of intelligence tests in the schools. *School Psychology Review, 26,* 189-210.

McGruder, J., Cors, D., Tiernan, A. M., & Tomlin, G. (2003). Weighted wrist cuffs for tremor reduction during eating in adults with static brain lesions. *American Journal of Occupational Therapy, 57,* 507-516.

McIntosh, V. V. W., Carter, F. A., Bulik, C. M., Frampton, C. M. A., & Joyce, P. R. (2011). Five-year outcome of cognitive behavioral therapy and exposure with response prevention for bulimia nervosa. *Psychological Medicine, 41,* 1061-1071.

Mead, M. (1928). *Coming of age in Samoa.* New York, NY: Blue Ribbon Books.

Meckler, L., & Hitt, G. (2010, March 24). Obama signs landmark health bill. *Wall Street Journal,* p. A4.

Meenan, R. B., Mason, J. H., Anderson, J. J., Guccione, A. A., & Kazis, L. E. (1992). AIMS–2: The content and properties of a revised and expanded Arthritis Impact Measurement Scales Health Questionnaire. *Arthritis and Rheumatism, 35,* 1-10.

Melzack, R. (1975). The McGill Pain Questionnaire: Major properties and scoring methods. *Pain, 1,* 277-299.

Melzack, R. (1987). The Short-Form McGill Pain Questionnaire. *Pain, 30,* 191-197. doi:10.1016/0304-3959(87)91074-8

Mercer, C. D. (1983). *Students with learning disabilities* (2nd ed.). Columbus, OH: Merrill.

Mercer, C. D., Mercer, A. R., & Pullen, P. C. (2011). *Teaching students with learning problems* (8th ed.). Upper Saddle River, NJ: Pearson/Merrill.

Merriam-Webster's Collegiate Dictionary (11th ed.). (2003). Springfield, MA: Merriam-Webster, Inc.

Merrill, S. C., & Mulligan, S. E. (2003). Neurological dysfunction in children. In E. B. Crepeau, E. S. Cohn, & B. A. B. Schell (Eds.), *Willard & Spackman's occupational therapy* (10th ed., pp. 699-720). Baltimore, MD: Lippincott, Williams & Wilkins.

Mey, G., & Gunther, H. (Eds.). (2015). *The life space of the urban child: Perspectives on Martha Muchow's classic study* (Vol. 1). Piscataway, NJ: Transaction Publishers.

Meyen, E. L., & Skrtic, T. M. (1988). *Exceptional children and youth* (3rd ed.). Denver, CO: Love Publishing.

Mikulic, M. A., Griffith, E. R., & Jebsen, R. H. (1976). Clinical applications of a standardized mobility test. *Archives of Physical Medicine & Rehabilitation, 57,* 143-146.

Miles, M. B., & Huberman, A. M. (1994). *Qualitative data analysis: An expanded sourcebook* (2nd ed.). Thousand Oaks, CA: Sage.

Miller, D. C. (Ed.). (2009). *Best practices in school neuropsychology: Guidelines for effective practice, assessment, and evidence-based intervention.* Hoboken, NJ: John Wiley & Sons.

Miller, L. H., Smith, A. D., & Mehler, B. L. (1988). *The Stress Audit manual.* Brookline, MA: Biobehavioral Institute.

Miller, L. J. (1988). *Miller Assessment for Preschoolers.* San Antonio, TX: Pearson/PsychCorp.

Miller, L. J. (2006). *Miller Function and Participation Scales: Examiner's manual.* San Antonio, TX: Harcourt Assessment, Inc.

Miller, L. J., & Oakland, T. (2013). *Goal-Oriented Assessment of Lifeskills (GOAL).* Torrance, CA: Western Psychological Services.

Miller, M. (1990). Ethnographic interviews for information about classrooms: An invitation. *Teacher Education and Special Education, 13,* 233-234.

Miller, N. E. (1969). Learning of visceral and glandular responses. *Science, 163,* 434-445.

Miller-Kuhanek, H., Henry, D., Glennon, T., Parham, L. D., & Ecker, C. (2008). *The sensory processing measure.* Los Angeles, CA: Western Psychological Services.

Millon, T., Green, C., & Meagher, R. (1982). *Millon adolescent personality inventory manual.* Minneapolis, MN: National Computer Systems.

Mills v. Board of Education of District of Columbia, 348 F. Supp. 866 (1972).

Milone, M. (2007). *THS-R: Test of Handwriting Skills, Revised.* Novato, CA: Academic Therapy Publications.

Minichiello, V., Aroni, R., Timewell, E., & Alexander, L. (1995). *In-depth interviewing: Principles, techniques, & analysis* (2nd ed.). Melbourne, Australia: Longman Cheshire.

Mitchell, P. (2009). Mental health care roles of non-medical primary health and social care services. *Health and Social Care in the Community, 17,* 71-82.

Modern Language Association of America. (2016). *MLA handbook* (8th ed.). New York, NY: Author.

Montessori, M. (1912). *The Montessori method* (A. E. George, Trans.). New York, NY: Frederick A. Stokes.

Montgomery, S. A., & Åsberg, M. (1979). A new depression scale designed to be sensitive to change. *British Journal of Psychiatry, 134,* 382-389.

Morris, W. (Ed.). (1973). *The American heritage dictionary of the English language.* Boston, MA: Houghton Mifflin.

Morrison, M. T., Giles, G. M., Ryan, J. D., Baum, C. M., Dromerick, A. W., Polatajko, H. J., & Edwards, D. F. (2013). Multiple Errands Test–Revised (MET–R): A performance-based measure of executive function in people with mild cerebrovascular accident. *American Journal of Occupational Therapy, 67*(4), 460-468.

Morse, J. M. (Ed.). (1994). *Critical issues in qualitative research methods.* Thousand Oaks, CA: Sage.

Moustakas, C. (1994). *Phenomenological research methods.* Thousand Oaks, CA: Sage.

Mulcahey, M. J., Smith, B. T., Betz, R. R., & Weiss, A. A. (1995). Outcomes of tendon transfer surgery and occupational therapy in a child with tetraplegia secondary to spinal cord injury. *American Journal of Occupational Therapy, 49*, 607-617.

Mullen, E. M. (1995). *Mullen Scales of Early Learning.* Circle Pines, MN: American Guidance Service.

Muñoz, J. P., Moreton, E. M., & Sitterly, A. M. (2016). The scope of practice of occupational therapy in U.S. criminal justice settings. *Occupational Therapy International, 23*, 241-254.

Nadolsky, J. M. (1974). The work sample in vocational evaluation: A consistent rationale. *Vocational Evaluation and Work Adjustment Bulletin, 7*(2), 2-5.

Naglieri, J. A., LeBuffe, P. A., & Pfeiffer, S. I. (1992). *Devereaux behavior rating scales—School.* San Antonio, TX: Pearson/PsychCorp.

Naglieri, J. A., LeBuffe, P. A., & Pfeiffer, S. I. (1994). *Devereaux scales of mental disorders.* San Antonio, TX: Pearson/PsychCorp.

Nasreddine, Z. S., Phillips, N. A., Bédirian, V., Charbonneau, S., Whitehead, V., Collin, I., ... & Chertkow, H. (2005). The Montreal Cognitive Assessment, MoCA: A brief screening tool for mild cognitive impairment. *Journal of the American Geriatrics Society, 53*(4), 695-699.

National Library of Medicine. (2018). *Medical subject headings.* U.S. National Library of Medicine. Retrieved from https://www.nlm.nih.gov/mesh/.

National Rehabilitation Information Center (.2018). *Information for independence.* Retrieved https://www.naric.com/?q=en/home.

Neistadt, M. E. (1987). An occupational therapy program for adults with developmental disabilities. *American Journal of Occupational Therapy, 41*, 433-438.

Neistadt, M. E. (1992). The Rabideau kitchen evaluation, revised: An assessment of meal preparation skill. *Occupational Therapy Journal of Research, 12*, 242-255.

Neistadt, M. E. (1993). The relationship between constructional and meal preparation skills. *Archives of Physical Medicine and Rehabilitation, 74*, 144-148.

Neistadt, M. E. (1994). A meal preparation treatment protocol for adults with brain injury. *American Journal of Occupational Therapy, 48*, 431-438.

Neistadt, M. E. (2000a). *Occupational therapy evaluation for adults: A pocket guide.* Baltimore, MD: Lippincott.

Neistadt, M. E. (2000b). Rabideau Kitchen Evaluation-Revised: An assessment of meal preparation skill. In M. E. *Neistadt, Occupational therapy evaluation for adults: A pocket guide* (pp. 136-137). Baltimore, MD: Lippincott, Williams & Wilkins.

Newton, S. (2007). The growth of the profession of occupational therapy. *U.S. Army Medical Department Journal, Jan-Mar,* 51-58.

Nighswonger, W. E. (1981). *Talent Assessment Programs.* Jacksonville, FL: Talent Assessment, Inc.

Noble, L. M., Noble, A., & Hand, I. L. (2009). Cultural competence of healthcare professionals caring for breastfeeding mothers in urban areas. *Breastfeeding Medicine, 4*, 221-224.

Northrop, F. S. C. (1981). *Science and first principles.* New York, NY: Macmillan.

Nowak, M., Preston, H., & Horoszewski, K. (2015). Validity and reliability of an iPod® forearm goniometer app. *American Journal of Occupational Therapy, 69.* doi: 10.5014/ajot.2015.69S1-PO5096.

Nunes, M. L., Carlini, C. R., Marinowic, D., Neto, F. K., Fiori, H. H., Scotta, M. C., ... da Costa, J. C. (2016). Microcephaly and Zika virus: A clinical and epidemiological analysis of the current outbreak in Brazil. *Jornal de Pediatria (Versão em Português), 92,* 230-240.

Oakley, F. M. (1988). *Role Checklist–Revised.* Bethesda, MD: National Institutes of Health.

Oakley, F. M., Kielhofner, G., Barris, R., & Reichler, R. K. (1986). The Role Checklist: Development and empirical assessment of reliability. *Occupational Therapy Journal of Research, 6,* 157-170.

O'Connor, J. (circa 1920a). *O'Connor Finger Dexterity Test.* Wood Dale, IL: Stoelting Company.

O'Connor, J. (circa 1920b). *O'Connor Tweezer Dexterity Test.* Wood Dale, IL: Stoelting Company.

Okuma, Y., & Nomura, Y. (1998). Senescence-accelerated mouse (SAM) as an animal model of senile dementia: pharmacological, neurochemical and molecular biological approach. *Japanese Journal of Pharmacology, 78*(4), 399-404.

Oliver, M. (1991). *Social work: Disabled people and disabling environments.* London, United Kingdom: Jessica Kingsley.

Oliver, R., Blathwayt, J., Brackley, C., & Tamaki, T. (1993). Development of the safety assessment of function in the environment for rehabilitation (SAFER tool). *Canadian Journal of Occupational Therapy, 60,* 78-82.

O'Neill, J., Brown, M., Gordon, W., & Schonhorn, R. (1985). The impact of deinstitutionalization on activities and skills of severely/profoundly mentally retarded multiply-handicapped adults. *Applied Research in Mental Retardation, 6,* 361-371.

Orley, J., Saxena, S., & Herrman, H. (1998). Quality of life and mental illness: Reflections from the perspective of the WHOQOL. *British Journal of Psychiatry, 172*(4), 291-293. doi: 10.1192/bjp.172.4.291

Osaro, E., & Chima, N. (2014). Challenges of a negative work load and implications on morale, productivity and quality of service delivered in NHS laboratories in England. *Asian Pacific Journal of Tropical Biomedicine, 4,* 421-429.

Osipow, S. H., & Spokane, A. R. (1987). *Occupational Stress Inventory manual: Research version.* Odessa, FL: PAR Inc.

Ottenbacher, K., & York, J. (1984). Strategies for evaluating clinical change: Implications for practice and research. *American Journal of Occupational Therapy, 38,* 647-659.

Ottenbacher, K. J. (1986a). *Evaluating clinical change: Strategies for occupational and physical therapists.* Baltimore, MD: Lippincott, Williams & Wilkins.

Ottenbacher, K. J. (1986b). Reliability and accuracy of visually analyzing graphed data from single-subject designs. *American Journal of Occupational Therapy, 40,* 464-469.

Ottenbacher, K. J., & Barrett, K. A. (1990). Statistical conclusion validity of rehabilitation research: A quantitative analysis. *American Journal of Physical Medicine and Rehabilitation, 69,* 102-107.

Ottenbacher, K. J., & Cusick, A. (1990). Goal attainment scaling as a method of clinical service evaluation. *American Journal of Occupational Therapy, 44,* 519-525.

Parker, R. I., Vannest, K. J., & Davis, J. L. (2011). Effect size in single-case research: A review of nine nonoverlap techniques. *Behavior Modification, 35,* 303-322.

Parkham, L. D, Ecker, C., Miller Kuhaneck, H., Henry, D. A., & Glennon, T. J. (2010). *The sensory processing measure.* Los Angeles, CA: Western Psychological Services.

Parsons, T. (1939). The professions and social structure. *Social Forces, 17,* 457-467.

Patterson, C. H. (1958). *Counseling the emotionally disturbed.* New York, NY: Harper and Brothers.

Patton, M. Q. (1990). *Qualitative evaluation and research methods* (2nd ed.). Thousand Oaks, CA: Sage.

Paul, S., & Orchanian, D. (2003). *Pocket guide to assessment in occupational therapy.* Clifton Park, NY: Delmar, Cengage Learning.

Pavlov, I. P. (1927). *Conditioned reflexes: An investigation of the physiological activity of the cerebral cortex.* London, United Kingdom: Oxford University Press.

Payton, O. D. (1988). *Research, the validation of clinical practice* (2nd ed.). Philadelphia, PA: F.A. Davis.

Pazzaglia, M., Haggard, P., Scivoletto, G., Molinari, M., & Lenggenhager, B. (2016). Pain and somatic sensation are transiently normalized by illusory body ownership in a patient with spinal cord injury. *Restorative Neurology and Neuroscience, 34,* 603-613.

Pearson, K. (1900). The grammar of science. Рипол Классик. London, United Kingdom: Charles and Black.

Pearson Assessments. (2010). *Qualification levels.* Retrieved from https://www.pearsonassessments.com/

Peloquin, S. M. (1991). Occupational therapy service: Individual and collective understandings of the founders, part 2. *American Journal of Occupational Therapy, 45*, 733-744.

Pennsylvania Ass'n, Retard. Child. v. Commonwealth of Pa, 334 1257 (Dist. Court, ED Pennsylvania 1971).

Perls, F. S. (1969). *Gestalt therapy verbatim.* Lafayette, CA: Real People Press.

Piaget, J. (1926). *The language and thought of the child* (M. Gabain & R. Gabain, Trans.). London, United Kingdom: K. Paul, Trench, Trubner.

Piaget, J. (1977). *Equilibration of cognitive structures.* New York, NY: Viking Press.

Pickens, S. Naik, A. D., Burnett, J., Kelly, P.A., Gleason, M., & Dyer, C. B. (2007). The utility of the KELS test in substantiated cases of elder self-neglect. *Journal of the American Academy of Nurse Practitioners, 19*, 137-142.

Pinninti, N. R., Rissmiller, D. J., & Steer, R. A. (2010). Cognitive-behavioral therapy as an adjunct to second-generation antipsychotics in the treatment of schizophrenia. *Psychiatric Services, 61*, 940-943.

Piper, M. C., & Darrah, J. (1994). *Alberta Infant Motor Scales (AIMS).* Philadelphia, PA: W. B. Saunders.

Piper, M. C., Pinnell, L. E., Darrah, J., Macquire, T., & Byrne, P. M. (1992). Construction and validation of the Alberta Infant Motor Scale (AIMS). *Canadian Journal of Public Health, 83*(Suppl. 2), 46-50.

Plantinga, L. C., Johansen, K. L., Schillinger, D., & Powe, N. R. (2012). Lower socioeconomic status and disability among US adults with chronic kidney disease, 1999-2008. *Preventing Chronic Disease, 9*, E12.

Polku, H., Mikkola, T. M., Portegijs, E., Rantakokko, M., Kokko, K., Kauppinen, M., ... Viljanen, A. (2015). Life-space mobility and dimensions of depressive symptoms among community-dwelling older adults. *Aging & Mental Health, 19*, 781-789.

Poole, J., Dunn, W., Schell, B., Tiernan, K., & Barnhart, J. (1991). Statement: Occupational therapy services management of persons with cognitive impairments. *American Journal of Occupational Therapy, 45*, 1067-1068.

Portney, L. G., & Watkins, M. P. (2009). *Single-subject designs* (3rd ed.). Upper Saddle River, NJ: Pearson Prentice Hall.

Post, S. G. (Ed.). (2004). *Encyclopedia of bioethics* (3rd ed.). New York, NY: Macmillan.

Potter, A. J., Mueller, K. J., Mackinney, A. C., & Ward, M. M. (2014). Effect of tele-emergency services on recruitment and retention of US rural physicians. *Rural Remote Health, 14*, 2787.

Powell, L. E., & Myers, A. M. (1995). The activities-specific balance confidence (ABC) scale. *Journals of Gerontology Series A: Biological Sciences and Medical Sciences, 50*(1), M28-M34.

Power, M., Bullinger, M., & Harper, A. (1999). The World Health Organization Quality of Life Group: The World Health Organization WHOQOL-100: Tests of the universality of quality of life in 15 different cultural groups worldwide. *Health Psychology, 18*(5), 495-505

Power, P. (2000). *A guide to vocational assessment* (3rd ed.). Austin, TX: Pro–Ed.

Power, P. (2006). *A guide to vocational assessment* (4th ed.). Austin, TX: Pro-Ed.

Pribram, K. H. (1958). Comparative neurology and the evolution of behavior. In A. Roe & G. G. Simpson (Eds.), *Behavior and evolution* (pp. 140-164) New Haven, CT: Yale University.

Radomski, M. V., Trombly-Latham, C. A. (Eds.). (2014). *Occupational therapy for physical dysfunction.* Philadelphia, PA: Wolters Kluwer Health/Lippincott Williams & Wilkins.

Radosevich, D. M., Wetzler, H., & Wilson, S. M. (1994). *Health Status Questionnaire (HSQ) 2.0: Scoring comparisons and reference data.* Bloomington, MN: Health Outcomes Institute.

Raison, C. L., Klein, H. M., & Steckler, M. (1999). The moon and madness reconsidered. *Journal of Affective Disorders, 53*, 99-106.

Ransford, A. O., Cairnes, D., & Mooney, V. (1976). The pain drawing as an aid to the psychologic evaluation of patients with low-back pain. *Spine, 1*, 127-134.

Rape, R. N. (1987). Running and depression. *Perceptual and Motor Skills, 64*(3 Pt 2), 1303-1310.

Rappaport, M. (2005). The Disability Rating Scale and Coma/Near Coma scales in evaluating severe head injury. *Neuropsychological Rehabilitation 15*, 442-453.

Rappaport, M., Hall, K. M., Hopkins, K., Belleza, T., & Cope, D. N. (1982). Disability Rating Scale for severe head trauma patients: Coma to community. *Archives of Physical Medicine and Rehabilitation, 63*, 118-123.

Reason, P. (1998). *Human inquiry in action: Developments in new paradigm research.* London, United Kingdom: Sage.

Reid, W. M., Seavor, C., & Taylor, R. G. (1991). Application of a computer-based zero-one methodology to the assignment of nurses to a clinical rotation schedule. *Computers in Nursing, 9*, 219-223.

Reitz, S. M. (1992). A historical review of occupational therapy's role in preventive health and wellness. *American Journal of Occupational Therapy, 46*, 50-55.

Remsburg, R. E., Bennett, R. G., Wendel, V. I., & Durso, S. C. (2002). Demographic and health characteristics of residents choosing to use on-site medical care in a newly opened continuing care retirement community (CCRC). *Journal of the American Medical Directors Association, 3*(5), 297-301.

Ren, X. S., Kazis, L., & Meenan, R. F. (1999). Shortform Arthritis Impact Measurement Scales: Tests of reliability and validity among patients with osteoarthritis. *Arthritis Care Research, 12*, 163-171.

Reynolds, C. R. (2008). RTI, neuroscience, and sense: Chaos in the diagnosis and treatment of learning disabilities. In E. Fletcher-Janzen & C. R. Reynolds (Eds.), *Neuropsychological perspectives on learning disabilities in the era of RTI* (pp. 14-53). Hoboken, NJ: John Wiley & Sons.

Reynolds, C. R., Kamphaus, R. W., & Vannest, K. J. (2015). *BASC3: Behavior Assessment System for Children.* San Antonio, TX: PscyhCorp.

Rice, M. S., Dusseau, J. M., & Miller, B. K. (2011). A questionnaire of musculoskeletal injuries associated with manual patient lifting in occupational therapy practitioners in the state of Ohio. *Occupational Therapy in Health Care, 25*, 95-107.

Rice, M. S., & Hernandez, H. G. (2006). Frequency of knowledge of results and motor learning in persons with developmental delay. *Occupational Therapy International, 13*(1), 35-48.

Richardson, G. A., & Day, N. L. (2018). Longitudinal studies of the effects of prenatal cocaine exposure on development and behavior. In W. Slikker, Jr., M. G. Paule, & C. Wang (Eds.), *Handbook of developmental neurotoxicology* (2nd ed., pp. 379-388). Pittsburgh, PA: Elsevier.

Rodger, S., Chien, C. W., Turpin, M., Copley, J., Coleman, A., Brown, T., & Caine, A. M. (2016). Establishing the validity and reliability of the Student Practice Evaluation Form-Revised (SPEF-R) in occupational therapy practice education: A Rasch analysis. *Evaluation & the Health Professions, 39*, 33-48.

Roeder, E. W. (1970). *Roeder Manipulative Aptitude Test.* Lafayette. IN: Lafayette Instruments.

Roid, G. H. (2003). *Stanford-Binet Intelligence Scales* (5th ed.). Itasca, IL: Riverside Publishing.

Rogers, J. C., & Holm, M. B. (1989). *Performance assessment of self-care skills.* Unpublished performance test. Pittsburgh, PA: University of Pittsburgh.

Roley, S. S., DeLany, J. V., Barrows, C. J., Brownrigg, S., Honaker, D., Sava, D. I., ... American Occupational Therapy Association Commission on Practice. (2008). *Occupational therapy practice framework: Domain and Process* (2nd ed.). American Journal of Occupational Therapy, 62, 625-683.

Roll, S. C., & Hardison, M. E. (2017). Effectiveness of occupational therapy interventions for adults with musculoskeletal conditions of the forearm, wrist, and hand: A systematic review. *American Journal of Occupational Therapy, 71*, 7101180010p1-7101180010p12.

Romana, H.-W. (2006). Is evidence-based medicine patient-centered and is patient-centered care evidence-based? *Health Services Research, 41*(1), 1-8.

Rosenthal, R., & Rosnow, R. (1991). *Essentials of behavioral research: Methods and data analysis* (2nd ed.). New York, NY: McGraw-Hill.

Ross, F. L. (1992). The use of computers in occupational therapy for visual-scanning training. *American Journal of Occupational Therapy, 46*, 314-322.

Ross, R. G., & LaStayo, P. C. (1997). Clinical assessment of pain. In J. Van Deusen & D. Brunt (Eds.), *Assessment in occupational therapy and physical therapy* (pp. 123-133). Philadelphia, PA: W. B. Saunders.

Rousseau, J.-J. (1883). *Emile: Or, concerning education: Extracts containing the principal elements of pedagogy found in the first three books* (J. Steeg, Ed.; E. Worthington, Trans.). Boston, MA: D. C. Heath & Co. (Original work published 1762)

Rushmer, R. F. (1972). *Medical engineering: Projections for health care delivery.* New York, NY; London, United Kingdom: Academic Press.

Rusk, H. A. (1971). *Rehabilitation medicine.* St. Louis, MO: Mosby.

Sachs, D., & Linn, R. (1997). Client advocacy in action: Professional and environmental factors affecting Israeli occupational therapists' behaviour. *Canadian Journal of Occupational Therapy, 64*, 207-215.

Sackett, D. L., Rosenberg, W. M., Gray, J. A., Haynes, R. B., & Richardson, W. S. (1996). Evidence based medicine: What it is and what it isn't. *British Medical Journal, 312*(7023), 71-72.

Sailor, W. (1991). Special education in the restructured school. *Remedial and Special Education, 12*(6), 8-22.

Sainsbury, A., Seebass, G., Bansal, A., & Young, J. B. (2005). Reliability of the Barthel Index when used with older people. *Age and Ageing, 34*, 228-232. doi: 10.1093/ageing/afi063

Salmoni, A. W., Schmidt, R. A., & Walter, C. B. (1984). Knowledge of results and motor learning: A review and critical reappraisal. *Psychological Bulletin, 95*, 355-386.

Salovey, P., & Mayer, J. D. (1990). Emotional intelligence. *Imagination, Cognition, and Personality, 9*, 185-211.

Sand, R. (1952). *The advance to social medicine.* London, United Kingdom: Staples Press.

Sarno, J. E., Sarno, M. T., & Levita, E. (1973). The functional life scale. *Archives of Physical Medicine and Rehabilitation, 54*, 214-220.

Sarno, M. T., & Marks, M. (1955). *Aphasia rehabilitation: Manual and work book.* New York, NY: Institute of Physical Medicine and Rehabilitation, New York University-Bellevue Medical Center.

Sattler, J. M. (1988). *Assessment of children* (3rd ed.). San Diego, CA: Author.

Sattler, J. M. (1992). *Assessment of children* (3rd ed., Rev.). San Diego, CA: Author.

Sattler, J. M. (2008). *Assessment of children: Cognitive foundations* (5th ed.). San Diego, CA: Author.

Schatzman, L., & Strauss, A. L. (1973). *Field research: Strategies for a natural sociology.* Englewood Cliffs, NJ: Prentice-Hall.

Schinka, J. A., Raj, A., Loewenstein, D. A., Small, B. J., Duara, R., & Potter, H. (2010). Cross-validation of the Florida Cognitive Activities Scale (FCAS) in Alzheimer's disease research center sample. *Journal of Geriatric Psychiatry and Neurology, 23*, 9-14.

Schmidt, R. A. (1988). *Motor control and learning: A behavioral emphasis* (2nd ed.). Champaign, IL: Human Kinetics.

Schmidt, R. A., Lange, C., & Young, D. E. (1990). Optimizing summary knowledge of results for skill learning. *Human Movement Science, 9*, 325-348.

Schmidt, R. A., & Lee, T. D. (2005). *Motor control and learning: A behavioral emphasis* (4th ed.). Champaign, IL: Human Kinetics.

Scholtz, J., Mannion, R. J., Hord, D. E., Griffin, R. S., Rawal, B., Zheng, H. ... Woolf, C. J. (2009). A novel tool for the assessment of pain: Validation in low back pain. *PLoS Med, 6*, e1000047. doi:10.1371/journal.pmed.1000047

Schrank, F. A., Miller, D. C., Wendling, B. J., & Woodcock, R. W. (2010). *Essentials of WJ III cognitive abilities assessment* (2nd ed.). Hoboken, NJ: Wiley.

Schuling, J., deHaan, R., Limburg, M., & Groenier, K. (1993). The Frenchay Activities Index: Assessment of functional status in stroke patients. *Stroke, 13*, 1173-1177.

Schwandt, T. A., & Halpern, E. S. (1988). *Linking auditing and metae-valuation: Enhancing quality in applied research.* Thousand Oaks, CA: Sage.

Séguin, E. (1848/1997). *Traitement moral, hygiène et éducation des idiots* [Moral treatment, hygiene and education of idiots]. Paris, France: Association pour l'étude de l'histoire de la sécurité sociale.

Selye, H. (1956). *The stress of life.* New York, NY: McGraw-Hill.

Shaffir, W., & Stebbins, R. A. (1991). *Experiencing fieldwork: An inside view of qualitative research.* Thousand Oaks, CA: Sage.

Sharpe, P. A., & Ottenbacher, K. J. (1990). Use of an elbow restraint to improve finger-feeding skills in a child with Rett syndrome. *American Journal of Occupational Therapy, 44*, 328-332.

Shaywitz, S. E., & Shaywitz, B. A. (2008). Paying attention to reading: The neurobiology of reading and dyslexia. *Development and Psychopathology, 20*, 1329-1349.

Shea, C. H., & Wulf, G. (2005). Schema theory: A critical appraisal and reevaluation. *Journal of Motor Behavior, 37*, 85-101.

Shea, T. M., & Bauer, A. M. (1994). *Learners with disabilities: A social systems perspective of special education.* Madison, WI: Brown & Benchmark.

Shrader, C. R. (2006). *History of operations research in the United States Army, Volume 1: 1942-1962.* Washington, DC: Office of the Deputy Under Secretary of the Army for Operations Research, United States Army.

Sibley, L., & Armbruster, D. (1997). Obstetric first aid in the community—Partners in safe motherhood. A strategy for reducing maternal mortality. *Journal of Nurse-Midwifery, 42*, 117-121.

Sidaway, B., Fairweather, M., Powell, J., & Hall, G. (1992). The acquisition and retention of a timing task: Effects of summary KR and movement time. *Research Quarterly for Exercise and Sport, 63*, 328-334.

Sigmon, S. B. (1987). *Radical analysis of special education: Focus on historical development and learning disabilities.* New York, NY: Falmer Press.

Sin, H., & Lee, G. (2013). Additional virtual reality training using Xbox Kinect in stroke survivors with hemiplegia. *American Journal of Physical Medicine & Rehabilitation, 92*, 871-880.

Singam, A., Ytterberg, C., Tham, K., & von Koch, L. (2015). Participation in complex and social everyday activities six years after stroke: Predictors for return to pre-stroke level. *PLoS One, 10*, e0144344.

Singh, A., & Misra, N. (2009). Loneliness, depression and sociability in old age. *Industrial Psychiatry Journal, 18*, 51-55.

Skinner, B. F. (1953). *Science and human behavior.* New York, NY: Macmillan.

Slade, C. (2003). *Form & style: Research papers, reports, theses.* Boston, MA: Houghton Mifflin Company College Division.

Slade, C., Campbell, W. G., & Ballou, S. V. (1997). Form and style: Research papers, reports, theses (10th ed.). Boston, MA: Houghton Mifflin.

Slade, C., & Perrin, R. (2007). *Form & style: Research papers, reports, theses* (13th ed.). Boston, MA: Houghton Mifflin.

Slavin, M. D., Ni, P., Tulsky, D. S., Kisala, P. A., Heinemann, A. W., Charlifue, S., ... Jette, A. M. (2016). Spinal Cord Injury-Functional Index/Assistive Technology Short Forms. *Archives Physical Medicine Rehabilitation., 97*, 1745-1752

Smith, D. D., & Tyler, N. C. (2010). *Introduction to special education: Making a difference* (7th ed.). Upper Saddle River, NJ: Merrill/Pearson.

Smith, L. M. (1994) Biographical method In N.K. Denzin & Y.S. Lincoln (Eds.), *Handbook of qualitative research* (pp. 286-305). Thousand Oaks, CA: Sage.

Snow, C. P. (1964). *The two cultures, and a second look.* Cambridge, United Kingdom: Cambridge University Press.

Söderback, I., & Paulsson, E. H. (1997). A needs assessment for referral to occupational therapy: Nurses' judgment in acute cancer care. *Cancer Nursing, 20,* 267-273.

Spearman, C. (1927). *The abilities of man.* New York, NY: Macmillan.

Speller, L., Trollinger, J. A., Maurer, P. A., Nelson, C. E., & Bauer, D. F. (1997). Comparison of the test–retest reliability of the Work Box™ using three administrative methods. *American Journal of Occupational Therapy, 51,* 516-522.

Spence, K. W. (1948). The postulates and methods of "behaviorism." *Psychological Review, 55,* 67-78.

Spielberger, C. D., Gorsuch, R. L., Lushene, R., Vagg, P. R., & Jacobs, G. A. (1983). *Manual for the State-Trait Anxiety Inventory.* Palo Alto, CA: Consulting Psychologists Press.

Spradley, J. P. (1979). *The ethnographic interview.* Fortworth, TX: Holt, Rinehart and Winston.

SPSS Inc. (2010). *SPSS industry solutions: Healthcare.* Retrieved from https://www.ibm.com/products/spss-statistics

Stainback, W., & Stainback, S. B. (1992). *Controversial issues confronting special education: Divergent perspectives.* Boston, MA: Allyn & Bacon.

Stamm, T., Geyh, S., Cieza, A., Machold, K., Kollerits, B., Kloppenburg, M., … Stucki, G. (2006). Research study: Measuring functioning in patients with hand osteoarthritis—content comparison of questionnaires based on the International Classification of Functioning, Disability and Health (ICF). *Rheumatology, 45,* 1534-1541.

Stecco, C., & Aldegheri, R. (2008). Historical review of carpal tunnel syndrome. *La Chirurgia degli organi di movimento, 92,* 7-10.

Steffe, L. P., & Gale, J. E. (Eds.). (1995). *Constructivism in education.* Hillsdale, NJ: Lawrence Erlbaum.

Stein, F. (1976). *Anatomy of research in allied health.* Cambridge, MA: Schenkman Publishing Company.

Stein, F. (1987). *Stress Management Questionnaire.* Unpublished questionnaire. Vermillion, SD: University of South Dakota.

Stein, F. (1988). Research analysis of O.T. assessments used in mental health. In B. J. Hemphill-Pearson (Ed.), *The mental health assessment in occupational therapy: An integrative approach to the evaluative process* (pp. 225-247). Thorofare, NJ: SLACK Incorporated.

Stein, F. (2008). Stress Management Questionnaire. In B. J. Hemphill-Pearson (Ed.), *Assessments in occupational therapy mental health: An integrative approach* (2nd ed., pp. 293-307). Thorofare, NJ: SLACK Incorporated.

Stein, F., Bentley, D. E., & Natz, M. (1999). Computerized assessment: The Stress Management Questionnaire. In B. J. Hemphill-Pearson (Ed.), *Assessments in occupational therapy mental health: An integrative approach* (pp. 321-337). Thorofare, NJ: SLACK Incorporated.

Stein, F., & Cutler, S. K. (2002). *Psychosocial occupational therapy: A holistic approach* (2nd ed.). Clifton Park, NY: Delmar, Cengage Learning.

Stein, F., & Smith, J. (1989). Short-term stress management programme with acutely depressed in-patients. *Canadian Journal of Occupational Therapy, 56,* 185-192.

Sternberg, R. J. (1985). *Beyond IQ: A triarchic theory of human intelligence.* Cambridge, MA: Cambridge University Press.

Stevens, S. S. (1951). *Handbook of experimental psychology.* New York, NY: John Wiley & Sons.

Strauss, A., & Corbin, J. (1998). *Basics of qualitative research: Techniques and procedures for developing grounded theory.* Newbury Park, CA: Sage.

Strauss, A. A., & Kephart, N. C. (1940). Behavior differences in mentally retarded children measured by a new behavior rating scale. *American Journal of Psychiatry, 96,* 1117-1124.

Strauss, A. A., & Lehtinen, L. E. (1947). *Psychopathology and education of the brain-injured child.* New York, NY: Grune & Stratton.

Strauss, A. A., & Werner, H. (1941). The mental organization of the brain-injured mentally defective child. *American Journal of Psychiatry, 97,* 1194-1203.

Strauss, A. A., & Werner, H. (1943). Comparative psychopathology of the brain-injured child and the traumatic brain-injured adult. *American Journal of Psychiatry, 99,* 835-838.

Strong, K. E., Campbell, D. P., & Hansen, J. (1985). *The Strong-Campbell Interest Inventory.* Minneapolis, MN: National Computer Systems.

Strunk, W., & White, E. B. (1979). *The elements of style* (3rd ed.). New York, NY: Macmillan.

Strunk, W., & White, E. B. (1999). *The elements of style* (4th ed.). Boston, MA: Allyn & Bacon.

Suchman, E. A. (1967). *Evaluative research: Principles and practice in public service and social action programs.* New York, NY: Russell Sage Foundation.

Swanson, H. L., & Watson, B. L. (1989). *Educational and psychological assessment of exceptional children: Theories, strategies, and applications* (2nd ed.). Columbus, OH: Merrill.

Tanta, K. J., Deitz, J. C., White, O., & Billingsley, F. (2005). The effects of peer-play level on initiations and responses of preschool children with delayed play skills. *American Journal of Occupational Therapy, 59,* 437-445.

Tate, R. L., Rosenkoetter, U., Vohra, S., Kratochwill, T., Sampson, M., Barlow, D. H., … Wilson, B. (2016). The single-case reporting guideline in behavioral interventions (SCRIBE) 2016 Statement. *Archives of Scientific Psychology, 4,* 1-9.

Teng, S.-Y. (1943). Chinese influence on the Western examination system: I. Introduction. *Harvard Journal of Asiatic Studies, 7,* 267-312.

Terman, L. M., & Merrill, M. A. (1960). *Stanford-Binet Intelligence Scale: Manual for the third revision, Form LM.* Oxford, United Kingdom: Houghton Mifflin.

Tesch, R. (1990). *Qualitative research: Analysis types and software tools.* New York, NY: Falmer Press.

Thomson, L. K. (1992). *The Kohlman Evaluation of Living Skills* (KELS, 3rd ed.). Rockville, MD: American Occupational Therapy Association.

Thomson, L. K. (1999). The Kohlman Evaluation of Living Skills. In B. J. Hemphill-Pearson (Ed.), *Assessment in occupational therapy mental health: An integrative approach* (pp. 401-409). Thorofare, NJ: SLACK Incorporated.

Thorndike, E. L. (1920). Intelligence and its uses. *Harper's Magazine, 140,* 227-235.

Thorndike, E. L., Bregman, E. O., Cobb, M. V., & Woodyard, E. (1926). *The measurement of intelligence.* New York, NY: Teachers College Bureau of Publications.

Thorwald, J. (1963). *Science and secrets of early medicine.* New York, NY: Harcourt, Brace and World.

Thurstone, L. L. (1938). Primary mental abilities (Psychometric Monographs, No. 1). In H. J. Eysenck (Ed.), *The measurement of intelligence* (pp. 131-136). Dordrecht, Germany: Springer.

Tiffin, J. (1948). *Purdue Pegboard.* Rosemont, IL: London House.

Tinetti, M. E. (1986). Performance-oriented assessment of mobility problems in elderly patients. *Journal of the American Geriatrics Society, 34*(2), 119-126.

Toglia, J. (1996). *The multicontext approach to cognitive rehabilitation* [Supplemental manual to a workshop]. New York, NY: New York Hospital-Cornell Medical Center.

Tomlin, G., & Borgetto, B. (2011). Research pyramid: A new evidence-based-practice model for occupational therapy. *American Journal of Occupational Therapy, 65,* 189-196.

Tona, J. L., & Schneck, C. M. (1993). The efficacy of upper extremity inhibitive casting: A single-subject pilot study. *American Journal of Occupational Therapy, 47,* 901-910.

Townsend, E. (1996). Institutional ethnography: A method for showing how the context shapes practice. *OTJR: Occupation, Participation and Health, 16,* 179-199.

Tracy, S. E. (1910). *Studies in invalid occupations: A manual for nurses and attendants.* Boston, MA: Whitcomb & Barrows

Tryon, W. W. (1982). A simplified time-series analysis for evaluating treatment interventions. *Journal of Applied Behavior Analysis, 15,* 423-429.

Tukey, J. W. (1977). *Exploratory data analysis.* Reading, MA: Addison-Wesley.

Turabian, K. L. (2013). *A manual for writers of research papers, theses, and dissertations* (W. C. Booth, G. G. Colomb, & J. M. Williams, Eds.; 8th ed.). Chicago, IL: University of Chicago Press.

Turnbull, H. R., & Turnbull, A. P. (1998). *Free appropriate public education: The law and children with disabilities* (5th ed.). Denver, CO: Love.

Twisk, F. N., & Maes, M. (2009). A review on cognitive behavioral therapy (CBT) and graded exercise therapy (GET) in myalgic encephalomyelitis (ME)/chronic fatigue syndrome (CFS): CBT/GET is not only ineffective and not evidence-based, but also potentially harmful for many patients with ME/CFS. *Neuro Endocrinology Letters, 30,* 284-299.

Tyson, P. (2009). Research in child psychoanalysis: Twenty-five-year follow-up of a severely disturbed child. *Journal of the American Psychoanalytic Association, 57,* 919-945.

Umeda, C., & Deitz, J. (2011). Effects of therapy cushions on classroom behaviors of children with autism spectrum disorder. *American Journal of Occupational Therapy, 65,* 152-159.

U.S. Department of Defense, Joint Services Steering Committee. (1963). *Human engineering guide to equipment design* (C. T. Morgan, Ed.). New York, NY: McGraw-Hill.

U,S, Department of Education. (1998). *To assure the free appropriate public education of all children with disabilities: Twentieth Annual Report to Congress on the Implementation of Education of the Individuals with Disabilities Education Act.* Washington, D.C.: U.S. Government Printing Office.

U.S. Department of Education. (2009). *2007 annual report to Congress on the Individuals with Disabilities Education Act, Part D.* Washington, DC. Retrieved from http://www2.ed.gov/about/reports/annual/osep/2007/part-d/idea-part-d-2007.pdf.

U.S. Department of Health and Human Services. (2009). *Code of federal regulations (CFR): Basic HHS policy for protection of human research subjects.* Retrieved from https://www.hhs.gov/ohrp/regulations-and-policy/regulations/common-rule/index.html

U.S. Department of Labor, Bureau of Labor Statistics. (2009). *Occupational outlook handbook 2010-2011 Edition, occupational therapists.* Retrieved from https://www.dol.gov

U.S. National Library of Medicine. (2018). *MEDLINE, PubMed, and PMC (PubMed Central): How are they different?* Retrieved from https://www.nlm.nih.gov/pubs/factsheets/dif_med_pub.html

University of Chicago. (2017). *The Chicago manual of style* (17th ed.). Chicago, IL: University of Chicago Press.

Uomoto, J. M., & Williams, R. M. (2009). Post-acute polytrauma rehabilitation and integrated care of returning veterans: Toward a holistic approach. *Rehabilitation Psychology, 54,* 259-269.

Vahabzadeh, M., Lin, J. L., Mezghanni, M., Epstein, D. H., & Preston, K. L. (2009). Automation in an addiction treatment research clinic: Computerised contingency management, ecological momentary assessment and a protocol workflow system. *Drug and Alcohol Review, 28,* 3-11.

Valpar International Corporation. (n.d.a.). *DOT—Dictionary Of Occupational Titles.* Retrieved from http://www.valparint.com/dot.htm

Valpar International Corporation. (n.d.b.). *RHAJ—Revised Handbook For Analyzing Jobs.* Retrieved from http://www.valparint.com/RHAJ.HTM

Valpar International Corporation. (1973). *Valpar component work samples.* Tucson, AZ: Author.

Van Boven, L., Kane, J., McGraw, A. P., & Dale, J. (2010). Feeling close: Emotional intensity reduces perceived psychological distance. *Journal of Personality and Social Psychology, 98,* 872-885.

Van Deusen, J., & Brunk, D. (1997). *Assessment in occupational therapy and physical therapy.* Philadelphia, PA: Saunders.

van Emmerik-van Oortmerssen, K., Vedel, E., van den Brink, W., & Schoevers, R. A. (2015). Integrated cognitive behavioral therapy for patients with substance use disorder and comorbid ADHD: Two case presentations. *Addictive Behaviors, 45,* 214-217.

Van Heest, K. N. L., Mogush, A. R., & Mathiowetz, V. G. (2017). Effects of a one-to-one fatigue management course for people with chronic conditions and fatigue. *American Journal of Occupational Therapy, 71,* 7104100020p1-7104100020p9.

van Manen, M. (1990). *Researching lived experience: Human science for an action sensitive pedagogy.* London, United Kingdom: State University of New York.

Vanderbeken, I., & Kerckhofs, E. (2016). A systematic review of the effect of physical exercise on cognition in stroke and traumatic brain injury patients. *NeuroRehabilitation, 40,* 33-48.

Velozo, C. A., Kielhofner, G., & Lai, J.-S. (1999). The use of Rasch analysis to produce scale-free measurement of functional ability. *American Journal of Occupational Therapy, 53,* 83-90.

Velozo, C. A., Magalhaes, L., Pan, A., & Weeks, D. K. (1993). Measurement qualities of the Level of Rehabilitation Scale-III (LORS-III). *Archives of Physical Medicine and Rehabilitation, 74*(6), 661.

Venes, D. (2017). *Taber's cyclopedic medical dictionary* (21st ed.). Philadelphia, PA: F.A. Davis.

Ventegodt, S., Clausen, B., & Merrick, J. (2006). Clinical holistic medicine: The case story of Anna. II. Patient diary as a tool in treatment. *The Scientific World Journal, 6,* 2006-2034.

Vergason, G. A., & Anderegg, M. I. (1992). Preserving the least restrictive environment. In S. Stainback & S. B. Stainback (Eds.), *Controversial issues confronting special education: Divergent perspectives* (pp. 45-54). Boston, MA: Allyn & Bacon.

Videler, A. C., van Royen, R. J., & van Alphen, S. P. (2010). [Treatment of personality disorders in older adults. Three case studies]. *Nederlandse Vereniging voor Gerontologie, 41,* 96-103.

Vidich, A. J., & Lyman, S. M. (2003). Qualitative methods: Their history in sociology and anthropology. In N. K. Denzin & Y. S. Lincoln (Eds.), *Handbook of qualitative research* (2nd ed., pp. 55-130). Thousand Oaks, CA: Sage.

Vocational Research Institute. (1980). VITAS: Vocational Interest, Temperament and Aptitude System. Philadelphia, PA: Author.

Vygotsky, L. S. (1961). *Thought and language.* New York, NY: Wiley. (Original work published 1934)

Vygotsky, L. S. (1986). *Thought and language* (Rev. ed.). Cambridge, MA: MIT Press.

Wade, D. T., Collen, F. M., Robb, G. P., & Warlow, C. P.(1992). Physiotherapy intervention late after stroke and mobility. *British Medical Journal, 304,* 609-613.

Wallace, M., & Shelkey, M. (2006). Katz Index of Independence in Activities of Daily Living (ADL). *Annals of Long Term Care, 14*(11). Retrieved from http://www.annalsoflongtermcare.com/article/6412

Wallas, G. (1926). *The art of thought.* New York, NY: Harcourt, Brace.

Wallis, W. A., & Roberts, H. V. (1962). *The nature of statistics.* New York, NY: The Free Press.

Walters, L., Kahn, T. J., & Goldstein, D. M. (2009). *Bibliography of bioethics* (Vol. 35). Washington, DC: Georgetown University, Kennedy Institute.

Wang, J., Kane, R. L., Eberly, L. E., Virnig, B. A., & Chang, L. H. (2009). The effects of resident and nursing home characteristics on activities of daily living. *Journals of Gerontology Series A: Biomedical Sciences and Medical Sciences, 64*(4), 473-480.

Watling, R., & Hauer, S. (2015). Effectiveness of Ayres Sensory Integration and sensory-based interventions for people with autism spectrum disorder: A systematic review. *American Journal of Occupational Therapy, 69,* 6905180030p1-6905180030p12.

Watling, R. L., & Deitz, J. (2007). Immediate effect of Ayre's sensory integration-based occupational therapy intervention on children with autism spectrum disorders. *American Journal of Occupational Therapy, 61,* 574-583.

Watson, J. D. (1968). *The double helix: A personal account of the discovery of the structure of DNA.* New York, NY: Atheneum.

Weaver, W. (1947). *The scientists speak.* New York, NY: Boni and Gaar.

Weber, M., Parsons, T., & Weber, A. M. (1964). *The theory of social and economic organization.* New York, NY: Free Press.

Webster's College Dictionary. (1992). New York, NY: Random House

Wechsler, D. (1939). *The measurement of adult intelligence.* Baltimore, MD: Lippincott, Williams & Wilkins.

Wechsler, D. (2003). *Wechsler Intelligence Scale for Children* (4th ed.). San Antonio, TX: PsychCorp.

Wechsler, D. (2014). *Wechsler Adult Intelligence Scale* (WAIS–IV; 4th ed.). San Antonio, TX: PsychCorp.

Weiner, D., Pieper, C., McConnell, E., Martinez, S., & Keefe, F. (1996). Pain measurement in elders with chronic low back pain: Traditional and alternative approaches. *Pain, 67,* 461-467.

Weiss, C. H. (1972). *Evaluation research: Methods for assessing program effectiveness.* Englewood Cliffs, NJ: Prentice-Hall.

Wernicke, C. (1970). The aphasic symptom-complex: A psychological study on an anatomical basis. *Archives of Neurology, 22,* 280-282.

Westby, C. E. (2000). A scale for assessing development of children's play. In K. Gitlin-Weiner, A. Sandgrund, & C. Schaefer (Eds.), *Play diagnosis and assessment* (pp. 15–57) New York, NY: Wiley.

Westby, M. D., & Backman, C. L. (2010). Patient and health professional views on rehabilitation practices and outcomes following total hip and knee arthroplasty for osteoarthritis: A focus group study. *BMC Health Services Research, 10,* 119.

White, R. W. (1952). *Lives in progress.* New York, NY: Holt, Rinehart and Winston.

Whiteford, G. E. (1995). Other worlds and other lives: A study of occupational therapy student perceptions of cultural difference. *Occupational Therapy International, 2,* 291-313.

Whiting, S., Lincoln, N., Bhavnani, G., & Cockburn, J. (1985). *Rivermead Perceptual Assessment Battery (RPAB).* United Kingdom: NFER-Nelson.

Wiener, N. (1948). *Cybernetics: Or control and communication in the animal and the machine.* Cambridge, MA: MIT Press.

Wightman, W. P. D. (1971). *The emergence of scientific medicine.* Edinburgh, Scotland: Oliver & Boyd.

Will, M. C. (1986). Educating children with learning problems: A shared responsibility. *Exceptional Children, 52,* 411-415.

Willard, H. S., & Spackman, C. S. (1971). *Occupational therapy* (4th ed.). Philadelphia, PA: J. B. Lippincott.

Willer, B., Ottenbacher, K. J., & Coad, M. L. (1994). The community integration questionnaire: A comparative examination. *American Journal of Physical Medicine & Rehabilitation, 73,* 103-111.

Williams, J. H., Drinka, T. J., Greenberg, J. R., Farrell-Holtan, J., Euhardy, R., & Schräm, M. (1991). Development and testing of the assessment of living skills and resources (ALSAR) in elderly community-dwelling veterans. *Gerontologisit, 31,* 84-91.

Williams, S., & Bloomer, J. (1987). *Bay Area Functional Performance Evaluation* (2nd ed.). Palo Alto, CA: Consulting Psychologists Press.

Williams, S. L., Bloomer, J. S., Houston, D., Managh, M. F., Cook, J. V., Mann, W. C., ... & Wolfe, A. (2004). *Bay Area Functional Performance Evaluation (BaFPE).* Ottawa, Canada: École des Sciences de la réadaptation, Sciences de la santé, Université d'Ottawa.

Wilson, B. A., Baddley, A., Cockburn, J., & Hiorns, R. (n.d.). *The Rivermead Behavioural Memory Test. Supplement 2: Validation study.* Titchfield Hants, England: Thames Valley Test Company.

Wilson, B. A., Greenfield, E., Clare, L., Baddeley, A., Cockburn, J., Watson, P., ... & Nannery, R. (2008). *Rivermead Behavioural Memory Test— Third Edition (RBMT-3).* San Antonio, TX: Pearson/PsychCorp.

Winkler, A. C., & McCuen, J. R. (1979). *Writing the research paper: A handbook.* New York, NY: Harcourt, Brace, & Jovanovich.

Winkler, A. C., & McCuen, J. R. (1998). *Writing the research paper: A handbook* (5th ed.). New York, NY: Harcourt, Brace, & Jovanovich.

Winkler, A. C., & McCuen-Metherell, J. R. (2011). *Writing the research paper: A handbook* (8th ed.). Boston, MA: Cengage Learning.

Winnie, A. J. (1912). *History and handbook of day schools for the deaf and blind: A bulletin of information concerning the origin, maintenance, advantages and standing of the day schools for the deaf and blind in Wisconsin.* Madison, WI: Democrat Printing Company.

Wolfensberger, W. P., Nirje, B., Olshansky, S., Perske, R., & Roos, P. (1972). *The principle of normalization in human services.* Toronto, ON, Canada: National Institute on Mental Retardation.

Wolpe, J. (1969). *The practice of behavior therapy.* New York, NY: Pergamon.

Woo, D. A., Olek, M. J., & Frohman, E. M. (2006). Diagnosis and management of multiple sclerosis: Case studies. *Neurologic Clinics, 24,* 199-214.

Woodcock, R. W., McGrew, K. S., Mather, N., & Schrank, F. A. (2003). *Woodcock-Johnson III diagnostic supplement to the tests of cognitive abilities.* Itasca, IL: Riverside.

Woods, K., Karrison, T., Koshy, M., Patel, A., Friedmann, P., & Cassel, C. (1997). Hospital utilization patterns and costs for adult sickle cell patients in Illinois. *Public Health Reports, 112,* 44-51.

Woodside, H. H. (1971). The development of occupational therapy 1910-1929. *American Journal of Occupational Therapy, 25,* 226-230.

World Health Organization. (2018). *About WHO.* Retrieved https://www.who.int/about-us.

Xakellis G. C., Jr., Frantz, R. A., Lewis, A., & Harvey, P. (1998). Cost-effectiveness of an intensive pressure ulcer prevention protocol in long-term care. *Advances Wound Care, 11*(1), 22-29.

Yerkes, R. M. (Ed.). (1921). *Psychological examining in the United States Army.* Washington, DC: US Government Printing Office.

Yerkes, R. M. (Ed.) (1930). Autobiography of Robert Mearns Yerkes. In C. Murchison (Ed.) *History of psychology in autobiography* (Vol. 2, pp. 381-407). Worchester, MA: Clark University Press.

Zinsser, W. (1990). *On writing well: An informal guide to writing nonfiction.*(4th ed.). New York, NY: HarperCollins.

Zung, W. K. (1965). A self-rating depression scale. *Archives of General Psychiatry, 12,* 63-75.

Zytowski, D. G. (n.d.). *Kuder® career search with person match: Technical manual* (ver. 1.2). Adel, IA: Kuder Inc.

Index

AbleData, 166

achievement tests, 296-297

alpha, 229

ambiguity, as research fallacy, 41-42

ambiguous terms, operationally defining, 42

American Journal of Occupational Therapy, 170

American Journal of Physical Medicine & Rehabilitation, 170

analysis of covariance, 205

analysis of variance, 254-258

    critical values, 392-395

Annals of International Occupational Therapy, 170

appeal to authority, as research fallacy, 40-41

approval of research problem, denial, 151-154

aptitude tests, 296-297. *See also* intelligence tests

    alternative tests to, 295

    influence of, 294-295

Archives of Physical Medicine and Rehabilitation, 170

Asian Journal of Occupational Therapy, 170

assumptions, research study, stating, 184-185

audio recorder use, in data collection, 135

Australian Occupational Therapy Journal, 171

bar graphs, 223-225

    constructing, 223-225

behavior rating scales, 303

bell-shaped curve, 214

Berman, Eric, 109

beta, 229

Bettelheim, Bruno, 109

bibliographic citations, 352-353

Binet, Alfred, influence of, 294-295

binomial distribution table, 413-414

Biological Abstracts, 167

biological description, 7-12

    Galen, 10

    Harvey, William, 11-12

    Hippocratic writings, 9

    Paracelsus, 11

    Renaissance medicine, 10

    scientific anatomy, 7-9

    Vesalius, Andreas, 11

biomedical engineering, 35

Blehar, Everett Waters, 109

Breuer, Josef, 109

British Journal of Occupational Therapy, 171

Canadian Journal of Occupational Therapy, 171

case studies, 111-113

    need for study, 111-112

    research methodology, 112

    results, 112-113

    review of literature, 112

chemotherapy, 16

chi-square, 262-263

    distribution, critical values, 411-412

Church, Joseph, 109

CINAHL, 163

citations, APA style, 354-355

classification of scales, research study, 198

The Cochrane Library, 167

Coles, Robert, 109

computer applications in diagnosis, 33

computer treatment applications, 33

constructivism, factors promoting, 40

continuous variables, 212

control group, usage of term, 57

convenience sample, research study, 193-194

correlated *t*-test, 251-253

correlation, definition of, 259

correlational research, 87-92

    data collection, 92

    example, 88-90

    hypotheses formulation, 90-91

    interpretation of results, 92

    purposes of, 87-90

    research variables, 90

    sample selection, 92

    variables, operational definitions, 91-92

correlational sample, 217

creativity, quality of researcher, 46

criterion-referenced test, 336-337

    applying to research, 337

crude mortality rate, calculation of, 240

CSA Sociological Abstracts, 166

cumulative frequency distributive polygon, 225-226

Printed in the United States
by Baker & Taylor Publisher Services